TECHNICAL NURSING
OF THE ADULT
Medical, Surgical, and Psychiatric
Approaches

TECHNICAL NURSING OF THE ADULT

Medical, Surgical, and Psychiatric Approaches

SANDRA B. FIELO
R.N., M.A. in Medical-Surgical Nursing
Middlesex County College, Edison, New Jersey

SYLVIA C. EDGE
R.N., M.A. in Psychiatric Mental Health
Middlesex County College, Edison, New Jersey

THE MACMILLAN COMPANY
Collier-Macmillan Limited • London

© Copyright, The Macmillan Company, 1970

All rights reserved. No part of this book may be reproduced or transmitted in any form or by any means, electronic or mechanical, including photocopying, recording or by any information storage and retrieval system, without permission in writing from the Publisher.

First Printing

Library of Congress catalog card number: 74–93724

The Macmillan Company
866 Third Avenue, New York, New York 10022
Collier-Macmillan Canada, Ltd., Toronto, Ontario

PRINTED IN THE UNITED STATES OF AMERICA

For their patience, encouragement,
and continuous delight in its preparation,
the authors dedicate this book to
their husbands
JOEL FIELO and WALDO EDGE
and to their children
JEFF and ERIC FIELO and PETER EDGE,
with love.

FOREWORD

TODAY's nursing education programs are preparing the practitioners who will meet tomorrow's needs for nursing services. The future is not a nebulous concept but a reality hard upon us, even before we have comfortably reckoned with the past. It is a promising, fertile field to every graduate and an exciting challenge to every teacher. One clear implication is that yesterday's methods will not be appropriate to tomorrow's needs.

The registered nurse is an essential part of the health industry, which is rapidly becoming the top industry in the nation. Numerous reports in current literature point to the shortage of nurses and urge the expansion of nursing education programs. The nursing profession is working toward meeting these growing needs not only by increasing numbers of graduates but in wiser utilization of nursing power.

Two significant trends toward meeting these future needs are the expansion and development of nursing education programs in colleges and universities and preparation geared for professional and technical nursing practice. A crucial factor in the success of this movement is a clear differentiation of these kinds of nursing practice, followed by utilization of graduates in nursing services on the basis of this differentiation. For nursing education this implies development of curricula to educate a clearly defined practitioner on each level of practice.

The dynamic growth of associate-degree nursing programs is one of the most promising developments toward providing larger numbers of qualified bedside nurses. The placement of these programs in community colleges is consistent with the philosophy of these colleges to meet community needs. It is also consistent with contemporary technologic advances. The age of technical practice has come into its own, and graduates of these programs will comprise a large part of the work force in other fields as well as in nursing.

Technical nursing practice is appropriate in a variety of patient settings; however, large numbers of nurses will be employed in hospitals. The degree of effectiveness of these practitioners will be in direct proportion to the degree of effectiveness of professional nursing practice in each situation. Nursing care teams with a professional nurse as the leader and several technical nurses as team members, along with ancillary personnel, promise better utilization of skills and knowledge, greater job satisfaction, and a higher quality of patient care.

Professional nursing practice is viewed as covering the broad, overall spectrum of nursing concerns, classically identified as care, cure, and coordination. General and professional education, obtained in baccalaureate and higher-degree nursing education programs in the social, physical, biologic, and nursing sciences, will enable the nurse to perform nursing skills in a variety of settings, to use the problem-solving approach, to analyze critically, to do long-range planning and evaluation, to anticipate the consequences of actions, to direct care toward maintenance and prevention, to teach patients and families, to be a leader in other nursing problems requiring further study, to engage in research, to represent nursing personnel on the health team, to identify nursing problems requiring further study, and to interpret health services in relation to the broader community.

Graduates of technical nursing programs with considerable knowledge and a high degree of skill obtained through general and technical nursing education at the associate-degree level are needed to assist professional nursing practitioners, who cannot meet all the nursing needs alone. Technical nursing practice is viewed as taking place in a more circumscribed and predictable setting. It includes carrying out nursing and medically delegated measures directly related to patient care, using principles as a basis for action with sufficient knowledge and a high degree of skill, using judgment in nursing situations and knowing when professional judgment is required, assisting in planning and evaluating ongoing patient care, directing personnel with less knowledge, and taking part in nurse-patient teaching.

In associate-degree nursing programs, one of the challenges facing instructors is the selection of content and learning experiences from the vast and complex store of information available, appropriate to curriculum objectives. Innovative and creative patterns of education and teaching techniques are in order.

The authors combine their expertise in teaching nursing with their experience in the associate-degree nursing program to produce this text, which should be of great assistance to teachers and students. Although the approach is to consider broad problems, the book contains the depth required to combine essential knowledge with the acquisition of skills in the areas of medical, surgical, and psychiatric nursing applicable to technical nursing practice.

> ROSE M. CHANNING, R.N., M.A.
> Chairman, Division of Health Technologies
> Middlesex County College

PREFACE

WE HAVE attempted to identify broad content areas from which the principles of safe, knowledgeable care of any adult can be delimited. Only those illnesses that are most frequently seen in the hospital are discussed in detail. However, the common aspects of the care of patients with innumerable illnesses can be identified through understanding and use of the broad-content areas.

Our approach is direct and concise. Major emphasis is on points to remember in caring for any patient with a related broad-area illness.

We believe that the response of persons to the stress of illness varies in degree, not in kind, and that an awareness of this fact is basic to nursing of all adults regardless of the setting. We also believe that every patient has the right to a nurse who can perceive his behavior nonjudgmentally and help him through the stressful period.

The authors are indebted to the following persons who read various portions of the manuscript and offered their expert opinions: Miss Eleanor A. Bates, Mrs. Corliss Henry, and Mrs. Jewel L. Nickens.

S. B. F.
S. C. E.

CONTENTS

UNIT I
THE INTERPERSONAL BASIS OF NURSING

CHAPTERS

1. The Communication Process — 2
2. The Therapeutic Environment and Relevant Concepts — 6
3. Learning and Living—A Progressive Process — 11
4. Personality Structure and Development — 20
5. Mental Illness — 25
6. Treatment Modalities — 40
7. Addiction: Alcohol and Drugs — 53
8. The Rights of the Mentally Ill — 59
9. The Bold New Approach — 61
10. The History and Development of the Care of the Mentally Ill — 63

UNIT II
THE PATIENT WITH INFECTION

11. The Patient with Infection: An Ecologic Approach — 72
12. Defense Mechanisms — 74
13. Hospital-Acquired Infection — 77
14. Venereal Diseases — 81

UNIT III
PROLIFERATION AND MATURATION OF CELLS

15. Cancer — 88
16. The Patient with Breast Cancer — 101

UNIT IV
WATER AND ELECTROLYTE BALANCE

17.	Basic Concepts	112
18.	Common Imbalances of Water and Electrolytes	126
19.	Water and Electrolyte Replacement	137
20.	Multiple Water and Electrolyte Problems: Burns	148
21.	Multiple Water and Electrolyte Problems: Urologic Dysfunction	165

UNIT V
THE PATIENT WITH A PROBLEM TRANSPORTING MATERIAL TO AND FROM CELLS

22.	The Cardiopulmonary Emergency	214
23.	Coronary Disease—Coronary Proneness	234
24.	Management of Patients with Cardiovascular Disease	255
25.	Cardiac Surgery	273
26.	Peripheral Vascular Disease	278
27.	Inadequate Composition of Material to Cells: The Patient with a Blood Dyscrasia	293

UNIT VI
THE PATIENT WITH A PROBLEM IN SUPPLY AND REMOVAL OF GASES

28.	The Respiratory System	306
29.	Diagnostic Tests	312
30.	Care of Any Patient with Respiratory Involvement	315
31.	Interference in Maintenance of a Patent Airway	326
32.	The Patient Having Chest Surgery	337

UNIT VII
THE PATIENT WITH HORMONAL IMBALANCE

33.	Biochemical Regulators and Adaptators	342
34.	Specific Endocrine Glands and Their Malfunction	346
35.	Diabetes Mellitus	367
36.	Sex Steroids	389

UNIT VIII
THE PATIENT WITH A PROBLEM IN NEUROLOGIC-ORTHOPEDIC CONTINUITY

37.	Rehabilitation	396
38.	Evaluation and Initial Management of Disorders of the Nervous System	413
39.	Increased Cranial Pressure	430
40.	Convulsive Disorders	437
41.	Vascular Diseases of the Brain	444
42.	Progressive Neurologic Diseases	451
43.	Some Specific Orthopedic Problems	455
44.	The Eye	479
45.	The Ear	496

UNIT IX
THE PATIENT WITH A PROBLEM IN CELLULAR NUTRITION

46.	The Cultural Meaning of Food	506
47.	Anatomy and Physiology of the Gastrointestinal System	512
48.	Principles in the Care of Any Patient with Imbalance in Cell Nutrition: Some Common Diagnostic Procedures	520
49.	The Patient with Peptic Ulcer	525
50.	The Patient with Intestinal Obstruction	537
51.	The Patient with Interference in Production and/or Passage of Bile	542
52.	Some Frequently Occurring Gastrointestinal Disorders	553

APPENDIXES

A.	Medic Alert	558
B.	Classification of Mental Illnesses	560
INDEX		565

UNIT I

THE INTERPERSONAL BASIS OF NURSING

1

THE COMMUNICATION PROCESS

IT IS not new for nurses to recognize that people relate to each other through communication, a process that can be observed and experienced. Communication, according to Jurgen Reusch, embraces all the modes of behavior that an individual employs consciously or unconsciously to affect others.[1]* Communication may be verbal or nonverbal.

Verbal communication is the spoken word. Verbal language is, by and large, our favorite form of conveying messages. Words usually inform the listener of our thoughts. Voice is more frequently used to express how we feel about our thoughts. Actions (gestures) help us get our ideas across. When gestures are eliminated from our conversation, there is a reduction in the fluency of oral speech with articulation becoming less precise. Nonverbal communication includes gestures, body movements, somatic signals, and symbolism in the arts. Most of us use gestures to help ourselves in speaking as well as to make our speech intelligible to others. Nonverbal communication is transmitted also via touch, smell, hearing, silence, and the written word.

Nonverbal communication is considered to be a more reliable expression of true feelings. This is because an individual has less conscious control over his nonverbal behavior.[2] Verbal and nonverbal communication can be observed simultaneously.

Vocal nonverbal communication consists of crying, wheezing, moaning, coughing, laughing, yelling, groaning, screaming, humming, and so forth. Following are some examples of nonverbal communication with their meanings:

1. Open hand with palm up indicates acceptance of an idea, friendship, a willingness to become friends.

2. Thumb down indicates an emphatic NO!

3. Pointed index finger might be used to point out a person or denote a single idea.

The crux of successful interpersonal relationships lies in successful communication. Successful communication is seldom accomplished imme-

* References for Unit I appear on pages 65–69.

diately, even in the "normal" world of human relationships. Therefore, nurses need to recognize that it takes limitless patience, experience, and some knowledge about the communication process to be therapeutic with the mentally ill.

A Communication Exercise

In your leisure time try to reveal an emotion or feeling through your voice without changing your facial expression. Try to do so through facial expression alone. Which is more successful?

Language

Language is the tool we use to communicate verbally. The words we use to designate objects and express thoughts in conventionally or socially acceptable ways are the *symbols*. *Reference* is the meaning of the symbol held in the mind of the user.[3]

The aim of effective communication is the selection of *symbols* that are similarly meaningful to the receiver as well as the sender. Thus, the receiver and the sender can effect a fusing of their communication. There can be a sense of "being on the same wave length," a sense of "being in tune with each other."

Effective communication helps to maintain mental health, overcome obstacles, and establish a basis for mutual understanding. To be able to communicate with others guards against intolerable loneliness.

In order to communicate with others the nurse must be equipped with the ability to *perceive*, that is, the ability to register incoming signals. The nurse must also be able to evaluate, to store previous impressions, to scan new impressions against the background of old ones, and to make decisions. Finally, she must be able to transmit messages verbally and nonverbally.

For the nurse, part of this communication process entails listening. Listening *is not* a passive exercise—it is active! When listening to patients the nurse should:

1. Be alert to ideas expressed in the verbal productions of the patients.
2. Listen to the words selected by others to express ideas.
3. Identify the feelings expressed in these words and the tone of voice.
4. Recognize that listening skill is related to what is heard with the *eyes* as well as the *ears*.
5. Recognize that the natural consequence of listening is a decision to act or not to act in relation to what is heard.

Observation

A second part of this communication process is observation. *Observation* is a method used by the nurse to help her look for signs that tell how the patient reacts to life's situations. Observation is an essential activity in establishing and maintaining a nurse-patient relationship.

Characteristics of good observation are:

1. It is purposeful.
2. It is planned.
3. It is objective.

Development of observational skills is essential in nursing. However, this is probably one of the most difficult skills for the nurse to acquire. The nurse observes behavior. Behavior is a mode of conducting oneself; it is the way in which a person acts in response to a stimulus.[4]

One method of learning this skill is to begin with gross observation, such as how the patient dresses, with whom he talks, and where he sits. Once the nurse feels she has noted gross behavior, she should move her focus toward more specific aspects of the patient's behavior, such as body movements, posture, and facial expressions.

Observational skills are very important when caring for the mentally ill because *all behavior has meaning and purpose and can be understood.* Therefore, it is particularly important for the nurse to observe any changes in the patient's behavior and what is happening in the situation to cause this change.

The behavior of the mentally ill does not differ in kind from that of the normal person. It differs only in degree.[5] Therefore, the nurse must recognize that her observations will provide the raw material with which she makes and implements plans for nursing care based on her observation of patient behavior.

Psychiatric nursing, on the technical level, involves purposeful interaction of the nurse with a patient or group of patients. She acts on what she hears, observes, and feels. The nurse should realize that there are always reservations in communication and that no one will be simply "frank."[6] Therefore, in her interaction with a patient she will have to set the initial goal based on her observation of his behavior.

The technical nurse should be able to use open-ended comments, such as, "You were saying . . . ," and reflection, such as "You want to go home," to give the patient a chance to express and explore his feelings. She should learn not to use clichés and automatic expressions, such as, "Don't worry," because they thwart exploration of feelings. In addition, the nurse needs to be aware that one chief handicap to communication is anxiety.[7] (See pp. 7–8.) The nurse must use her skills to prevent and avoid unnecessary anxiety in order to facilitate meaningful communication.

A basic ingredient in the nurse-patient relationship is the capacity of the nurse to give to another person in a thoughtful way without expecting something in return. Thus, the nurse-patient relationship is the core of nursing practice.[8]

The technical nurse engages in supportive nurse-patient relationships with selected patients under the supervision of a nurse with broad professional preparation.[9] This technical nurse recognizes that every nurse-patient relationship has phases. There are the orientation phase, the working phase, and the termination phase.[10] A portion of the nurse-patient relationship embodies interview. It is a planned, purposeful, time-limited interaction in which nurse and patient progress through these phases. During orientation and throughout the nurse-patient relationship, the nurse functions primarily in the counseling subrole. She may, at times, assume one of the other roles, serving as a resource person, a mother surrogate, a socializing agent, a technical expert, or a manager. Assuming these roles is not the primary focus in psychiatric nursing. They are secondary to the counseling subrole.[11] The phase of orientation also begins termination as the nurse sets limits regarding the length of time she will be spending with the patient. She sets a date for termination.

During the working phase the nurse and patient begin talking about the patient's experiences. The nurse tolerates silence, is selective in her verbal responses, and continually revises her plan for the relationship as necessary. The technical nurse recognizes her limitations and seeks appropriate assistance as she accumulates data from the patient.

The termination phase is started during orientation. The last meeting of the nurse and patient is considered to be the "termination." Together, they summarize areas discussed and evaluate the progress that has been made. Separation is not easy, and this phase may be difficult.

2

THE THERAPEUTIC ENVIRONMENT AND RELEVANT CONCEPTS

The Therapeutic Environment

THE concept of a therapeutic environment (milieu) began when Maxwell Jones, M.D., published a book called *Social Psychiatry*, later called *The Therapeutic Community: A New Treatment Method in Psychiatry*. This was a report of efforts in Belmont Hospital in England during and after World War II to rehabilitate neurotic service patients through the creation and use of a therapeutic community (environment, milieu).

In the therapeutic environment concept the emphasis is on activities that foster emotional growth. It means having therapeutic people in a patient's environment. The goal of the therapeutic environment is to help patients develop new and more effective patterns of behavior throughout a 24-hour period. This is done by promoting wholesome interaction between staff and patients and by promoting patient-centered activities.

Basic characteristics of a therapeutic environment include the following factors:

1. Absence of serious conflict among personnel.
2. A friendly, warm atmosphere throughout the unit.
3. A feeling of security on the part of all, especially nursing personnel, who deal with patients.
4. A maximum of individualization in dealing with the patient.
5. Opportunity to discuss interpersonal relationships on the unit—provision for ward conferences.
6. Opportunity for the patient to take real responsibility for himself and for other patients.
7. Sufficient comfort, food, and cleanliness.
8. Sufficient perceptual stimulation and activity to prevent regression and withdrawal.
9. Deliberate efforts toward resocialization of the patient.
10. An air of optimism about prognosis of mental disorders.

A Word About Permissiveness

Permissiveness in a therapeutic environment is based on the unconditional acceptance of the patient by the nurse.[12] This means the nurse accepts the patient as a human being even if at times she cannot accept his behavior. For example, every time Mrs. Smith rinses her dentures in the water fountain, the nurse assists her to the women's washroom, stating, "This is where you may rinse your dentures, Mrs. Smith. I will not allow you to rinse them in the drinking fountain."

Permissiveness does not imply that the nurse does not set limits. Set limitations facilitate growth and healthy living.

Anxiety

Two key psychiatric concepts are anxiety and fear. According to Peplau,[13] "anxiety is a response to unknown danger that is felt, experienced as discomfort, and that arms the human organism for mobilizing resources to meet the difficulty." This feeling results from a *perception*, on the part of the individual, that the situation is going to be, is about to become "out of hand" in some way. This loss of equilibrium, the "getting out of hand," is felt and can be observed by the various physiologic changes that go on within the anxious individual. Respirations become rapid and more shallow, the pulse accelerates, flushing or pallor occurs. Some common gastrointestinal symptoms include cramps, diarrhea, vomiting, nausea, and "butterflies in the stomach." Dryness of the mouth is often reported. Perspiration usually increases on the palms of the hands and the soles of the feet and in the axillae. As the discomfort of anxiety increases, *perception* decreases. Any threat to the security of an individual produces anxiety to some degree.

Degree of Anxiety

1. *Mild Level.* Person is alerted, sees, hears, grasps more than previously.

2. *Moderate Level.* Person's perceptual field is narrowed; he sees, hears, grasps less, but can attend to more if asked to do so.

3. *Severe Level.* Person's perceptual field is greatly reduced—the focus is on detail or on many scattered details ("tunnel vision").

4. *Panic Level.* Panic, awe, dread, terror, detail previously focused upon is "blown up." [14]

How does a person gain relief from anxiety?

1. Acting out behavior—overt: anger, crying; covert: hostility, displacement.

2. Somatizing behavior—using the body to express feelings of anxiety.
3. "Freezing to the spot"—immobilized by the anxiety.
4. Using anxiety beneficially, enduring it while in the process of searching for its causes.
5. In the service of learning. Mild anxiety "sharpens" our intellect and readies us for learning.

Anxiety often leads to a feeling of fatigue regardless of whether the individual has been very restless or immobilized. Talk may be coherent or incoherent, relevant or irrelevant.

An interesting aspect of anxiety is that it spreads from one person to another. It is always communicated *interpersonally*.[15] For example, a mother can unwillingly communicate it to her child, a lecturer throughout a class, a nurse to the patient. Anxiety is an *affect*. Affect means an emotion or feeling tone.[16]

As nurses we should be able to recognize anxiety in our patients, because one of our roles is to minimize anxiety or at least not increase it unnecessarily. We should also help the patient tolerate his anxiety and channel it into productive activity. Anxiety is a prevalent occurrence in nursing. We deal with birth, illness, and death. These situations will normally generate anxiety. In addition, the many situations and stresses that we react to individually produce degrees of anxiety. Therefore, the nurse must make every effort not to use her standards in determining whether a situation is stressful or not for another person. We can, however, strive to view the situation from the patient's vantage point.

Fear

Fear is aroused by a concrete, external immediate danger. The person who is fearful is fearful of something of which he is definitely consciously aware. For example, when a boy crossing the street does not see a car that "comes from out of nowhere" and from whose path he must jump out of the way, he probably gets a fright. This feeling of fright will make his heart beat faster and perspiration increase. In this case it is something definite that caused the specific temporary changes in his body. This is fear. In fear the individual faced with a threatening situation has two choices: flight or fight. In the example given above the choice was flight.

Both fear and anxiety have similar functions. Both are signals to the person that he is in some serious danger. The difference is that in anxiety we do not know why we feel the discomfort. Anxiety is present in every mental disease.[17] It is most important for the nurse to remember that anxiety is a very *distressing* state. The suffering from it can be worse than the suffering from a physical illness because it can last so long and relief is difficult to obtain. Once the cause of *fear* in a patient is identified and removed, the feeling of fear is relieved.

Conflict

Another important concept in psychiatric nursing is conflict. Conflict is an experience that increases tension and is said to be present only when tendencies for avoidance are present.[18] Avoidance, "keeping away," in the nurse-patient relationship is an action, verbal or nonverbal, in which the patient "keeps away" from the counseling situation.[19] In conflict there are two opposing goals. This concept can be recognized when the patient shows hesitation, vacillation, and/or blocking and an inability to decide on a course of action.[20] The nurse can help the patient in conflict by helping him clarify his goals and take action based on this clarification. When we say, "You cannot have your cake and eat it too," we are acknowledging the existence of a conflict.

Grief

Grief is a universal phenomenon among human beings, and the period of active grief is a very stressful one. The sequence of events characterizing normal grief and the meaning of each is essential knowledge for the nurse. Recognition of what is normal will enable the nurse to identify the pathologic and intervene in this process when necessary.

Normal Grief Sequence [21]

1. SHOCK AND DISBELIEF

Here the person refuses to accept the diagnosis or the death. The initial reaction of "It can't be" may be followed by a stunned, numbed feeling with the individual trying to carry out everyday activities. This phase may last a few minutes, hours, or days. This behavior is an attempt to protect oneself against stress. Grief occurs in response to the loss of a person or a body part or its function. It occurs when a person realizes he is dying.

2. DEVELOPING AWARENESS

In this phase the anguish of the loss with its accompanying feelings becomes more conscious. The surroundings seem empty and frustrating. Anger may appear directed toward the helping people in the environment, i.e., the doctor, nurses, family members. Crying with tears is typical. The patient may "bargain" with a superior being, e.g., "I'll be religious in exchange for extra time." There is always hope for a miracle.

3. RESTITUTION

This is the work of mourning. The family gathers, and ritualistic funeral activities emphasize the reality of the death. Depression is present in the dying patient.

4. RESOLVING THE LOSS

Here the mourner tries to deal with the loss intrapsychically. Thoughts are constantly with the deceased. Negative and hostile feelings are repressed in order to reduce guilt feelings. This process may continue for many months.

5. THE OUTCOME

Successful work of mourning takes a year or more. Healthy resolving of the loss is evidenced by the ability of the mourner to remember comfortably and realistically the pleasures and disappointments of the lost relationship. Many factors influence the eventual outcome:

a. The importance of the lost object as a source of support
b. The age of the lost object
c. The nature of the relationship
d. The degree of preparation for the loss
e. The physical and emotional health of the mourner at the time of the loss

The perceptive nurse can best serve the patient and his family when she uses her knowledge of the grief process along with her intuition and empathic feelings to guide and support them through this stressful period. Interrupting the phases of grief interferes with progress toward successful resolution.

3

LEARNING AND LIVING—A PROGRESSIVE PROCESS

Learning and Living

THE tasks the individual must learn—the developmental tasks of life, according to Havinghurst [22]—are those tasks that arise at or about certain periods in the life of the individual, successful achievement of which leads to his happiness and to success with later tasks. Failure leads to unhappiness in the individual and difficulty with later tasks.

Some tasks arise from physical maturation, such as learning to walk, learning to behave appropriately to the opposite sex in adolescence, and learning to accept the menopause. Developmental tasks also arise from the personal values and aspirations of the individual that are part of his personality or self. The self emerges from the interaction of internal and environmental forces.

Developmental tasks are closely related. Difficulty in one task, which may show up, for example, in school, is closely tied up with difficulty in another task. There are special times in life for the achievement of each developmental task.

Some tasks are recurrent. Learning to get along with one's age group is an example. This remains the same from the time school begins to puberty, when the nature of the task changes as one has to learn to get along with members of the opposite sex. The same task develops later when one learns to get along with age-mates of both sexes. Even then the task is not completed. The older person often faces it when he has to learn to accept the fact that he will be associating with other "elders."

Success with a recurring task in its earlier phases accounts for success in the later phases. Therefore, the central period for learning the task is when it first appears. New learnings are added, however, as the task changes in later life. For early tasks refer to Table 3–1.

The developmental tasks of adolescence, ages 12 to 18, are primarily centered about physical changes and emotional growth. It is a period when young people strive for emancipation from parents and when peer acceptance is of paramount importance. Adolescents vacillate between dependence and independence. They learn to handle more complex situa-

TABLE 3–1. DEVELOPMENTAL TASKS IN 10 CATEGORIES

	Infancy (Birth to 1 or 2)	Early Childhood 2–3 to 5–6–7	Late Childhood 5–6–7 to pubescence
I *Achieving an appropriate dependence-independence pattern*	1. Establishing one's self as a very dependent being 2. Beginning the establishment of self-awareness	1. Adjusting to less private attention; becoming independent physically (while remaining strongly dependent emotionally)	1. Freeing one's self from primary identification with adults
II *Achieving an appropriate giving-receiving pattern of affection*	1. Developing a feeling for affection	1. Developing the ability to give affection. 2. Learning to share affection	1. Learning to give as much love as one receives; forming friendships with peers
III *Relating to changing social groups*	1. Becoming aware of the alive as against the inanimate, and the familiar as against the unfamiliar 2. Developing rudimentary social interaction	1. Beginning to develop the ability to interact with age-mates 2. Adjusting in the family to expectations it has for the child as a member of the social unit	1. Clarifying the adult world as over against the child's world 2. Establishing peer groupness and learning to belong

OF BEHAVIOR OF THE INDIVIDUAL FROM BIRTH TO DEATH

Early Adolescence (pubescence to puberty)	Late Adolescence (puberty to early maturity)	Maturity (early to late active adulthood)	Aging (beyond full powers of adulthood through senility)
1. Establishing one's independence from adults in all areas of behavior	1. Establishing one's self as an independent individual in an adult manner	1. Learning to be interdependent—now leaning, now succoring others as need arises. 2. Assisting one's children to become gradually independent and autonomous beings	1. Accepting graciously and comfortably the help needed from others as powers fail, and dependence becomes necessary
1. Accepting one's self as a worthwhile person really worthy of love	1. Building a strong mutual affectional bond with a (possible) marriage partner	1. Building and maintaining a strong and mutually satisfying marriage relationship 2. Establishing wholesome affectional bonds with one's children and grandchildren 3. Meeting wisely the new needs for affection of one's own aging parents 4. Cultivating meaningfully warm friendships with members of one's own generation	1. Facing loss of one's spouse, and finding some satisfactory sources of affection previously received from mate 2. Learning new affectional roles with own children, now mature adults 3. Establishing ongoing satisfying affectional patterns with grandchildren, and other members of the extended family 4. Finding and preserving mutually satisfying friendships outside the family circle
1. Behaving according to a shifting peer code	1. Adopting an adult-patterned set of social values by learning a new peer code	1. Keeping within reasonable balance activities in the various social, service, political, and community groups and causes that make demands upon mature adults 2. Establishing and maintaining mutually satisfactory relationships with the in-law families of spouse and married children	1. Choosing and maintaining ongoing social activities and functions appropriate to health, energy, and interests

TABLE 3–1.

	Infancy (Birth to 1 or 2)	Early Childhood 2–3 to 5–6–7	Late Childhood 5–6–7 to pubescence
IV *Developing a conscience*	1. Beginning to adjust to the expectations of others	1. Developing the ability to take directions and to be obedient in the presence of authority 2. Developing the ability to be obedient in the absence of authority where conscience substitutes for authority	1. Learning more rules and developing true morality
V *Learning one's psycho-socio-biological sex role*		1. Learning to identify with male adult and female adult roles	1. Beginning to identify with one's social contemporaries of the same sex
VI *Accepting and adjusting to a changing body*	1. Adjusting to adult feeding demands 2. Adjusting to adult cleanliness demands 3. Adjusting to adult attitudes toward genital manipulation	1. Adjusting to expectations resulting from one's improving muscular abilities 2. Developing sex modesty	

[Continued]

Early Adolescence (pubescence to puberty)	Late Adolescence (puberty to early maturity)	Maturity (early to late active adulthood)	Aging (beyond full powers of adulthood through senility)
	1. Learning to verbalize contradictions in moral codes, as well as discrepancies between principle and practice, and resolving these problems in a responsible manner	1. Coming to terms with the violations of moral codes in the larger as well as in the more intimate social scene, and developing some constructive philosophy and method of operation. 2. Helping children adjust to the expectations of others and to conform to the moral demands of the culture	1. Maintaining a sense of moral integrity in the face of disappointments and disillusionments in life's hopes and dreams
1. Strong identification with one's own sex mates 2. Learning one's role in heterosexual relationships	1. Exploring possibilities for a future mate and acquiring "desirability" 2. Choosing an occupation 3. Preparing to accept one's future role in manhood or womanhood as a responsible citizen of the larger community	1. Learning to be a competent husband or wife, and building a good marriage 2. Carrying a socially adequate role as citizen and worker in the community 3. Becoming a good parent and grandparent as children arrive and develop	1. Learning to live on a retirement income 2. Being a good companion to an aging spouse 3. Meeting bereavement of spouse adequately
1. Reorganizing one's thoughts and feelings about one's self in the face of significant bodily changes and their concomitants 2. Accepting the reality of one's appearance	1. Learning appropriate outlets for sexual drives	1. Making a good sex adjustment within marriage 2. Establishing healthful routines of eating, resting, working, playing within the pressures of adult world	1. Making a good adjustment to failing powers as aging diminishes strengths and abilities

TABLE 3–1.

	Infancy (Birth to 1 or 2)	Early Childhood 2–3 to 5–6–7	Late Childhood 5–6–7 to pubescence
VII *Managing a changing body and learning new motor patterns*	1. Developing physiological equilibrium 2. Developing eye-hand coordination 3. Establishing satisfactory rhythms of rest and activity	1. Developing large muscle control 2. Learning to co-ordinate large muscles and small muscles	1. Refining and elaborating skill in the use of small muscles
VIII *Learning to understand and control the physical world*	1. Exploring the physical world	1. Meeting adult expectations for restrictive exploration and manipulation of an expanding environment	1. Learning more realistic ways of studying and controlling the physical world
IX *Developing an appropriate symbol system and conceptual abilities*	1. Developing preverbal communication 2. Developing verbal communication 3. Rudimentary concept formation	1. Improving one's use of the symbol system 2. Enormous elaboration of the concept pattern	1. Learning to use language actually to exchange ideas or to influence one's hearers 2. Beginning understanding of real causal relations 3. Making finer conceptual distinctions and thinking reflectively
X *Relating one's self to the cosmos*		1. Developing a genuine, though uncritical, notion about one's place in the cosmos	1. Developing a scientific approach

[Continued]

Early Adolescence (pubescence to puberty)	Late Adolescence (puberty to early maturity)	Maturity (early to late active adulthood)	Aging (beyond full powers of adulthood through senility)
1. Controlling and using a "new" body		1. Learning the new motor skills involved in housekeeping, gardening, sports, and other activities expected of adults in the community	1. Adapting interests and activities to reserves of vitality and energy of the aging body
		1. Gaining intelligent understanding of new horizons of medicine and science sufficient for personal well-being and social competence	1. Mastering new awareness and methods of dealing with physical surroundings as an individual with occasional or permanent disabilities
1. Using language to express and to clarify more complex concepts 2. Moving from the concrete to the abstract and applying general principles to the particular	1. Achieving the level of reasoning of which one is capable	1. Mastering technical symbol systems involved in income tax, social security, complex financial dealings and other contexts familiar to Western man	1. Keeping mentally alert and effective as long as is possible through the later years
	1. Formulating a workable belief and value system	1. Formulating and implementing a rational philosophy of life on the basis of adult experience 2. Cultivating a satisfactory religious climate in the home as the spiritual soil for development of family members	1. Preparing for eventual and inevitable cessation of life by building a set of beliefs that one can live and die with, in peace

Reprinted with permission from Caroline Tryon and Jesse W. Lillenthal III, "Guideposts in Child Growth and Development," *NEA Journal*, 39:189, March 1950.

tions and become responsible for decision making. They begin to realize the unique nature of their own personality. It can be a turbulent period because of hormonal upheaval.

The period of early adulthood, ages 18 to 30, is a time when the individual presents a special readiness and sensitivity to learn. This is a most individualistic period because the person must select his work role. This decision making is stressful. It is sometimes a frustrating period because young people are kept in the student role when they are actually ready for more independent undertakings. Often, marriage must wait until school is finished.

Middle age (the adult years) occurs between 30 and 55 years of age. It is significant to note that this is a family-oriented task period. The developmental tasks of family members are reciprocal; they overlap and interchange at times. It is a period of marital adjustment and parenthood. The mature adult has the ability to respond differently to various situations. He channels his tensions into constructive behavior leading to accomplishment of long-term goals. This is a period of work productivity. The biologic changes of aging make themselves known. This is the period in which menopausal changes develop, and a woman's reaction to menopause often mirrors her prior reaction to adolescent changes. (See pp. 13–17.)

The developmental tasks of later maturity, age 56 and on, differ in only one respect from those of other ages. They involve the strategy of holding on to life rather than seizing more of it. Limitations in the mental, physical, and economic spheres are evident; the older person has to work hard to hold on to what he already has. He develops many of the chronic diseases of aging. He must often accept enforced retirement and find new occupational satisfaction. He helps growing and grown children become responsible adults. He may increase his social and civic activities and must make advantageous use of his leisure time.

The time of onset of old age is difficult to define. It is different for each individual. Biologic signs include lowered metabolic rate, changes in the circulatory system, decreased neuromuscular coordination and gradual muscle and tissue atrophy. "Good health" becomes precarious. The fundamental needs for affection, love, security, and respect are more intensely felt. He bears witness to the death of many friends. Acceptance of the life-span is essential.

It is important for the nurse to understand developmental tasks so that normal changes will not be confused with pathologic changes. This involves a knowledge of physical and psychologic growth as it occurs at the various task levels since personality develops simultaneously.

Mental Health and Mental Illness

In mental illness the abnormality is in the mind, the emotions, and the overall behavior. It is the kind of behavior that causes others to say: "He is not in his right mind," or "There is something wrong with the way he acts." Mental illness should be viewed as part of a continuum. The difference between illness and health is a matter of degree. The observable mental and emotional symptoms are only a part of the illness—the external part. There are also abnormalities in the internal machinery of the mind and emotions. The mind and emotions do not exist apart from the body.

The fact that both the mind and body are involved in the manifestation of mental illness does not necessarily give us any indication as to the cause of mental illness. Whether the basic cause is psychologic or physical or a combination of both, the result is a personality that behaves in an abnormal way. The situation in which the individual finds himself and the people with whom he interacts play an important part in triggering off the onset of illness.

A reasonable approach to the study of the etiology of mental illness would be to consider the individual's total life experiences. Emphasis would then be placed on cultural, biologic, physiologic, interpersonal, and intrapersonal factors.[23] Interpersonal relationships, therefore, play a very important part in the development of mental illnesses—as an original cause in the formation of the abnormal response and as a contributing factor later. A mentally healthy individual, as distinct from the maladjusted person, lives creatively rather than merely passively. This means that he is not unduly distressed by the conflicts he faces. He attacks his problems in a realistic manner and understands and accepts his shortcomings and those with whom he must deal.

It would be a misunderstanding to assume that the mentally healthy individual is without emotional conflict or that he must be a social conformist. Ideally, a mentally healthy person is a productive person. He is a good friend, roommate, or neighbor. He may not be perfect or brilliant, but he can be adequate. Ask yourself how many people you know have no skin blemishes, no colds, and no cavities in their teeth.

The criteria for mental health include:

1. The setting of realistic goals
2. Harmonious interpersonal relationships
3. Self-acceptance
4. A sense of self-satisfaction
5. Productivity
6. Creativity

4

PERSONALITY STRUCTURE AND DEVELOPMENT

VARIOUS schools of thought exist in the field of psychiatry. In America the trend has been *eclectic* in nature. This means that concepts from more than one school of thought have been used in developing a usable theory of personality development. All are based on the views originating with Sigmund Freud. It is important for the nurse to understand Freud's theory of personality structure because it is the basis for others in use today. Freud described personality as consisting of three basic parts: the id, the ego, and the superego. These three basic parts are the factors that produce what we call behavior.

The id is a collective name for the unconscious. It contains everything that is inherited, that is present at birth.[24] Logic does not exist for the id; it cannot be modified by experience because it is not in contact with the external world. The id only wishes or acts. It can be controlled by the ego. The goal of the id is to obtain satisfaction.

The ego is one portion of the id that has undergone special development. It serves as an intermediary between the id and the external world. The ego attempts to do this by permitting the id to express itself in socially acceptable ways that are appropriate for the world of reality. It has the task of self-preservation.[25]

The superego is the moral or judicial branch of one's personality. It represents the ideal rather than the real and strives for perfection. The chief function of the superego is a limitation of satisfaction. The superego maintains its authority over the ego by creating anxiety and stimulating feelings of guilt and remorse.[26] It is the "conscience." The superego operates at the unconscious level.

Freud popularized the concept that the mind consists of three overlapping divisions: the conscious, the subconscious, and the unconscious. The conscious is that part of the mind that is in awareness. It functions only when the individual is awake. The preconscious, or subconscious, includes those thoughts, memories, and ideas that, although not conscious at the moment, can readily be brought into consciousness if the individual concentrates on recall. The unconscious portion of the mind is vast, and only a small part of the content of mind is conscious at any given time.[27] The unconscious is the storehouse for all the feelings, responses, and memories experienced by the individual during his entire life. These feelings, responses, and memories cannot be recalled at will. Material stored here has a powerful influence on behavior because it acts as a motivating force.

Parts of the id, the ego, and the superego are in all areas of the conscious and unconscious. The larger part of the id is in the unconscious. Behavior occurs because of conflict between or among the id, ego, and superego. The behavior that results resolves the conflict. The method may be unhealthy and lead to further conflict. Resolution may be through the use of certain methods of thinking, or *defense mechanisms* (sometimes called mental mechanisms). The defense mechanisms protect the ego and lessen anxiety.

Defense Mechanisms

There are many mechanisms that are important to an understanding of behavior, but because several overlap it is not feasible or necessary to identify all of them in detail.

REPRESSION. This is thought of as the *basic mechanism* in severe psychoses. In repression the individual walls off intense feelings so that they cannot enter awareness. Repression solves the situation by not solving it. These walled-off thoughts, feelings, needs, or fantasies would be dangerous, disturbing, or painful if permitted to remain conscious. Repression acts on an unconscious level.

DENIAL. This might be considered plain, ordinary rejection. All people use this to some extent. When using denial, the individual simply refuses to face facts as they are. Example: Inability of a wife to accept the death of her husband as she regularly sets a place for him at the table. Often the fact that something is being denied is unconscious.

REGRESSION. In regression the individual attempts to obtain gratification in a way that he found satisfactory when he was younger. He regresses. Use of this defense mechanism can take extreme forms and degrees. Example: Untidy excretory habits and/or the fetal posture sometimes seen in schizophrenic patients indicates regression.

CONVERSION. This is a condition in which strong emotional conflicts are expressed as, or converted into, physical symptoms. Example: The girl who hates her mother and is torn between the desire to strike her and fear of the consequences develops a paralyzed arm. The conflict is resolved, albeit unrealistically.

RATIONALIZATION. This is simply finding a logical reason for the things one is doing or wants to do. It is self-deception. Example: The student who buys a miniskirt that she could do without and cannot really afford explains its purchase satisfactorily to herself and her parents.

PROJECTION. This is an unconscious process in which the individual denies an unacceptable idea or emotion by attributing its origin to someone else. In its milder form, the person may severely criticize faults in others that are actually his own weak points. In its severe form, if the need for self-protection becomes very great, the disowned impulses and motives may be projected through delusions or hallucinations, particularly delusions of persecution.[28] For example, the person may feel the FBI is after him.

REACTION FORMATION. In reaction formation the original attitude or set of feelings is replaced in consciousness by the opposite attitude or feelings. Example: A young man who became a chronic alcoholic eventually lost his job, family, and friends and dropped out of sight for a few years. When he returned, he had become a teetotaler and a preacher. His favorite theme was the punishment that the person who drank alcoholic beverages would receive in the world to come.

There are many other defense mechanisms, such as compensation, undoing, sublimation, dissociation, and displacement. Some of these mechanisms serve the individual well, some serve as purposeful crutches, and some may lead to personality disorganization and self-destruction.

Defenses serve a purpose for an individual and are needed. If, through the psychotherapeutic process, the patient's pathologic defenses are removed, he is left "naked," as it were, and something must replace the defenses removed. Hopefully, if they were truly destructive ones, more healthy ones replace them.

Personality Development

The stages of growth and differentiation of the personality may be traced in several frames of reference. The most widely known is the Freudian psychoanalytic approach which traces the stages of psychosexual (psychosocial) development from the oral, through the anal, phallic, latency, and genital phases.[29]

The personality of an individual grows and matures from birth on. This takes place through a series of orderly, fairly predictable stages. According to Erik H. Erikson,[30] these stages of psychosexual (psychosocial development) are trust versus mistrust, autonomy versus shame, initiative versus guilt, industry versus inferiority, identity versus role confusion, intimacy versus isolation, generativity versus stagnation, and ego integrity versus despair.

Sullivan saw these stages of psychosexual (psychosocial) development as learning to count on others to gratify needs and wishes, learning to accept interference to wishes in relation to comfort, learning to form satisfactory relationships with peers, learning to relate to chums of same sex, learning to become independent, and learning to establish satisfactory relationships with members of the opposite sex.[31]

The transition from each stage of psychosexual development to the next is gradual. The personality evolves gradually and in a successful, satisfactory sequence of development. The passing of one stage does not end the gratifications associated with it. Traits from different stages blend and combine in various ways. In some people traits from one stage may dominate so that one may speak of "the oral character" or "the anal character." These may represent adaptive or maladaptive personality patterns. Some interests and desires from each stage of development must be inhibited, modified, or given up because of internal (superego) pressure and environmental pressure.

These stages, as presented by each theorist, overlap and blend. For example, one can see manifestations of one stage, i.e., oral, trust versus mistrust, and learning to count on others to gratify needs and wishes, throughout childhood and into adult life. This first stage is most important because it is the basic element on which emotional maturity is built. The failure of basic trust and mutuality has been recognized in psychiatry as the most far-reaching failure, undercutting all development.[32]

Many a patient becomes emotionally disturbed because he has never learned to trust himself or others or even to feel worthy of trust. Bridging this gap, making up for this tremendous unmet need in early experience, places a great challenge before the nurse. Gently and gradually she has to show the patient that he can trust her and that she can accept his needs and will try to meet them in a realistic manner. In the trusting relationship that develops the nurse should help the patient trust himself and his own feelings, freeing him to grow emotionally as well as intellectually. Through these learning situations the nurse will encourage him to trust others—patients, staff, and family. Why do this? Because as long as the patient cannot trust himself, the nurse, or his environment, he will be an "emotional cripple." He will remain sick, unable to relate to people or situations in a healthy fashion.

Building trust is a nebulous, intangible endeavor. It may be nothing more than providing a comb for the patient, giving a reassuring pat, or just making yourself available. It means keeping promises. Whatever the nurse does, she must keep in mind the general principles of psychiatric nursing.

General Principles of Psychiatric Nursing *

1. Accept each patient as you find him and his illness as it exists.
2. Nurses can use self-understanding as a therapeutic tool.

* Adapted from: Ruth V. Matheney and Mary Topalis, *Psychiatric Nursing*, 4th ed. C. V. Mosby Company, St. Louis, 1965, pp. 76–94.

3. Consistency can be used to contribute to patient security.

4. Reassurance must be given subtly and in an acceptable manner.

5. Anything that produces or increases patient anxiety is usually not good for the patient.

6. Patient's behavior should not be interpreted to him.

7. Verbal and physical force should be avoided if possible.

8. Patients need to be allowed the expression of negative emotion.

9. Nursing care should center on the patient as a person, not on the control of symptoms.

10. Explanation of routines and procedures should be given at the patient's level of understanding.

11. Intimate relationships with patients are not conducive to a therapeutic atmosphere.

12. Modification of procedures to meet the needs of the mentally ill should follow basic principles.

13. An intellectual approach to the patient's problem is useless.

14. Personal values and personal relationships should be initiated only by the patient.

5

MENTAL ILLNESS

Psychoneuroses

THE person with a psychoneurotic disorder, the "neurotic," suffers either from intolerable anxiety or from some symptom that protects him from his feelings of anxiety. He maintains contact with reality; therefore, the degree of distortion and disorganization is not as great as that seen in psychosis. The difference between neurosis and psychosis is mainly a matter of degree.

Although he remains in contact with reality, the individual with a neurosis shows a handicap that he and the people around him recognize as being unnecessary, unusual, or sick. The form of neurosis depends on the success with which the various stages of psychosexual development, described in Chapter 4, were achieved.[33]

A neurosis does not necessarily stem from one specific thing. It may stem from several things, for example:

1. Deprivation of love and interest as a child
2. An inadequate acquaintance with the realities of the world
3. Inability to love and hate effectively [34]

Women are about ten times as subject to neuroses as men.[35] This is thought to be due, in part, to the fact that more rigid repressions of instinctual wishes is required of women with less opportunity to seek gratification aggressively.

Anxiety as a symptom may be found in a variety of disorders, if not all. A certain amount of anxiety is a perfectly normal reaction to any stressful situation.

In the condition called *acute anxiety neurosis,* the patient does not primarily complain of anxiety. He confronts his physician with somatic complaints. He experiences a feeling of impending death because he has shortness of breath, palpitations, constriction of the chest, and headache. In addition he also experiences diarrhea, constipation, disturbed appetite, epigastric pains, and urinary frequency.[36] These symptoms usually frighten the patient. He cannot work. He is miserable and depressed. Many of these symptoms appear at one time causing the patient to respond with a *panic reaction*. Everything is blown out of proportion.

The treatment of the patient with an acute anxiety reaction depends, to a large extent, on the behavioral history. It is important for the physician to know *what* the patient says as well as *how* he says it. Knowledge of past as well as current behavior and events is essential. The physical examination is also significant because certain physiologic factors are observed via instruments, i.e., blood pressure, temperature, and the appearance of the pupils.

Treatment of a patient with acute anxiety neurosis is possible with tranquilizers. With large initial dosage the patient obtains symptomatic relief. Smaller maintenance doses alter the basic physiologic disturbance, and a therapeutic effect is obtained. The patient and his relatives should be warned at the onset of treatment that to be most effective, treatment may have to be continued for some time. The neurotic person usually has poor health most of the time. He likes to go to doctors. The psychotic most often is brought in by relatives.

Protection against anxiety is seen most directly in the so-called *hysterical conversion* reaction in which the anxiety and conflict are converted into a physical symptom that is without physical cause. This is a very dramatic type of neurosis and as such is one of the easiest to recognize.[37] The symptoms, either sensory or motor or both, that develop in the hysterical patient help to resolve his anxiety. The symptoms represent the unconscious conflict from which the patient is suffering. In stress situations these patients may become paralyzed, blind, deaf, or mute, thus avoiding the demands made on them. This physical symptom, which the patient finds nonthreatening, has been called by French psychiatrists *la belle indifférence* (the beautiful indifference). The primary gain is *defense against* anxiety. The secondary gain is the temporary advantage that the symptomatology affords.

In contrast to the agitated anxiety neurotic, the hysterical neurotic presents a calm demeanor. This symptom is out of proportion to the stress or cause alleged to be involved.[38] A physical examination is very helpful because the symptomatology has no accurate relation to the nervous system.

Treatment is difficult. This patient has no desire to surrender his symptom. Often the physician must present a cure in such a way that it is not humiliating to the patient. The patients are not good candidates for tranquilizer therapy because they have a tendency to overreact to the side effects of drugs. Intense psychotherapy, in which the physician attempts to find out why the patient slipped into a specific hysterical reaction and what can be done about it, has worked. Restoration of self-respect and self-esteem is essential in this process.

Phobic reactions are those that occur when a relatively harmless situation is reacted to as though it were dangerous or when the danger is grossly overestimated. These neurotic fears are transferred, unconsciously, to some external object or situation.[39]

Many situations and objects can become the center for the formation of a phobia. A *phobia* is a persistent, pathologic *fear* out of the proportion to the stimulus. The common ones have been given names, such as acrophobia, fear of heights; claustrophobia, fear of closed-in places; zoophobia, fear of animals. The phobic object usually symbolizes the original object or situation. In effect, the patient substitutes fear for anxiety.

The phobia serves as a means for the patient to conceal and exclude from conscious awareness the internal or unconscious source of the fear. The loss of a neurotic phobia would bring back intolerable anxiety. Psychotherapy is necessary to help the patient work through his fears.

OBSESSION. The persistent recurrence of an unwelcomed and often distressing thought. This thought has unconscious significance. An example would be the patient who is tormented by recurrent thoughts and fears of dirt and germs.

OBSESSIVE PERSON. This is often the type of individual who is very prompt, precise, meticulous, the "perfectionist." Most obsessive patients are extremely concerned about what others think of them. In addition, this person has a repetitive urge to carry out ritualistic acts such as compulsive hand washing.

COMPULSION. An unwelcomed urge to perform an act or series of acts: for example, the person who needs to wash his hands repeatedly for fear of becoming contaminated. A compulsion is, in effect, an obsession in action. The compulsive does not *want* to act upon his compulsion; he *has* to act. If he is prevented from the action(s) by force or other circumstances he experiences extreme anxiety.

A wide range of disability is associated with obsessive-compulsive reactions, and patients may be totally or mildly disabled. These obsessive-compulsive reactions are often among the most severe of the psychoneurotic disorders, and they offer the poorest prognosis. The obsessive-compulsive person is very sick and is resistive to treatment. He is most often helped by the physician who offers sympathetic counsel and pharmacologic relief of his anxiety.

Nursing Expectations

When caring for the psychoneurotic patient the technical nurse can:

1. Attempt to become aware of her attitude toward patients suffering from neurotic problems.

2. Recognize that the physical complaints of the neurotic patient are real to him and respond accordingly.

3. Develop an awareness of the significance of unconscious conflicts as they relate to a patient's neurotic symptoms.

4. Demonstrate sympathy and empathy with patients who experience emotionally conditioned pain.

5. Develop a therapeutic nursing care plan for the neurotic patient with the assistance of staff members.

6. Assist the anxious patient to develop an interest outside himself.

7. Recognize that most psychoneurotic patients are treated in the doctor's office or in the general hospital.

8. Identify and record change in patients' anxiety levels.

In addition, see pages 23–24 for general principles of psychiatric nursing.

Psychoses

Psychoses are generally considered the most severe psychologic disorders. They are characterized by an extensive disorganization of the personality accompanied by a break from reality. The psychotic becomes incapable of making social adjustment, and this results in the need for hospitalization. The psychotic disorders include:

1. Involutional psychotic reactions
2. Schizophrenic reactions
3. Affective reactions
4. Paranoid reactions

As the ego in a psychotic breaks down, unconcious material is expressed in its rawest form. This expression is disorganized, bizarre, and difficult to understand. Psychotics usually have one or more of the following symptoms: delusions, hallucinations, or illusions.

DELUSION. A *fixed false* belief maintained by the patient without appropriate evidence.[40] These beliefs cannot be altered by reason or experience. Example: A patient believes he is Napoleon.

HALLUCINATION. An imaginary sensory perception without external stimuli regarded by the patient as real; it may occur in any of the five senses; it can be chemically or emotionally induced.[41] For example, when a schizophrenic patient talks aloud to "someone," that "someone" is actually there to him.

ILLUSION. A false response to sensory perception.[42] Example: The shadow of a tree looks like a person.

The two major subdivisions of the psychoses are the schizophrenias and the affective psychoses. The former can be characterized as primarily disorders of thought and mental function, the latter as primarily disorders of feeling and mood.

Schizophrenia is one of our major medical problems. It has been determined that approximately 54 per cent of all hospital beds in the United States today are occupied by psychiatric patients. About one half of these beds are occupied by schizophrenics.[43]

The major incidence of schizophrenia is during the most productive periods of life, roughly between the ages of 15 and 44. The schizophrenic psychoses are the chief causes of prolonged and serious disability. They rarely kill, but they are significantly destructive by claiming their victims among people during their most productive working ages.

Common characteristics of schizophrenia include:

APATHY. This is a feeling in which emotion is minimal or seemingly absent. Often the feelings manifested by the patient are out of keeping with the event.

ASSOCIATIVE LOOSENESS. This is a peculiarity occurring in the thought processes and in the handling of words that makes it difficult, if not impossible, to follow the trend of the patient's conversation; e.g., he may use "word salad," in which sentences sound garbled, or he may use perseveration, in which he involuntarily repeats answers to a previous question in response to new questions.

AUTISTIC THINKING. This is thinking that is so subjective and so private that it is undecipherable to others. Autism is manifested by a preponderance of daydreaming and fantasy. Only the patient is aware of its meaning. Meaning can be inferred if one has familiarized himself with the patient, his history, and some of the symbolic ways in which he uses words. An example would be a schizophrenic patient who "invents" words of his own, i.e., sound combinations that have no linguistic meaning. Such words are called neologisms.[45]

AMBIVALENCE. This is an attitude that is highly developed in the schizophrenic. It consists of a mixture of feelings of hate, fear, and love toward those people whom one might expect only to love. The schizophrenic is ambivalent toward almost everything. These opposing feelings neutralize each other, making it difficult for the patient to express either.

The first signs of schizophrenia show up many years before the actual breakdown. There appears an early tendency toward *withdrawal*, accompanied by extreme sensitivity to feelings of being unloved, rejected, and unworthy. These feelings are generally followed by loneliness, suspiciousness, moodiness, aloofness, and separation from others. In addition, less attention is given to the family, work, school, personal appearance, and responsibilities. Emotional responses become flat and shallow; this is sometimes referred to as "flattened affect." Total apathy may also occur, or there is silly laughing and smiling about nothing. When the final break with reality comes, delusions and/or hallucinations usually make their appearance. Emotions and thoughts become more unrelated and speech more irrelevant. The patient feels that people in his environment are hostile and threatening. His words and manner are used more to conceal than to reveal feeling.

There is no proof that schizophrenia is a disease entity that has a single cause. Some authorities believe that schizophrenia is best considered a group of interrelated disease states, and others feel schizophrenia is a disease with a number of different forms or types, each type characterized by distinctive symptoms.

The prevailing practice today is to speak of "schizophrenia" as a single disease and to differentiate a number of types according to the dominant symptom pattern. This practice will be followed here.

Brief Description of the Major Types of Schizophrenia

SIMPLE

The simple schizophrenic begins to withdraw early in life, becoming almost reclusive with constricted interests. The patient eventually becomes a passive burden to his family. This condition is marked by apathy, failure of human relationships, and deterioration over a long period of time with obvious delusions or hallucinations. This type is rarely seen in its pure form today.

HEBEPHRENIC TYPE

This type of schizophrenia is characterized by silly, inappropriate smiling, unpredictable giggling, hallucinations, and some delusional thought. There is personality disintegration. These patients also demonstrate profound regression with neglect of personal habits, bizarre language, and inappropriate fluctuating emotions. They may be denudative (they strip off their clothes) or wear bizarre costumes and carry bundles filled with strange mementos. Response to the surroundings is just about nil, separation from reality nearly complete.

CATATONIC TYPE

The characterizing symptoms of this type have to do with *motion*. In one phase, catatonic stupor, there is little or no motion at all. The patient remains mute, stuporous, and in one fixed position for long periods of time (waxy flexibilitas).

In catatonic excitement, there is uncontrolled, excessive movement and activity. There is aggressive, hostile moving about and destructiveness. Objects may be smashed, clothing torn, and people attacked. Delusions and hallucinations are common along with posturing, grimacing, and meaningless speech. Negativism prevails. Often there is a refusal to eat or sleep to the point of physical exhaustion.

PARANOID TYPE

The characteristic feature of the paranoid type is delusions of persecution. People are out to "get" him, to capture him, to kill him, to poison him, and he has hostile, aggressive behavior in "defense" against his persecution. The paranoid schizophrenic experiences frequent hallucinations in which voices "accuse" him of wicked actions or thoughts. Sexual anxiety and concerns about homosexuality are common in this condition. The paranoid patient is frequently assaultive or may be violent. He often talks about magical "rays" or "powers" that control him.

The nurse needs to recognize that the behavior of the schizophrenic is unpredictable and may fluctuate and that schizophrenic reactions are characterized by marked difficulty in interpersonal relationships and usually involve a strong tendency to *withdraw* from reality. To replace reality the patient creates a fantasy world that is less tense and threatening to him. Creation of his schizophrenic world limits the patient's interaction with others in the real world. Attempts to build up a relationship with him often meet with failure because he seems to retreat to his world before every approach. This is a process known as regression. Sullivan felt that the schizophrenic is shy, low in self-esteem, and rather convinced that he is not highly appreciated by others.[46]

Nursing Expectations

When caring for the patient who demonstrates symptoms of withdrawal, the technical nurse can:

1. Direct her care toward the prevention of regression by
   a. Maintaining a therapeutic environment,
   b. Demonstrating an accepting attitude of the patient.
2. Assist the patient to maintain good personal hygiene and, whenever possible, wear his own clothes.
3. Initiate toileting routine to assist regressed patients with excreta problems.
4. Record and report, when necessary, daily bowel habits.
5. Make sure the patient is receiving a balanced diet.
6. Be alert to the physical condition of patients.
7. Demonstrate patience, tact, and tolerance toward hostile attitudes and aggressive behavior.
8. Design a nursing care plan for the withdrawn patient with other staff members and modify it as necessary.
9. Recognize that insulin shock treatment is an effective somatic treatment for schizophrenia.

32] THE INTERPERSONAL BASIS OF NURSING

10. Know the pharmacologic agents used in the treatment of the psychoses.

11. Protect against aggressive behavior by being aware of clues that indicate its coming arrival.

The Affective Disorders

The affective disorders are those known as the manic-depressive psychoses. From the name of the disease it is clear that it consists of opposite emotional states—mania and depression. In these disorders the pathologic state of mind is usually circumscribed and self-limited. The patient suffers from an exaggerated mood of depression or elation, which lasts an average of three months to two years if untreated. The alternation, or swing from one mood to the other, may be quite sudden and frequent. One phase can occur with the other. Generally speaking, the people who have manic-depressive attacks are extroverts. They are sociable, outgoing people. Sometimes this extroversion conceals shyness and feelings of inadequacy. This illness is seen more often in women than men and more often in the upper socioeconomic classes.

In the depressive state the patient complains of fatigue, anorexia, and insomnia. The depressive state may range from mild to deep stuporous depression. Worries, doubts, and fears are numerous. Gloominess, indecision, and isolation from social contact are common. As the depression becomes more intense, the physical attitude of the patient becomes one of despondency, hopelessness, and desperation. Often there is a sense of terrible dread and impending disaster. There may be attempts at suicide.

In the manic phase the patient is overactive and excessively alert, sleeps little, writes long letters, is overtalkative, makes numerous phone calls, is sometimes destructive, and is full of plans. Often there is poor judgment in the spending of money. This manic patient can be amusing for a period of time; then he becomes tiresome. He is euphoric and a "busybody."

Both phases of the manic-depressive psychosis respond well to electroconvulsive therapy. Once the immediate psychotic state has improved, psychotherapy should be utilized to effect a better functioning of the individual. Pharmacologic agents are also used in the treatment of the affective disorders.

Nursing Expectations

Technical nursing care of patients with affective disorders includes the ability to:

1. Remove the patient, in the manic phase, from all exciting and disturbing influences.

2. Demonstrate reserve at the patient's unconventional behavior.

3. Exhibit firmness in her approach to the manic patient.
4. Arrange to make her observations of the manic patient as unobtrusive as possible.
5. Be alert to the patient's desires to escape because they usually do not wish to be hospitalized.
6. Initially review requests made by patient with staff before permission is granted or denied.
7. Segregate manic patients, because one stimulates another.
8. Recognize and provide nourishment for the manic patient, especially liquids.
9. Recognize the need for and promote rest and sleep.
10. Direct the manic patient's activities toward constructive goals.
11. Recognize the danger of *suicide* during the depressive phase.
12. Provide adequate nutrition for the depressed patient.
13. Observe, record, and report changes in patient behavior, verbal and nonverbal.

Depression

The nurse may find herself quite drained emotionally after being with the depressed patient for a time. The feelings of loneliness and emptiness that pervade are exhaustive. Despair, loss of self-esteem, the real or imagined loss of a loved object, a health or financial disaster, loss in social status, and separation or divorce could cause such depressed feelings. According to Freud's psychoanalytic theory, "the ego sees itself deserted by the superego and lets itself die." [47]

Depression is serious. Everyone is depressed at times, and this is "normal." We may experience "Monday blues," be sad because we have a cold, have a gloomy spell, or feel remorse because of financial worries. Provided these blue feelings do not interfere with our daily tasks, we accept them as a natural part of living.

The following is a brief description of three types of depression, showing manifestations of each in several areas.

Suicide

Karl Menninger, in his book *Man Against Himself*, outlines the following dynamic theory of suicide:

A. Impulses derived from primary aggressiveness are crystallized as "a wish to kill,"
B. Impulses derived from a modification of this primitive aggressiveness are crystallized as "the wish to be killed,"
C. Impulses from primary aggressiveness plus other motives are crystallized as the "wish to die."

First there exists a conscious hate for someone, which yields conscious guilt feelings. These guilt feelings are intolerable, and as a result there

TABLE 5–1

	Neurotic Depression	Reactive Depression	Internal Depression (Endogenous)
Cause	Severe or prolonged stress; unresolved conflicts; chronic anxiety, fear, anger. Self-pity, impatience, and anger at the world. Blames others for his unhappiness, will accuse and distrust almost everyone. Family members usually react with sympathy, pity, annoyance	A meaningful loss of a loved one; an opportunity or material things, etc. Sense of emptiness is present here—felt outside self and in the environment. As a rule the person's self-esteem remains intact. This depression invites empathy	Sadness characterized as a sense of emptiness within the person. Something is wrong with her. Out of this grows convictions of unworthiness, guilt. Her twisted thoughts urge her to blame others. Relatives cannot understand this and do not recognize this as depression. They see and feel hostility
History of depression in family	Sometimes related to depression in family	No relationship to depression in family	Commonly other members in family have had depressions
Onset	Gradual, several weeks—builds up slowly	Sudden—related to a loss	Rapid (1–4 weeks). Seems to come from nowhere
Nature	Mixed—sometimes slowed, other times agitated	Tends to be retarded and slowed down	Usually agitated type, restlessness, "nervousness"
Sleep	Restless, morning sleep is deep	Difficulty falling asleep—but sleeps through	Falls asleep easily, up 4–5 A.M. not to return
Crying	Some crying spells	Steady tearfulness, sobbing	Intense, spontaneous crying spells
Mood	Unpredictable—optimistic A.M., depressed P.M.	Constant feeling of sadness	Worse in the morning, better in the evening

TABLE 5-1. [*Continued*]

	Neurotic Depression	Reactive Depression	Internal Depression (Endogenous)
Self-esteem	High and low fluctuates	No loss of self-esteem, environment empty	Complete loss; emptiness in self
Anxiety	Constantly present, may rise to panic state	Present—tends to diminish with time	Present—tends to increase with progression of illnesss
Memory	Variable, unreliable	Poor	Poor
Recurrence	Frequent with remissions	With a new loss	Common with varied periods of remission
Suicidal thoughts	Frequently present, covered up by desire to live	May be present and intense	Present and intense fear of death expressed
Suicide attempts	Frequent, attention gathering, hopes to be rescued	Occasional, meaningful; related to loss of hope	Common, should be anticipated, related to desire for relief from mental pain

is the development of conscious hopelessness, fatigue, fear, despair, and eventually depression. The danger of suicide is greatest as the patient goes into and comes out of his depression. Factors to consider in the evaluation of suicide risk include:

1. Degree of depression. The greater the depression the greater the suicide risk.
2. Amount of agitation. The more agitated and restless the patient is, the more likely he is to attempt suicide.
3. Use of alcohol or sedatives. These agents decrease cortical control and add to chance of impulsive behavior.
4. Family history of suicide.
5. Religion. Some religious beliefs are a deterrent to suicide.

The prevention of suicide is a task of great importance for the nurse as she cares for the depressed patient. Suicidal attempts are rarely made without some previous clue from the patient. For instance, a skier may give away his favorite skis. It is believed that suicide is motivated by sociologic, cultural, psychologic, and ecologic factors. Seventy-five per cent of the subjects who have committed suicide had a history of having previously threatened or attempted suicide.[48]

SUICIDE PREVENTION

According to the National Institute of Mental Health, suicide is the twelfth most frequent cause of death in this country. This is probably an understatement since there is no way of knowing how many apparently accidental deaths are concealed suicides.

Many of the current suicide prevention crisis programs were originally stimulated or implemented by concerned clergy. Psychiatrists and other mental health professionals quickly became involved in these programs which are located in 22 states and the District of Columbia. The second edition of the *Directory of Suicide Prevention Facilities* (1968) lists over 60 facilities.

These suicide prevention programs operate under two important principles: (1) someone should be available to persons in crisis and (2) the someone who is available should be able to respond to the person in crisis with resourcefulness and competency. It is felt that these programs provide a service oriented to reaching out and holding on to suicidal persons. Life-saving or holding-on is their *first order of business*.

Psychophysiologic Autonomic and Visceral Disorders (Psychophysiologic/Psychosomatic Disorders)

It is now well recognized that emotional problems can lead to disturbances of physical functions and even to physical disease.[49] For example, fear can cause increased secretion of urine, increased peristalsis, and increased sweating. Psychophysiologic medicine does not neglect the physical problems in diseases of the body but includes a consideration of the role of psychologic or emotional factors in their development and perpetuation.

Psychosomatic symptoms are real even though their causes may be obscure. Well-known conditions with psychosomatic connections include:

1. Peptic ulcer
2. Asthma
3. Urticaria
4. Ulcerative colitis
5. Some cardiac arrhythmias and hypertension

Therefore, the nurse must attempt to establish a nurse-patient relationship of therapeutic value. The patient will need emotional and physical support. The nurse communicates to the staff any clues she discovers.

The person who develops a psychosomatic illness has usually suffered serious feelings of insecurity early in life and has not developed the usual mechanism of defense to protect him against the insecurity. The defense developed is on a physiologic level, the affect being expressed through the viscera. Psychosomatic reactions to stress, over long periods of time, often produce structural organic changes leading to the development of a chronic disease.

Superficially, the individual may seem like a reasonably stable person who relates well to others. However, when he is subjected to an emotion as it was experienced earlier in life, and his defenses have broken down, there can occur intense physiologic activity. For example, when the patient with a peptic ulcer, who has defended himself against feeling his dependency needs by being very self-sufficient, has a business setback, he may become overwhelmed and have an exacerbation of his condition even though he is already wealthy.

Treatment of the patient with a psychosomatic illness is directed toward helping him gain an understanding of the sources of unhappiness and emotional turmoil. The somatic aspects must also be treated as they occur. Thus the psychiatrist and the internist work together. Many factors are inherent in the etiology of psychophysiologic illness; however, stress is the one most amenable to preventive measures. The nurse must recognize that the discomfort is real to the patient, and when medication is prescribed, the nurse should administer it without hesitation. Making light of the patient's symptoms can intensify his somatic reaction.

Organic Brain Disorders

Organic brain disorders are so called when they are produced by definite organic lesions in the nervous system and when they are due to actual destruction of brain cells and their fibers. The resultant mental deterioration is usually dependent on the degree of pathology present and the site of the disease entity. Patients with stable premorbid personalities often show remarkably few symptoms despite relatively extensive brain damage.

Acute. Organic syndromes from which the patient recovers; usually the result of temporary, reversible, diffuse impairment of brain tissue function. *Examples:* acute alcoholic intoxication and acute brain syndrome associated with barbiturate intoxication. See also Appendix B.

Organic. Results from relatively permanent, more or less irreversible impairment of cerebral tissue function. *Examples:* chronic brain syndrome associated with alcoholism and senile brain disorder.

It is significant to note that as science discovers new ways to extend life, the problems of senility become increasingly important. Senility has increased because medicine has been able to prolong the life-span but it has not been able to protect the brain from the effects of hardening of the arteries and deterioration of brain cells.

Organic brain disorders are characterized by a basic syndrome consisting of:

1. Impairment of memory
2. Impairment of judgment
3. Impairment of orientation
4. Impairment of comprehension
5. Fluctuation in levels of attention
6. Labile and shallow affect

Prognosis is variable and depends on the extent and location of the pathology. A disorder that appears reversible, hence acute, at the beginning may prove later to have left permanent damage and a persistent organic brain syndrome. As an example, senile patients suffer from a clouding of consciousness, concentration is impaired, and confabulation often occurs. Confabulation is the filling in of memory gaps with detailed but inaccurate accounts derived from fantasy. These accounts vary with each telling and are a defense against anxiety and the embarrassment caused by a failing memory and disorientation.

Senility not only is deterioration of the brain, but brings with it a time of loss; loved ones die, physical capacities become limited, the past has more to offer than the future, one's vocation ends, and death is imminent. Each of these factors is a stress of the highest order and occurs when the personality has become hardened and rigid.

The treatment for patients with senile brain disease, chronic brain syndrome associated with cerebral arteriosclerosis, includes vitamin therapy, supportive care, occupational therapy, group therapy as in "over 60" clubs, senior citizens' groups, and shock therapy for acute symptoms. Prevention is *education for old age!*

Nursing Expectations

In rendering technical nursing care the nurse should:

1. Strive to establish and maintain a therapeutic environment recognizing that these types of patients are extremely sensitive to their environment.
2. Not threaten, scold, or argue with the patients.
3. Listen to but not focus on the patient's incorrect ideas. Any attempt to change them will give the nurse feelings of inadequacy and helplessness in addition to adding to the patient's anxiety and feelings of insecurity.
4. When the patient is suffering from delirium, protect him against injury or suicide.

5. For patients in fearful states, protect them by removing unnecessary stimulation, reducing noise, and preventing anxiety-producing interactions.

6. Encourage the patient to eat and maintain the necessary activities of daily living.

7. When possible, help the patient avoid daytime naps.

8. Demonstrate consistency in routine.

9. Recognize that the individual's previous personality will, in part, determine how he will react to stress.

Sociopathic Personality Disturbances

Those who live by the pleasure principle alone without regard for the demands of society present a problem for themselves and the community. Disorders included under this heading are

1. Antisocial reactions
2. Dyssocial reactions
3. Sexual deviations
4. Addictions (see Chap. 7)

Before adolescence, the antisocial individual demonstrates symptomatic behavior such as truancy, behavior problems, and delinquency. The antisocial person wants his pleasure at once—he wants what he wants when he wants it. He does not tolerate frustration and does not modify behavior as a result of punishment. He is often described as having an outwardly pleasing personality, but he usually has no close interpersonal relationships. This individual uses flattery and makes promises that are not meant to be kept.

The antisocial personality does not see himself as sick and rarely seeks treatment voluntarily. Prognosis is poor. These patients are seldom seen in a facility caring for the mentally ill. More often they are imprisoned in other institutions. The antisocial personality is loyal to no one but himself. In contrast, the dyssocial personality may be loyal to a group.

Individual and group therapy have been used. The therapist working with these patients is cautioned against allowing them to manipulate, to "con" him.

When the antisocial individual is hospitalized, the nurse must be aware of his skill at manipulating people and exercise positive, consistent control when necessary. In addition, the nurse should be aware of those patients in the environment who could be easily affected by the antisocial patient's behavior, and she should intervene as necessary.

The sexual deviant achieves sexual gratification in ways considered undesirable by society; examples include rape, homosexuality, voyeurism, and exhibitionism.

6

TREATMENT MODALITIES

The Physical Therapies (Somatic Therapies)

Insulin Coma Therapy

INSULIN coma therapy was the first of the modern shock therapies. It was introduced in Vienna about 1932 by the Polish psychiatrist Manfred Sakel. Sakel initially began using insulin in the treatment of drug addiction. It was only after observations of accidental hypoglycemia that resulted in an improvement in the mental state that Sakel undertook this therapy for the treatment of schizophrenia. Sakel's theory was that under the influence of shock treatment sick and defective cell connections in the brain would be separated. He believed these defective connections were caused by psychologic influences on cells.[51]

Insulin coma therapy is considered the most widely accepted somatic treatment for schizophrenia.[52] In recent years its use has decreased because it is potentially dangerous and medically complicated.[53] The advent and widespread use of tranquilizers have also contributed to the decreased use of insulin coma therapy.

The technique of insulin coma therapy involves the administration of daily increasing doses of regular insulin via intramuscular injection until a hypoglycemic coma develops. These doses of insulin sharply reduce the level of sugar in the blood. The brain is deprived of its chief foodstuff, and the patient sinks into coma. The average coma dose varies from 200 to 400 units of regular insulin.[54] The physiologic reaction of the patient is the primary concern, not the amount of insulin.

Termination of coma depends on its depth. If the patient responds to command, glucose is given by mouth. If he does not respond to command, glucose can be given by nasal gastric gavage or by intravenous injection.

The results of treatment have included improvement in the patient's mood, reduction of delusional material, and active participation in group activities. The most serious side effect is prolonged or irreversible coma.

Following insulin coma therapy the patient should shower and have a substantial meal (because he fasts before treatment) making sure that sodium is included to replace that lost from diaphoresis during the treatment. The nurse assisting with this treatment has to learn about the great number of symptoms that may arise and about the various complications that may result. Nurses must be in constant attendance during this treatment.

Electroconvulsive (Shock) Therapy

This form of therapy began in 1935 with Meduna in Hungary who used a pharmacologic means to produce convulsions. Meduna used a camphor preparation which proved unreliable and was later replaced by pentylenetetrazol (Metrazol).[55] In 1938 Cerletti and Bini replaced pharmacologic convulsive treatment with electricity in small amounts.

Electroconvulsive therapy is thought to interrupt the abnormal electrical pathways and produce a convulsion similar to a grand mal seizure. It was discovered that the best results were obtained not in schizophrenia but in depression and other affective disorders.[56] Electroconvulsive therapy involves use of an alternating electric current controlled by the doctor. *The current* is conducted through electrodes placed on both temples. Electrojelly or saline solution is used on the simple metal disks that are attached with a rubber band to the patient's *head.*

Some authorities believe the electroshock therapy works by producing a grand mal seizure that represents a well-deserved punishment for the patient's sins. Others follow the assumption that a convulsion eliminates toxic substances from the nerve cells.[57] In either case it gives good results in the treatment of some depressions and, to a lesser degree, overactivity.[58]

Special permission is needed for the patient to receive this treatment. The patient is usually fasting before the treatment and is alert to events going on around him. Very often fears and resistance to treatment may be evident through verbal and nonverbal expression. It is at this time that the nurse must support the patient and recognize some of the reasons for these fears and anxieties.

The fears and anxieties may be based on several factors:

1. Childhood training to avoid electrical outlets, wiring, and electric appliances
2. The association of electroconvulsive therapy with the harmful effects of electricity in general (pain, burns, shock, electrocution)
3. Anxiety about the unknown and an air of secrecy and isolation surrounding the procedure
4. Fear of being unconscious with the possibility of death or loss of control of one's faculties
5. Recall of previous treatment complications to oneself or others

Electroconvulsive therapy is usually given three days a week until approximately 20 treatments have been given. It is a relatively safe procedure with few contraindications. Prior to the treatment the patient should be taken to the toilet, and his temperature, pulse, respiration, and blood pressure should be checked and recorded. If premedication is given, such as a drug to decrease secretions, the patient should be informed that his mouth will feel dry but that this is desired. The nurse is responsible for having a padded tongue blade on hand and an airway and oxygen tank available in case the patient has respiratory difficulty. During and after treatment the care of the patient should follow the principles of caring for any unconscious patient who has had a seizure.

Nurses should avoid using the term "electric shock" when talking with patients. When answering questions and reassuring patients about this, the nurse can honestly say that there will be no pain and that the patient will remember nothing about the treatment but that he will have a desire to sleep. It is advisable for the nurse to remain with the patient throughout the experience.

Complications most feared from electroconvulsive therapy are fractures and cardiovascular problems. These are rare today thanks to a refinement of the treatment process and careful taking of the history and physical data prior to treatment along with careful selection and administration of premedication by the physician.

Psychotherapy

Psychotherapy is the art of treating mental disorders utilizing interview approach.[59] It deals with the thoughts and emotions of individuals. There are many different kinds of psychotherapy. In each the basic method involves a verbal and emotional interchange between the patient and the therapist.

The two major classes of psychotherapy are supportive psychotherapy and reconstructive psychotherapy.

In supportive psychotherapy little emphasis is placed on the underlying unconscious factors that may have caused the illness. Instead the physician focuses on current problems and the way the patient handles them. Together, he and the patient explore problem areas. Ultimately, through suggestion, reassurance, and guidance, the patient gains insight, and his behavior can be changed. The physician may find that additional therapies enhance the process. He may use drugs, hypnosis, and/or shock therapy. The patient must actively participate in this process.

In reconstructive therapy emphasis is placed on the unconscious conflicts that may have caused the illness. The physician focuses on the unconscious, repressed emotions. The patient's troublesome feelings and emotions are probed, taken apart, looked into, and analyzed. These feelings and emotions are traced back to their origins to find out what caused them to develop in this way and to understand them in the light of past experiences.

Techniques Used in Reconstructive Therapy

The physician can often determine significant areas by observing the sequence in which the patient presents his thoughts. Some techniques utilized in reconstructive therapy include free association, dream analysis, and hypnosis.

In free association the patient says everything that comes to mind, and eventually, as conscious controls relax, the patient speaks about thoughts and feelings that have been part of his unconscious. In dream analysis the physician interprets the often disguised content that presents itself in dreams. In hypnosis the physician alters conscious awareness, and the patient is more receptive to suggestion and direction.

Treatment time in both supportive and reconstructive psychotherapy varies with the individual's progress. Emergency psychotherapy is done in a brief time. More lasting treatment often takes more than one year.

Psychoanalysis

Traditional psychoanalysis was developed by Sigmund Freud in the early 1890's in Vienna. The patient meets with the psychoanalyst for several sessions each week. The focus is on exposure of unconscious conflicts often stemming from childhood experience with significant people, especially parents. Sessions are unstructured, and little direction is given by the psychoanalyst. Not all patients make good candidates for psychoanalysis.

An essential factor during the psychoanalytic process is the strong feeling called *transference,* which is a shifting toward the doctor of feelings and desires originally experienced by the patient for his parents and other significant people. As transference proceeds, the patient reenacts with the psychotherapist (the "parent") the original struggle or conflict of childhood.[60] A favorable attitude toward the psychotherapist by the patient is regarded as positive transference. Resistant attitudes of the patient toward the psychotherapist are regarded as negative transference.

Group Therapy

Group therapy is a method of treatment through which a number of persons with emotional problems meet with a therapist, in an organized, structured situation, to achieve better understanding of themselves and others.[61] Group psychotherapy has several advantages:

1. Expediency. It conserves the therapist's time and permits him to serve more patients.
2. It affords an opportunity for the patients to develop skills in interacting with others.
3. For a few patients the group gives a feeling of safety.

In group therapy the patient interacts with a number of other patients as well as the therapist. The patients and therapist may deal with questions about anxiety, sex, hostility, fears, phobias, loneliness, dread, and shyness. The group session is often focused on the observable behavior patterns of its members, who collectively try to resolve the attitudes aroused.

The role of the therapist in a group setting is primarily supportive. He guides the conversation and facilitates expression of feeling while the patients themselves provide the raw material. They are the workers. Sometimes, the members fail to focus on essential material; they concentrate on material that is peripheral to the central focus. For example, they may talk about the weather or a news event. It is the job of the therapist to redirect the focus.

Nursing Expectations

The technical nurse can be expected to demonstrate an understanding of and an ability to carry out the following tasks when working with mentally ill patients who are participating in the aforementioned forms of psychotherapy:

1. Contribute to the nursing team as a team member in planning nursing care for individual and small groups of patients.
2. Modify nursing goals as the patient needs change.
3. Plan and organize her nursing care to facilitate the participation of patients in their prescribed therapy.
4. Assist small groups of patients in activities of daily living so that a therapeutic milieu is maintained.
5. Demonstrate an awareness of the possible effects of her own behavior on patients.
6. Intervene directly or seek appropriate assistance in destructive patient interaction.[62]
7. Identify and discuss her feelings about the patients and their milieu with a nurse who has broad professional preparation and other significant staff members.

Adjunctive Therapies

The adjunctive therapies are those planned mental or physical activities for a patient that run concurrently with other therapies. They are specifically prescribed.

They are planned to hasten recovery from illness by providing an environment free of pressure in which patients

1. Can develop healthier interpersonal relationships through socialization.

2. Can improve and maintain good work habits and adequate work tolerance.
3. Can develop and improve self-esteem and self-confidence.
4. Can develop and nurture a hobby.
5. Can explore vocational aptitudes.
6. Can enjoy leisure time.

Examples of Adjunctive Therapies
OCCUPATIONAL THERAPY

The objective of occupational therapy for the mentally ill is to provide for each patient an opportunity to function—to "do things"—with other people. Most of the activities are manual. Some relate to the person's work interests or hobbies. Occupational therapies provide one way of expressing feelings; for instance, the patient may bang his hammer in an aggressive manner, yet be making a copper ashtray. A well-done task supports a patient's self-esteem.

Examples of occupational areas include woodworking, arts and ceramics, needlework, printing, typing, weaving, greenhouse activities, and other miscellaneous crafts.

RECREATIONAL THERAPY

The objective of recreational therapy is to provide a medium through which people can express their feelings and relate to others. Recreation helps to get the patient's thoughts away from himself and directs them toward others in a way that gives him pleasure and helps him to make friends. Recreational therapy affords release of tension. It helps re-establish interaction with others.

Recreational therapy may include games (active and passive, team or individual), dances, movies, and cooking instruction.

MUSIC THERAPY

The objective of music therapy is to provide a medium for the expression of feelings. In psychiatric facilities that have a trained music therapist, creative dance is included as an integral part of this therapy. In addition, music therapy includes music appreciation, choir, private instruction, and general music activities. Music therapy provides a means for self- and group-expression.

The Technical Nurse's Responsibility in the Adjunctive Therapies

The nurse should

1. Participate in staff conferences so that comments and suggestions may be made regarding which patient is ready for an adjunctive therapy and how patients in a therapy are progressing.

2. When referral is made by the doctor, expedite getting the patient to his assignment.

3. Encourage regular attendance at therapy sessions.

4. Notify the department concerned when a patient is unable to attend.

5. Keep abreast of the patient's progress.

6. Seek assistance from staff in the adjunctive therapies when simple activities are needed for patients who cannot leave the units and provide same to encourage patient interaction.

Dynamically Oriented Art Therapy

Dynamically oriented art therapy has been an established form of psychotherapy for over 26 years. It is based on the recognition that man's fundamental thoughts and feelings are derived from the unconscious and often reach expression in images rather than in words. By means of pictorial projection, art therapy encourages a method of symbolic communication between patient and therapist. The images may also deal with data of dreams, fantasies, daydreams, fears, conflicts, and childhood memories.[63]

Art therapy accepts as basic to its treatment methods the psychoanalytic approach to the mechanisms of repression, projection, identification, sublimation, and condensation.[64] It is thought that every individual has a latent capacity to project his inner conflicts into visual form, and as patients picture such inner experiences, they often become more verbally articulate.

Art therapy was originally applied to the treatment of individual patients, but it is now also being used as a supplementary technique in various forms of psychiatric group therapy.[65]

According to authorities in the field, a wide range of neurotic and psychotic adult patients, as well as emotionally disturbed adolescents and children, have been treated successfully by means of dynamically oriented art therapy. These various types of patients have been treated in private practice, psychiatric hospitals, and clinics.[66]

The art therapist does not interpret the symbolic art expression of his patient, but encourages the patient to discover for himself the meaning of his art productions. Spontaneity is encouraged; however, a more direct approach may be used for some patients.[67]

The Psychotropic Drugs [*]

In the past 14 years psychopharmaceutic agents have revolutionized the treatment and care of the mentally ill. By making patients more manageable they have transformed the prison-like, antiquated atmosphere

---

[*] Drugs that affect the functioning of the mind.

of mental hospitals into the more dignified environment of therapeutic communities. They have made it possible to maintain patients in the community without hospitalization. Use of drugs places an increased responsibility on the nurse because drugs bring the patients into closer touch with reality. They make patients more accessible to psychotherapy. Thus nurses, who are closer to the patients, who see them more consistently, and who are more aware of their behavior, have the opportunity and obligation to reinforce the treatment program as well as communicate changes in behavior to appropriate people.

Second, these drugs are highly active and must be accurately and precisely administered. Their effects on the patients must be constantly observed and recorded. The rules for administering medication are the same in the psychiatric setting as in any other nursing situation. The fact that many patients are ambulatory makes it imperative that the nurse know her patients by name. It is most important for the nurses to realize that drugs control abnormal behavior and lessen symptoms, but that they, in themselves, do not change ideas. People are needed to implement change. Drugs cannot change heredity, family structure, or socioeconomic situations. Therefore, drugs alone are not the answer. They must be used in conjunction with other therapies to significantly influence patient behavior and produce in the once sick individual a degree of health.

In the early years of psychiatry drugs were used primarily to calm the "violent" patient by putting him to sleep. Paraldehyde is an example. It is a powerful sedative and hypnotic drug with a disagreeable odor and taste. It is given orally, rectally, or intramuscularly.

The tranquilizing (ataractic) drugs have introduced a new regime in the management of the mentally ill. These drugs

1. Calm the patients without putting them to sleep.
2. Have a longer lasting effect than sedatives.
3. Make it possible to keep severely disturbed patients in an open ward.
4. Give hope to the "hopeless" patients.
5. Appear to decrease the number of patients who must be kept in hospitals.
6. Make mental hospitals more attractive places to work.
7. Have proved useful outside of the hospital as prescribed by doctors in their offices to relieve anxiety.
8. Are palliative, not curative, agents.

The major tranquilizers used in the United States may be divided into two primary groups: the *rauwolfia* derivatives and the phenothiazines.[68]

Tranquilizers are those drugs that relieve or prevent uncomfortable emotional feelings. Some characteristics of tranquilizers are:

48] THE INTERPERSONAL BASIS OF NURSING

1. They are considerably less addicting than narcotics.
2. They are most effective in patients who have not been overtly sick for a long time.
3. Some have sedative and/or hypnotic effects.
4. *No* uniform dosage exists for these drugs.

An example of a *Rauwolfia* derivative is *reserpine,* a derivative of an Indian plant with long, tapered, crooked roots that contain most of the *Rauwolfia* alkaloids. The first modern reference to its use in psychiatric conditions was made in 1931. Reserpine (Serpasil) exerts a calming effect and induces a sense of well-being in tension, anxiety, and stress. It has been used as a substitute for electroconvulsive therapy and to control delirium tremens in acute alcoholism. Severe mental depression has appeared in a small percentage of patients in a dosage over 1 mg daily.[69] The advent of the phenothiazines has largely replaced the use of the *Rauwolfia* alkaloids because the same desirable tranquilizing effects can be obtained with synthetic chemicals of the phenothiazine group.

There are many drugs that fall into the phenothiazine group (Table 6–1), but we shall concern ourselves with chlorpromazine (Thorazine), which will serve as a model for all others in this group.

TABLE 6–1. THE MAJOR TRANQUILIZERS *

Generic Name	Trade Name	Outpatient Psychiatric Dose Range (mg)	Inpatient Psychiatric Dose Range (mg)
RAUWOLFIA DERIVATIVES			
Reserpine	Serpasil	0.5–2.0	3–20 (for psychotics)
PHENOTHIAZINES			
Chlorpromazine	Thorazine	30–400–800	400–2000
Thioridazine †	Mellaril	50–400	400–800
Prochlorperazine	Compazine	15–60	75–150
Perphenazine	Trilafon	8–24	16–64
Trifluperazine	Stelazine	4–10	6–80

* Dosage will vary according to the disorder being treated, the age and general condition of the patient, the drug used and the severity of the symptoms.
† Extrapyramidal symptoms are rare with this medication.[73]

Chlorpromazine (Thorazine) was first synthesized in 1883, with its first reported treatment of mental illness made in 1952.[70] It was found that, generally speaking, the phenothiazines are much quicker acting drugs and are more effective than many other drugs when given orally. They produce a considerable degree of sedation when given for the first time in doses of 5 to 100 mg [71] along with an indifference or slowing of responses to external stimuli. There is also a diminution of initiative and of anxiety without a change in the state of waking and consciousness.

The three major properties of chlorpromazine (Thorazine) are:

1. Capacity to alleviate anxiety, tension, apprehension, and agitation without clouding consciousness or depressing mental activity
2. Ability to potentiate central nervous system depressants
3. Profound antiemetic effect

The pharmacologic actions and effects of chlorpromazine (Thorazine) are:

1. It acts mainly on the hypothalamus and reticular substance, which may account for its sedative effects.
2. It acts on other areas of the diencephalon including the basal ganglia, which may account for its tranquilizing effects.[72]

The uses of chlorpromazine in psychiatry include control of agitation, anxiety, tension, disorders, and confusion seen in the psychoses, severe personality disorders, and neuroses. After the symptoms are controlled, the sedating effect usually disappears and the tranquilizing action continues.

The dosage and route of administration will vary according to the disorder being treated, the age and general condition of the patient, the drug used, and the severity of the symptoms (Table 6–1). These drugs can be administered orally, rectally, and intramuscularly.

The phenothiazines are capable of causing many kinds of side effects and toxic reactions. As a result the phenothiazines are reserved for treatment of more severe mental illnesses, and a "minor" tranquilizer is used to manage the less severe anxiety states.

SIDE EFFECTS OF PHENOTHIAZINES (Not all listed have been observed with every phenothiazine derivative)

1. Drowsiness—common during early stages of therapy
2. Dryness of the mouth, nasal congestion, some constipation
3. Mild fever (99° F.) during the first days of therapy with large intramuscular doses
4. Increased appetite and weight gain
5. Postural hypotension (experienced as fainting, dizziness)
6. Tachycardia
7. Jaundice (incidence has been low)

8. Agranulocytosis (rarely occurs but may be seen more often in women than in men, evidenced by sore throat or signs of infection)

9. Dermatologic reactions (most of a mild urticarial type)

10. Extrapyramidal symptoms. On high doses some patients exhibit symptoms that closely resemble those of parkinsonism

   a. *Akathisia*—motor restlessness—incessant movement or tapping of feet, inability to sit still, chewing movement of jaw, rolling of tongue

   b. *Akinesia*—weakness and muscle fatigue

   c. *Dyskinesia*—abrupt onset of facial grimacing, distortion, and involuntary muscle control; also, torticollis, lordosis, or scoliosis, plus others

Phenothiazine-caused parkinsonism can be relieved by reducing the dosage or by adding an antiparkinsonian drug.

11. Photosensitivity (this is a reaction in which certain chemicals present in drugs and other substances cause the skin to become abnormally sensitive to light). This reaction resembles the reaction seen with severe sunburn. The patient is to be well covered outdoors. Some photosensitizing agents are antibiotics, sulfa drugs, sedatives, tranquilizers, some barbiturates, and perfumes and colognes that contain bergamot or other oils

12. Convulsions—may be precipitated by phenothiazines especially in epileptics

The minor tranquilizers (Table 6–2) are useful in the management of acute anxiety and tension as seen in the psychoneuroses and in emotional disturbances precipitated by physical illness. They, too, are palliative, not

TABLE 6–2. THE MINOR TRANQUILIZERS

Generic Name	Trade Name	Daily Psychiatric Adult Dose Range (mg)
Meprobamate	Equanil	400–1600
Chlordiazepoxide	Librium	15– 300
Diazepam	Valium	4– 40

curative. One important side effect that is most significant in the minor tranquilizers is a lessening of normal caution, ambition, and judgment, which studies have shown has led to an increase in the accident-proneness of the individual taking these drugs.[74]

Antidepressant Drugs

The first of the antidepressants to be used in this country was iproniazid (Marsilid), which was introduced as a tuberculostatic drug. It is no longer commonly used because it produced quite undesirable side effects, one being postural hypotension. Its desirable effect of lifting the spirits was generally not noticed for ten days to three weeks.

Some antidepressants are monoamine oxidase inhibitors. These interfere with enzyme activity in the brain cells, increasing or prolonging the action of serotonin, a substance produced by cell metabolism, and counteracting depression. The use of these drugs should be confined to moderate to severe depressive reactions. The side effects of the antidepressants (MAO) include headache, dizziness, blurred vision, dry mouth, increased appetite, vomiting, insomnia, and nightmares. Hypertensive crises have occurred in patients on the MAO inhibitors after the ingestion of strong or aged cheese. These symptoms may appear at any time on any dosage, and use of more than one antidepressant drug at a time is considered a serious risk.

The nonenzyme inhibitors are short-acting and not cumulative. They seldom, if ever, potentiate other commonly prescribed drugs and may be used with tranquilizers.

Antidepressants—The Amphetamines

Other preparations utilized to modify depressive psychoneurotic and psychotic states are combinations of a quick-acting barbiturate and dextroamphetamine sulfate. (See Table 6–3.) These preparations give

TABLE 6–3. ANTIDEPRESSANT DRUGS

Generic Name	Trade Name	Daily Dose Range (mg)
MONOAMINE OXIDASE INHIBITORS (psychic energizers)		
Phenylzine dihydrosulfate	Nardil	10– 75
Nialamid	Niamid	15–200
Isocarboxazide	Marplan	10– 75
IMINODIBENAL DERIVATIVES (no MAO inhibitors) * (psychostimulants)		
Amitriptyline hydrochloride	Elavil	75–150
Imipramine	Tofranil	75–225

* These drugs should never be administered with any monoamine oxidase inhibitors.

the patient a feeling of energy and well-being and in essence are psychic stimulants. An example is Dexedrine, with a dose range of 15 to 30 mg. The toxic effects include jitteriness, insomnia, increased susceptibility to accidents, and some addiction.

Another mild stimulant and antidepressant is methyl phenidate (Ritalin), which brightens mood and improves performance. Nervousness and insomnia, the most common side effects, are readily controlled by reducing dosage. Average dosage is 20 to 30 mg daily with a maximum of 40 to 60 mg daily. The drug may be administered orally, intravenously, intramuscularly, or subcutaneously.[75] Ritalin overcomes drug-induced lethargy caused by tranquilizers, particularly anticonvulsants, or other sedative drugs.

Caffeine is considered another mild central nervous system stimulant that, to a limited extent, allays fatigue and has a fleeting effect on the mood. Caffeine is present in tea, cocoa, and cola beverages, with its therapeutic dose being 150 to 250 mg, which corresponds to one cup of coffee.

Lithium Carbonate

Lithium carbonate, a simple salt, is coming into wide use in American psychiatry. This drug is one of several compounds classified as being "profitless" as it is relatively cheap and is readily available in raw form. However, recent studies in the United States have produced ample evidence that lithium, when used with proper clinical and laboratory precautions, is a safe and effective treatment for acute mania.[76] The most impressive feature of lithium is its ability to normalize pathologic mood without producing sedation or impairment of intellectual functioning.[77]

According to recent studies, lithium is also an effective prophylaxis against recurrent episodes of mania, but its effectiveness in depression is not clear.[78] Two groups of side effects of lithium have been identified: (1) gastrointestinal irritation, tremor of the hands, thirst, and polyuria; and (2) lithium intoxication or poisoning with signs of sluggishness, drowsiness, coarse tremor or muscle twitching, anorexia, vomiting and diarrhea, and severe impairment of consciousness.

Lithium is administered orally in capsules of 300 mg with an average dose of 900 mg per day. Collaborative studies by the National Institute of Mental Health and the Veterans Administration will provide detailed and extensive evidence about this drug and its future use in psychiatry.

7

ADDICTION: ALCOHOL AND DRUGS

Alcohol Addiction

THERE are many definitions of alcoholism but they all agree on one point—alcoholism is characterized by excessive ingestion of alcoholic beverages. Controlled drinking is not alcoholism.[79]

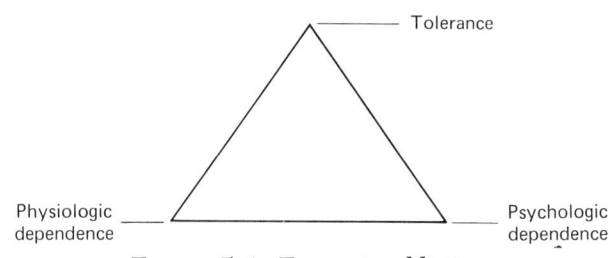

FIGURE 7-1. Factors in addiction.

Alcoholic beverages have been part of man's diet since the beginning of recorded history and may date back to primitive times. Almost any type of vegetation can be fermented and later distilled. For example, grain and potatoes yield whiskey or vodka; corn yields bourbon; sugar cane yields rum; and a Mexican cactus yields tequila. Geography and local agriculture determine the native beverage.

Alcohol is continuously acting as a nervous system depressant. First, it acts on the higher centers of the forebrain, and second, it depresses the forebrain and midbrain affecting the cerebellar center for movement.[80] Alcohol slows and hampers motor performance (speech and eye movements) and mental function.

Alcoholism is considered a mental and a physical illness. The desired effect produced by the ingestion of alcohol is the feeling of euphoria. Alcoholics as a rule are sick, miserable, sad people seeking solace and escape in a readily available and socially acceptable drug.

The alcoholic has been described as an individual who has a low capacity for handling tensions; he is self-centered and dependent (but very resentful of his dependency). It sometimes appears as if the alcoholic is determined to destroy himself, alienate his family and friends, and ruin his reputation and career.

Karl Menninger in *Man Against Himself* wrote that alcoholism serves many purposes: it is a passive form of aggression toward others; it punishes the individual for his own repressed hostilities; and it keeps him from the greater self-punishment of total self-destruction.

Progressive symptoms of alcoholism are

1. Prealcoholic
   a. Gross drinking behavior
   b. Blackouts
   c. Gulping or sneaking drinks
2. Early stages of alcoholism
   a. Loss of control
   b. Alibi system
   c. Drinking alone
   d. Changing the pattern
   e. Antisocial behavior
   f. Loss of friends and job
   g. Hospitalization
3. Later stages of alcoholism
   a. Benders
   b. Unreasonable resentments
   c. Tremors
   d. Nameless fears, anxieties
   e. Protecting the supply
   f. Collapse of alibi system [81]

Treatment of Acute Alcoholism

The amount of alcohol that must be consumed for the individual to have the desired effect grows steadily. When the alcoholic stops drinking, a host of symptoms appear which often warrant hospitalization. They experience "the shakes"—a state of tremulousness, irritability, nausea, and vomiting. Delirium tremens is a severe form of this condition with greater psychomotor and speech overactivity accompanied by dilated pupils, fever, tachycardia, diaphoresis, and auditory and visual hallucinations. Death may occur from peripheral circulatory collapse or hyperthermia. The first state is associated with a high level of alcohol in the blood and the second state with a low or negligible level.

Typical treatment of the alcoholic having delirium tremens (DT's) consists of (1) intramuscular or oral doses of a psychopharmaceutical drug such as Librium; (2) intravenous feedings of 1,000 ml of 15 per cent glucose in saline plus liberal amounts of fruit juice to correct dehydration;

(3) regular insulin to hasten the metabolism of alcohol; and (4) parenteral vitamin-B complex to combat avitaminosis. Chronic drinking causes degeneration of the cerebrum and peripheral nerves because of a dietary and vitamin B deficiency. This is called Korsakoff's psychosis.

Antabuse Therapy

Antabuse is a drug designed to keep the alcoholic from drinking. It makes the taste of alcohol obnoxious and leaves the patient feeling sick and miserable. It comes in pill form and its effects last 24 hours or longer. It must never be given without the patient's knowledge. The discomfort is very severe and may last one, two, or four hours depending on the amount of alcohol ingested. There are flushing of the face and down the neck and chest, pounding headache, sudden faintness, and nausea and vomiting, followed by a cold sweat. Antabuse patients should carry a card stating "I am taking Antabuse: DO NOT GIVE ALCOHOL." The disadvantage of such treatment is that use of drugs does not effect a real cure. Psychotherapy and other adjunctive measures are also needed to effect lasting cure.

Drug Addiction (Abuse)

Drug abuse has three distinct aspects: psychologic, pharmacologic, and sociologic. Present in most cases of drug addiction is a kind of psychic dependence on the drug. The abuser wants and likes the feeling he gets from the drug, he feels he cannot function normally without the drug, and thus he develops a physical dependence on the drug. Physical dependence occurs when the body learns to live with the drug and tolerates increasing doses. The body also reacts with certain withdrawal symptoms when deprived of the drug. The three components of addition are tolerance, psychologic dependence (habituation), and physiologic dependence. (See Fig. 7-1.)

The five categories of substances with abuse potential (though any drug can be abused) are (1) narcotics, (2) sedatives, (3) tranquilizers, (4) stimulants, and (5) hallucinogens.[82]

Narcotics

These drugs have a depressant effect on the central nervous system and consist of opium and its derivatives (morphine, codeine, heroin) and synthetic opiates (meperidine, methadone). Federal law also includes coca leaf and its derivative, cocaine. Pharmacologically cocaine is a stimulant. Marihuana, although not a narcotic drug as considered medically or under law, is under the control of the Federal Bureau of Narcotics.[83]

Heroin appears to be the narcotic used by most addicts today. The first emotional reaction from heroin is usually an easing of fears and a relief from worry followed by a state of inactivity bordering on stupor. This drug reduces hunger, thirst, and the sex drive.

Medical authorities say the addict is a sick person. He needs treatment for his physical addiction and withdrawal sickness. Then he needs help to keep him from going back to drug use after his withdrawal. At present, treatment of narcotic abuse requires hospitalization. Some authorities advocate abrupt withdrawal ("cold turkey"), although this is considered inhumane and potentially dangerous. Gradual withdrawal has been effected through the use of morphine and methadone.

Synanon is an example of a self-help program run by ex-addicts. Synanon was started in California by Chuck Dederick, a former addict, in 1958. The basic philosophy of Synanon is that a person must become independent rather than rely on a superior being as held in AA. Group therapy sessions are held. They are led by former addicts. All verbal expression is allowed. No physical violence is tolerated.

Residents in a Synanon house live together in an autocratically run house with a father figure. All members are or were addicts. Members usually stay in Synanon two and a half years, but one can personally elect to make it his life's work.

The most difficult time for the addict comes after his discharge from the hospital, for during remission the addict needs supportive psychotherapy. A number of rehabilitation approaches to the problem are being tested such as rehabilitation through community clinics, halfway houses, and self-help programs run by ex-addicts.

Sedatives (Depressants)

The abuser takes sedatives orally, intravenously, or rectally. Barbiturate intoxication closely resembles alcohol intoxication but is far more dangerous because an unintentional overdose can easily occur, and convulsions that may follow withdrawal can be fatal. Examples of barbiturates are pentobarbital (Nembutal) and secobarbital (Seconal).

Chronic use of the barbiturates encourages the development of tolerance (gradual increase in dose of the drug to obtain an effect equal to that from the initial dose) plus a psychologic dependence on the drug. Withdrawal should always be supervised by a physician.

Tranquilizers

See pages 46–50.

Stimulants

The most widely known stimulant is caffeine, an ingredient in coffee, tea, cola, and other beverages. Effects of caffeine are relatively mild; usage is socially acceptable and not an abuse problem.

The amphetamines, commonly used in the treatment of obesity, are frequently abused. There is no physical dependency on these drugs, but after the drugs are withdrawn there can be mental depression and fatigue. Psychologic dependence is common. An example of an amphetamine is Benzedrine.

Hallucinogens

At present there is no general medical use for these drugs except in research. LSD (lysergic acid diethylamide) is being used in research on alcoholism.

The hallucinogens affect the central nervous system as evidenced by changes in mood and behavior, dilated pupils, tremors, and hyperactive reflexes. Perceptual changes also occur, especially those involving sight, hearing, touch, and body images.

Other less known but powerful hallucinogens or psychedelic (mind-altering) drugs include peyote, mescaline, psilocybin, and DMT (dimethyltryptamine). Marihuana is also considered a hallucinogen. These drugs are considered dangerous because panic and paranoid ideas can result from their use. Days, weeks, or even months after the individual has stopped using these drugs the things he saw and felt while on the drug may recur. Accidental deaths, suicide, and murder have been traced directly to the use of these drugs.[84]

Solvents

Inhalation of solvent fumes from glue, gasoline, paint thinner, and lighter fluid results in an effect similar to alcoholic intoxication. The sniffer feels euphoric, excited, and exhilarated and slurs his words. There can also be blurring of vision, ringing in the ears, and staggering. Physical dependence does not develop although there is a tendency to increase the amount inhaled. The danger here lies in the inhaling—the danger of suffocation. Development of psychotic behavior can also occur, and a severe type of anemia has been observed in glue-sniffers who have an inherited defect of the blood cells (sickle-cell disease).[85]

Nursing Implications

The nurse needs to be aware that individuals who use emotional "crutches," i.e., drugs and alcohol, to relieve tension and emotional discomfort have many needs and anxieties. They are usually viewed as unstable individuals with strong dependency needs and underlying feelings of inadequacy and inferiority. Morally, physically, and socially they regress.

When such patients are hospitalized, the nurse may expect withdrawal symptoms such as anxiety, tremors, gastric complaints, insomnia, muscle cramps, and irritability. The patients must be supervised carefully, and external stimuli should be reduced as much as possible during this time. Serious reactions such as diarrhea, vomiting, and convulsions must be reported immediately.

The nurse should know the rehabilitation agencies for drug addiction, such as Narcotics Anonymous and Synanon, along with the agencies for alcoholics, Alcoholics Anonymous, Alanon for adult family members, and Alateen for teenage family members, plus the many regional, state, and federal agencies.

8

THE RIGHTS OF THE MENTALLY ILL

THE two objectives of mental health legislation are protecting the interests and health of the mentally ill and decreasing the disruptive effects of such persons on our society. Hospitalization of the mentally ill, which is governed by state law, has several purposes: (1) to protect society, (2) to cure or rehabilitate the patient, and (3) to relieve the patient's family of a heavy burden.

In order to assist state legislators in drafting commitment statutes, the National Institute of Mental Health drew up the Draft Act [86] to be used as a model. A summary of its provisions regarding hospitalization of the mentally ill include:

1. Informal Admission. The patient applies at the hospital and says he wants help. No papers are signed. Many states do not have this type of admission.

2. Voluntary Admission. This admission is instigated by the patient. He "admits" himself, and this circumvents the problems of publicity, coercion, and ill feelings. Voluntary admission also encourages early admission, thus increasing the likelihood of an early cure. The patient may leave at any time provided he gives the hospital several days' notice (customarily three to ten). Almost all states encourage voluntary admissions. In most states, hospital authorities may detain a voluntary patient if, in the hospital director's opinion, the patient would benefit from continued hospitalization. At this time papers are signed, and the patient is committed to the hospital.

3. Medical Certification. Medical certification is a form of commitment in which the person is examined by a physician (in some states two physicians are required) upon presentation by the petitioner. (The applicant or petitioner is the person who starts the process, usually a relative, but it can be a police officer, an overseer of the poor, a sheriff, or an executive head of an institution.) If in the physician's judgment the individual should be hospitalized, the physician will issue medical certification. The judge *commits* the patient to the hospital.

4. Short-Term Admission. Short-term commitment is a procedure used to hospitalize mentally ill persons for short, definite periods of time. This procedure is used primarily for observation of the patient or for intensive short-term treatment. It is compulsory commitment. At the end of a fixed period (no longer than six months in any state) the patient must be released or recommended for hospitalization for an indefinite period.

5. *Emergency Commitment.* Emergency commitment provides a method for the hospitalization of persons dangerous to themselves, to property, and to others, for a short period of time. If necessary, emergency commitment allows time for the preparation of the usual commitment procedures.

Recently, statutes have provided certain personal rights to patients, which include the right of the patient to communicate with persons outside the hospital and the right to be free from publicity. How these rights have been adopted varies from state to state.

Certain medical rights are also provided for patients, such as the use of mechanical restraints. Use of restraints has been restricted by the Draft Act with the provision that they must be medically necessary and indicated as such on the patient's record.

Periodic examination is another important right because this procedure ensures that patients will not be detained longer than necessary. About 20 per cent of the states and the Draft Act provide for examination shortly after admission as an additional safeguard against an illegal admission and to provide more information about the patient.[87] Regardless of the admission procedure, there exist legal safeguards to assure that no patient will be subjected to forced commitment.

Nurses caring for the mentally ill should be familiar with the statutes of the state in which they are working.

9

THE BOLD NEW APPROACH

In the past 20 years it has become increasingly evident that some of the traditional patterns for caring for the mentally ill have acted to impede recovery from mental illness rather than accelerate it. One example would be the facilities used to care for the mentally ill. The state hospital has long been central in the distribution of psychiatric care. This facility has characteristically been removed from the community geographically as well as in the psychologic and philosophic orientation of the staff. The treatment in these institutions for the most part has been custodial rather than rehabilitative. Facilities for evaluation or treatment outside the state hospital have been limited in variety and inadequate in number.

In 1955 the Mental Health Study Act directed the Joint Commission on Mental Illness and Health to analyze and evaluate the needs and resources of the mentally ill in the United States and make recommendations for a national mental health program. This five-year study sets forth concrete steps to be taken by federal and state governments to strengthen mental health resources. The report of this study, *Action for Mental Health*, presents these steps.

New philosophies of psychiatric care have brought new understanding, along with the recommendations of the Joint Commission. Thus, today we see an encouraging shift from the custodial attitude to that of active community treatment and rehabilitation. Psychiatric service in the general hospital is viewed as evidence of this shift. It is believed that a majority of the patients who are treated in the psychiatric units of the general hospital might otherwise go untreated. Many patients are those who are willing to come to a general hospital but who would be unwilling to go either to a private mental hospital or to a state hospital. A majority are in the middle and lower-middle income bracket and do not have sufficient funds to permit long-term care.

Communities are now bringing a wide variety of mental health services within easy reach of patients who require treatment. Events really began moving in 1963 when President John F. Kennedy sent a message to congress calling for "a bold new approach" to the problems of mental health and mental retardation.[88]

What is community mental health? It means providing treatment for the mentally ill and preventing mental illness in local communities. A comprehensive community health center differs in several important ways from the traditional public mental hospital. A center should offer five essential services:

1. Inpatient treatment
2. Outpatient treatment
3. Partial hospitalization (day and night care)
4. Emergency services (24 hours a day)
5. Consultation with and education of individual and group leaders in the community [89]

A community mental health center provides for continuity of care.

This bold new approach indicates a trend toward comprehensive planning for comprehensive services. The technical nurse must be aware of this trend and of her role as a team member in a community mental health center.

10

THE HISTORY AND DEVELOPMENT OF THE CARE OF THE MENTALLY ILL

Persecution

THIS early period was governed by man's superstitious attitude toward his environment.

1552 B.C.	Magic and demons.
860 B.C.	Brief interlude of kindness and help.
560 B.C.	Magic and demons.
476 B.C.	To the thirteenth century, considered the Dark Ages. Persecution of doctors. Witchcraft.

Segregation

1450–1600	Renaissance (fifteenth and sixteen centuries).
1545	Origin of the word "bedlam." Monastery of St. Mary of Bethlehem in London converted into an *insane asylum*.
1709	Society of Friends in Philadelphia attempted to found a hospital. Hospital established in 1756 with the aid of Benjamin Franklin. First Chief of Service, Dr. Benjamin Rush, called the "Father of American Psychiatry."
1733–1815	Franz Anton Mesmer made popular the theory of animal magnetism (hypnosis).
1750–1800	Founding of St. Luke's Insane Asylum, London; Quaker Asylum (York Retreat), York; Lunatic Towers, Vienna; Eastern State Hospital, Virginia; and many others.

Humanitarian Period

1745	Birth of Philippe Pinel of France. He later recognized the need to rehabilitate the mentally ill and became physician at

Bicêtre Asylum for men and the Sâlpetrière Asylum for women in Paris. Here he worked to prove the fallacy of cruel and inhuman treatment of the mentally ill.

1841 — Dorothea L. Dix, a retired schoolteacher, began a crusade to remove mental patients from the jails and almshouses into mental hospitals.

Humanitarian Period and Beginning Scientific Attitudes Moving into the Twentieth Century

1825–1893 — Jean Martin Charcot, a French neurologist, was the most prominent person to place hypnotism on a scientific basis.

1850 — Piney Earle, an American, urged the use of occupational therapy in treating the mentally ill.

1856–1929 — Emil Kraepelin classified types of mental illness. He believed in an organic basis for each form of mental disorder. Introduced term "dementia praecox."

1856–1939 — Sigmund Freud (born in Vienna in 1856), a pupil of Charcot, formulated the theory and technique of psychoanalysis.

1857–1939 — Eugene Bleuler, the Swiss psychiatrist, introduced the term "schizophrenia."

1875–1961 — Carl Gustav Jung, a Swiss psychiatrist, was closely associated with Freud during the early days of psychoanalytic psychology.

1870–1937 — Alfred Adler, an Austrian psychiatrist, was an early student of Freud and coined the term "inferiority complex."

1892–1949 — Harry Stack Sullivan, an American psychiatrist, emphasized the interpersonal aspects of behavior and the significance of the concept of anxiety.

1908 — Clifford W. Beers founded the Mental Hygiene Society of Connecticut.

1909 — National Committee for Mental Hygiene formed.

1932–1957 — Manfred Sakel, a Polish psychiatrist, introduced in Vienna his hypoglycemic insulin treatment of schizophrenia.

1933–1935 — Egas Moniz (1874–1955) of Lisbon performed the first surgical operation on the intact brain for the relief of mental symptoms—prefrontal lobotomy. Moniz received a Nobel Prize in Medicine in 1949 for work in this area.

1935 — Meduna introduced in Hungary a treatment for mental depressions using a convulsion-producing drug, pentylenetetrazol (Metrazol).

1938 — Electroconvulsive therapy introduced by Cerletti and Bini.

1949 — Public Health Service, Federal Security Agency, under the National Mental Health Act of 1946 established the National Institute of Mental Health.

1950   Merger of the Psychiatric Foundation and the National Mental Health Foundation to form the National Association for Mental Health.

What follows in this twentieth century is a *bold new* approach utilizing new medical scientific and social tools now available to seek the causes, treatment, and prevention of mental illness and mental retardation.

The most recent contribution to the above has been the development of new drugs, particularly tranquilizers, that relieve or prevent uncomfortable emotional feeling. It is important to recognize that drugs control abnormal behavior and lessen symptoms but that people and ideas exercise a much greater influence. Therefore, psychotherapy, in some form, is an adjunctive necessity to treatment with drugs.

Emphasis is also being placed on the provision of skilled manpower to work in the mental health field as comprehensive community mental health centers are being constructed and community services increased.[90] Psychiatric mental health nursing has moved forward during this period with the election in 1968 of an Executive Committee for the Division on Practice of the American Nurses' Association. This body is working in the area of identifying further areas of concern for those in psychiatric nursing, as well as formulating standards for psychiatric nursing practice.[91]

REFERENCES

1. Davis, A., "The Skills of Communication," *Amer. J. Nurs.*, **63**:66–67, Jan. 1963.
2. *Ibid.*, p. 67.
3. Peplau, H., *Interpersonal Relations in Nursing*. G. P. Putnam's Sons, New York, 1952, p. 289.
4. Walsh, J., and Taylor, C., *An Approach to the Teaching of Psychiatric Nursing in Diploma and Associate Degree Programs: A Method for Content Integration and Course Development In The Curriculum*. National League for Nursing, New York, 1968, p. 52.
5. Matheney, R., and Topalis, M., *Psychiatric Nursing*, 3rd ed. The C. V. Mosby Co., St. Louis, 1961, p. 54.
6. Sullivan, H., *The Psychiatric Interview*. W. W. Norton & Co., New York, 1954, p. 217.
7. *Ibid.*, p. 217.
8. Orlando, I., *The Dynamic Nurse-Patient Relationship*. G. P. Putnam's Sons, New York, 1961, pp. 31–36.
9. Walsh, *op. cit.*, p. 21.
10. Ujhely, G., *Determinants of the Nurse-Patient Relationship*. Springer Pub. Co., New York, 1968, pp. 103–26.
11. Peplau, H., "The Crux of Psychiatric Nursing," *Amer. J. Nurs.*, **62**:52, Jan. 1962.
12. Trail, I., *Establishing Relationships in Psychiatric Nursing*. Springer Pub. Co., New York, 1966, p. 13.
13. Peplau, *op. cit.*, p. 127.
14. Peplau, H., "A Working Definition of Anxiety," in *Some Clinical Approaches to Psychiatric Nursing*, Burd and Marshall (eds.), The Macmillan Co., New York, 1963, pp. 323–26.
15. *Ibid.*, p. 325.
16. English, O., and Pearson, G., *Emotional Problems of Living*, 2nd ed. W. W. Norton & Co., New York, 1955, p. 25.
17. *Ibid.*, pp. 27.

18. Peplau., *op. cit.*, pp. 103–106.
19. Oden, G., "Avoidance," in *Some Clinical Approaches To Psychiatric Nursing*, Burd and Marshall (eds.), The Macmillan Co., New York, 1963, p. 105.
20. Peplau, *op. cit.*, p. 116.
21. Engel, G., "Grief and Grieving," *Amer. J. Nurs.*, **64**:93–98, Sept. 1964.
22. Havinghurst, R., *Developmental Tasks and Education*, 2nd ed. David McKay Co., New York, 1966, p. 2.
23. Mereness, D., *Essentials of Psychiatric Nursing*, 7th ed. The C. V. Mosby Co., St. Louis, 1966, pp. 126–31.
24. Freud, S., *An Outline of Psychoanalysis*. W. W. Norton & Co., New York, 1949, p. 14.
25. *Ibid.*, p. 15.
26. Noyes, A., Camp, W., and von Sickel, M., *Psychiatric Nursing*, 6th ed. The Macmillan Co., New York, 1964, pp. 4–6.
27. *Ibid.*, p. 3.
28. *Op. cit.*, p. 23.
29. Noyes, *op. cit.*, pp. 9–16.
30. Erikson, E., *Childhood and Society*. W. W. Norton & Co., New York, 1963, pp. 247–74.
31. Sullivan, H., *The Interpersonal Theory of Psychiatry*. W. W. Norton & Co., New York, 1953, pp. 49–310.
32. Erikson, E. *Insight and Responsibility*. W. W. Norton & Co., New York, 1964, p. 231.
33. Noyes, *op. cit.*, p. 190.
34. English, *op. cit.*, p. 6.
35. Alverez, W., *The Neuroses*. W. B. Saunders Co., Philadelphia, 1964, p. 39.
36. Ayd, F., "Treatment of the Neurotic," *Clinical Symposia*, Ciba, New Jersey, Nov.–Dec., 1957, pp. 151.
37. *Ibid.*, p. 159.
38. *Ibid.*, p. 159.
39. Noyes, *op. cit.*, p. 194.
40. Hofling, Co., Leininger, M., and Bregg, E., *Basic Psychiatric Concepts in Nursing*, 2nd ed. J. B. Lippincott Co., Philadelphia, 1967, p. 548.
41. *Ibid.*, p. 550.
42. *Ibid.*, p. 551.
43. *Ibid.*, pp. 313–14.
44. Jackson, D., *The Etiology of Schizophrenia*. Basic Books, New York, 1960, p. 3.
45. Hofling, *op. cit.*, p. 317.
46. Sullivan, *op. cit.*, p. 206.
47. Sheidman, S., and Farberow, N., *Clues to Suicide*. McGraw-Hill Book Co., New York, 1957, p. 5.
48. *Ibid.*, p. 2.
49. Noyes, *op. cit.*, p. 183.
50. *Ibid.*, p. 185.
51. Rinkel, M., and Hemroick, H. (eds.), *Insulin Treatment in Psychiatry*. Philosophical Library, New York, 1959, pp. 10–11.
52. Horowitz, W., "Insulin Shock Therapy," in *American Handbook of Psychiatry*, Vol. II. Basic Books, New York, 1959, p. 1485.
53. *Op. cit.*, p. 47.
54. *Op. cit.*, p. 1487.
55. Kalinowsky, L., "Convulsive Shock Treatment," in *American Handbook of Psychiatry*, Vol. II. Basic Books, New York, 1959, p. 1499.
56. *Ibid.*, p. 1510.
57. *Ibid.*, p. 1515.
58. Mereness, *op. cit.*, p. 77.
59. Hinsie, L., and Campbell, R., *Psychiatric Dictionary*, 3rd ed. Oxford University Press, New York, 1960, p. 615.
60. Milt, H., *Basic Handbook on Mental Illness*. Scientific Aids, New York, 1965, p. 61.
61. Bueker, K., and Warrick, A., "Can Nurses BE Group Therapists?" *Amer. J. Nurs.*, **64**:114, May 1964.
62. Walsh, *op. cit.*, p. 23.
63. Naumberg, M., *Dynamically Oriented Art Therapy; Its Principles and Practices*. Grune & Stratton, New York, 1966, p. 1.
64. *Ibid.*, p. 2.
65. *Ibid.*, p. 2.
66. *Ibid.*, p. 6
67. *Ibid.*, p. 4.
68. Ayd, F., "Major Tranquilizers," *Amer. J. Nurs.*, **65**:70, Apr. 1965.
69. ———, "Serpasil (Reserpine)." Ciba Pharmaceutical Company, Summit, N.J., Nov. 1967, pp. 1–4.
70. Goodman, L., and Gilman, A., *The*

Pharmacological Basis of Therapeutics, 3rd ed. The Macmillan Co., New York, 1966, p. 163.
71. *Ibid.*, p. 166.
72. ———, "The Psychiatric Nurse's Guide to Therapy with Thorazine, Stelazine, Compazine." Smith Kline & French Laboratories, Philadelphia, pp. 2–3.
73. Goodman, *op. cit.*, p. 170.
74. *Ibid.*, pp. 724–27.
75. ———, "Ritalin" Ciba Pharmaceutical Co., Summit, N.J., No. 6707, Sept. 1968.
76. Cole, J. (ed.), "Lithium Carbonate—Special Section," *Amer. J. Psychiat.*, **125**:487–557, Oct. 1968.
77. *Ibid.*, p. 556.
78. Bunny, W., et al., "A Behavioral-Biochemical Study of Lithium Treatment," *Amer. J. Psychiat.*, **125**:499–512, Oct. 1968.
79. Block, M., *Alcoholism*. John Day Co., New York, 1965, p. 19.
80. *Ibid.*, p. 27.
81. ———, "Progressive Symptoms of Alcoholism," National Council of Alcoholism, *Nurs. Outlook*, **65**:34, Nov. 1965.
82. ———, *Drug Abuse: Escape to Nowhere—A Guide for Educators*. Smith Kline & French Laboratories, Philadelphia, 1967, pp. 27–43.
83. *Ibid.*, p. 38.
84. *Ibid.*, p. 40.
85. ———, "Glue-Sniffing," National Clearing House for Poison Control Centers. U.S. Dept. of Health, Education, and Welfare, 1964.
86. ———, "A Draft Act Governing Hospitalization of the Mentally Ill." Public Health Service Publication No. 51. Government Printing Office, 1952.
87. Farmer, R., *The Rights of The Mentally Ill*. Arco Publishing Co., New York, 1967, p. 51.
88. Kennedy, J., "Special Message to Congress on Mental Illness and Mental Retardation—1963, Feb. 5," *Public Health News*, N.J. State Department of Health, June 1963, pp. 139–46.
89. ———, "The Community Mental Health Center, Bold New Approach." Public Health Service Publication, No. 1643, 1968.
90. *Op. cit.*, p. 142.
91. ———, "Psychiatric/Mental Health Nursing, Division on Practice," *American Nurses' Association*, New York, Dec. 1968, pp. 1–4.

ADDITIONAL READINGS

ALEXANDER, F., *Psychosomatic Medicine*. W. W. Norton and Co., New York, 1960.

ANGRIST, S., "The Mental Hospital; Its History and Destiny," *Pers. in Psych. Care*, **1**:20–26, 1963.

ARIETI, S., *Interpretation of Schizophrenia*. Robert Brunner, New York, 1955.

ARMSTRONG, S., and ROUSLIN, S., *Group Psychotherapy in Nursing Practice*. The Macmillan Co., New York, 1963.

AYD, F., "The Chemical Assault on Mental Illness," *Amer. J. Nurs.*, **65**:70–78, Apr. 1965; **65**:89–94, May 1965; **65**:78–84, June 1965.

BEERS, C., *A Mind That Found Itself*. Doubleday & Co., Garden City, N.Y., 1966, revised.

BELLAK, L., and SMALL, L., *Emergency Psychotherapy and Brief Psychotherapy*. Grune & Stratton, New York, 1965.

BLOCK, M., "Alcoholism Is Many Illnesses," *Nurs. Outlook*, **13**:35, Nov. 1965.

BOCKHOVEN, J., *Moral Treatment in American Psychiatry*. Springer Pub. Co., New York, 1963.

BOWLY, J., *Child Care and the Growth of Love*. Penguin Books, Baltimore, 1959.

BRAY, R., and BIRD, T., *The Principles of Psychiatric Nursing*. The Williams & Wilkins Co., Baltimore, 1964.

BROWN, D., "Nurses Participate in Group Therapy," *Amer. J. Nurs.*, **62**:68–69, Jan. 1962.

BUEKER, K., and WARRICK, A., "Can Nurses Be Group Therapists?" *Amer. J. Nurs.*, **64**:114–16, May 1964.

CLAWSON, G., "Nursing Care of Psychiatric Patients Receiving Insulin Therapy," *Amer. J. Nurs.*, **49**:621–26, Oct. 1949.

DEUTSCH, A., *The Mentally Ill in America*, 2nd ed. Columbia University Press, New York, 1949.

DYE, M., "Clarifying Patient's Communication," *Amer. J. Nurs.*, **63**:56, Aug. 1963.

EPPS, R., and HANES, L., *Day Care of Psychiatric Patients*. Charles C Thomas, Publisher, Springfield, Ill., 1964.

FARNSWORTH, D., "Mental Health—A Point of View," *Amer. J. Nurs.*, **60**:688, May 19, 1960.

FELDMAN, S., *Mannerisms of Speech and Gestures In Everyday Life*. International Universities Press, New York, 1965.

GILBER, I., "Drug Addiction—The Addict and His Drugs," *Amer. J. Nurs.*, **63**:53, July 1963.

HIMWICH, H., "The New Psychiatric Drugs," *Sci. Amer.*, Oct. 1955, pp. 2–6.

HOLMES, M., and WERNER, J., *Psychiatric Nursing in a Therapeutic Community*. The Macmillan Co., New York, 1966.

JAHODA, M., *Current Concepts of Positive Mental Health*. Basic Books, New York, 1959.

JELLINEK, E., *The Disease Concept of Alcoholism*. Hillhouse Press, New Haven, Conn., 1961.

Joint Commission on Mental Illness and Health, *Action for Mental Health.*. Science Editions, Inc., New York, 1962.

JONES, M., *The Therapeutic Community: A New Treatment Method in Psychiatry*. Basic Books, New York, 1953.

———, *Let Your Light So Shine*. Roche Laboratories, Nutley, N.J., 1967.

KÜBLER-ROSS, E., *On Death and Dying*. The Macmillan Co., New York, 1969.

MAHONEY, E., "The Fears and Feelings of the Patient on Electroconvulsive Therapy," *Amer. J. Nurs.*, **58**:560–62, 1958.

MARSHALL, H., *Dorothea Dix, Forgotten Samaritan*. Russell & Russell, New York, 1937.

MECHANIC, D., "Some Factors in Identifying and Defining Mental Illness," *Ment. Hyg.*, **46**:66, Jan. 1962.

MELAT, S., "The Development of Trust," *Perspect. Psychiat. Care*, **3**:28, 1965.

MONROE, R., *Schools of Psychoanalytic Thought*. Henry Holt & Co., New York, 1955.

National Institutes of Health, U.S. Dept. of Health, Education, and Welfare, Public Health Publication No. 81, 1967.

NEYLAN, M., "Anxiety," *Amer. J. Nurs.*, **62**:110, May 1962.

Osnos, R., "A Community Counseling Center for Addicts," *Nurs. Outlook,* **13**:38, Nov. 1965.

Overholder, W., *Major Principles of Forensic Psychiatry.* Basic Books, New York, 1959.

Peplau, H., *Basic Principles of Patient Counseling,* 2nd ed. Smith Kline & French Laboratories, Philadelphia, 1964.

Pullinger, W., "Remotivation," *Amer. J. Nurs.,* **60**:682–85, May 1960.

Ramirez, E., "Help for the Addict," *Amer. J. Nurs.,* **67**:2348, Nov. 1967.

Roche, P., "Legal Requirements for Hospitalization," *Ment. Hosp.,* **12**:16, Oct. 1961.

Schneck, J., *A History of Psychiatry.* Charles C Thomas, Publisher, Springfield, Ill., 1960.

Schuurmans, M., "Five Functions of the Group Therapist," *Amer. J. Nurs.,* **64**:108–10, 1964.

Shneidman, E., "Preventing Suicide," *Amer. J. Nurs.,* **65**:111–16, May 1965.

Shockley, E., and Schwartz, M., *The Nurse and the Mental Patient.* Science Editions, John Wiley & Sons, New York, 1956.

Stone, A., and Stone, S., *The Abnormal Personality Through Literature.* Prentice-Hall, Englewood Cliffs, N.J., 1966.

Taylor, S., "Addicts as Patients," *Nurs. Outlook,* **13**:41, Nov. 1965.

Ulett, G., and Goodrich, D., *A Synopsis of Contemporary Psychiatry.* The C. V. Mosby, Co., St. Louis, 1960.

von Mering, O., and King, S., "Remotivating the Mental Patient." Russell Sage Foundation, New York, 1957.

Wolberg, L., *The Technique of Psychotherapy.* Grune & Stratton, New York, 1954.

Wolf, N., "Setting Reasonable Limits on Behavior," *Amer. J. Nurs.,* **62**:104, Mar. 1962.

Zwerling, I., *The Psychiatric Day Hospital.* Basic Books, New York, 1966.

UNIT II

THE PATIENT WITH INFECTION

11

THE PATIENT WITH INFECTION: AN ECOLOGIC APPROACH

ECOLOGY is the study of the "economics" of living organisms. It encompasses all aspects of the way an organism interacts with its environment so that it can live and reproduce. It focuses on ways in which organisms learn to survive; what grows most rapidly and avoids death most successfully will survive.[1*] Ecology includes the way in which an animal gets his food, on the one hand, and the way he prevents being "used as food," on the other. Insufficient food and the predatory activity of a species' enemies function as devices that control what would otherwise be an astronomic reproduction rate. Overcrowding makes it difficult to obtain food and easy for infection to spread. Human beings fit into this ecologic scheme, too. Population rates have, in the past, been controlled by wars, famine, and epidemic spread of infectious disease. Millions died in the plagues of the past. Today, technologic and medical advances make it possible to provide sufficient food for the world, to regulate population density through family planning, to provide adequate available housing to prevent overcrowding, and to control infection and the vectors of infection. Survival is possible. Still, many people succumb to infectious disease.

An ecologic approach helps to control and prevent the disease by considering the natural history of the particular organisms and then by intervening somewhere in the life cycle to interrupt it. Here are some things the physician and nurse must consider:

1. What is the microorganism's reservoir: Does it live on animals? Rodents? In the soil? On man?

2. How is it transmitted: Is it air-borne? Does it get to man by a rodent vector? Insect? Is it milk-, water-, or food-borne? Is it transmitted directly from man to man (direct contact) or is it likely to be transmitted indirectly via an intermediate inanimate object (fomite)?

3. What is its incubation period (period between time of infection and appearance of first symptoms of illness)?

---

* References for Unit II appear on pages 84-85.

What Is Infection?

Microorganisms are part of the structure of our lives. They live with us and within us all the time. They are on our skin, in our noses and mouths, on our genitalia, and so forth. It is estimated that about half the bulk of feces consists of bodies of bacteria.[2] Most common diseases are due to organisms very like those normally found throughout our bodies. Yet, something "tips the balance" in favor of the infecting organisms, and disease is produced. This is called infection. It is a chemical contest between the invading organisms and the infected host. It can be caused by relatively large unicellular animals called protozoa (e.g., amebic dysentery), by bacteria (e.g., staphylococcal pneumonia), by rickettsia (e.g., Rocky Mountain spotted fever), or by viruses (e.g., influenza). Rickettsia and viruses can be reproduced only in living cells. Particular microorganisms have a predilection for particular invasion sites. This is called tissue affinity and is the reason why symptoms appear at particular sites. For instance, the streptococci might lodge in the throat, the influenza virus in the respiratory passages. The primary objective of the organisms is to use the host as a means of survival and propagation.[3] When the body is invaded by microorganisms, one of three things may happen:[4] the organisms can multiply without restraint and cause death; they may establish themselves in the host's tissues and they may persist there indefinitely; or they may provoke a defensive action that walls off and destroys the invading organisms leaving the individual healthy. The two most important internal defense mechanisms are the inflammatory response and the antigen-antibody reaction.

12

DEFENSE MECHANISMS

The Inflammatory Response

THIS response is invoked whenever the body is injured or is invaded by a foreign substance. It does not require a break in the skin. The reaction can be limited and local. A mosquito bite and a cut are examples. Or, the reaction can be widespread and general. A systemic infection and an anaphylactic reaction to penicillin or whole blood are examples. The latter can cause so violent a reaction that instead of defending the person, circulatory shock occurs and his life is threatened.

The inflammatory process attempts to wall off and localize the effects of the injury or the invading microorganisms. The inflamed part is red, swollen, hot, and painful. Here are the steps in the inflammatory process:

1. Histamine, liberated by damaged cells, causes capillary vasodilation.
2. Increased blood is delivered to the involved area causing it to feel hot and appear red.
3. Capillary membranes become more permeable, and fluid seeps out. There is swelling and discomfort as the nerves are impinged upon.
4. Leukocytes converge upon the area and ingest bacteria and dead cells (phagocytosis). The material is returned to the circulation for excretion by the kidneys. Leukocytes surround and wall off bacteria, preventing their spread. If bacteria are not adequately trapped at the local site, they can be picked up later in lymph nodes where they are destroyed by phagocytosis. The nodes become swollen and tender (lymphadenitis). Or, they can be destroyed by phagocytic cells along the course of the blood vessels or in the spleen, liver, lungs, bone marrow, or adrenal glands.[5]

Antigen-Antibody Response

Immunity

Antibodies are the body's fighters. They are individual globulin molecules that are produced by the reticuloendothelial system of the liver, spleen, and bone marrow, and in the lymph nodes. They are produced in response to specific foreign substances called antigens. A specific antibody is produced to render a specific antigen inactive. The antigen and antibody form a unique pair, much the way a key fits into a lock. Antibodies are produced to handle pathogens (disease-producing microorganisms). Antitoxins are produced to handle toxins. As long as antibodies are present in the blood and tissues, the person has a degree of protection against the disease.

A natural immunity is one that results because of heredity. More important, though, is acquired immunity, which develops during the life of the individual. Acquired immunity is considered *active* if the patient's system develops its own circulating antibodies to counteract the antigen. This results because the person has had the disease (symptoms may have been so minimal that he is not aware that he has had it) or it may result from the use of artificial agents that stimulate the person's system to develop specific antibodies. This artificial active immunity comes from the injection or ingestion of pathogenic but attenuated microorganisms or other products. Virulence is decreased so that these antigens do not cause the disease but do stimulate the production of disease specific antibodies. Vaccines are made from the microorganisms responsible for the diseases. Toxoids are made from the toxins secreted by some bacteria.

Acquired immunity is passive if the immunologic product contains antibodies obtained from blood of animals or humans who have been exposed to infectious organisms or toxins and thus contain antibodies or antitoxins. Hyperimmune serum globulin is an example. Passive immunity provides the person with an immediate but short-lasting immunity. He does not produce his own antibodies in response to the serum. Passive immunity is used in an emergency. It is usually followed by a dose of an active product in response to which the patient develops a long-lasting immunity. Length of protection varies with the product. Often, periodic "reminder" doses of the agent must be given. These are called booster doses.

Some tests are used to determine whether a person has been exposed to a disease and therefore carries antibodies for that disease. A positive reaction indicates that antibodies are present, not that the person has the disease. The tuberculin test is an example.

Some immunologic agents that produce active immunity include: [6] cholera vaccine, diphtheria toxoid, influenza virus vaccine, measles virus vaccine, rubella virus vaccine, mumps virus vaccine, pertussis vaccine, poliomyelitis vaccine (oral or injectable), rabies vaccine, smallpox vaccine, tetanus toxoid, BCG vaccine for tuberculosis protection, typhoid vaccine, typhus vaccine, and yellow fever vaccine.

Some immunologic agents that produce passive immunity include botulism antitoxin, diphtheria antitoxin, measles immune globulin, mumps immune globulin, pertussis immune globulin, antirabies serum, and tetanus antitoxin.

Why Does Infection Occur?

Many factors determine whether or not a person will develop an infection. His own state of health is of prime importance. If he is not chronically ill and is in good nutritional balance, the chances are less likely that he will become infected. If he is infected, the disease is less likely to be life-threatening. Susceptibility involves the state of all of the body's external and internal defense mechanisms, e.g., an intact skin and mucous membrane, acid gastric and vaginal secretions, an acid urinary pH, and adequate levels of circulating antibodies with adequate circulation to transport them. Other factors include the virulence (capability of producing illness) of the particular strain of organism, its density in numbers (the greater the number, the greater the chance of infection), the availability of susceptible hosts, and the number of people who have already been exposed to the organisms (the greater the number already exposed, the fewer the number of new cases).

If the number of new cases of the disease (incidence) strikes many people in a given region in the same span of time, it is called an *epidemic*. If the disease is continuously present to some extent in a given region, it is said to be *endemic*. An epidemic can occur in an endemic area.

13

HOSPITAL-ACQUIRED INFECTION

Staphylococcus Aureus

How sad it is to come to the hospital for treatment of one condition and be detained there because of an infection contracted there! Patients are under considerable risk of acquiring infections in the hospital. No tissue is exempt from possible invasion. The patient may develop a wound infection, a respiratory or urinary infection, or a generalized, life-threatening systemic infection. Symptoms depend on which tissue is affected. Hospital-acquired infection with gram-positive and gram-negative bacteria is on the rise. Because *Staphylococcus aureus* is frequently a causative organism, it will be considered as an example.

Staphylococcus aureus is the major cause of wound infection. The organism is a spherical, gram-positive bacterium that tends to occur in grapelike clusters. Staphylococci live primarily on dead organic matter (saprophytic) and on other living organisms (parasitic); however, they are not primarily parasitic, and their nutrient requirements are easily satisfied by nonliving organic media or even inorganic media.[7] The organisms are about one seventh the diameter of a red blood cell.[8] They grow in aerobic or anaerobic conditions. They are widely distributed in nature and are commonly found on the skin and mucous membranes, especially the nose and the nasopharynx of man. Man is their chief reservoir. The pathogenic and nonpathogenic strains are very similar.[9] They infect when resistance is decreased. They cause symptoms of illness when they leave the skin and nose and penetrate into deeper tissues.

Pathogenic species of staphylococci usually have these common properties:

1. They produce a golden pigment.
2. They produce pus.
3. They multiply at any temperature between 10° C. and 45° C. (50° to 113° F.).
4. They produce coagulase, an enzyme that causes coagulation of blood.
5. They produce toxins that destroy red blood cells (hemolysin),

destroy white blood cells (leukocidins), and attack the intestinal mucosa (enterotoxins).

6. They usually enter the body through the respiratory tract or mouth or through a break in the skin.

7. They are carried in the nose and throat of some people who exhibit no symptoms of illness, but who can spread the disease to others who are susceptible. Hospitalized patients are high-risk "susceptible others."

Some staphylococcal infections include pimples and sties, boils and carbuncles, abscesses, cystitis, food poisoning, osteomyelitis, and bronchopneumonia. Antibiotics are the drugs of choice; however, infections may be extremely difficult to cure because of resistance of the microorganisms to the drug. The microorganism has the ability to "genetically mutate"— change from a less virulent to a more virulent strain to aid survival. It can even change from a nonpathogen to a pathogen. This is why a culture and sensitivity test are ordered. The first indicates the microorganism. The second shows which antibiotic will be most effective in controlling it. A sensitivity tests guides the selection of antibiotic for use. Semisynthetic antibiotics like Staphcillin are frequently more effective than natural antibiotics to which a resistance has developed.

Application of moist heat in the form of hot soaks and compresses or dry heat in the form of lamps or diathermy may be used for local infection. Heat increases vasodilation in the inflamed area and thus augments this defense mechanism.[10] The patient with a staphylococcal infection is isolated. A staphylococcal infection interferes with normal wound healing, and a first-intention wound can become a second-intention wound. In a first-intention wound edges can be approximated and cells similar in structure to normal skin are laid down. In a second-intention wound dissimilar cells are laid down and scar tissue develops.

A Word About Food Poisoning

Staphylococcus aureus can be ingested. The microorganism produces an enterotoxin that attacks the intestinal mucosa. It incubates for about two hours. Then, the patient experiences headache, nausea, violent vomiting, severe diarrhea, and prostration. The patient usually recovers within 24 hours. Fatalities are rare. If, however, patients are infected with the exotoxin (toxin released by a living bacterium) of *Clostridium botulinum,* fatalities are frequent! This microorganism grows as a result of improper food processing with inadequate sterilization time. It is seen when foods are improperly canned at home, jarred, or pickled; it is sometimes seen when commercially canned foods are improperly processed. The incubation period is less than 24 hours. The patient vomits, is constipated, and is thirsty. There is secretion of a thick, viscid saliva and paralysis of the pharynx. There may be double vision. The exotoxin acts like an extremely powerful poison in the body. Recovery time is six to eight weeks.

Major Points in the Prevention and Spread of Infection and Care of the Infected Patient

Hospitalized patients are susceptible individuals. They may be old or chronically ill. They may have been treated with drugs that reduce resistance, e.g., steroids, anticancer drugs. They may have undergone the stress of surgery. In any case, their biologic integrity is threatened and resistance is lowered.

Most infectious disease is transmitted from person to person, especially by contaminated hands. Inanimate objects (fomites) play a less important part. They seem to be involved primarily when heavily contaminated. Spread of infection presents a vicious cycle in which an infected patient transmits pathogens to the nurse. If she does not follow the proper handwashing technique before and after caring for the patient, she can transmit the pathogens to another patient under her care. This cycle must be interrupted. (See Fig. 13–1.)

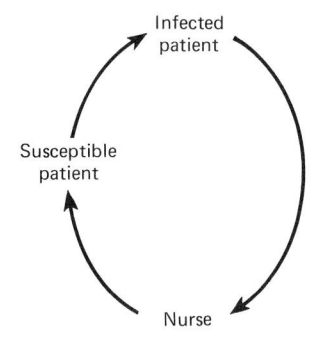

FIGURE 13–1. Vicious cycle of infection.

The two major nursing goals in caring for infected patients are adequate technique and continuous surveillance.[11] Here are some major points to remember:

1. Develop an "aseptic conscience." Regard any patient as if he had a potential infection: wash hands carefully before and after direct contact. Follow disinfection instructions carefully: soak thermometers in an appropriate disinfectant for an appropriate length of time. Time it! Make sure forceps are used properly and are resting in adequate disinfectant solution. Handle all dressings as if they were contaminated.

2. *Be on the alert for signs of beginning infection.* Review laboratory slips carefully and report significant findings to the physician. Note and report any temperature elevations or symptoms of inflammation (pain, heat, swelling, etc.).

3. *Know the disease a patient is being isolated for.* Learn its routes of entry and exit and protect against spread from these routes; e.g., use stool disinfection precautions if the route of exit is the bowel; use a dry mask if the pathogen is a highly virulent organism through the respiratory passages.

A handy reference source of information pertaining to individual communicable diseases is the report of the American Public Health Association, *Control of Communicable Diseases in Man.* It can be purchased from the American Public Health Association, 1790 Broadway, New York, New York, 10019.

4. *Be consistent in following the hospital's isolation technique procedure.* Make sure all people entering the isolation room (auxiliary personnel, housekeepers, visitors, physicians) are guided in use of the prescribed technique.

5. *Be on the alert for the presence of insects.* They should be exterminated immediately. They may be vectors of disease.

14

VENEREAL DISEASES

VENEREAL diseases are those diseases that are transmitted through sexual contact. They are called social or behavioral diseases. Their incidence has recently risen throughout the world, especially in the teen-age groups. This rise in incidence that has occurred among people of all walks of life is partly attributable to a "laissez-faire" attitude that developed since the advent of penicillin, the "cure drug." It also results from change in standards regarding sexual behavior, increase in premarital and extramarital sexual contacts, increase in homosexual transfer, and an overall increase in population mobility. It is not unusual for one infected individual to spread his disease to many nonsuspecting contacts. It is also possible to harbor the pathogen without obvious symptoms, and this asymptomatic carrier does not seek medical attention. Women frequently do not know they have a venereal disease because their anatomy may "hide" obvious signs. Instability of the home is repeatedly mentioned as a basic cause of sexual promiscuity and the consequent increase in venereal disease.

Although venereal diseases are considered "notifiable" in most states, many cases go unreported because of the stigma that people feel is attached to knowledge that they have had the disease. This means that likely contacts are not searched out and treated, and they, in turn, continue the vicious chain of infection. Case finding with treatment and education of the public remains the core of venereal disease control programs.

Syphilis (Lues)

Syphilis is the most deadly of the venereal diseases. Once blood-borne, the microorganisms can affect and damage every organ in the body. The disease is caused by the spirochete *Treponema pallidum*. This very fragile microorganism is a highly motile parasite that cannot live long without its human host. The pathogen is easily destroyed by heat, drying, and antiseptics. Its extreme delicacy makes it dependent on direct or nearly direct transfer.[12] It is transmitted sexually through contact with mucous membrane (genitalia, mouth, anus) or through minute breaks in the skin. Indirect transmission by means of clothing, towels, drinking cups, or a toilet seat rarely occurs because this is only possible while the organisms remain in moist secretion, and they are very vulnerable to quick dehydration. Syphilis can be transmitted to a fetus through the blood of a pregnant woman, and a newborn infant can be born with congenital disease. The organisms can also be transmitted through whole-blood infusions, but this is not likely if the blood is stored in a refrigerator for at least three hours. Refrigerated storage kills the pathogens. One infection does not produce an immunity to subsequent infections, although it is unlikely for a second infection to occur during the course of the initial infection. No artificial immunization is available to protect against syphilis.

Stages in the Disease [13]

PRIMARY SYPHILIS

This is the initial stage of the disease. The microorganism incubates for two to four weeks. Then, a chancre (sore) develops at the site of infection, usually the genitalia. The lesion begins as a dull red macule, becomes papular, and soon ulcerates and produces a serous exudate that is loaded with the spirochete. It is highly infectious. The chancre is painless and may remain unnoticed, e.g., if it is at the cervix. As the organisms move from the local site and become blood-borne, the chancre heals. A thin scar remains. The patient may think the disease "is over with" when its more serious stages are just beginning! The organism travels via the lymphatics to other parts of the body. Six to eight weeks after the beginning of the primary stage the secondary-stage symptoms begin.

SECONDARY SYPHILIS

During this stage there is a general tissue reaction to the dissemination of the spirochetes. Signs are likely to come and go. They last three to nine months and may be so inconspicuous that the patient is not aware of them. He may complain of headache, malaise, anorexia, loss of weight, low-grade fever, and aching pain in long bones, muscles, and joints. Lymph nodes swell. Hair may fall out. There are skin eruptions, and a rash may cover the entire body. Lesions called "mucous patches" develop on mucous membranes. The moist lesions of secondary-stage syphilis are also highly infectious. Together, the primary and secondary stages last three months to one year. They are followed by an asymptomatic "latent stage." Infection is still present, but there are no symptoms. The patient may again mistakenly believe he is cured. Sometimes the disease undergoes a recurrent phase in which lesions reappear, alternating with periods of latency.

LATE (TERTIARY) SYPHILIS

During this stage all body organs may be damaged. The patient adequately treated with a suitable antibiotic never reaches this stage! At first, the covering structures of the body (skin, mucous membrane, subcutaneous tissue) and the supporting structures (bone, joint, muscles, and ligaments) are involved. Later, the cardiovascular and neurologic tissues are involved. The characteristic lesion of the tertiary stage is a cellular, hard, fibrotic "gumma." The body is diffusely infiltrated with these gummata. The patient is usually noninfectious during the tertiary stage.

Briefly, the stages are: [14]

Stage one: chancre.
Stage two: rash, constitutional symptoms.
Latent phase: no symptoms.
Stage three: gummata of heart and nervous system, permanent damage.

Diagnosis of Syphilis

The most frequently used screening test is the VDRL (*Venereal Disease Research Laboratory*) serology test. It does not diagnose syphilis in the early stage before blood involvement. It is an antigen-antibody test in which flocculation (precipitation) occurs when the syphilis antibodies are present. It is usually performed routinely on all patients admitted to the hospital. The Kline and Kahn tests are similar. They too are negative during the incubation period. They become positive within 9 to 14 days after appearance of the chancre.

The Wassermann and Kolmer tests are complement-fixation tests. They indicate the presence of an antibody-like substance called reagin in infected serum. In most states, the Wassermann test is required before a couple is allowed to marry. These tests do not diagnose the disease while it is incubating.

The spirochete is best diagnosed by either microscopic dark-ground examination of exudate taken from a chancre or by the specific *Treponema pallidum* immobilization test (TPI) in which the patient's serum is mixed with a sample of live organisms. If the serum contains suitable antibodies, the live organisms lose their mobility and the test is positive.[15]

Treatment of Syphilis

Treatment of syphilis is specific: 600,000 units of procaine penicillin is injected each day for 10 to 12 days.[16] Sometimes, a physician will administer a very large initial dose to protect against the possibility that the patient may not return for subsequent injections. If the organism is penicillin-resistant, one of the tetracyclines is usually effective. The patient is not permitted to drink alcohol or to have sexual intercourse while the treatment is in progress. Relapse is possible if treatment is not adequate. Treatment is most effective if it is started early and is thorough.

Gonorrhea

This disease is more prevalent than syphilis and is a less potentially dangerous disease. It, too, is curable with an adequate regimen of penicillin. Gonorrhea is caused by the gram-negative diplococcus *Neisseria gonorrhoeae*. The organism is a nonmotile, nonspore-forming parasite that requires man as a host. The disease is usually transmitted by direct contact through sexual relations, although it may occasionally be transmitted from an object to man. It is frequently "hidden" in women when it is trapped in Skene's glands on either side of the urinary meatus or in Bartholin's glands in the lower part of the labia majora. The disease is diagnosed by a smear of material taken from the site of infection. The organisms are cultured and then studied with a microscope. The test is positive if the gram-negative diplococci are present.

Symptoms include burning on urination, urethritis with a thick yellowish-green discharge in men and women, and with a vaginal discharge.[17] There may be tenderness and pain. If the disease is untreated, the pathogens spread throughout the urogenital system attacking the epididymis, seminal vesicles, prostate, and bladder in the male; and the bladder, fallopian tubes, ovaries, and peritoneum in females. Vaginitis is usually not present in adult women [18] because of the resistant epithelium there. It may be present in young girls, however. If the microorganism enters the blood, septicemia may develop. An attack of gonorrhea does not confer immunity to subsequent infections.

A dose of 300,000 units of procaine penicillin is administered daily for three to four days, or until there are three negative cultures. Then, cultures are repeated every week for three months because organisms may have been harbored and "walled off" somewhere in the genitourinary tract.[19] The patient is considered cured if the repeat cultures are negative over this extended period of time. During the treatment period he must be careful not to reinfect himself by hands contaminated with the discharge. Careful hand washing is vital.

REFERENCES

1. Burnet, M. F., *Natural History of Infectious Disease*, 2nd ed. Cambridge University Press, 1953, p. 28.
2. *Ibid.*, p. 46.
3. Taylor, I., and Knowelde, J., *Principles of Epidemiology*. Little, Brown and Company, Boston, 1957, p. 84.
4. *Ibid.*, p. 84.
5. Shafer, K. N., Sawyer, J. R., McCluskey, A. M., and Beck, E. L., *Medical Surgical Nursing*. The C. V. Mosby Co., St. Louis, 1967, p. 55.

6. Rodman, M. J., and Smith, D. W., *Pharmacology and Drug Therapy in Nursing.* J. B. Lippincott Co., Philadelphia, 1968, pp. 646–47.
7. Carpenter, P. L., *Microbiology.* W. B. Saunders Co., Philadelphia, 1967, p. 437.
8. Smith, I. M., "Death from Staphylococci," *Sci. Amer.*, **218**:85, Feb. 1968.
9. Burnet, *op. cit.*, p. 62.
10. Shafer, *op. cit.*, p. 63.
11 Streeter, S., Dunn, H., and Lepper, M., "Hospital Infection—A Necessary Risk?" *Amer. J. Nurs.*, **67**:527, Mar. 1967.
12. Thompson, L. R., *Microbiology and Epidemiology.* W. B. Saunders Co., Philadelphia, 1962, p. 470.
13. King, A., and Nicol, C., *Venereal Diseases.* Cassell and Company Ltd., London, 1964, pp. 13–43.
14. Brooks, S. M., *Basic Facts of Medical Microbiology.* W. B. Saunders Co., Philadelphia, 1962, p. 140.
15. French, R. M., *Nurses' Guide to Diagnostic Procedures.* McGraw-Hill Book Company, New York, 1967, p. 165.
16. King, *op. cit.*, p. 110.
17. Shafer, *op. cit.*, p. 529.
18. Brooks, *op. cit.*, p. 102.
19. Shafer, *op. cit.*, p. 529.

ADDITIONAL READINGS

ALLANACH, W. G.: "Problems in Venereal Disease Control as Seen by a Private Practitioner," *Canad. J. Public Health*, **56**:140, Apr. 1965.

BENT, W. I., "Problems in Venereal Disease Control as Seen by a Medical Officer of Health," *Canad. J. Public Health*, **56**:137, Apr. 1965.

CATTERALL, R. D., "The Venereal Diseases," *Nurs. Times*, **64**:1041, Aug. 2, 1968.

ELLIOTT, H., and RYZ, K., "Venereal Disease Clinic," *Nurs. Times*, **64**:827, June 21, 1968.

GEBHARDT, L. P., and ANDERSON, D. A., *Microbiology.* The C. V. Mosby Co., St. Louis, 1965.

KLINE, P. A., "Isolating Patients with Staphylococcal Infections," *Amer. J. Nurs.*, **65**:102, Jan. 1965.

MORTON, R. S., "Health Education and Venereal Diseases," *Nurs. Times*, **63**:957, July 21, 1967.

ROBERTSON, E. A., "Problems in Venereal Disease Control as Seen by a Public Health Nurse," *Canad. J. Public Health*, **56**:142, Apr. 1965.

———, "Hands Spread More Infection Than Air, Physician Report in California," *Mod. Hosp.*, **104**:174, Mar. 1965.

UNIT III

PROLIFERATION AND MATURATION OF CELLS

15

CANCER

LIVING tissue is made up of millions of cells. Each cell has a prominent central structure, known as the nucleus. The nucleus regulates the activities of the cell. It carries the chromosomes that determine its hereditary characteristics, and it undergoes a complicated series of changes, at periodic intervals, known as mitosis. This occurs prior to cell division.

The cell, as the ultimate unit of living matter, performs all the functions that we think of as characteristic of the organism as a whole. Thus, cells that comprise the various organs of the body have specialized functions. For examples, we have muscle cells and nerve cells; digestive cells of the stomach and excretory cells of the kidney; protective cells of the skin; oxygen-carrying cells of the blood; male and female cells for reproduction; and so on.

The cells from different tissues and organs differ from one another in size, shape, and detailed structure. As a rule, each cell breeds true to type, so that new muscle tissue is produced by multiplication of pre-existing muscle cells, new skin from pre-existing "epithelial" cells, and so on. When a cell divides into two, the resulting daughter cells can, on maturing, divide into two, and these in their turn can divide again so that whole colonies and even whole organs can arise as descendants of a single cell.

Normally, this process does not proceed haphazardly. Growth develops according to an orderly plan controlled by the innate characteristics of the cells themselves and by the influence of circulating hormones. Therefore, when a tissue or organ, in the process of development, reaches a particular size and shape, growth automatically ceases.

But growth does not end there. There are at least two other conditions in which cellular division, or "proliferation," plays a vital part. These are called anabolism and catabolism. Throughout life cells are continually being destroyed. This process is called *catabolism*. Catabolism occurs in the body after cells have outlived their function. If these destroyed cells were not replaced, most of our protective and other functions would quickly deteriorate and we would succumb to the slightest harm. The perpetual replacement of destroyed calls, called *anabolism,* constitutes one of the most important functions of normal life. This replacement of destroyed cells is achieved by division of existing cells in a manner identical with that described in connection with general growth.

Cell division is a basic attribute of living tissue. It is called into play under varying conditions of health and disease and serves a vitally useful purpose. The extent of the proliferation is determined by the precise needs of the body, and when the particular task is completed, the proliferation ceases. There is normally a constant balance between the number of cells being destroyed and the number of new cells being produced. This purposefulness and self-limiting characteristic of cellular proliferation applies to all conditions in health and disease except one: tumor growth does not obey these laws.

Tumors

Here we come to the tumor or cancer problem. Tumor is Latin for *a swelling*. When a tumor is present in the body, the enlargement that is seen may be due to an increased number of cells in a tissue or organ or due to an inflammation or accumulation of blood or fluid in a localized area. Tumor cells are actually derived from normal cells by some process of transformation. What makes the problem so distinctive is that, unlike other changes that normal cells can undergo, the change into a tumor cell is immutable. "Once a tumor cell, always a tumor cell." After division into two, the daughter cells will continue to show the newly acquired characteristics, and so on ad infinitum.

Tumor cells may be described as "normal cells gone wild." One of the features that all tumors have in common is continuous growth. In addition to the rate of growth that characterizes a tumor, there is the fact that, as opposed to normal and reparative growth, which is limited in extent, tumors apparently have no controlling mechanism. Regardless of whether the rate is rapid or slow, the growth is progressive, without any ultimate limit other than that imposed by time and the length of survival of the host. Therefore, it is this *progressive feature* as distinct from *speed* that characterizes a tumor.

Tumors possess other properties. Tumors that demonstrate nothing other than the growth pattern described above are known as *benign*. Benign tumors are relatively harmless, and when they are found to be harmful, it is because of location and the amount of space they occupy.

Malignant tumors demonstrate aggressive tendencies against normal tissues. These tendencies are serious and a menace to life. In malignant and benign tumors there is growth by expansion, but in addition the malignant tumors are capable of penetrating normal tissues and destroying it. In more popular language, malignant tumors are called "cancers."

Cancer is a generic name for a variety of malignant neoplasms (new growths or tumors), due to unknown and probable multiple causes, arising in all tissues composed of potentially dividing cells.[1*] In cancer the "aggressive tendencies" are the truly harmful influences even though the rate of growth is important.

What are the "aggressive tendencies" of malignant tumors? There are two of them: the first is the ability of the malignant cells to *invade* and *destroy* surrounding normal tissue; the second is their capacity to produce secondary centers of tumor growth—or "metastases," as they are technically called.

Metastases are cancer colonies that form when a cell or chunk of cells drops off the primary tumor (neoplasm) and is carried in lymphatic channels or blood vessels to other parts of the body. Metastases can also occur by direct extension into adjacent tissue.[2] In the new part of the body the cancer takes up residence, if you will, and grows into new tumors. When metastasis formation develops, the condition is more serious than when the primary growth has only invaded locally. (See Fig. 15–1.)

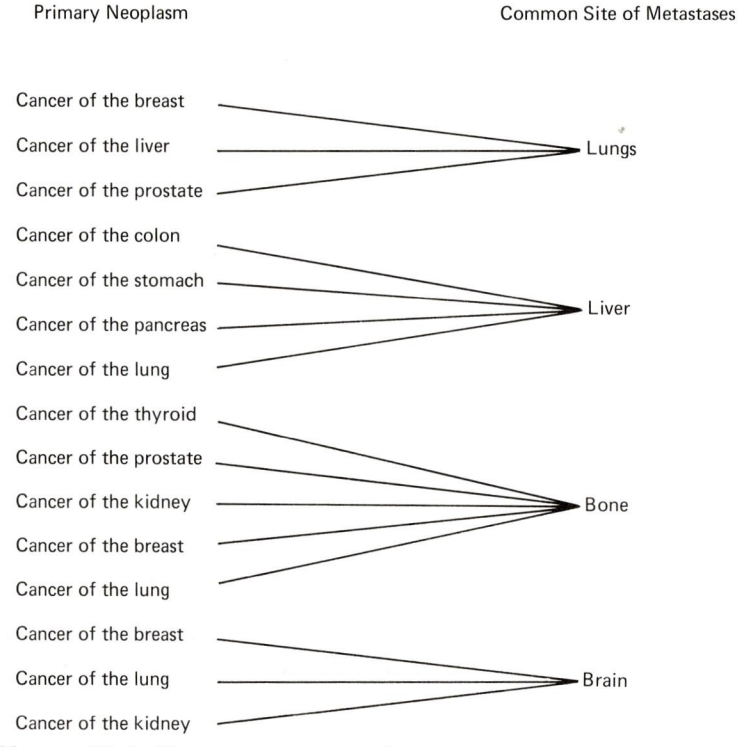

Primary Neoplasm — Common Site of Metastases

- Cancer of the breast
- Cancer of the liver — Lungs
- Cancer of the prostate
- Cancer of the colon
- Cancer of the stomach
- Cancer of the pancreas — Liver
- Cancer of the lung
- Cancer of the thyroid
- Cancer of the prostate
- Cancer of the kidney — Bone
- Cancer of the breast
- Cancer of the lung
- Cancer of the breast
- Cancer of the lung — Brain
- Cancer of the kidney

FIGURE 15–1. Four common sites of metastases and the primary-site neoplasms.

* References for Unit III are on pp. 108–109.

Cancer cells generally are rounded and plump, but not necessarily large. They contain king-sized nuclei; they store little material; they are mobile, adaptable to various environments, poorly regulated by the cell community, highly individualistic, antagonistic to cells of other cancers, and may be poison-producing.[3]

Malignant neoplasms are usually of two types: *carcinomas* which occur primarily in epithelial tissue such as the skin and lining of body cavities, organs, and glandular tissue such as the breast or prostate gland; *sarcomas,* which occur in connective tissue, i.e., bone. *Leukemia,* which is a neoplastic disease involving blood-forming tissues characterized by an overproduction of white blood cells, also falls under this type. *Melanoma,* one rare type of skin cancer, is the most dangerous of all cancerous skin lesions and is considered to be an epithelial sarcoma. It is called "black cancer" because it originates in pre-existing dark-colored moles. Other skin cancers have a high cure rate.

Look at the name of the tumor to determine what tissue it involves and whether it is benign or malignant. For example, myoma is a benign tumor (*oma*) of connective tissue (*my*); adenocarcinoma is a malignant tumor (*carcinoma*) of epithelial (*gland*) tissue.

Cancer is the second major cause of death in the United States, following cardiovascular diseases.[4] There were about 600,000 new cancer cases (diagnosed for the first time) in 1968, with one of every six deaths from all causes in the United States due to cancer.[5] Of every six persons who get cancer today, two will be saved and four will die.[6] It is significant to note that with our increased life expectancy and lowering of the number of deaths from infectious agents, the incidence and number of deaths from cancer have risen.[7]

Precise causes of abnormal cell growth are not known for the majority of human tumors. Two factors that are important when considering causes are (1) the susceptibility of the host and (2) the agent or group of possible causative agents.

The susceptibility of the host has to do with hereditary factors. When cancer strikes one member of a family, it is natural for other members to ask, "Is it inherited?" The most common answer is that humans do not inherit cancer. Some, however, may inherit a susceptibility, or predisposition, to certain tumors.[8] The only human cancer known to be directly inherited is that rare malignancy of the eye retinoblastoma.[9]

It is not easy to distinguish hereditary from environmental influences. Reference to occupational or other environmental influences playing a part in the development of human cancer can be found in writing as far back as the sixteenth century. In 1775 an English physician observed that cancer of the skin of the scrotum was unusually common among chimney-sweeps. Evidence pointed to soot as the responsible agent.[10]

The fact that sunlight is responsible for skin cancer in farmers and fishermen has been recognized for over a half-century. It has been observed that skin cancer affects blond people more readily than darkly colored people. Skin pigment acts as a protection against "sun rays." [11]

There are several other agents that researchers are investigating for possible carcinogenic effects (carcinogens are cancer causers). For example, certain agents have been found to be carcinogenic, i.e., arsenic, flavoring agents, safrol, and DDT. Water pollutants are also being investigated as to their carcinogenic effects. For example, some detergents have been found to cause cancer in animals,[12] and their concentration in drinking water has steadily increased. Regarding tobacco and cancer no responsible authority to date contends that cigarette smoking is the *sole* cause of lung cancer among men. However, most studies do indicate that cigarettes are the *principal* cause.

Cancers are often associated with disturbances of glands and the hormones manufactured by these glands. Humans with certain kinds of cancers can often be helped greatly but not cured by removing glands or giving hormones. The question about hormones is (1) are they inciting agents or (2) do they prepare the host (tissue) so that it responds to carcinogenic agents?

There is a lack of clear reliable information on environmental carcinogens as well as knowledge about intrinsic factors that may cause cancer in humans. Thus, additional and ongoing research is needed to lead the way to effective prevention and cure of cancer.

Cancer Detection

Cancer detection is emphasized as a way for individuals to protect themselves against cancer. The American Cancer Society, in a long-term campaign of public education, has publicized "seven warning signals" in the hope that individuals having any of them will consult their physician if the symptoms last more than two weeks. They are: (1) unusual bleeding or discharge; (2) a lump or thickening in the breast or elsewhere; (3) a sore that does not heal; (4) change in bowel or bladder habits; (5) hoarseness or cough; (6) indigestion or difficulty in swallowing; and (7) change in a wart or mole.

In addition, the American Cancer Society emphasizes that individuals should have a medical checkup annually; should avoid heavy cigarette smoking, overexposure to sunlight, and other known causes of cancer; and should learn the seven warning signals of cancer.

X-ray examination has been used to detect various kinds of cancer, but this technique has not been very successful in reducing cancer mortality. On the other hand, the "Pap" smear, which is a cytologic examination of a body fluid, has been extremely beneficial in detecting early cancer. Named after Dr. George N. Papanicolaou, its developer, it has been used successfully to detect cervical cancer. This procedure has also been used to detect cancer in other areas, for instance, lung cancer from sputum and bronchial washings, bowel cancer from cells in feces, breast cancer from cells in breast secretions. In addition to these measures, a carefully taken history and physical examination are essential in cancer detection.

In the case of cancer the body defenses are helpless. These defenses do not destroy the growth; instead, they nourish it at the expense of healthy organs and tissues. Thus, successful treatment of cancer is that which ensures the elimination of all the cancer cells.

Surgery

Surgery is one method used to effect a cure of cancer. Surgery can get right down to the "roots" of the invading malignant growth and remove those parts of the surrounding normal tissues that harbor the outlying cancer cells and the cancer mass itself. The important thing about the surgical approach is the removal of surrounding tissue to ensure that none of the outlying malignant cells are left behind. When metastasis has occurred, the chances of cure by surgery are remote.

Treatment by radiation, directed toward elimination and control of malignant cells, has advantages and limitations. The rays emitted during radiation therapy have the property of killing living cells mainly through their action on the nucleus. This killing action varies in degree according to the cells acted upon. Healthy cells can be destroyed in this process. The appropriate dose, carefully selected by the physician, can destroy cancer cells without appreciably harming the surrounding normal cells.

Some cancers can be treated equally well by either surgery or radiation. Where there is a choice of surgery or radiation therapy, the general advantage of radiation is that properly conducted treatment is less maiming and disfiguring. It usually requires less hospitalization, involves less strain and trauma, and eliminates the risk of spreading cancer at operation. Surgery and irradiation constitute the most common combination and most effective method of treating patients with malignant neoplasms.

Anticancer Drugs

Drugs used to slow the advance of cancer and provide symptomatic relief have been classified as anticancer drugs. (See Table 15–1.) These include:

Hormones, gland-secreted and artificial. Chemical messengers by which control is exerted against the growth and function of various kinds of body cells. An example would be an adrenocortical steroid such as cortisone acetate.

Antimetabolites. These are drugs that block normal cell processes, such as methotrexate, which inhibits the intracellular enzyme, folic acid.

Alkylating agents, which are cell poisons affecting normal and malignant cells. They react with, or "alkylate," a number of chemical groupings vital to cell function. They are toxic to cell nuclei. An example would be nitrogen mustard.

TABLE 15-1. SUMMARY OF SPECIFIC AGENTS USED IN CANCER CHEMOTHERAPY

Name	Routes of Administration	Indications	Nausea and Vomiting	Major Late Toxic Manifestations
STEROID HORMONES				
Androgen				
Testosterone propionate	IM, PO	Carcinoma of breast	None	Fluid retention, masculinization
Estrogen				
Diethylstilbestrol dipropionate	PO, IM	Carcinoma of prostate and breast	Occasional	Fluid retention, feminization, uterine bleeding
Adrenocortical Hormone				
Cortisone acetate Meticorten	PO	Acute leukemia, carcinoma of breast lymphomas	None	Fluid retention, hypertension, diabetes, increased susceptibility to infection
ANTIMETABOLITES				
5-Fluorouracil (5-FU)	IV	Carcinoma of breast, colon, thyroid, ovary, liver, bladder	None	Stomatitis, bone marrow depression
Methotrexate	PO, IM Intrathecally	Acute leukemia, choriocarcinoma	Occasional	Oral and digestive tract ulcerations, bone marrow depression, thrombocytopenia, and bleeding

TABLE 15-1. [*Continued*]

Name	Routes of Administration	Indications	Nausea and Vomiting	Major Late Toxic Manifestations
ALKYLATING AGENTS				
Mechlorethamine hydrochloride (Mustargen hydrochloride)	IV	Carcinoma of lung, ovary, breast, chronic leukemias Hodgkin's disease	Yes	Depressed blood count yields severe bone marrow depression, leukopenia, thrombocytopenia, bleeding
Cyclophosphamide (Cytoxan)	PO, IV	Lymphomas, carcinomas of ovary and lung Hodgkin's disease	Occasional	
ANTIBIOTIC				
Actinomycin D (Cosmegen)	IV	Wilms's tumor, testicular tumors	Yes	Stomatitis, diarrhea, dermatitis, alopecia, bone marrow depression

Several substances have been demonstrated to produce a reduction in the threshold of cancer cells to the injurious effects of irradiation. Some agents that have demonstrated this ability to "potentiate" x-rays are the alkylating agents and actinomycin D.

Radiation

Radiation medicine, also known as radiotherapy, is the treatment of disease, most frequently cancer, by means of x-ray and radioactive substances. Damage in tissue from radiation is produced by ionization of molecules into smaller parts, each acquiring an electrical charge in the process. Such charged particles are called ions. When produced in the body, they result in altered and abnormal tissue.

The principal types of radiation that can cause ionization are alpha, beta, and gamma rays. Of the three types, alpha radiation is the most strongly ionizing but the most weakly penetrating. Alpha rays do not penetrate unbroken skin. Alpha rays can travel only a few inches in air and are stopped by a sheet of paper. Beta radiation is intermediate between alpha and gamma radiation as far as ionizing power and penetration are concerned. Beta particles can travel as much as several feet in air and penetrate thin sections of such material as paper, plastic, and body tissue. Gamma rays ionize sparsely, but are capable of penetrating considerable thicknesses of such dense materials as iron, lead, and concrete.

These radiations are measured by the amount of ionization that accompanies their absorption, commonly expressed in terms of *roentgens* or *milliroentgens*.

The sources of ionizing radiation may be from machines such as the cobalt unit or from supervoltage equipment such as betatron and cyclotron units. Isotopes, too, may be used. These are atoms of an element that are chemically identical but are distinguishable by their weight. In dealing with isotopes it is important to know the specific one used, because each is characterized by a half-life peculiar to itself, and each emits characteristic ionizing radiation. The half-life is one measure of the instability of a radioisotope and is the length of time it takes a given quantity of the isotope to lose one half of its activity. For example, a physician injects radioactive gold, which has a half-life of three days, into the thoracic cavity of a patient on

March 1—
March 4—half of its activity is gone
March 7—one quarter of its activity remains
March 10—one eighth of its activity remains
March 13—one sixteenth of its activity remains

Hazard and Control

It is generally agreed that exposure to ionizing radiation is basically harmful and may produce tissue changes that will affect the health of those exposed. The nurse must realize that damage does result from the absorption of ionizing radiation! External exposure can be controlled by the use of shielding, timing, and safe-distance specifications for the operations involved. In addition, the nurse must be aware that two particular properties of radiation damage make it essential to maintain adequate records. One is the complete failure of the human senses to warn of the presence of radiation of any kind. The other is the fact that no constant clinical symptoms have yet been identified that reliably warn of latent radiation injury, injury that may not show up for months or years. A basic rule is that *any unnecessary exposure to radiation is too much for the radioisotope worker.*[14]

Palliative treatments constitute a major portion of radiation therapy, and the benefit the patient receives has to be determined by careful observation. The nurse needs to be aware that the relief of pain, of pressure symptoms, of obstruction, and of malaise in general cannot be expressed readily in figures but is of great importance to the patient. To regain a feeling of "well-being" and the ability to work and partake in normal activities is of great importance to the patient, even if the improvement lasts only a short time. If the treatments are too severe, they will not be beneficial but only add to the suffering of the patient.[15]

Usually diagnostic procedures utilizing radiation do not require special handling; however, the nurse taking care of the patient receiving radiation for therapy should: (1) check the patient's chart to find out what he is receiving, the dosage, and when treatment was started; (2) use soap and water only with physician's permission, (3) do not use powder or ointment on the area, or wash off the area outlined on the patient where treatment is given; (4) arrange for special disposal and handling of contaminated materials, if necessary; (5) wash her hands with soap and water after caring for a patient; (6) refrain from touching her hands to her face while caring for the patient; (7) if the patient dies, tag him sufficiently; and (8) discontinue measures after the decay rates of isotopes has progressed to a safe point.

When any part of the body, such as the hand, is contaminated with a small amount of radiation, it is best not to wash the part because this would result in spreading the contamination. The surrounding areas should be washed, and the affected spot should be cleaned with cotton-tipped applicators.[16]

TABLE 15–2. NURSING INSTRUCTIONS FOR PATIENTS RECEIVING RADIOACTIVE MATERIALS *

1. Nurses may spend whatever time is necessary near the patient for ordinary nursing care unless special restrictions have been established.

2. If the patient's clothes or bed linens are contaminated by fluid originating in the patient, notify the radiologist.

3. Wear rubber gloves while handling contaminated objects. Place gloves in special container after use.

4. Nurses or other attendants shall not remain in the immediate proximity of the patient longer than instructed by the radiologist.

5. Visitors must remain more than 6 ft. away from the patient, and the patient must remain in bed while visitors are in the room.

6. Unless otherwise notified, all excreta may be disposed of in the normal manner.

7. The patient may be released from the hospital when released by the radiologist.

8. In the event of death, immediately notify the physician in charge of radiology and do not remove the body from the room.

9. When the patient is discharged, his room should be surveyed for contamination before being remade.

* Refer to the radiation department in the hospital for specific instructions concerning care of the patient receiving treatment.

TABLE 15–3. NURSING AND VISITOR PRECAUTIONS REGARDING PATIENTS RECEIVING RADIOACTIVE ISOTOPES IN THERAPEUTIC AMOUNTS *

1. Nurses may spend whatever time is necessary near the patient for ordinary nursing care. It is preferable not to employ private-duty nurses, but to use circulating general floor nurses for these patients.

2. Patients are allowed visitors in accordance with usual hospital rules unless otherwise notified. Children and pregnant women are prohibited.

3. No special precautions are needed for dishes, utensils, or instruments except as noted.

4. With radioactive gold (Au^{198}) no special precautions are needed for vomitus, urine, stools, or sputum.

5. With radioactive iodine (I^{131}) the vomitus in the first 8 hours will be highly radioactive. Call the Radioisotope Department at once! The urine will also be highly radioactive—the patient should have bathroom privileges and be advised to flush the toilet several times after each use.

6. Following intracavity administration of radioactive gold there may be a certain amount of drainage at the puncture site for a few days. It is advisable to change the dressings only when necessary. Disposable gloves should be worn. The gloves and dressing should be placed in a labeled bag. Since the radioactive gold is purple, contamination is easily noticed. Any contaminated linens should be bagged and labeled. The radioisotope technician will check the room daily and remove any contaminated material.

7. The radioisotope technician will be responsible for monitoring the area for radiation and will advise the nurses when precautions no longer need be taken.

8. For any special instructions call the Radioisotope Department.

* To be placed on the front of the patient's chart. A notice should also be placed on the patient's door advising all visitors to check with the charge nurse before entering.

Sheets, pillowcases, rubber sheets, pajamas, and other materials in contact with patients receiving radiation therapy, especially intracavity instillations, should not be placed in the hospital laundry system. These materials should be stored in suitable containers until the activity becomes reduced to the normal amount by the decay process.

The Meaning of Cancer to Patient and Family

The patient with cancer is fearful. His life is threatened, and he fears the loss of his job and the burden he may be to his family. The family of the patient with cancer is also fearful. They fear the loss of a loved one and the effects of treatment on the loved one—be it surgery, radiation, chemotherapy, or a combination of all three. They are anxious about the outcome of treatment and want to know if treatment will result in a return to "normal" for the loved one.

All patients fear disfigurement.[17] This is a threat to the body image and is closely bound up with their feelings of self-esteem. Many fears are related to "old wives' tales" about cancer and may be dispelled when the patient is informed about the whys and wherefores as treatment plans are made and carried out.

The patient may express these fears verbally and nonverbally as feelings of doom, anger, helplessness, shame, disgrace, or abandonment. The aim of the nurse is not to avoid these feelings but to take note of when they are demonstrated and how they are expressed. The patient should be encouraged to discuss his feelings and helped to look at events as realistically as possible. Good communication between the nurse and family could also help the patient.

The nurse working with the cancer patient and his family needs to realize that many cancer patients will have to endure physical anguish, that great expense is involved, and that the time of acute illness and convalescence may be extensive. Therefore, a false cheerful attitude with comments such as, "You haven't a thing to worry about," or "You look just fine!" are not helpful to the patient or his family. We need not weep with them or be "crepe hangers" either. As nurses we can have empathy for and interest in our patients with cancer and their families. We will at times fulfill the roles of technical expert, mother surrogate, or resource person as the occasion requires.

The patient's reaction to "terminal" cancer care (that form of cancer that begins when it is accepted that the patient's disease cannot be controlled) depends on his chronologic age, his emotional maturity (developmental task level), his typical reaction to stress and crisis, and his general pattern of behavior. Most families need help in accepting terminal aspects of the illness, and in letting the patient share in the responsibility of taking practical steps to arrange his affairs. The family should be helped in their efforts not to overprotect the patient.

Religious faith has sustained both patients and families. Early contact with the proper clergyman is important to prevent the frightening feeling of "last rites" at his appearance. People are most satisfied in their own homes, and whenever possible, adjustment should be made to facilitate home care. The clergyman should be notified as changes are planned and carried out.

Kindness, acceptance, and support, especially from professional persons, have been proved to be of great significance to the patient. They give him the kind of security he needs to face his problem. The nurse should examine her feelings about cancer and not avoid them because they will affect her approach to the patient.

Community Action

The *Sword of Hope* is the symbol that to most Americans means, "Help Fight Cancer." It is the registered trademark of the American Cancer Society. This society has for more than a decade supported a program of research in the causes, treatment, prevention, and diagnosis of cancer.

In addition, it provides an information and counseling service regarding existing facilities and services related to cancer within a given community. This program also provides assistance to the cancer patient and his family with the help of community resources (medical and social), along with the loan of sickroom equipment and transportation services. The national headquarters of the American Cancer Society is in New York City, and there are many local chapters throughout the United States.

Local health agencies (such as the local public health nursing agency and the local homemaker service) also contribute to the care of the cancer patient.

Pain

One common manifestation of illness is pain and fear of pain. Pain is a sensory perception. Pain impulses are transmitted from receptors to spinal tracts by way of mixed peripheral nerves. One system, which consists of large, myelinated fibers, conducts impulses rapidly. A second system of small, unmyelinated fibers conducts pain impulses slowly. The first system alerts the individual to the presence of pain and localizes it. The second system contributes to the suffering experienced in the presence of pain. The thalamus functions in the awareness of the pain and has connections with many areas of the brain. The cerebral cortex is thought to function in the localization of pain and in the recognition of its nature, severity, and significance.

The nurse's role in prevention and relief of pain is to:

1. Make the necessary observations that serve as a basis for arriving at an appropriate course of action,
2. Institute appropriate action to prevent or to alleviate pain,
3. Observe the effects of measures used to relieve pain.

In order to carry out the above, the nurse should know the nature of the patient's pain, such as the location, intensity, and length of time the pain has been and is being experienced. It is also necessary to recognize some of the words used to describe pain, such as crushing, boring, burning, gnawing, and pricking. Fatigue, sickness, debility, and repeated painful procedures reduce tolerance to pain to a low level.

Treatment of pain by the physician is carried out by the use of medication to decrease and relieve the pain as well as by medication to decrease the anxiety caused by pain, which, in some instances, markedly decreases the pain a patient experiences. Surgical procedures may also be performed when relief is not given by the use of these other agents. A *chordotomy* is the most satisfactory procedure for the relief of pain. This procedure is often performed in the treatment of diffuse pain caused by a malignant disease, often referred to as intractable pain.

16

THE PATIENT WITH BREAST CANCER

CARCINOMA of the breast is the most common form of cancer occurring in white women over 40 years of age in the United States.[18] Cancer of the breast is rarely seen in women under 25 years of age and is rare among men.

There few early symptoms of carcinoma of the breast. The most important, single presentation sign is a *lump*, usually painless.[19] Other symptoms are local pain, enlargement of lump, lump in axilla, soreness in nipple, discharge from nipple, retraction of nipple, ulceration, enlargement of breast, puckering from attachment of tumor to skin, weight loss, and hemorrhage.

The most important measure a woman can take for early detection is breast self-examination. This examination is best carried out once a month, in the middle of the menstrual cycle, when mammary engorgement is minimal. (See Fig. 16–1.) If a lump is felt, the woman should see a physician immediately. Immediate hospitalization will be recommended, and the patient will be scheduled for surgery. At this time a frozen section of the lump is taken. Frozen section diagnosis is a rapid method of taking fresh tissue and cutting and staining it for microscopic examination. In this manner a number of slides can be looked at in a short period of time. Frozen-section diagnosis is a highly accurate method of diagnosis.[20] A frozen section helps the physician make a therapeutic decision. The surgeon decides on the basis of the report to carry out further surgery or to close the incision.

Mammography, soft-tissue roentgenography of the breast, is an adjunctive procedure that may offer assistance in the diagnosis of breast disease. There is now a satisfactory roentgenographic technique, which is highly accurate, safe, simple, inexpensive, nontraumatic, and acceptable to the patient; it was developed at the University of Texas, M. D. Anderson Hospital.[21]

Mammography, a gross diagnostic procedure, is not a substitute for physical examination; the two are complementary. Nor is either method a substitute for biopsy examination. However, mammography has proved to be the only means by which breast cancer can be determined before clinical signs and symptoms are present.[22]

1

Sit or stand in front of your mirror, with your arms relaxed at your sides, and examine your breasts carefully for any changes in size and shape. Look for any puckering or dimpling of the skin, and for any discharge or change in the nipples.

2

Raise both your arms over your head, and look for exactly the same things. See if there's been any change since you last examined your breasts.

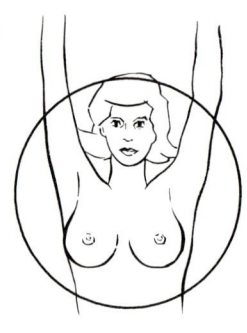

3

Lie down on your bed, put a pillow or a bath towel under your left shoulder, and your left hand under your head. (From this Step through Step 8, you should feel for a lump or thickening.) With the fingers of your right hand held together flat, press gently but firmly with small circular motions to feel the inner, upper quarter of your left breast, starting at your breastbone and going outward toward the nipple line. Also feel the area around the nipple.

4

With the same gentle pressure, feel the lower inner part of your breast. Incidentally, in this area you will feel a ridge of firm tissue or flesh. Don't be alarmed. This is perfectly normal.

5

Now bring your left arm down to your side, and still using the flat part of your fingers, feel under your armpit.

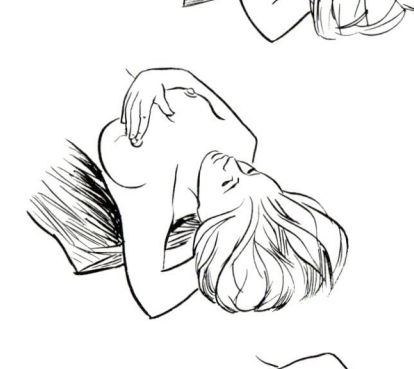

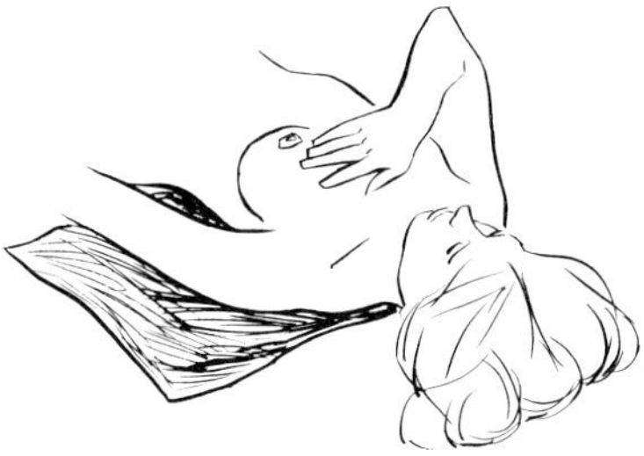

6

Use the same gentle pressure to feel the upper, outer quarter of your breast from the nipple line to where your arm is resting.

7

And finally, feel the lower outer section of your breast, going from the outer part to the nipple.

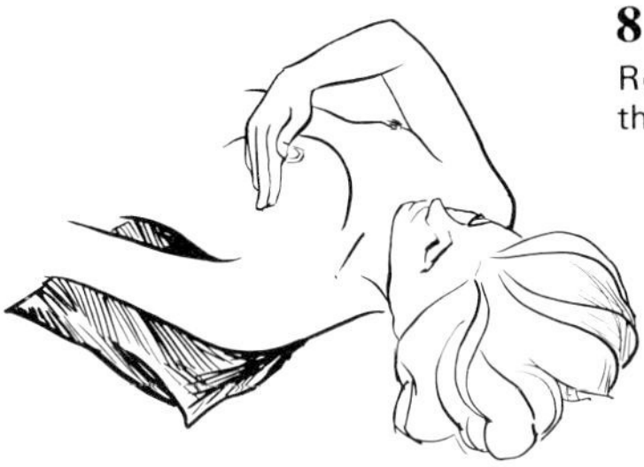

8

Repeat the entire procedure, as described, on the right breast.

- Your own doctor may want you to use a slightly different method of examination. Ask him to teach you that method.

- Examine your breasts every month, just after your period. Be sure to continue these checkups after your change of life.

- If you find a lump or thickening, *leave it alone* until you see your doctor. Don't be frightened. Most breast lumps or changes are *not* cancer, but only your doctor can tell.

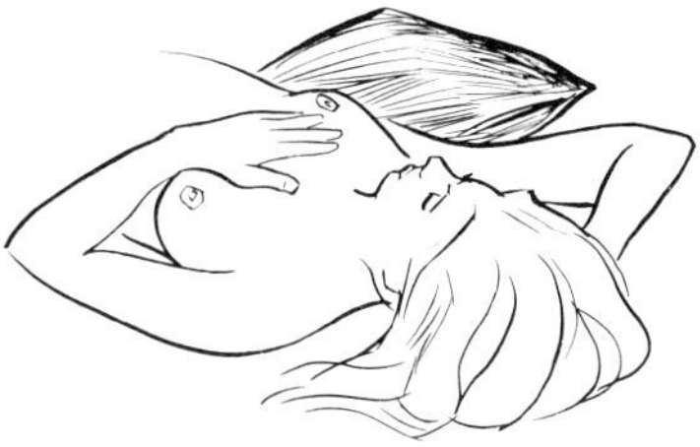

FIGURE 16-1. Breast self-examination (Courtesy, American Cancer Inc.)

INDICATIONS FOR MAMMOGRAPHY *

1. Signs and symptoms of breast cancer
2. Study of opposite breast following mastectomy
3. Strong family history of breast cancer
4. Pendulous or lumpy breasts
5. Cancerophobia
6. Adenocarcinoma in women, primary site undetermined [23]

If the lump shows malignant properties, the treatment is usually a radical mastectomy. This procedure involves removal of the pectoralis major and minor muscles, the adjacent lymph nodes, and the entire breast.

* Indications are generally for breasts exhibiting definite or questionable signs of disease.

When a large amount of skin is removed, the defect over the chest wall is covered with a skin graft. Therefore, if the surgeon suspects a malignancy, he will often request a thigh prep, along with the prep of the trunk—front and back, because grafting will be necessary and grafts are usually taken from the patient's thigh.

Preoperative Care

Preoperative care of the patient about to have breast surgery should focus on her feelings. Loss of a breast may seriously jeopardize her body image. As the nurse is not usually aware of the amount of surgery the patient will have, it can be harmful to project concrete ideas of how the patient will look when she returns from surgery. The nurse best serves as a listening, interested individual at this period, refraining from making comments that will increase the patient's anxiety. In addition, routine preoperative procedures will need to be carried out, making sure that these are explained to the patient.

Postoperative Care

Postoperative care focuses chiefly on the prevention of complications. The surgery is usually long and involves the traumatization of a large amount of tissue. Shock must be watched for and prevented. Dressings must be observed frequently for signs of bleeding. If drainage apparatus is used, this must be checked frequently and emptied when necessary, making sure the amount, color, and time are recorded on the patient's chart.

Position and early mobilization of the arm on the affected side are directed toward prevention of postoperative deformity. A sling may be used the first day or the arm elevated at right angles to decrease edema. The rate of mobilization depends, to some degree, on the presence or absence of a skin graft and the amount of tension on the wound site. Passive motion is started as early as possible.

X-ray therapy may be combined with surgery in an attempt to kill any errant cells. This treatment is frequently followed by anorexia, nausea and vomiting, and fatigue. The nurse should report and record these symptoms if they occur and pay special attention to the diet and fluid balance of this patient.

When exercises are started in the hospital, they may consist of informal activities, such as combing and brushing the hair and assisting with bathing, or a set of definite exercises performed at specific intervals. The nurse must consult with the physician before instituting any regimen for the patient. Whatever method is used, it is important that, once exercises have been started, the patient continue to move her arm because it is difficult to regain range of motion once it is lost. The patient should not be pushed past the point recommended by the physician. (See Fig. 16-2.)

Prosthesis

After the operative site has healed, the patient will be ready for a prosthesis, or artificial breast form. Many are available in department stores. The physician is the one to decide when the patient is ready to begin wearing a prosthesis.

The patient should have the opportunity to try on several prostheses and brassieres. To assure the patient's comfort and peace of mind, it is important that both fit well. The three types most commonly utilized are sponge rubber, cotton-filled, and water-filled. The brassiere should provide firm support and not be of stretchable material or have cutting straps.

For more specific information the patient may be referred to Reach to Recovery, a unit of the American Cancer Society. This is a voluntary organization made up of women who have had mastectomies. They are specifically trained to give support and helpful hints to the woman with a new mastectomy. (Reach to Recovery, 1841 Broadway, New York, New York, 10023, 212-582-7888.)

Lymphedema

The lymphatic drainage of the operative site is drastically interfered with in the operative procedure. As a result fluid may accumulate in "pockets" or storage spaces. In the hospital these "pockets" are usually emptied by means of drains or suctioned off by mechanical means. At home the dressing will need to be re-inforced by adding gauze pads to the outside. The inside dressing should not be changed unless this is ordered by the physician. If the arm becomes heavy and swollen, an arm bandage may be applied, preferably at the first sign of swelling. Elevation of the arm is also helpful whenever the patient is sitting.

Control of the Spread of Breast Cancer

Ovariectomy (oophorectomy) yields temporary regression by destroying the main source of estrogens, the ovaries, which are thought to stimulate the malignant cells. This procedure usually gives a one-year remission.

Adrenalectomy may be performed when the ovariectomy ceases to be effective. The adrenal glands are removed. This procedure is sometimes performed at the same time as an ovariectomy. The adrenalectomized patient will have to take cortisone in some form for the remainder of her life. This is called replacement therapy. There may also have to be some dietary modification because cortisone has sodium-retaining properties and thus will have to be restricted if complications arise or limited to prevent complications.

Total hypophysectomy is a procedure used to deprive the body of its normal hormones in an effort to arrest cancer. The pituitary gland is removed. The only tumor thus far favorably affected has been cancer of the breast. Removal of every vestige of the pituitary is a requisite for the securing of a remission. This operation is less hazardous and annoying than a bilateral adrenalectomy. However, removal leads to many possible complications:

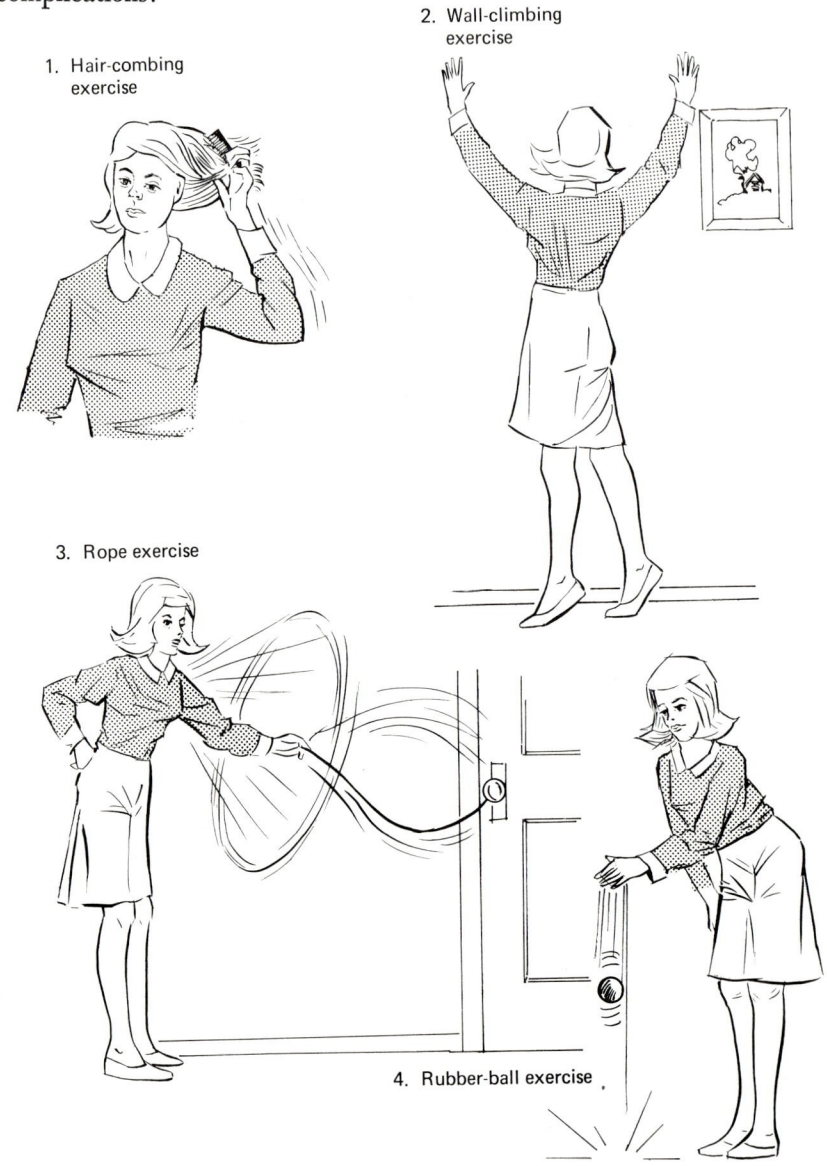

1. Hair-combing exercise

2. Wall-climbing exercise

3. Rope exercise

4. Rubber-ball exercise

5. Pulley exercise

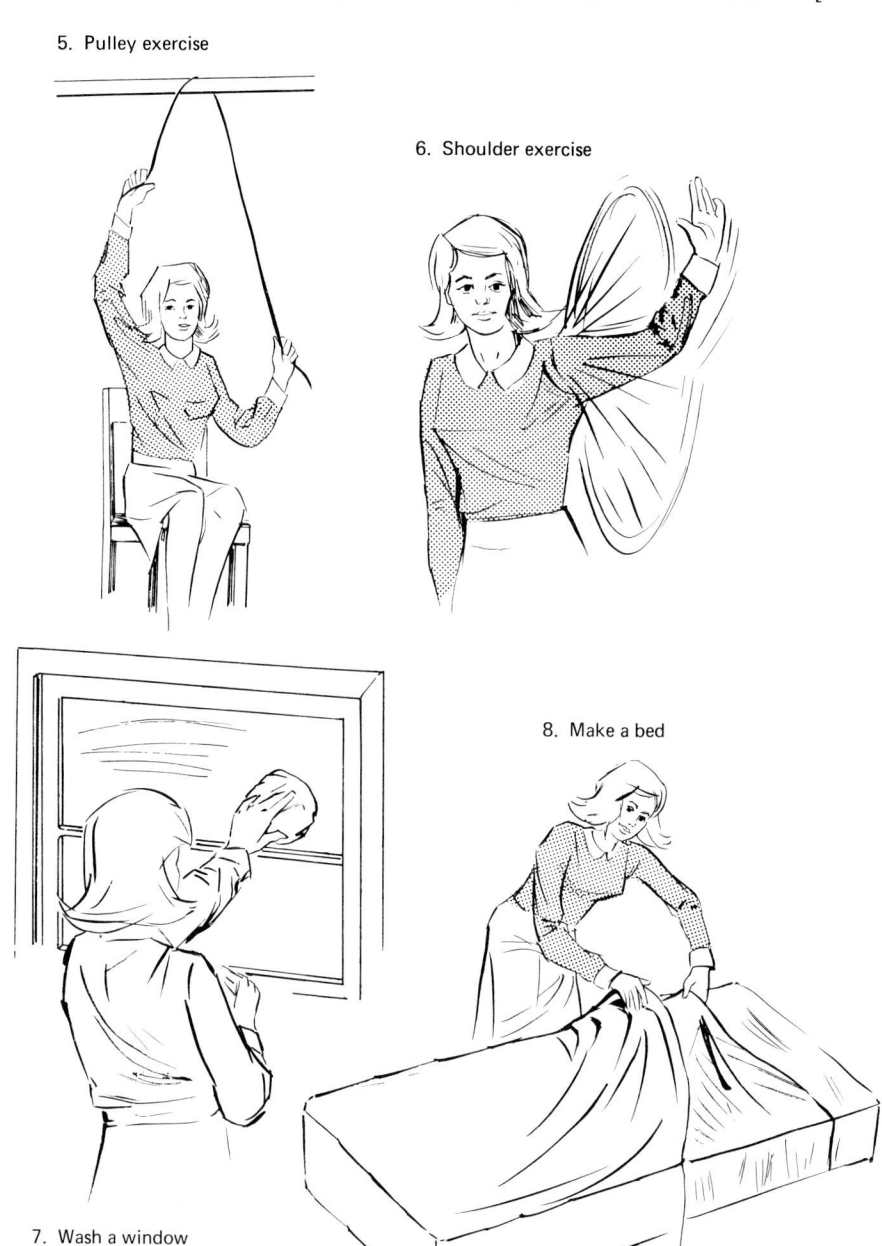

6. Shoulder exercise

7. Wash a window

8. Make a bed

Figure 16–2. In postmastectomy exercises try to work naturally using the arms in all positions.

1. Anorexia
2. Diabetes insipidus (disappears in a few days or weeks)
3. Cessation of growth of skeletal and soft tissues
4. Atrophy of the thyroid, adrenal cortex, and gonads
5. Hypertrophy of liver, spleen, and kidneys
6. Decreased basal metabolic rate
7. Decreased life-span

After this procedure the patient must take cortisone and thyroid for the rest of her life.

REFERENCES

1. Ackerman, L., *Cancer Diagnosis, Treatment and Prognosis*, 3rd ed. The C. V. Mosby Co., St. Louis, 1962, p. 11.
2. *Ibid.*, p. 75.
3. McGrady, P., *The Savage Cell*. Basic Books, New York, 1964, pp. 5-6.
4. *Op. cit.*, p. 17.
5. ———, *1968 Cancer Facts and Figures*. American Cancer Society, New York, 1968, No. 7008, p. 3.
6. *Ibid.*, p. 4.
7. *Ibid.*, p. 4.
8. McGrady, *op. cit.*, p. 160.
9. *Ibid.*, p. 164.
10. Birenblum, I., *Man Against Cancer*. The Johns Hopkins University Press, Baltimore, 1952, p. 42.
11. *Ibid.*, p. 43.
12. McGrady, *op. cit.*, p. 40.
13. Ackerman, *op. cit.*, p. 102.
14. Fields, T., and Seed, L., *Clinical Use of Radioisotopes*. Year Book Publishers, Chicago, 1957, p. 327.
15. *Ibid.*, p. XX.
16. *Ibid.*, p. 326.
17. Barkley, V., "What Can I Say to the Cancer Patient?" *Nurs. Outlook*, **6**: 316–118, June 1958.
18. Thomas, A. "Typical Patient Family Attitudes," *Public Health Rep.*, **67**: 960–62, Oct. 1952.
19. Ackerman, *op. cit.*, p. 1063.
20. *Ibid.*, p. 1081.
21. Egan, Robert, "The Role of Mammography in the Diagnosis of Breast Tumors," in *Recent Advances in The Diagnosis of Cancer* (A Collection of Papers Presented at the Ninth Annual Clinical Conference, 1964, at the University of Texas M. D. Anderson Hospital and Tumor Institute at Houston Texas). Year Book Publishers, Chicago, 1966, p. 210.
22. *Ibid.*, p. 214.
23. *Ibid.*, p. 216.

ADDITIONAL READINGS

ALEXANDER, S., "Nursing Care of a Patient After Breast Surgery," *Amer. J. Nurs.*, **57**:157–72, 1957.

BARD, M., "Emotional Control in Mastectomy Nursing," *RN*, **21**:76–87, Oct. 1958.

CANTRILL, S., "The Care of the Patient with Advanced Cancer of the Breast," *Radiology*, **66**:46–54, Jan. 1956.

PEARSON, O., "Hypophysectomy in Treatment of Advanced Cancer," *J.A.M.A.*, **161**:17–21, May 1956.
SHAFER, *et al.*, *Medical-Surgical Nursing*. The C. V. Mosby Co., St. Louis, 1967.
SMITH, D., and GIPPS, C., *Care of the Adult Patient*. J. B. Lippincott Co., Philadelphia, 1968.

UNIT IV

WATER AND ELECTROLYTE BALANCE

17

BASIC CONCEPTS

THE maintenance of equilibrium inside the body is like the functioning of an intricate piece of machinery. When all of its interrelated parts are running smoothly, there is optimum function. But let one part become disrupted, and every other part will be affected, too. Body equilibrium is much the same. Its balance involves the superb blending of many different processes all aimed at one major goal—to maintain a life-sustaining internal environment for the cells.

Homeostasis or homeokinesis are the all-encompassing terms that are used to describe these continuous, ongoing, dynamic processes aimed at maintaining equilibrium. Homeokinesis is a newer term that implies a nonstatic more "on-the-move" set of processes. Either term can be used.

What Is an Electrolyte?

An electrolyte is a tiny substance that carries an electric charge when placed in solution. Dry table salt is an example. It carries no electric charge in its dry, molecular form. If it is dissolved in water, it ionizes (dissociates) into two independent ions (Na^+ and Cl^-) each carrying an electric charge. If the NaCl is placed in a wet cell, the positively charged Na^+ ion would travel to the negative pole of the cell (the cathode) and the negatively charged Cl^- ion would travel to the positive pole (anode). (See Fig. 17-1.) Substances capable of dissociating into ions when in solution are called electrolytes. Those that do not ionize in solution are called nonelectrolytes. Glucose, urea, and creatinine are examples of nonelectrolytes.

Why Is Body Water Important?

All physicochemical activities of life take place in a water solution. Water is the largest single constituent of all living organisms and is essential for the proper functioning of cells. It is needed for transport of nutrients to and waste products from cells; it collects heat produced by

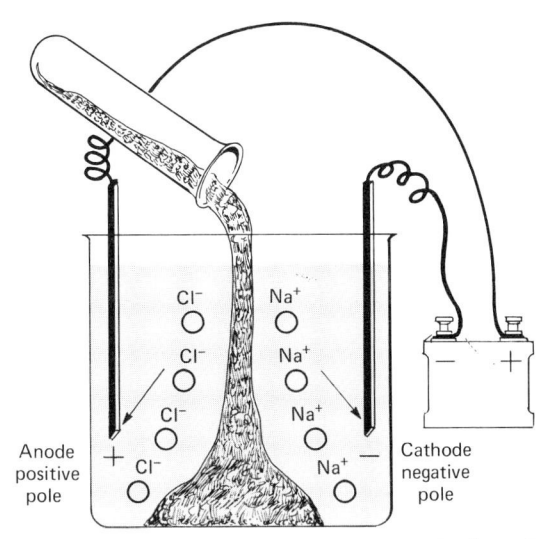

FIGURE 17-1. Table salt dissociates into Na+ and Cl− when placed in wet cell. Na+ migrates to the cathode; Cl− migrates to the anode.

the cells and carries it to the body surface for dispersal; and it is involved in maintenance of the concentrations of water and electrolytes needed to support life.

Electrolytes do their work in a water solution. Sixty per cent of the total body weight of a lean adult is water: 40 per cent of this water is within the cells; 20 per cent is outside the cells. Adipose (fat) tissue is relatively free of water; therefore, the percentage of body weight that is water is less in an obese person.

A solution that contains both water and electrolytes is called a fluid.

What Are the Sources of Water?

Water is derived from oral liquids, from the oxidation (burning) of foods, and from the water content of solid food. A lean piece of meat contains about 75 per cent water weight. A normal mixed diet yields 300 to 350 gm of water when it is oxidized; 12 ml of water is derived from the burning of 100 mixed calories. More specifically, 100 gm of fat yields 107 gm of water; 100 gm of carbohydrate yields 55 gm of water; and 100 gm of protein yields 41 gm of water.

How Is Water Lost?

About 1,500 ml of water is lost through the urine each day; about 600 to 1,000 ml is lost through vaporization from the skin and lungs; and about 150 ml is lost through the stool. Water lost through vaporization from the lungs and skin is not visible and is called "insensible" loss. It does not contain electrolytes. That which can be seen and felt over and above insensible loss is called "sensible" loss. It is the product of sweat gland activity (perspiration) and constitutes a method for increased heat loss when there is increased heat production, e.g., fever, exercise, and increased environmental temperature and humidity. Sensible water loss contains both water and electrolytes.

Water lost through feces and through vaporization from the lungs and skin is called obligatory loss. It goes on regardless of environmental temperature.

There must be a daily balance between the amount of water taken in and the amount excreted. Usually, the volume of fluid consumed equals the volume of urine excreted, and the volume of water derived from oxidation and from solid foods equals the amount lost through vaporization from the lungs and skin and in feces.

Intake	Output
1,500 ml ingested as fluids	1,500 ml as urine
800 ml water content of food	⎰ 1,000 ml vaporization from lungs and
350 ml water of oxidation	⎱ skin
2,650 ml	150 ml stool
	2,650 ml

Where Are Water and Electrolytes Found?

The Fluid Phases

For convenience, the physiologist has designated two major "fluid phases" within the body. They are the intracellular phase (fluid within all cells) and the extracellular phase (fluid outside the cells). The extracellular phase is further divided into an intravascular (plasma) space and an interstitial (tissue) space. Fluids located in ducts, the gastrointestinal tract, the urinary collecting system, and so forth are called transcellular. (See Fig. 17–2.) Fluids are not static. They do their work within and between the various phases. There is continuous movement. Water and smaller electrolytes can pass freely across the semipermeable membranes separating the fluid phases. There is a great deal of movement between the interstitial (tissue) and intravascular (plasma) phases, and there is some movement between the intracellular and intravascular phases. Two thirds of the total body fluid is found in the cell phase; one third is in the extracellular phase. The terms "contraction" and "expansion" of fluid phases are used to indicate, respectively, a decrease and increase in fluid volume.

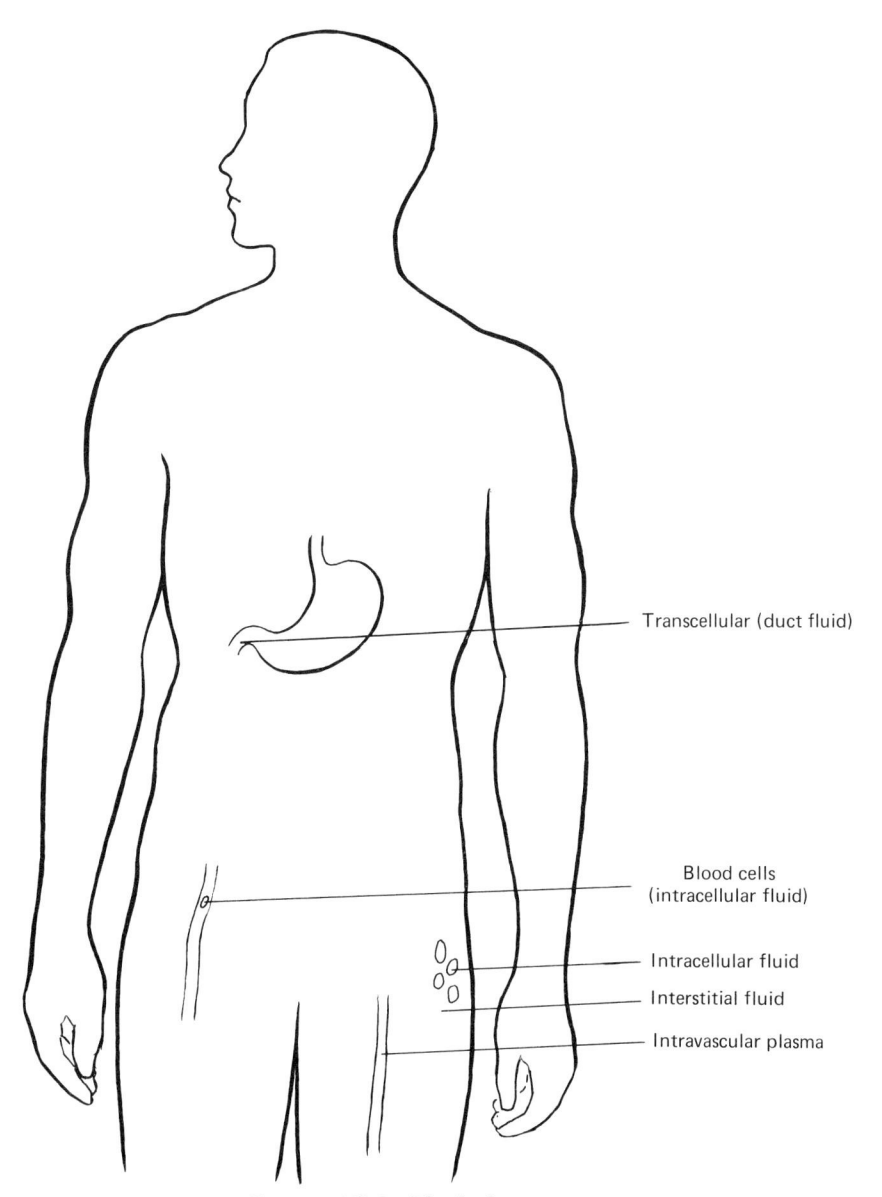

FIGURE 17-2. Fluid phases in man.

How Is an Electrolyte Measured?

Electrolytes are important because of their total number, because of their weight, and because of their ability to combine (cations and anions) and form electrically neutral molecules. Weight, by itself, is not indicative of the ability of the ion to combine, or "act." Chemical combining power is best indicated by a measurement called "equivalent value." An equivalent is defined as the chemical-combining power of an ion equal to the chemical-combining power of 1 gm of hydrogen. It is derived by dividing the atomic weight of an ion by its valence. For instance, sodium has an atomic weight of 23. Its valence is 1. Its equivalent value is 23. Calcium has an atomic weight of 40 with a valence of 2. Its equivalent value is 20.

Because quantities of molecules are measured in such tiny amounts, the milliequivalent value is used. This is 1/1,000 of the equivalent value. Now, let's look at the milliequivalent measurement more carefully!

We are most interested in the ability of a cation and anion to combine and form an electrically neutral molecule. This chemical-combining power is best indicated by the milliequivalent measurement, which involves not only atomic weight, but valence as well. Valence is the power of an ion to combine with other ions. For instance, sodium combines readily with chloride to form the molecule sodium chloride. (See Fig. 17–3.) It con-

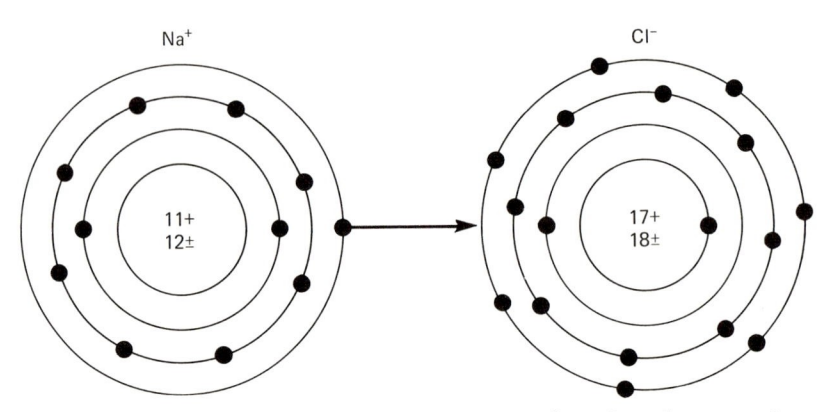

FIGURE 17–3. Valence is the property an atom has of combining with other atoms. Comparison is often made with hydrogen, which is the lightest element and has a "holding power" of 1.

tains 11 positively charged protons and 11 negatively charge electrons. It has an atomic weight of 23 (the sum of the protons and neutrons in its nucleus) and an atomic number of 11 (number of protons). There is a single negatively charged electron in its outer ring (valance 1) that readily moves over to complete the outer ring of chloride. Thus, we see the ability of the cation Na^+ to combine with the anion Cl^- to form the molecule NaCl.

It is interesting to compare the "action power" of various electrolytes. One milliequivalent of chemical activity is exerted by 1 mg hydrogen,

23 mg sodium, 39 mg potassium, 40 mg calcium, and 35 mg chlorine. One milliequivalent of any cation is, therefore, equivalent in action power to 1 mEq of any anion.[1*] Electrolyte balance means an equal milliequivalent value (chemical activity) of cations and anions in a fluid phase. *Equilibrium means "milliequivalent sameness."* There are charts available to convert milligram values to milliequivalents-per-liter values. A text in water and electrolytes should be consulted to see the mathematical formula used to convert milligrams per cent to milliequivalents per liter. (See Fig. 17–4.)

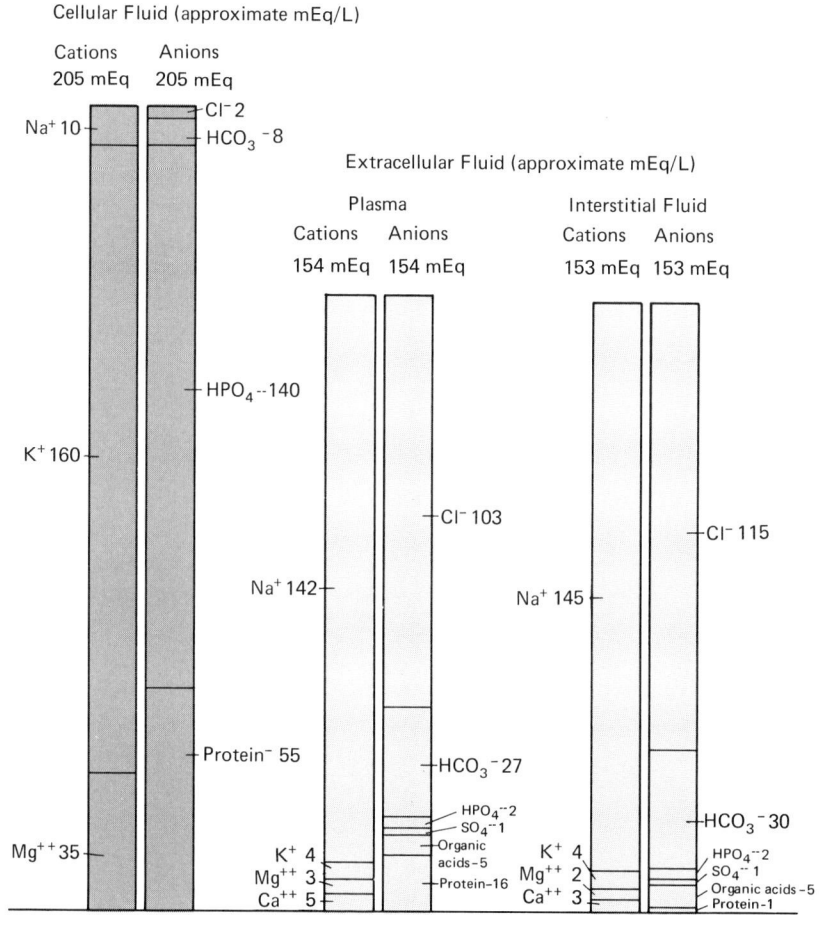

FIGURE 17–4. Cations and anions in each fluid phase (milliequivalents per liter).

* References for Unit IV are on pp. 210–11.

What Forces Cause Water and Electrolytes to Move?

Diffusion

Diffusion is the simplest type of fluid movement. Water and electrolytes move from the area of their highest concentration toward the area of their least concentration, across semipermeable membranes, until equilibrium is reached.

Osmosis and Osmotic Pressure

Osmosis is, by far, the most important force causing water and electrolyte activity. The "force" is a pressure created by the random movement and bumping of electrolytes against each other. The greater the concentration of electrolytes, the greater the bumping of particles, and the greater the osmotic pressure created.

In order to maintain pressure balance between the fluid phases, water freely seeps across semipermeable membranes toward the area of greatest electrolyte concentration and osmotic pressure. Water helps to equalize the electrolyte concentration on either side of the semipermeable membrane. Osmosis, then, is the movement of water (and some solutes) toward the area of greatest particle concentration. *Said more simply: water goes where the particles are; water goes where the salt is.*

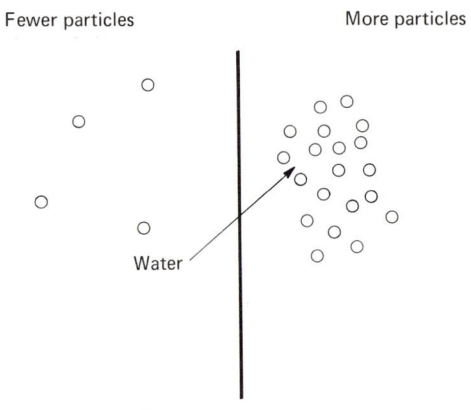

FIGURE 17-5. Osmosis. Water moves across a semipermeable membrane toward the greatest concentration of particles.

The principal osmotic effects are exerted by sodium and chloride ions in the extracellular fluid, and by potassium, magnesium, phosphates, and proteinates in the intracellular fluids. (See Fig. 17-5.)

A Word About Tonicity

Tonicity refers to the osmotic effect of constituents of one phase on another. It is very important because of the changes it can cause within and between the fluid phases. An *isotonic* fluid has the same amount of solute or osmotic pressure as the fluid to which it is compared and will not cause change between the phases. Isotonic saline (0.9 per cent) is an example. A *hypotonic* solution has a smaller amount of solute or less osmotic pressure than the solution to which it is compared; because water goes where the particles are, it will move toward areas of higher concentration across semipermeable membranes. Half-strength saline (0.45 per cent) is an example. A hypertonic solution has a greater amount of solute or greater osmotic pressure than the solution to which it is compared and will pull water from other areas toward itself. Five-per-cent saline is an example.

Hormonal Response to Changes in Fluid Volume

When the plasma volume decreases or its tonicity increases, a hormonal response is triggered. Called "the stress response," it calls into play a series of endocrine activities designed to protect the organism from the decrease in volume.

The hypothalamus stimulates the pituitary gland. Antidiuretic hormone (ADH) is secreted by the posterior pituitary. It causes the kidney tubules to reabsorb more water. The person does not void as much. The pituitary gland also sends messages to the adrenal cortices (cortex of the adrenal glands), and aldosterone is secreted. Aldosterone is called "the electrolyte hormone." It protects the organism from loss of fluid volume by causing retention of sodium and excretion of potassium. Retention of sodium conserves the water that would normally have been required to excrete the sodium. Potassium is believed to be excreted to offset the increased tonicity of extracellular sodium. (See Fig. 17–6.)

Stress Response Following Surgery

This hormonal response to stress is particularly evident for two to five days after surgery. It is all too easy to overhydrate a patient during this stress response period by allowing him too large a volume of liquids either by mouth or by vein.

Acid-Base Regulation

The body maintains a remarkable balance between the hydrogen ion–hydroxyl ion concentration of its fluids. A solution is considered "acid"

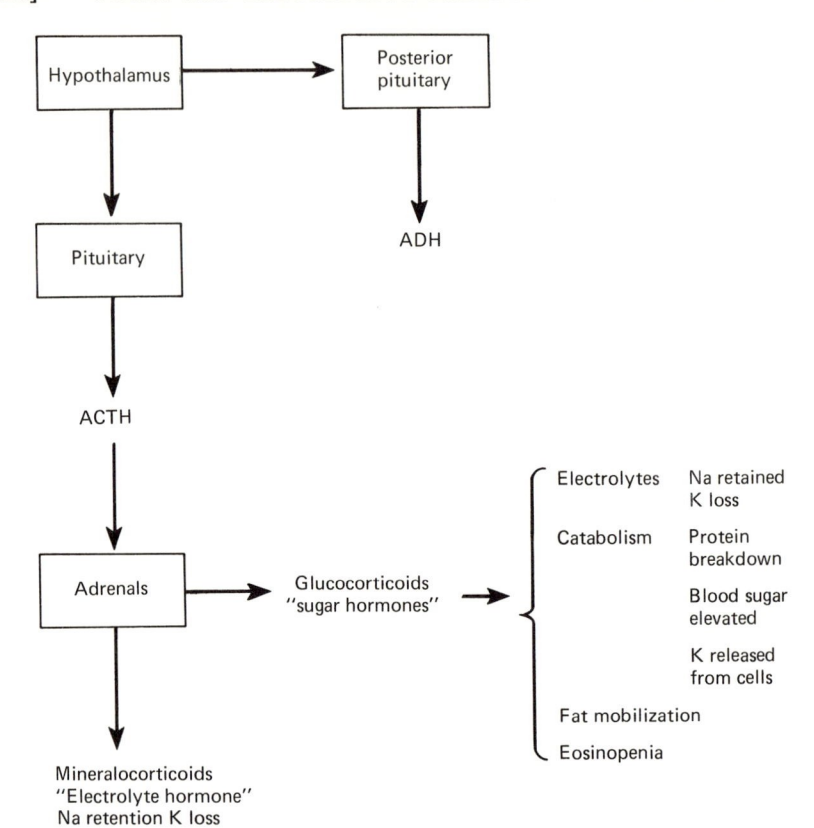

FIGURE 17–6. The stress reaction. (Modified from H. Statland, *Fluid and Electrolytes in Practice*, 1957. Reprinted with permission of J. B. Lippincott Company, Philadelphia.)

when the concentration of hydrogen ions exceeds the concentration of hydroxyl ions; it is alkaline when the concentration of hydroxyl ions exceeds that of hydrogen ions. It is neutral when both are equal. *The key ion in the acid-base story is hydrogen.* An acid gives hydrogen to solutions making them more acid (hydrogen donor), whereas a base accepts hydrogen from solutions making the solution less acid (hydrogen acceptor.) The more readily an acid relinquishes its hydrogen, the stronger it is as an acid; the more readily a base accepts the hydrogen, the stronger it is as a base. Usually, the amount of hydrogen is so small that it can only be expressed in tiniest (and longest!) numbers, e.g., 0.0000001 gm per liter. This is an inconvenient number to write or to say (try it!); so an easier method using the pH notation is used. pH is the simplified expression of the hydrogen ion concentration using the logarithm calculation. Logarithm conversion tables are available. Logarithm deals with powers

FIGURE 17-7. pH ranges.

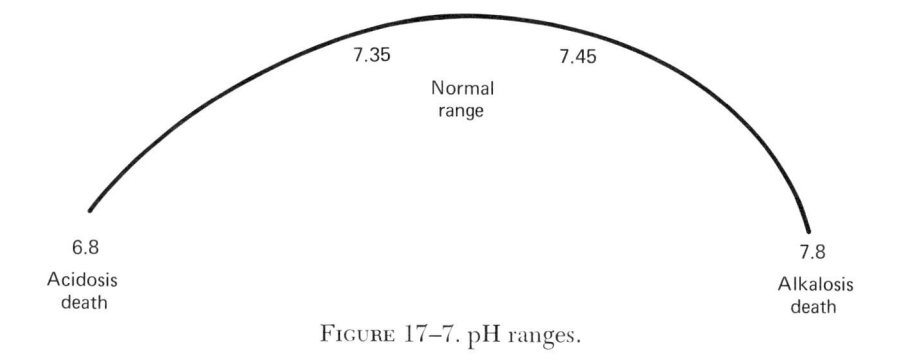

of 10. Thus, the inconvenient number 0.0000001 gm hydrogen per liter becomes 10^{-7} (count the number of places to the right of the decimal point); the minus sign is automatically dropped, and 10^{-7} becomes pH 7. A pH of 8 would indicate a tenfold decrease in the amount of hydrogen; a pH 6 would indicate a tenfold increase (10^{-6}) in the amount of hydrogen.

The pH of pure water is a neutral 7.0. The pH of blood is 7.35 to 7.45 (average 7.40). The body has a survival range between pH 6.8 and pH 7.8. *The smaller the number, the greater the amount of hydrogen and the greater the acidity; the larger the number, the less the amount of hydrogen and the greater the alkalinity.* (See Fig. 17-7.)

How Is Acid-Base Balance Regulated?

There are three major regulatory mechanisms that control acid-base equilibrium. They are called compensatory mechanisms. They include body buffer systems, respiratory regulation, and kidney regulation.

Buffers

A buffer is a solution that can take up or discard hydrogen or hydroxyl ions with little change in its own pH. A buffer is like a chemical sponge that can hoard or discard hydrogen ions. The two principal buffer systems of the extracellular fluid are the carbonic acid:base bicarbonate system and hemoglobin. The former is more important quantitatively.

Carbonic Acid:Base Bicarbonate Buffer System

Carbon dioxide unites with water in the extracellular fluid to form carbonic acid: CO_2 plus $H_2O \rightarrow H_2CO_3$. Cations Na, K, Ca, and Mg unite with bicarbonate to form "base bicarbonate," e.g., Na plus $HCO_3 \rightarrow NaHCO_3$. *A ratio of 1 mEq H_2CO_3 to 20 mEq base bicarbonate must be* *maintained to keep normal acid-base equilibrium.* The carbonic acid:base bicarbonate system resists major changes in pH even if very strong acids or bases are added to it. As long as the ratio of carbonic acid to base bicarbonate remains 1:20 (2:40; 0.5:10), the pH of blood stays within its normal range.

Respiratory Regulation

The lungs influence acid-base regulation by removing carbon dioxide from the blood and eliminating it in expired air. Because the expired air is moist, the CO_2 is in the form of carbonic acid (H_2CO_3), and as a result, hydrogen ions are eliminated.

Kidney Regulation

The kidneys are the master chemists of the body. By the time the hydrogen gets to them for excretion it is in an array of different salts and is removed by indirect methods. For example, the kidney tubules "exchange" hydrogen of carbonic acid for sodium, send the newly formed $NaHCO_3$ back to the blood, and excrete the hydrogen.

Is the Hydrogen Imbalance of Metabolic or Respiratory Origin?

Acidosis and alkalosis are further described by the manner in which the hydrogen ion is produced. In metabolic acidosis or alkalosis the hydrogen ion is the product of metabolic activity. It is not gaseous or volatile. Metabolic disturbances primarily affect the base-bicarbonate side of the carbonic acid:base bicarbonate buffer system by adding to or subtracting from it.

Examples of conditions causing metabolic acidosis include starvation, thyrotoxicosis, infections with fever, and diabetes mellitus. In each instance, the cells have insufficient use of carbohydrate for energy. As a result, fats and proteins are excessively burned. Their by-products, ketone bodies, require base for their excretion, and the body stores of base are depleted.

Examples of conditions causing metabolic alkalosis include vomiting, gastrointestinal suction without replacing electrolytes, drinking tap water while automatic suction is operating, and ingesting large amounts of milk and readily absorbable alkali in the form of Sippy powders, sodium bicarbonate (baking soda), milk of magnesia, and calcium and magnesium carbonate. Some antacids are not absorbed from the intestinal tract and therefore do not cause alkalosis. Aluminum hydroxide gel is an example. In each of these conditions alkali reserve is increased with an upset in the hydrogen ion–hydroxyl ion concentration.

The body is peculiarly vulnerable to base bicarbonate excess (alkalosis) if there is potassium loss,[2] for example, when a patient takes a potent diuretic or adrenocortical hormones for long periods of time. Although potassium loss does not cause metabolic alkalosis directly, it makes the body vulnerable if chloride loss should also occur, as when the patient vomits.

In respiratory acidosis or alkalosis the hydrogen ion is the product of respiratory processes. It is gaseous or volatile. Respiratory disturbances primarily affect the carbonic acid side of the carbonic acid:base bicarbonate buffer system by adding to or subtracting from it. Respiratory acidosis can occur in any condition in which the ventilatory efficiency of the lungs is diminished. Examples of such conditions include emphysema, bronchiectasis, pneumothorax, hemothorax, inadequate ventilation during surgery, bronchial pneumonia, neuromuscular diseases such as poliomyelitis, lung edema, depression of respiratory neurons by drug intoxication, acute alcoholism, and wounds or burns of the respiratory tract. The patient who is brought to the hospital for cardiac resuscitation is in respiratory acidosis.

Respiratory alkalosis occurs when there is hyperventilation not primarily resulting from an interference with pulmonary gaseous exchange. It is caused by central nervous system respiratory stimulation. Carbon dioxide (in the form of carbonic acid) is excreted at a faster-than-normal rate resulting in a deficit of carbonic acid. The condition is seen in hysteria and anxiety reaction, or it may result after prolonged strenuous exercise. Other conditions that may produce respiratory alkalosis are fever, meningitis, encephalitis, intracranial surgery, and anoxia at high altitudes. (See Table 17–1.)

TABLE 17–1. ACIDOSIS AND ALKALOSIS

	Symptoms	Lab Reports	Treatment	Conditions Causing
Metabolic acidosis	Disorientation Shortness of breath on exertion Deep, rapid Kussmaul respirations Nausea, vomiting Dehydration Weakness	Urine pH below 6.0 Plasma pH below 7.35 Plasma bicarbonate below 25 mEq/L	Re-establish adequate blood volume; re-establish proper carbohydrate oxidation Correct extracellular and intracellular losses of water and electrolytes, e.g., 0.9% NaCl; K; solium lactate or sodium bicarbonate	Diabetes mellitus Starvation Thyrotoxicosis Vomiting Infections with fever Ingestion abnormal organic acids Salicylate intoxication

TABLE 17-1. [*Continued*]

	Symptoms	Lab Reports	Treatment	Conditions Causing
Metabolic alkalosis	Hypertonic muscles Tetany from decreased Ca ionization Hypopnea: slow, shallow breathing Cyanosis Personality change	Urine pH above 7.0 Plasma pH above 7.45 Plasma bicarbonate above 29 mEq/L	Correct primary abnormality Correct electrolyte losses, e.g., with K, Cl Only give ammonium chloride IV slowly at 2-3 ml per minute to prevent metabolic acidosis Give 0.9% saline if extracellular chloride deficit	Vomiting with loss of chloride and reattachment of Na to bicarbonate Suction GI tract without electrolyte replacement; drinking while suction is in operation; excess ingestion soluble alkaline powders Excess parenteral administration NaCl without K. Long-term use of potent diuretics with K loss; long-term use adrenocortical hormones
Respiratory acidosis	Disorientation Respiratory embarrassment; later respiratory hyperventilation; dyspnea; wheezing; tachycardia; cyanosis; suprasternal retraction; coma; weakness	Urine pH below 6.0 Plasma pH below 7.35 Plasma bicarbonate below 29 mEq/L	Improve underlying pulmonary insufficiency through antibiotics, postural drainage, bronchodilators and detergents, inhalation therapy with nebulization; intermittent positive pressure breathing, mechanical respirators; tracheostomy	Emphysema, bronchiectasis, pneumothorax, hemothorax, inadequate ventilation during surgery, bronchial asthma, pneumonia, neuromuscular disease affecting chest, lung edema, depression respiratory neurons from drug or alcohol intoxication, wounds or burns of upper respiratory tract

TABLE 17–1. [*Continued*]

	Symptoms	Lab Reports	Treatment	Conditions Causing
Respiratory alkalosis	Unconsciousness Deep rapid breathing may become slow to compensate for decreased H_2CO_3 Tetany Convulsions	Urine pH above 7.0 Plasma pH above 7.45 Plasma bicarbonate below 25 mEq/L	Treat underlying cause of hyperventilation Rebreathe CO_2 from paper bag	Central respiratory stimulation; hysteria; anxiety; disease of central nervous system, fever, intracranial surgery; anoxia at high altitudes; extreme emotional apprehension; oxygen lack; salicylate poisoning; intentional overbreathing

Tests to Determine pH of Blood

To evaluate the acid-base status of blood, the respiratory component may be determined by the pressure of carbon dioxide in blood or plasma (pCO_2), and the metabolic component may be determined by plasma bicarbonate (HCO_3^-). Normal pCO_2 is 35 to 50 mm Hg. An elevation indicates respiratory acidosis; a decrease indicates respiratory alkalosis. The normal plasma bicarbonate range is 22 to 26 mEq per liter in arterial blood and 24 to 28 mEq per liter in venous blood. An elevation indicates metabolic alkalosis. A decrease indicates metabolic acidosis. Sometimes, carbon dioxide–combining power is ordered. It actually indicates [3] bicarbonate value. Normal serum combines with 56 to 65 volumes per 100 ml of carbon dioxide; that is, 100 ml of serum will absorb 56 to 65 ml of gas. An increase in carbon dioxide–combining power means more bicarbonate is formed. Alkalosis results. A decrease in the carbon dioxide–combining power means less bicarbonate is formed and acidosis results. Carbon dioxide content may be measured. It is the sum of minimal amounts of carbon dioxide and bicarbonate plus carbonic acid. Normal range is 20 to 30 mEq per liter. An elevation indicates an increase in bicarbonate, or alkalosis, and a decrease indicates a decrease in bicarbonate or acidosis.

18

COMMON IMBALANCES OF WATER AND ELECTROLYTES

What Are the Common Imbalances of Water and Electrolytes?

IMBALANCES result from too much or too little of an electrolyte, or too much or too little water, which changes the concentration of the electrolyte. Although single electrolyte losses are rarely seen, one predominant deficit can usually be picked out.

Sodium

Sodium is the dominant cation of the extracellular phase. About 3 to 7 gm of sodium are ingested in the United States per person per day, and this intake is considered to be more than sufficient to meet daily needs. The primary physiologic function of sodium is the control of the distribution of water throughout the body (see "Osmosis," pp. 118–19). Sodium is also involved as a buffer base in maintenance of acid-base balance, in the conduction of nerve impulses, in the maintenance of neuromuscular irritability, and in muscle contractility.

Sodium and Water Deficit in the Extracellular Phase
DEHYDRATION

In this imbalance there is a deficit of sodium and water in roughly the same proportion as they exist in the extracellular fluid. This is true dehydration. The overused term has become a catchall to indicate a variety of losses and/or gains. Dehydration is encountered in any acute condition in which there is loss of water and electrolytes. Severe vomiting is an example.

Water Deficit Plus Sodium Excess in the Extracellular Phase

In this imbalance there is too little water and too much sodium salt. We speak of sodium salts because sodium latches on to a variety of anions, along with chloride, in the body. One of the major causes for this imbalance is a failure to heed the thirst mechanism. The patient simply "does not get that drink of water" when he is thirsty. The patient who does not care for "just plain water" and who receives cold coffee and warm juice may acquire this imbalance, as may the semiconscious or psychotic patient, the geriatric patient, and the patient who cannot swallow without pain. Solute loading is another hospital-acquired cause of this imbalance. Increasing the tonicity of the extracellular phase with added solute load and not balancing it with additional water is common. The patient receiving nasogastric feedings of dextrose and amino acids or concentrated milk drinks is an example. Other conditions causing this imbalance are impeded kidney conservation of water as in diabetes insipidus and salt poisoning and after swallowing seawater.

Swallowing seawater imposes an increase in solute load. The ingestion of salt water, three times as salty as body fluid, increases the tonicity in the stomach. Water is drawn from the plasma in an attempt to dilute it. When the increased pressure becomes unbearable, the stomach contents are vomited. Loss of fluid through vomiting further increases sodium concentration. The kidney is unable to keep up with this massive addition of solute.

Sodium Deficit

This is an imbalance in which there is a water and sodium deficit, but with a relatively greater loss of sodium. The tonicity of the extracellular phase is decreased causing water to move out of the extracellular phase and into the intracellular phase. The deficit occurs when there is inadequate sodium ingestion coupled with use of a diuretic; when sodium is lost through drainage, especially gastrointestinal body secretion (e.g., from fistulas or vomiting or diarrhea), or through a mechanically induced deficit such as when the gastrointestinal secretions are suctioned and the patient is given water or ice chips while the suctioning is in progress (electrolytes are "washed out"); or through diluting sodium stores. On a very hot day we lose sodium and water through perspiration but we tend to replace only water. In the absence of sweating a person needs about 0.5 gm sodium a day. The addition of extra salt at the table or one 0.5-gm tablet of sodium chloride is advisable on very hot days.

All these deficits are treated by combating shock through replacement of lost fluids, volume for volume. Electrolyte deficits are replaced. Very often glucose is used with saline solution. It is a "protein sparer." It is burned for energy in place of protein.

Signs of sodium and water deficit include: [4]

FROM A DECREASE IN CIRCULATING VOLUME

Thirst
Loss of weight

Flushed, dry skin
Dry mouth and mucous membranes
Decreased tissue turgor (when the skin is pinched it remains in the pinched position one-half minute or more)
Eyes that appear sunken
Cold extremities
Drop in body temperature (there is an elevation when volume deficit progresses to very severe phases)
Generalized weakness
Drop in blood pressure
Tachycardia
Syncope (fainting) with postural changes
Personality changes, disorientation, delirium, coma

FROM LOSS OF SODIUM

Thirst is usually absent
Weakness
Apathy
Anorexia
Nausea, vomiting
Feeling of faintness on standing
Muscle fatigue from usual exercise (e.g., it becomes a physical effort to shave or brush the hair)
Muscle cramps if water is suddenly ingested
Tremors
Muscle twitching and rigidity
Hyperirritability to stimuli
Dull headache, which becomes marked in the standing position
Mental confusion
Convulsions

A Word About Heat Exhaustion

Heat exhaustion is a most serious condition caused by prolonged heat exposure, a loss of sodium chloride in sweat, and water replacement without salt. The loss of sodium decreases the osmotic pressure of the extracellular phase and water then leaves this phase and swells the cells. Symptoms begin insidiously as the plasma volume decreases. The patient complains of headache, fatigue, and muscle cramps. He is giddy and may faint. He is nauseated and may vomit. Ultimately, he can have circulatory collapse.

Heat exhaustion can also stem from inadequate water replacement during heat and sweating. In this case, there is a sodium excess. The patient is thirsty. If the water deficit progresses, the thirst becomes intense, the skin and mouth dry, and the urine scanty and highly concentrated.

The temperature begins to rise to dangerous levels. The pulse and breathing quicken. Coma and death can follow circulatory failure.

The patient should be put to bed in a cool place and given a high salt and/or water intake. Twenty grams of sodium chloride are given until the deficit is corrected. Six to eight liters of water are given rapidly if exhaustion is from water deficit.

Heatstroke

This is the most serious of these kinds of conditions. The production of sweat apparently fails, and the rectal temperature rises to 105° F. and more. Cells die at 106° F. Pulse and respirations increase with the elevated temperature, and there may be projectile vomiting and incontinence of liquid feces. Most important, there are petechial hemorrhages in the brain, heart, kidney, and liver. Central nervous symptoms develop. The patient becomes disoriented and he may convulse.

The high body temperature must be reduced quickly. As an emergency measure clothes should be removed and the patient should be immersed in whatever water is available. His skin should be massaged vigorously as this aids in accelerating heat loss through peripheral vessels and helps return cool blood to internal organs. At the hospital, the patient may be immersed in a tub of ice water with his temperature taken every five minutes, or he may be placed on a hypothermia blanket. Salt and water losses are replaced slowly until there is adequate renal function. After one to three days of intensive treatment sweat glands again function.

Water Excess in All Fluid Phases

WATER INTOXICATION

Too much water can be just as dangerous as too little water! This imbalance occurs when there is a gain in volume of water in all fluid phases. Because water is able to permeate membranes to each fluid phase, there is no change in tonicity and no electrolyte imbalance. Water intoxication is seen when there is diminished blood flow through the kidneys and sufficient volumes of water fail to be excreted (congestive heart failure; cirrhosis of the liver) or when there is an excess of production of antidiuretic hormone, as following severe stress.

The symptoms depend on how quickly the water excess occurs. If it is rapid, there is extreme progression of symptoms from muscle weakness, sleepiness, and loss of attention, to incoordination, changes in behavior, confusion, and delirium. If the water excess builds up slowly, the symptoms begin gradually. There are weight gain, weakness, apathy, sleepiness, anorexia, nausea, vomiting, marked salivation, and lacrimation though there is no unusual sweating. The skin is warm, moist, and flushed. Fingerprinting occurs. (When the finger is rolled over the sternum or tibia, the mark remains.) There may be a moist, gurgling sound to the respiration and isolated muscle twitching. Voiding decreases.

Treatment includes withholding water for 24 hours, and administering a hypertonic solution. The added solute requires water for its excretion.

Water and Sodium Excess in the Extracellular Phase

OVERHYDRATION

In this imbalance there is an increase in the concentration and volume of the extracellular phase, often because of administration of hypertonic sodium chloride by vein. With the increased tonicity of the extracellular phase, there is movement of water from the cells, ultimately causing a contracted intracellular phase of an expanded extracellular phase. Symptoms come from increased blood volume. There are a rise in blood pressure, rapid weight gain, dyspnea, hoarseness, and edema.

Edema

Edema is a common condition in which the volume of the interstitial (tissue) phase is increased. There is an increase in water volume and sodium concentration. Edema usually stems from a disruption in the normal pressure gradients within the capillaries. (See Fig. 18–1).

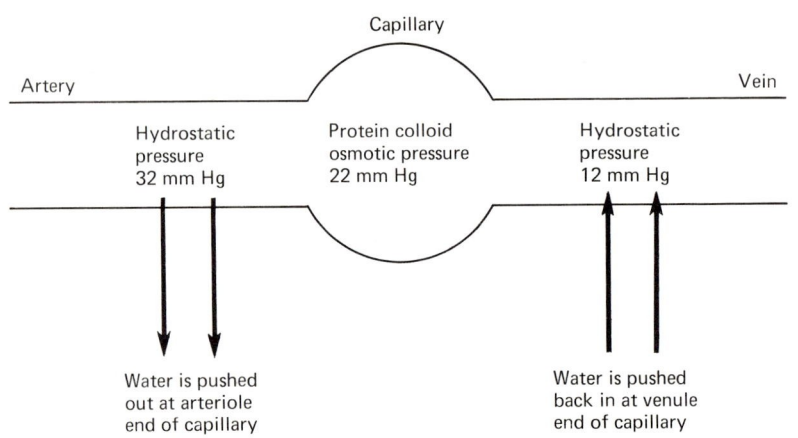

```
                              Capillary

     Artery                                                      Vein

              Hydrostatic      Protein colloid    Hydrostatic
              pressure         osmotic pressure   pressure
              32 mm Hg         22 mm Hg           12 mm Hg


              Water is pushed                    Water is pushed
              out at arteriole                   back in at venule
              end of capillary                   end of capillary
```

FIGURE 18–1. Pressure gradients within the capillaries.

Normally, fluid is pushed out of the capillary at the arteriole end because the pressure there is greater than the "pullback" pressure exerted by large protein molecules (colloids) in the center of the capillary. Fluid is pushed back into the capillary at the venule end because the pressure is less than that of the protein osmotic pressure. In edema, these pressure gradients are disrupted and fluid remains in the tissue phase.

Edema fluid cannot be adequately used to meet body needs. The edematous patient may actually be in a depleted water and electrolyte state!

WHY DOES EDEMA OCCUR?

Edema occurs whenever capillary membranes are damaged and their permeability increased. Water and electrolytes seep out and remain in the tissues. This happens whenever the body's inflammatory response is triggered by trauma, burns, infection, sunburn, allergy, and so forth. It happens when there is a decrease in plasma protein. Fluid is not "pulled back" into the capillary. A deficit of body protein is seen with some kidney disease, with starvation (recall the edematous children who are malnourished), and so forth. It is also seen whenever venous flow is interfered with. In the horizontal position the osmotic pull of plasma protein exceeds the venous hydrostatic pressure, and fluid is returned to the capillaries; however, the venous pressure rises in the standing position, and the massaging action of muscles on veins is needed to push fluid back into the capillaries. Exercise, rather than standing still in one position, helps this massaging action. The obese person tends to be edematous because fat pads interfere with the massaging action of muscles on veins. There is also an increase in venous hydrostatic pressure in persons with thrombophlebitis, varicose veins, and lymphatic obstruction, and when wearing constricting circular garters or constricting long-leg panty girdles.

WHERE DOES EDEMA OCCUR?

Edema occurs first in areas of low tissue tension such as the eyelids and the genitalia. It is called "pitting" edema if the indentation made following pressure with the finger remains. This indentation looks like a pitted area. Edema is called "dependent" when it occurs in areas in which gravity and position are the determining factors. Dependent edema occurs in the ankles when the person is standing, in the sacral area when he is sitting. Edema is "refractory" if it remains after a full therapeutic regimen.

Edema is treated by restricting salt to the amount that is normally lost daily, usually 2 gm or less each day. This allows for a gradual diuresis and avoidance of symptoms of sodium deficit (low-salt syndrome). Water intake is restricted to the amount needed to meet obligatory losses (that lost through vaporization from the lungs and skin and in the stool). Cation-exchange resins, diuretics, rotating tourniquets, and paracentesis may be used.

Potassium

Potassium is the most abundant cation in the body. It is the dominant intracellular cation. It is ingested as part of the daily diet, from whence it is absorbed through the intestinal tract, to the extracellular phase, and from here to the cells. Potassium is to the cell phase as sodium is to the extracellular phase! It is the chief regulator of intracellular osmolarity; it is necessary for the action of certain enzyme systems associated with the production of energy and cellular growth, and it is essential for conduction of nerve impulses. Nerve impulses may be blocked by either high or low concentrations of potassium. Skeletal muscle function is also related to potassium metabolism. Potassium is involved, along with sodium, in normal muscle contractility. During muscle contraction potassium moves out of the muscle cell and sodium moves in; when muscle relaxation occurs, the potassium and sodium regain their normal positions. *Potassium affects the myocardium.* In high concentrations it depresses the myocardium so that the heart stops in diastole. In low concentrations the heart stops in systole.

POTASSIUM DEFICIT

The average normal intake of dietary potassium is 0.8 to 1.5 gm every day. There is no storage of potassium; instead, any excess is eliminated through the urine.

The kidney does not have as precise a mechanism for conservation of potassium as for sodium. Thus, potassium continues to be excreted in the urine, regardless of intake. The two principal avenues of potassium loss are through the gastrointestinal tract and in urine. A deficit occurs when there has been no ingestion of potassium for several days; when there has been vomiting, diarrhea, ulcerative colitis, or fistula drainage; when renal disease is present; when there is metabolic change as in diabetic acidosis (there is cell damage with loss of potassium); or as a result of medically induced loss. Potassium deficit is seen when potent diuretics, especially thiazides, are used and potassium is not replaced; when large doses of corticosteroids are used; when there is prolonged intravenous feeding without added potassium; and when there is continuous gastrointestinal suction without replacement. It can be self-induced by the chronic use of laxatives and enemas.

SYMPTOMS OF POTASSIUM DEFICIT

The majority of clinical signs of potassium deficit are nonspecific in the early stage. Deficits result in disturbances in cellular function involving many organ systems.

Neuromuscular. Apathy, depression, muscle weakness, muscles feel like "half-filled water bottles," cyanosis, shallow respirations

Cardiovascular. Irregular, weak pulse, hypotension, cardiac arrhythmias

Gastrointestinal. Progressive anorexia, nausea, decreased intestinal motility with resulting distention and paralytic ileus

Treatment includes replacement of losses as well as therapy for the underlying disorder. An oral potassium salt may be given as a dietary supplement, e.g., 5 to 10 gm potassium chloride per day. If gastric irritation results, the dosage may be changed to 2 gm every four hours. If the patient cannot take anything by mouth, parenteral replacement is indicated, e.g., 40 mEq potassium per liter of replacement fluid, per day. The rate of infusion of a solution containing added potassium should not exceed 15 ml per minute, and the patient should be watched for signs of potassium intoxication. Potassium is relatively safe once it gets into the cells, but has lethal effects if its extracellular (plasma) level is too high. Normal kidney function is the key to safe potassium therapy. The physician will probably make frequent serum potassium level studies and may monitor the patient with an electrocardiograph.

POTASSIUM EXCESS [6]

This imbalance is often seen in advanced kidney disease, as a result of adrenal insufficiency, or after a severe burn or massive crushing injury. It may develop as a result of parenteral administration of potassium salts. Early symptoms include irritability, nausea, intestinal colic, and diarrhea. Later, there are weakness, paralysis of the extremities and sometimes the muscles of respiration, difficulty in phonation, and absence of deep reflexes. The patient may experience sensations of tingling about the mouth, tongue, hands, and feet. Cardiac arrhythmias may occur (especially bradycardia), and cardiac arrest must be watched for.

Treatment involves management of the underlying condition and regulation of the water and electrolyte intake. Hemodialysis or peritoneal dialysis is often used.

Calcium Imbalance

Serum levels of calcium are controlled by the action of parathyroid hormone and the adrenal glands. The adrenal steroids tend to depress serum calcium, and the parathyroid hormone tends to increase it. Serum calcium levels are also regulated by a small percentage of body calcium that is not in the highly mineralized form essential to bony support. This "metabolic, highly ionizable" calcium responds to serum levels, regardless of parathyroid activity. It is "fast-acting."

CALCIUM DEFICIT

Calcium deficit can be caused by loss of excessive quantities through diarrhea of sprue or in acute pancreatitis, massive subcutaneous infection, or hypofunction or surgical removal of the parathyroid glands. Symptoms of hypocalcemia include fatigue, grimacing, muscular weakness, constipation, palpitation, and numbness of the extremities; or there may be overt signs of tetany with neuromuscular hyperirritability (increased reaction of motor and sensory nerves to stimuli) with painful tonic spasms of groups of muscles. Facial spasm produces stiffness and rigidity, with typical "tetany facies." Cardiac muscle is stimulated. There are carpopedal (foot) spasms and laryngospasm and paresthesias (unusual sensations), frequently followed by convulsions. Carpal spasm may be produced to help make a diagnosis. A blood pressure cuff is inflated on the arm for one to five minutes. A positive reaction consists of production of typical contraction of the fingers and hand. This is called Trousseau's phenomenon and is indicative of tetany.

A positive Chvostek sign is also indicative of tetany. When the face is tapped, there is contraction of the lip, nose, or entire side of the face.

Hypocalcemia is corrected by the administration of calcium orally, intramuscularly, or by vein. It is given in conjunction with large doses of vitamin D, which aides in its absorption.

HYPERCALCEMIA

In the normal adult excessive ingestion of calcium does not cause hypercalcemia. Calcium not needed for metabolism is excreted; however, excessive ingestion of calcium by a person with a condition that causes increased calcium absorption or decreased renal excretion may cause excess serum levels. This is seen in hyperparathyroidism, tumors of the parathyroid glands, thyrotoxicosis, malignant metastases to bone, adrenal insufficiency, excess administration of vitamin D for arthritis therapy, and prolonged excessive intake of milk with alkali. This last condition is reversible. Symptoms include hypotonic muscles (ultrarelaxed), kidney stones, flank pain, deep bony pain, anorexia, nausea, polyuria, thirst, nitrogenous bodies in the blood, and weight loss. The cause of the hypercalcemia must be located and treated.

Calcium is also affected by alkalosis and acidosis. Calcium ionization is decreased in the presence of alkalosis and increased in the presence of acidosis. Therefore, though there may be no loss of calcium in alkalosis, there is a decrease in calcium ionization (chemically and metabolically usable calcium), and the patient demonstrates symptoms of tetany.

Imbalance of Magnesium

Magnesium, like potassium, is predominantly an intracellular ion. It seems to be essential to the proper functioning of the neuromuscular system. It is found in all green plant foods, and deficits are not common. The deficit occurs in chronic alcoholics who have grossly inadequate diets; with prolonged parenteral therapy lacking in magnesium; in prolonged severe diarrhea; and so forth. Signs include tremors, aimless plucking at the bedclothes, hyperactive reflexes, disorientation, and convulsions. Intravenous administration of magnesium quickly relieves the symptoms.

Magnesium excess is seen when there are renal insufficiency and severe dehydration. Symptoms include respiratory embarrassment, lethargy, and coma. Treatment is aimed at correction of the primary disorder.

Water and electrolyte imbalance is the common denominator of most illness. Anticipate the type of loss: look for symptoms of the loss. (See Table 18-1.)

TABLE 18-1. AMOUNT AND CONCENTRATIONS OF ELECTROLYTES IN BODY SECRETIONS AND EXCRETIONS IN 24 HOURS

Fluid	mL	Na (mEq/L)	K (mEq/L)	Cl (mEq/L)	HCO3 (mEq/L)	pH	Imbalance Results in
Saliva	1,500	9	25.8	10	10–15		
Gastric juice	2,500	20–120	5–25	84	0–14	Acid	EC volume deficit; metabolic alkalosis with tetany; Na,K deficit;
Bile	500	120–160	3–12	100.6	40	Alkaline	Na deficit; metabolic acidosis
Pancreatic juice	700	110–160	4–15	76.6	121	Alkaline	EC volume deficit; Na,K deficit; metabolic acidosis
Intestinal juice (includes pancreatic juice and bile)	3,000	110–165	15–70	104	31	Alkaline	EC volume deficit; Na, K deficit; metabolic acidosis
Urine	1,500	40–90	20–60	40–120	None	Acid	
Plasma		137–147	4–5.6	98–106	None		
Transudates		130–145	2.5–5	90–110	None		
Sensible perspiration							EC volume deficit; Na deficit

If the nurse understands the components of water and electrolytes in the various body fluids, she can anticipate symptoms that might occur if that body fluid is being abnormally depleted. Loss of gastrointestinal secretions is the most common cause of water and electrolyte problems. About 8 L of fluid pass back and forth across the gastrointestinal mucosa every day. Normally, these secretions perform their function in digestion and absorption and are almost entirely reabsorbed; however, if there is inadequate intake or excess loss through vomiting, suction, T-tube drainage, fistulas, diarrhea, and so forth, imbalance occurs rapidly. Imbalance also occurs if there is excessive sweating, open wounds, burns, or increased body temperature.

19

WATER AND ELECTROLYTE REPLACEMENT

How Are Water and Electrolytes Replaced?

ONCE the need for replacement therapy is determined, action must be taken promptly. Replacement must be instituted quickly, must be adequate to meet the needs of the patient, and must be sustained long enough for the body to re-establish water and electrolyte balance. The three main aims of therapy are:

1. To replace previous losses
2. To provide maintenance requirements
3. To meet concurrent losses

Although sugar solutions, salt, and water were the mainstays of therapy not long ago, the goal today is a more sophisticated replacement of electrolytes as well as salt, water, and sugar.

Estimates of the amount of fluid to be administered are made according to age, body weight, or body surface area, which includes weight and height. (See Table 19–1.)

To keep a continuous check on the effectiveness of therapy, weight is checked daily; intake and output are recorded carefully; and laboratory studies, including determinations of red blood count, hemoglobin, hematocrit, serum sodium, potassium, bicarbonate, and chloride, are done frequently. An SMA 12 may be done. This is a series of 12 tests of blood serum done on one sample of blood. It is a "simultaneous multiple analysis." (See Fig. 19–1.)

TABLE 19–1. WATER AND ELECTROLYTE NEEDS PER SQUARE METER OF BODY SURFACE IN 24 HOURS

	Minimal Need	Average	Maximal
K	10 mEq	50–70 mEq	250 mEq
Na	10 mEq	50–70 mEq	250 mEq
H_2O	700 ml	1,500 ml	2,700 ml

138] WATER AND ELECTROLYTE BALANCE

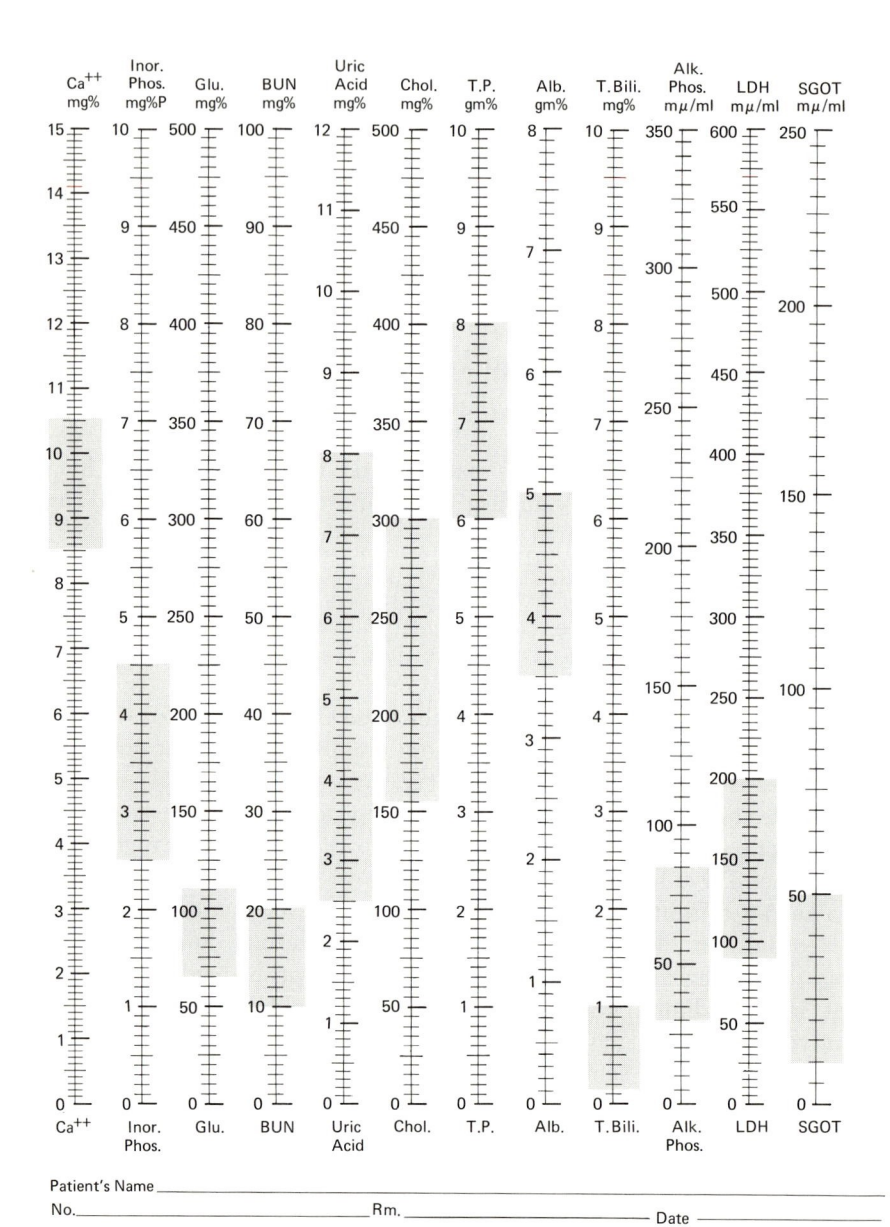

FIGURE 19-1. Simultaneous multiple analyses of blood. Twelve tests are performed with a single blood specimen. "SMA" as used on the chart is a registered trademark of the Technicon Corporation. (Redrawn from Chart 011-0019, Technicon Corporation, Ardsley, N.Y., © Copyright 1965, 1966, 1967, and 1968, with permission.)

Methods of replacement fall into two broad classifications. The enteral route involves all feedings within the alimentary tract through oral, nasogastric, and rectal routes. The parenteral route involves all feedings outside the alimentary tract, including intradermal, subcutaneous, and intravenous feedings, and intraosseous (into the red marrow of the sternum or tibia), intra-arterial, and intraperitoneal feedings.

The oral route is the method of choice. It is the natural route and is safest because it does not involve feedings directly into the blood stream with the ever-present possibility of overloading the circulatory system or causing an antigen-antibody reaction. Oral feedings must be planned and observed just as carefully as parenteral feedings!

Tube feedings are used if the patient is unable to take food and fluid by mouth. Tube feedings are called gastric gavage. The tube is passed through the nose or mouth into the stomach while the patient is lying on his side or sitting with his head tilted slightly forward, to help pass it along the floor of the nasal cavity. The physician makes sure the tube is in the stomach and not the trachea by placing the tip in a glass of water (if it is in the trachea, bubbles appear when the patient exhales) or by attaching a syringe to the tube and withdrawing gastric contents. Special formulas made up of eggs, milk, salt, vitamins, and dextrimaltose, diluted with warm water, are dripped through the tube slowly. The feeding is preceded and followed by an ounce of warm water to clear the tubing. No more than 500 ml is fed at one time. Usually 150 to 200 ml is given every three to four hours. The patient is fed while he is in an upright or semiupright position to decrease the possibility of aspiration if the tube becomes displaced. Mouth and nostril care with glycerin or half-strength peroxide should be given four to six times a day. (See Fig. 19-2.)

Proctoclysis (feeding by rectum) is not used too frequently as it is difficult to ascertain what has been absorbed.

Hypodermoclysis is the subcutaneous route of administration, used when a vein cannot be entered, or when infusion of fluid directly into the circulatory system would be dangerous. Fluids are administered through one or two needles directly below the layers of skin, but outside muscle tissue. Injection sites include the lateral chest, the abdomen midway between the navel and the anterior superior spine, the anterior and lateral aspects of the thighs, the buttocks, and the loose tissue below each breast and below the axillae.

Clysis is fairly safe if the fluid administered resembles plasma in tonicity and is administered at a rate of 30 to 40 drops per minute. Only isotonic or hypotonic solutions can be used. Sometimes 150 units of the enzyme hyaluronidase is injected into the tubing to enhance the absorption of the clysis solutions.

Intravenous administration (venoclysis) is used when rapid absorption of a calculated quantity of fluid is required. Fluids can be given for short or long periods of time at a rate of 30 to 60 drops per minute or 60 to 120

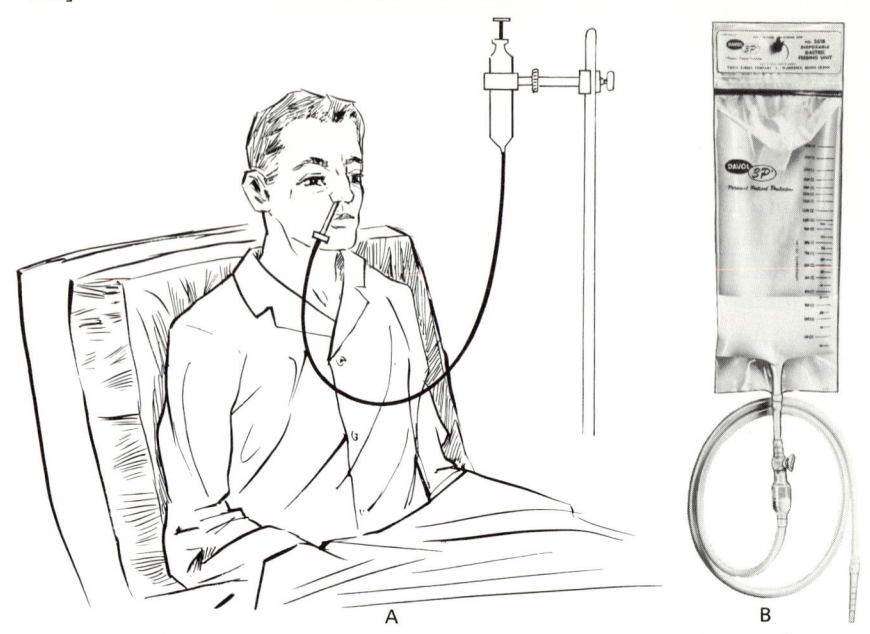

FIGURE 19-2. Nasogastric feeding. A. Feeding is poured into the Asepto syringe. Patient is in sitting position. B. Commercial apparatus is hung from an IV standard. (Courtesy, Davol, Inc., Providence, R.I.)

drops per minute if the patient is in shock. *All infusions are given slowly to patients with cardiovascular disease* (not over 60 drops per minute). The physician should determine the number of drops per minute or the length of time a solution is to run. If he orders 2,000 ml of solution to be given in 12 hours, here is how it can be calculated:

1. Read the information on the commercial apparatus to see how many drops are in each milliliter. There are usually 10 to 15 drops per milliliter in adult infusion sets. There are 15 drops in each milliliter in the set being used for this calculation.

2. There are 15 drops in 1 ml.; therefore, there are 30,000 drops in 2,000 ml.

3. 30,000 gtt : 720 min :: X drops : 1 min
    30,000 : 720 :: X : 1
    720 X = 30,000
    X = −30,000 divided by 720
    X = 42

4. To have 2,000 ml infused in 12 hours, regulate the drops at 42 per minute.

Volume may be ordered by milliliter per minute. This can be converted to drops per minute once the number of drops in each milliliter is determined.

The rate of flow is influenced by the size of the needle, the height of the flask, the viscosity of the fluid, a shift in the patient's position, or anchoring tape that is too tight. If possible, the patient should be completely bathed, should have a clean hospital gown, and should have his treatments completed before the infusion is started. It is also a good idea, if possible, to schedule the infusion so that it does not interfere with the patient's normal nighttime sleep. *Only an administration set with a filter can be used if blood is to be administered.* A small flask of normal saline is used to flush the tubing before and after the blood is administered. Blood cannot be preceded by a calcium-containing solution or hemolysis (clumping) of cells will occur. Isotonic sodium chloride or dextrose 5 per cent in quarter- or half-strength saline (not plain 5 per cent dextrose) is compatible with blood.

Types of solutions used for venoclysis include carbohydrate solutions to supply calories and prevent excessive burning of fats and protein (e.g., glucose in water); protein solutions to provide amino acids and nitrogen (e.g., amigen); solutions providing specific electrolytes (e.g., Ringer's solutions; Butler's solutions); and colloidal (large molecular particles) solutions used to increase circulating blood volume (e.g., whole blood, plasma, packed red cells, concentrated salt-poor albumin, plasma expanders such as dextran). Fats are still in the experimental stage for intravenous use.

There are hazards involved in the use of venoclysis. Local reactions arising from trauma at the administration site are most frequently seen. If the wall of the vein is inadvertently pierced, discoloration and edema appear at the injection site, with infiltration of infused fluid into the tissue spaces and possible hematoma formation. The area around the injection site feels hard and is painful.

Thrombophlebitis occurs when the same vein is injected over and over again, when irritating or highly concentrated substances are injected, or when a hooked needle is used. The vein hardens and the patient experiences pain in the direction of the flow of blood. When any local reaction occurs, the fluid should be stopped and a new injection site found.

Systemic reactions in which the patient feels chills and has an elevated temperature are caused by improperly sterilized equipment or by pyrogen products of dead bacteria remaining in distilled water after being killed by sterilization.

Speed Shock

If fluids are administered too rapidly, speed shock may occur. The patient experiences pounding headache, chest constriction, chills, back pain, subcutaneous edema, rapid pulse, apprehension, dyspnea, and cardiac embarrassment. *The fluid should be stopped immediately* with the needle left in the vein, and the physician should be called.

Air Embolism

Though not seen too frequently, an embolus (moving particle in the blood) may result from failure to clear apparatus of air before administration of the fluid. The effect of the embolus will depend on which vessel is occluded by it and on which tissues are then deprived of blood.

Hazards of Blood Administration

A special word must be said about the dangers of blood administration. The bloods of different persons have different antigenic and immune properties, so that antibodies in the plasma of one person's blood react with antigens in the red blood cells of another. Furthermore, the antigens and the antibodies are almost never precisely the same in one person as in another. When cells from one person are infused into another, antibodies will be developed in response to the antigens not present in the recipient's own blood. For this reason, regardless of the matching procedure, it is easy for the blood to be mismatched. This results in varying degrees of red cell agglutination (clumping) and hemolysis (bursting) in the recipient.

At least 30 commonly occurring antigens have been found in human blood cells, but two particular groups are more likely to cause reaction than others. These are the O-A-B- system of antigens and the Rh-Hr system. Bloods are divided into different groups according to the antigens (agglutinogens) present in the red blood cells and the antibodies (agglutinins) present in the plasma. Group O has no agglutinogens. It is very weakly antigenic. Group A and B are strongly antigenic and can cause severe clumping and cell bursting if given to a person with A or B agglutinins (anti-A; anti-B). (See Table 19–2.)

TABLE 19–2. BLOOD GROUPS

Type	Agglutinogen Antigen Red Blood Cell	Agglutinin Antibody Plasma
O	No agglutinogens	Alpha and beta (anti-A and anti-B)
A	A	Beta (anti-B)
B	B	Alpha (anti-A)
AB	A and B	No agglutinins

In addition to type O-A-B antigens, red blood cells contain other antigenic substances including the Rh factor. If this factor is present, the person is said to be Rh-positive. Eighty-five per cent of the white population are Rh-positive; 95 per cent of American Negroes are Rh-positive. Blood that does not contain the Rh factor is called Rh-negative. Antigenic reactions occur when Rh-positive blood is injected in Rh-negative recipients. The first infusion may merely sensitize the patient; subsequent infusions cause severe reactions.

Before an infusion is administered, donor and recipient blood are typed. Then, they are "cross-matched." This consists of mixing the two bloods in the laboratory to determine whether or not clumping or hemolysis occurs.

Special Hazards of Blood Administration

All the mentioned hazards of venoclysis can occur when blood is administered. In addition there are several other hazards caused by the unique nature of the substance to be infused—blood is the human tissue of another person. It is very much like a transplant.

INCOMPATIBILITY (HEMOLYSIS)

Incompatibility is the most dreaded of transfusion reactions. It usually comes from giving the patient even the tiniest amount of the wrong blood. Symptoms of hemolysis occur within the first 10 to 15 minutes of transfusion. They include lumbar (back) pain, feeling of coldness, fullness in the head, chest constriction, fever, chills, flushed face, the urge to defecate and urinate, and later hemoglobinemia and hemoglobinurea. Because of the speed of the reaction, the first 50 ml of blood should be administered slowly over a 30-minute period. The nurse should remain with the patient during the first 15 to 30 minutes and should observe him frequently thereafter. After the first 30 minutes, the blood is given at a rate of 30 to 60 drops per minute, depending on the physician's order. Blood is never given unless the patient is identified carefully (check wristband and bedcard; have the patient state his name) and his name and the name on the slip with the blood are identical. Other data found on the slip (blood type, Rh factor, and so forth) should be checked against data in the chart. The expiration date on the label should be noted. The blood should be dark red and should not contain air bubbles. It must always be given with a filter administration set. A baseline temperature should be taken before the infusion. Fever often heralds an adverse reaction.

Hemolysis also occurs if the blood is administered with a calcium-containing solution or with 5 per cent dextrose in water, which contains no electrolytes and can cause hemolysis when mixed with blood. Blood can be administered safely with isotonic sodium chloride or dextrose 5 per cent in quarter- or half-strength saline. A small flask of normal saline is hung with the blood, using a Y-type administration set. It is run into the tubing before and after the blood infusion.

POTASSIUM EXCESS FROM AGED BLOOD

Whole blood must be refrigerated (39° to 50° F.) and used within 21 days. As it ages, the cells tend to break down, and they release potassium into the plasma. Severe symptoms of potassium excess may occur. They include nausea, diarrhea, intestinal colic, muscular weakness with flaccid paralysis, paresthesias (odd sensations) of the hands, feet, tongue, and face, slowed or irregular pulse rate, cardiac arrest, and death.[6]

ALLERGIC REACTIONS

Usually not as rapid or as serious as hemolytic reactions, allergic reactions occur as a result of blood hypersensitivities of the donor. The recipient may experience hives, asthma, or a more serious anaphylactic (antigen-antibody) reaction. If the reaction is mild, antihistamines control the symptoms. Otherwise, adrenal seroids must be used.

VIRAL HEPATITIS (HOMOLOGOUS SERUM JAUNDICE)

Viral hepatitis is transmitted through whole blood and through plasma. Despite careful screening of donors, it must still be considered a calculated risk of blood infusion. Donors may never have had viral hepatitis diagnosed; they may withhold the information; or they may be incubating the disease (two to six months). Also, the incidence of serum hepatitis is increased by the use of "pooled plasma" (plasma collected from many people). Its incidence can be reduced by pooling only a few units of plasma and by storing it at room temperature for six months. The virus lives indefinitely in frozen plasma but loses much of its activity when kept at room temperature. Incidence can also be decreased by checking the bilirubin content of blood-bank blood before it is distributed for use. If the bilirubin content is elevated, the blood is discarded because liver disease may have been present.

CIRCULATORY OVERLOADING

Once in the circulatory system, the large molecules of blood cannot seep out. The heart must continue to pump the additional volume. Circulatory overload occurs when too much blood is given too fast, especially in patients with known cardiovascular, renal, or hepatic disease. Symptoms include dry cough, engorged jugular veins, dyspnea, and cyanosis. The rate of administration should be checked carefully with the physician.

Reactions from Use of Anticoagulants

The customary anticoagulant used to prevent blood from clotting is citrate. The anticoagulant-preservative combination is acid citrate dextrose. Citrate ions combine with calcium ions of plasma to prevent clotting.

The difficulty lies in the fact that normal nerve, muscle, and heart function cannot occur in the absence of ionized calcium. If very large quantities of citrated blood are used, this calcium deficiency becomes evident. Hemorrhage due to prolonged clotting time is also a danger. Heparinized blood may be selected if large amounts of infusions are needed.

Hypothermia

If large volumes of cold blood are rapidly transfused, the patient may develop hypothermia and cardiac arrest. To prevent this, the blood may be warmed through a special blood-warming coil submerged in a 99° F. water bath before it is infused.

Again, the rules for safe administration of blood are:

1. Store blood in refrigerator. Check expiration date on label.
2. Do not use if discolored or if it contains gas bubbles.
3. Administer with a filter set.
4. Identify patient with extreme care.
5. Make sure label information and chart information concur.
6. Do not air-vent a plastic container.
7. Gently mix blood before administration.
8. Do not give blood with calcium-containing solutions or with 5 per cent dextrose in water. Do not hang these solutions parallel to blood.
9. Administer the first 50 ml slowly over a 30-minute period.
10. Stay with the patient during the first 15 to 30 minutes. If any complication occurs, stop the blood immediately.
11. Do not allow container to empty fully. This increases the chance of air embolism.

A text on water and electrolyte balance should be reviewed for detailed methods of intravenous replacement.

Emphasis for Nursing Practice

Because most diseases engender some form of water and electrolyte disruption, the nurse must be constantly on the alert for symptoms heralding imbalance. Here are some major pointers:

1. Know what the disease is and what kinds of imbalance may be caused by it. Anticipate the loss. For example, gastric secretions are normally acid. A loss through drainage, suction, or vomiting might cause metabolic alkalosis. Intestinal secretions are normally alkaline and contain potassium. Loss might cause metabolic acidosis and potassium deficit. Realize that stress reactions occur following surgery and the patient has sodium retention and potassium excretion for two to five days.

2. Pay particular attention to intake and output. Even in the absence

of an order, measure, estimate, and record loss through urine, drainage, perspiration, vomiting, and so forth. Keep a readily available intake-and-output sheet at the bedside with a description of containers in use in the particular hospital and the volumes they contain. Remind and instruct the patient to record even the smallest sips of water. If an intravenous infusion is running when it is time to record an eight-hour total, the amount already absorbed is listed for that shift; the amount still in the bottle is listed for the next shift. Realize that the desire for or lack of desire for food or fluids go hand in hand with water and electrolyte imbalance. Never ignore the statement, "I am thirsty."

3. Know exactly what the physician means if he orders "fluids ad lib." Can the patient have up to 3,000 ml? Tap water? Should liquids be of a more physiologic make-up, e.g., bouillon, fruit juice?

4. Weight is a good indicator of fluid status. Weigh the patient at the same time every day, preferably before breakfast with an empty bladder, and wearing similar clothing.

5. If an intravenous infusion is running, observe it frequently. Time the drops for a full minute. Changes in position, kinked or compressed tubing, and so forth may alter the rate. Make sure the fluid is not infiltrating. Stop the infusion if signs of complications develop (see pp. 141–142) but leave the needle in the vein.

6. Do not allow a patient to suck ice chips or drink water while suction is in operation. If ice chips are ordered, estimate the quantity of water derived from them.

7. Pay particular attention to observation of vital signs and compare with the previous vital signs record. Changes indicate a variety of water and electrolyte imbalances. For instance, temperature drops when there is sodium and water deficit and increases when there is sodium excess with water deficit. Pulse becomes bounding and easily obliterated, then rapid and weak, during circulatory (plasma volume) collapse and becomes weak, rapid, and irregular during potassium deficit. Respirations become deep and rapid in the presence of metabolic acidosis and shallow and slightly irregular in the presence of metabolic alkalosis. Hyperventilation occurs in metabolic acidosis; shortness of breath and dyspnea occur when there is fluid volume excess or pulmonary edema. Blood pressure falls when circulatory collapse is impending, when there is sodium deficit or severe potassium deficit or excess; blood pressure rises when there is fluid volume excess or magnesium deficit.

8. Pay particular attention to changes in skin and mucous membranes. Poor skin turgor, pallor or flushing, cold clamminess, dryness, pitting edema, and fingerprinting on the sternum are all indicative of fluid volume deficit or excess.

9. Pay particular attention to skeletal muscle changes. Hypotonus (flabbiness) is seen with potassium deficit and calcium excess; hyper-

tonus is seen with calcium deficit. Cramping is seen with sodium deficit, and so on.

10. Observe behavioral changes. Emotional lability, inability to concentrate, errors in judgment, mental confusion, and belligerence out of proportion to the cause may indicate hypoxia from hypovolemia, and so on. Never ignore the statement, "I just don't feel right."

20

MULTIPLE WATER AND ELECTROLYTE PROBLEMS: BURNS

IMBALANCES of single elements are discussed for ease of presentation. Often, though, patients present multiple water and electrolyte imbalances, frequently complicated by acidosis or alkalosis. These imbalances are categorized as "mixed excesses and depletions." The burned patient falls into this category.

What Are Burns?

Burns are tissue injuries caused by thermal, electrical, or chemical agents, and by most forms of radiant energy.[7] They are classified according to depth and percentage of body involvement.

Depth of Burns (Thickness)

First-degree burns are superficial, partial-thickness injuries involving only the epidermis. With first-degree burns there is redness (erythema), edema, and pain. The skin feels hot and blanches with pressure. It heals spontaneously, with peeling. Sunburn and a burn from a low-intensity flash are examples.

Second-degree burns involve the epidermis and the dermis. The skin is red, hot, and painful. There are vesicles (blisters) with oozing. The surface seems "to weep." Second-degree burns heal in two to three weeks with some scarring and depigmentation. Infection may convert second-degree burns to more serious third-degree states. Scalds and flash-flame burns are examples.

Third-degree burns involve the epidermis, the dermis, and the subcutaneous tissue. The skin is charred or pearly white and dry. Fat may be exposed. There is injury to the nerve fibers, sweat and sebaceous glands, and hair follicles. Red blood cells may be damaged by the heat and cause anemia and hematuria. An eschar forms over the area. This is a tough covering of dead tissue. It sloughs, and grafting over the area is necessary. There is scarring, and this scarring may prevent easy movement of the part. Contractures may develop. Because of nerve destruction there is no pain. Third-degree burns are called "anesthetic." Fire causes third-degree burns.

It is often difficult to differentiate second- and third-degree burns because they may look very much alike, and they may blend with each other. Although many tests have been devised to differentiate depth (e.g., a hair lifts out of its follicle easily in third-degree burns), none has proved completely accurate.

While normal skin serves as a relatively impermeable shield to water and electrolytes, second- and third-degree burns act like semipermeable membranes through which water and electrolytes can seep out of and into the body. Therefore, burned patients often have serious fluid problems.

Percentage of Body Involvement

The well-known "rule of nines" is used to determine percentage of area involved. (See Fig. 20–1.) Burns are considered "critical" if there is more than 30 per cent partial-thickness involvement, if there is more than 10 per cent full-thickness involvement,[8] or if the burn is complicated by respiratory tract injury, fractures, or major soft-tissue injury.

What Do You Do If the Patient Is Burned at Home?

Burns can impose a serious threat to life. Because it is so difficult to estimate the extent of the injury, any burned person should seek medical attention.

At home:

1. If flame is involved, roll the burning person in a blanket or coat on the ground to put the fire out. Do not allow the person to stand because this increases the danger of breathing flames and smoke into the respiratory passages.

2. Cover the burned area with a clean, preferably ironed cloth (e.g., a pillowcase). Keep the patient lying down.

3. Do not apply any burn ointment or greasy substance until the patient is seen by the physician. Ointment "covers up" the area and makes it more difficult for the physician to appraise and treat the wound.

4. If a small area is burned, immerse the part in ice water until the pain disappears.

5. Do not give anything by mouth if the patient is nauseated or vomiting. If a long interval is anticipated before medical attention can be obtained, let the patient sip warm salty liquids, e.g., bouillon, if he can tolerate them.

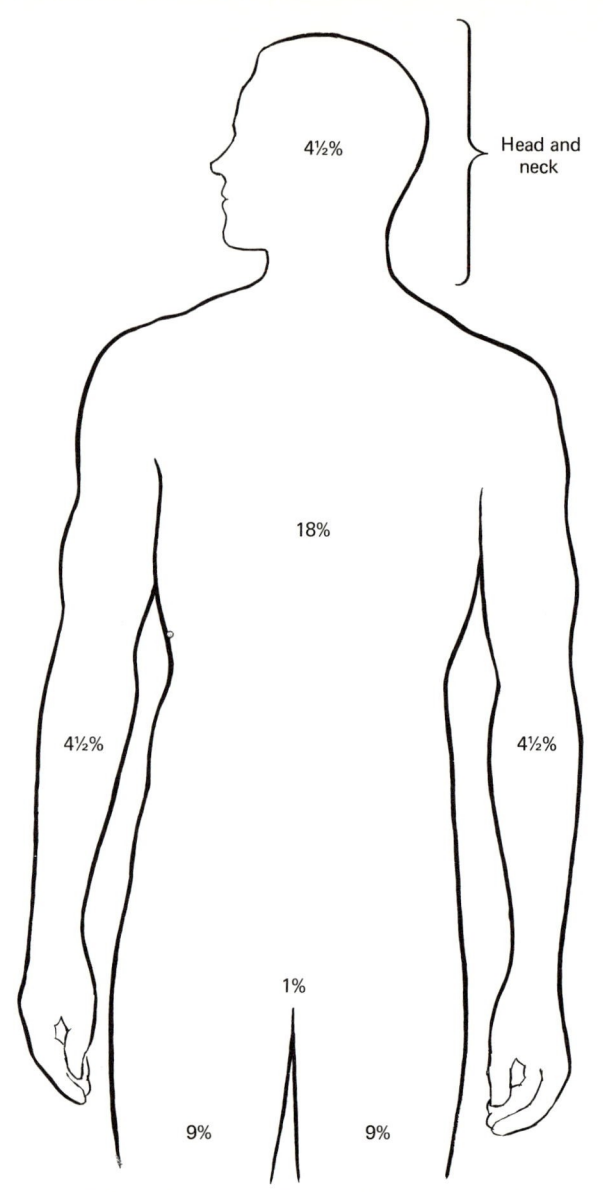

FIGURE 20-1. The "rule of nines" is used to estimate the percentage of burn involvement. Percentages shown are for the anterior surfaces of the body. Posterior surfaces are identical.

Use of Ice Water for Treatment of Minor Burns

There is some evidence [9,10] that ice water is an effective therapeutic measure in burns of less than 20 per cent. Use of the ice water results in an immediate alleviation of pain and an apparent decrease in the usual burn sequelae. The cooling is continued, sometimes for several hours, until the pain does not recur when the part is withdrawn from the cold bath. Ice-cold towels are used if it is not feasible to immerse the part. Evidently the time factor plays an important part in the effectiveness of the treatment. The sooner the immersion, the better the result.

At the Hospital

Clothing is removed or cut off, and gross burn debris removed. The patient's total condition is appraised by the physician. Burns are tolerated poorly if the patient is over 50 or if there is pre-existing renal or cardiovascular disease. If there are burns of the respiratory tract, an immediate tracheotomy is done. A retention catheter is inserted. A specimen of blood is obtained for baseline studies of hematocrit and electrolytes. Analgesics such as morphine sulfate or meperidine hydrochloride (Demerol) are administered for the pain. They are usually given intravenously rather than subcutaneously because subcutaneous injections are poorly absorbed when a patient is severely burned (there is extensive subcutaneous tissue damage) and repeated doses of the medication may accumulate in the areas and result in fatality! Large doses of analgesics are not given because of the danger of respiratory depression and because they mask other symptoms. A prophylactic dose of penicillin may be given. An estimate of the extent of the burn is made and recorded on a burn diagram. Intravenous fluids are always started if there is 20 per cent or more body involvement or if circulatory shock is evident. "When considerable body surface is involved, the intravenous pathway is the patient's lifeline." [11]

Tetanus Immunization

Tetanus (lockjaw) is a serious communicable disease that can cause fatal contractions of the muscles of the neck and mandible. The causative microorganism is *Clostridium tetani*. Its spores live in the intestinal canals of animals (especially horses) and man. Although it is not transmitted directly from man or animal to man, the organism is deposited in the soil and dust through excreta. It is transmitted as an infective agent through puncture wounds, burns, and similar injuries. *Clostridium tetani* is anaerobic. It lives in the absence of atmospheric oxygen. Puncture wounds in which openings to the air "close over" rapidly and burns in which large amounts of necrotic tissue form provide this anaerobic medium. Therefore, any burned patient requires some form of tetanus immunization.

One milliliter of tetanus toxoid is administered to patients who have been previously immunized. This provides an antibody "reminder dose."

It is an active form of immunization. At least 5,000 units of tetanus antitoxin or 250 units of tetanus human immune globulin (Hyper-Tet) is administered deep into the muscle if the patient has not been previously immunized. This provides passive immunization that lasts about ten days. It should be followed by use of the toxoid so that the patient can begin to develop an active immunity. There is always the danger of an allergic response if the antitoxin is used because it comes from horse serum. For this reason, most hospitals are currently using the pooled tetanus–human immune globulin instead of the antitoxin. Skin testing is not required when human immune globulin is used.

Information Needed in the Emergency Room

The nurse must begin to obtain pertinent information in the emergency room. This information may have to be obtained from the family. It should include: [12]

1. When did the burn occur?
2. What was the burning agent?
3. How long was the patient exposed to the agent?
4. Were any medications given prior to hospitalization? Narcotics?
5. Was the burn sustained in a closed area where heat and fumes may have been inhaled? (Is respiratory edema a possibility?)
6. Are there any pre-existing illnesses?
7. What is the usual preburn weight?
8. Is pain present?
9. Is the patient known to have any drug allergies?

The following is a list of the initial treatment given to a severely burned patient: [13]

1. Remove clothes and cover patient with sterile sheet.
2. Estimate the percentage of body surface burned and the depth of the burn.
3. Calculate fluid replacement.
4. Initiate shock therapy if needed.
5. Perform tracheotomy if respiratory distress is noted or probable, e.g., from steam burns of the head and neck.
6. Insert urinary catheter for hourly urine measurements.
7. Insert catheter or cannulas for central venous pressure monitoring and intravenous fluid administration.
8. Draw blood for study.
9. Administer intravenous analgesics for pain.
10. Culture burn area.

11. Insert nasogastric tube if nausea, vomiting, or distention is present.
12. Weigh patient and record this baseline weight.
13. Take temperature, pulse, respirations, blood pressure, and record.
14. Administer tetanus toxoid, antitoxin, or human immune globulin.
15. Place patient in warm, humid room and bathe burn area with copious amounts of tepid water containing pHisoHex, in a 3 per cent bath, to remove dirt, grease, and aid in débridement. Rinse with distilled water.
16. Place patient on special bed if necessary, e.g., Stryker frame, Circ-O-Electric bed. (See pp. 404–406.)

EMERGENCY EQUIPMENT NEEDED

1. Intravenous equipment: needles, syringes, tourniquet, arm board, tape.
2. Cutdown equipment.
3. Intravenous solutions (plasma, dextran, lactated Ringer's, isotonic saline, 5 per cent dextrose in water or saline).
4. Tracheotomy set.
5. Catheterization equipment: indwelling retention catheter, collection bag, collection device to measure small amounts of urine.
6. Sterile linen, gowns, gloves.
7. Sterile swabs and culture tubes.
8. Liter bottles of sterile sodium chloride and sodium bicarbonate solutions.
9. Instrument set for débridement.
10. Burn diagram.

Personnel may be required to wear a sterile gown, gloves, and mask as a reverse-isolation "protection for the patient." Sterile precautions depends on the philosophy of the physician and must be clarified so that they are used consistently by all personnel, if required.

To understand the rationale of therapy for major burns, the inflammatory response to trauma and specific burn phases will be discussed.

The Inflammatory Response

This response occurs whenever the body is injured. (See also p. 74.) There is an immediate release of histamine from the damage tissue. Histamine causes the capillaries to dilate. Their membranes become more permeable, and there is seepage of water, plasma, plasma proteins, and electrolytes (especially sodium) across the capillary membranes and into the burned area. If the injury is large, there is great seepage of plasma out of the vascular phase, and shock may occur. Fluids converge upon the burn area. They pool there. The most rapid exudation occurs in the first six to eight hours. It may continue for 48 to 72 hours and may reach 1,000 to 2,000 ml a day.[14] Cells are damaged and potassium is released from them into the extracellular phase. Increased serum potassium can reach intolerable levels. There is damage to the red blood cells, with clotting of cells in the burn area and a generalized anemia. Red blood cells have a shortened life because the heat trauma makes them more fragile, and infection depresses the blood-forming organs. This contributes to the anemia.[15]

The Burn Phases

Circulatory Shock and Tissue Edema

The shock phase lasts between 48 and 72 hours. It is an extremely life-threatening period when there is a dramatic shift of fluids from the intravascular (plasma) phase to the interstitial (tissue) phase at the burn site. The greater the shift, the greater the loss of circulating volume, and the more profound the shock! Sodium is lost from the plasma and causes tissue edema; however, the edema only masks a generalized body dehydration as fluids pour toward the injured site. More water is lost as vapor through the damaged skin. Damaged cells release their major cation, potassium, and the level of circulating potassium becomes extremely dangerous, especially to the heart. Arrhythmias develop. The kidneys suffer from the decreased blood volume. They cannot secrete an adequate volume of urine, and body wastes accumulate. Along with this, they must often excrete hemoglobin from heat-damaged red blood cells. Hemoglobinuria, with damage to the kidneys, develops. Renal shutdown is a grave possibility. Patients who feel well one minute suddenly become apathetic, nauseated, and weak. Urinary output becomes dangerously low as blood volume drops. The skin is cold and clammy, and there is a drop in blood pressure with an increase in pulse rate. Patients may vomit blood. They may become disoriented.

The sequence of events is something like this:

Heat injury → damage to capillaries → increased capillary permeability → loss of water and electrolytes → decreased intravascular fluid → increased interstitial fluid → circulatory shock

The nurse must watch for symptoms of burn shock. They include: [16]

1. Extreme thirst
2. Restlessness
3. Tachycardia
4. Pallor, cold perspiration (however, skin may be pink and dry)
5. Disorientation
6. Oliguria
7. Vomiting blood
8. Sleepiness

Healing

The burn exudate dries in these initial 48 to 72 hours. Along with dehydrated, dead skin, it forms a tough covering to protect the wound. This covering is called the burn eschar. Healing takes place underneath this eschar. The area is filled up with new capillaries, fibroblasts, and collagen. This is called granulation, and it occurs in all degrees of burns. If enough normal tissue remains, as in partial-thickness burns, granulation and epitheliazation occur. Cells similar in structure to the normal skin cells are laid down, and skin grafting is usually unnecessary. If, however, there is extensive full-thickness destruction, epitheliazation with laying down of similar skin cells does not occur, and only granulation tissue remains. This is tough, fibrous scar tissue. It is numb. As it heals, it shrinks, and contraction of the surrounding tissue may lead to malfunction and deformity.[17] Grafting is always necessary.

Management During the Shock Phase

MAINTAINING CIRCULATION

The goal of treatment during this initial phase is to prevent circulatory collapse and to maintain kidney output. Intravenous fluids are administered in amounts capable of maintaining the circulation, yet in volumes small enough to prevent increasing the interstitial edema. This is a delicate task. Clinical shock is believed to be preventable if fluid therapy can be instituted as soon after injury as possible. Fluids are always administered intravenously for moderate and severe burns. A polyethylene catheter is inserted into a peripheral vein such as one at the ankle or shoulder. If a peripheral vein is not available, the femoral vein can be used. In this case, the catheter must be removed and inserted into the opposite femoral vein in a week to prevent thrombosis. (See Fig. 20-2.)

Choice of fluids includes colloid substances such as plasma, dextran, or whole blood; or saline solutions such as lactated Ringer's solution or isotonic saline. For example, 600 ml of plasma and 1,000 ml of lactated Ringer's may be given until full therapy is determined.

The Brooke Army Medical Center Formula is an example of a formula used to estimate amounts of water and electrolytes to be administered. Formulas only serve as guides; the patient's condition and response to therapy are the main determining factors. The Brooke Formula includes: Colloid, 0.5 ml per kilogram body weight × per cent of body burns; electrolytes (lactated Ringer's solution), 1.5 ml per kilogram body weight × per cent of burn; water (glucose in water), 2,000 ml. Half of the total is administered in the first eight hours, and one fourth in the second and third 8-hour periods. Glucose is used as a protein sparer. In the second 24 hours, half the amount of colloid and electrolytes plus 2,000 ml of water is used. Potassium may be administered after the first 48 hours, if kidney function is adequate.

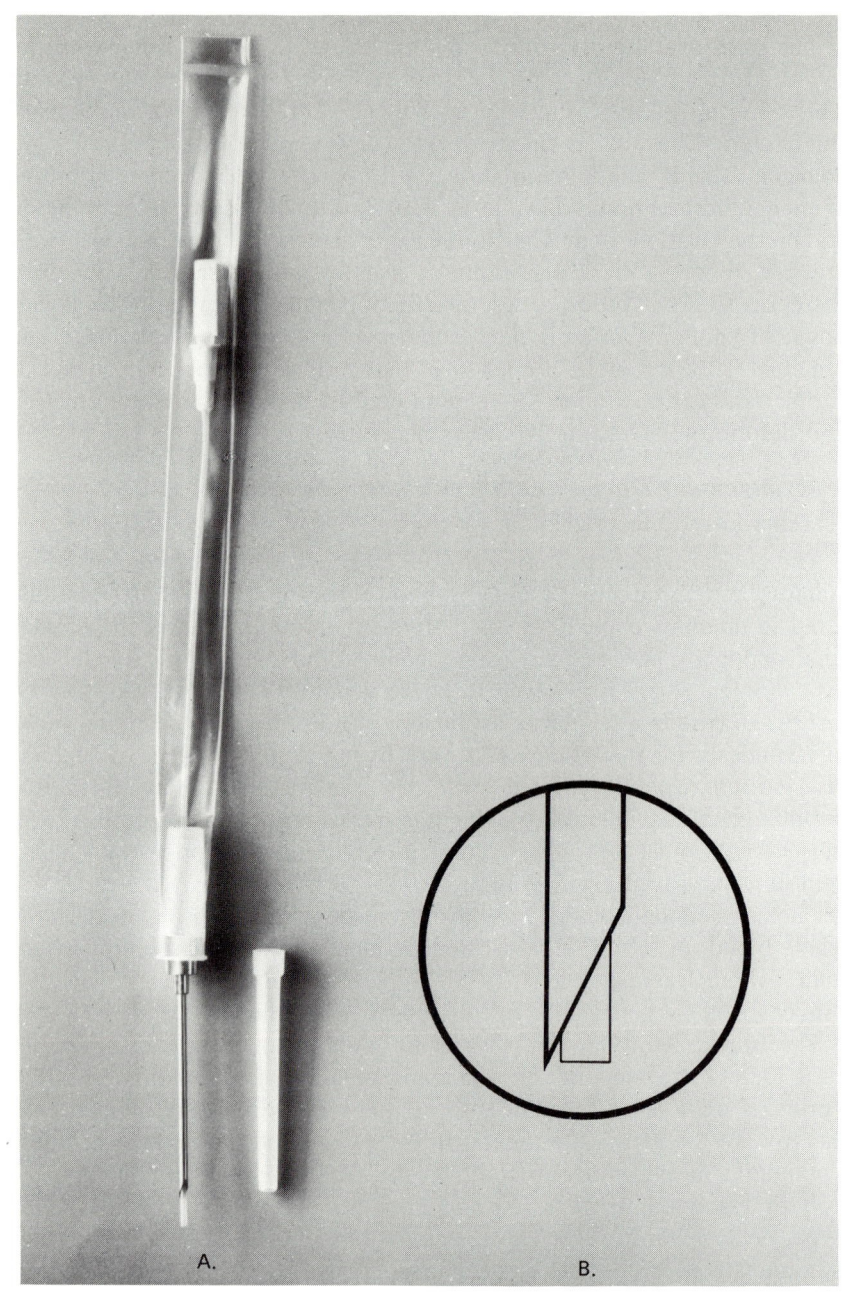

FIGURE 20–2. *A.* An inside-needle catheter. (Courtesy, C. R. Bard, Inc., Murray Hill, N.J.) *B.* The catheter is advanced through the needle into the vein. The needle is pulled back and taped to the skin.

MONITORING KIDNEY OUTPUT

An indwelling uretral catheter is inserted when burns are moderate or severe. Urinary output is the best indicator of the adequacy of fluid replacement. The goal for urinary output is usually 25 to 50 ml per hour (1 ml per minute), although in some instances the physician may desire an output of 2 to 3 ml per minute.[18] He will specify desired urinary volume. The nurse must report deviations and regulate intravenous drops

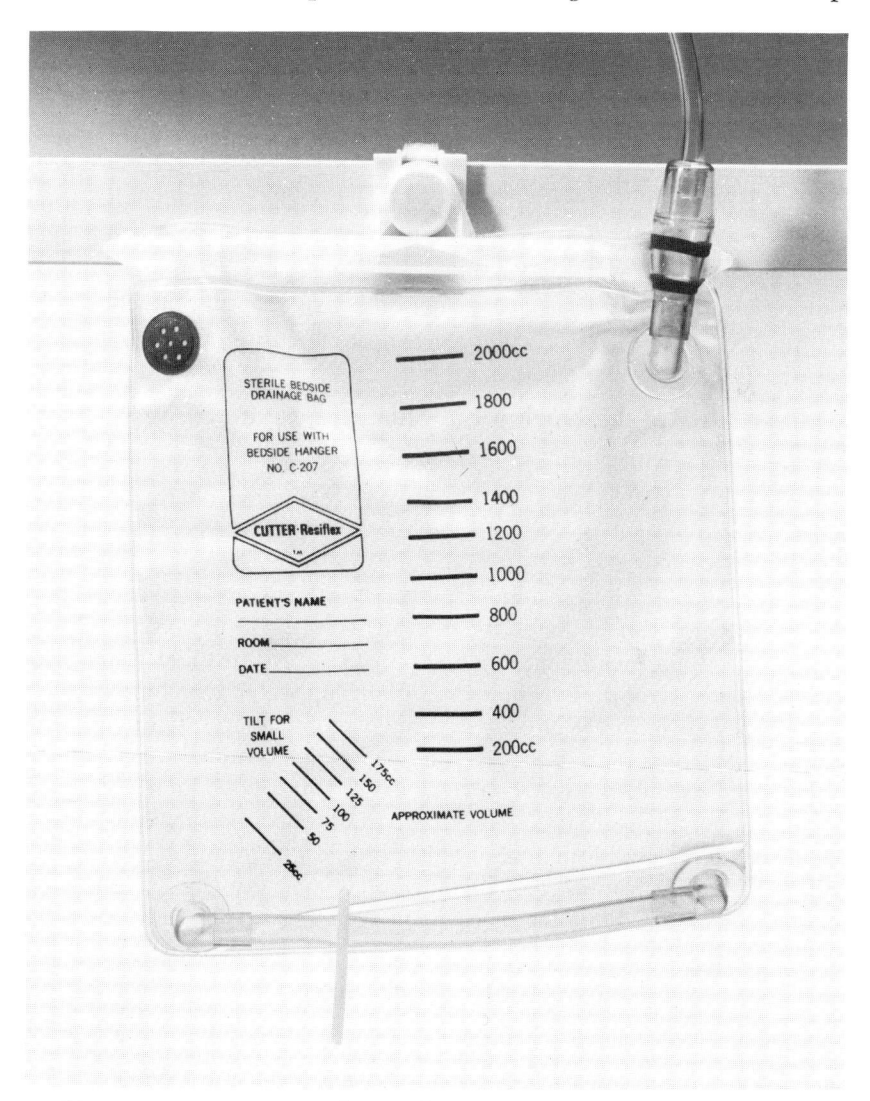

FIGURE 20-3. Urinary collection bag can be tilted to see small volumes. (Courtesy, Cutter Laboratories, Berkeley, Calif.)

per minute in accordance with her findings. The rate is increased if urinary output falls below 25 ml per hour and decreased if output is above 50 ml per hour. Output is measured every half- to one hour during the early postburn phase. A commercial collection device with small calibrations can be used. (See Fig. 20–3.) If the catheter is to be irrigated, the volume of irrigant should be measured and the amount returned measured and recorded.

The patient should be weighed at the same time, in the same state of dress, every day for seven days; twice a week for two weeks; and then once a week through convalescence.[19]

MEASURING INTAKE AND OUTPUT

An intake-and-output record should be placed in a prominent place. All intake should be recorded, e.g., oral and intravenous fluids, irrigating solutions that remain in the body, and ice chips. All output should likewise be recorded, e.g., loss through burn drainage, perspiration, vomiting, sputum, bleeding, and stools. Urine not only is measured, but is observed for appearance, gross blood, color, concentration or dilution, and so forth.

Oral Intake During the Shock Phase and Later

The patient is allowed nothing by mouth during the first postburn day. He experiences extreme thirst and must be reminded not to drink tap water. On the second postburn day he is usually permitted oral electrolyte solutions. These should not contain potassium because of the increased blood level of potassium resulting from release from damaged cells. Electrolyte ice chips can be made by freezing 1 teaspoon of salt and 3 teaspoons of sodium bicarbonate in 1,000 ml (1 qt) of distilled water. The patient should suck these rather than plain tap-water ice chips because tap water tends to dilute already decreased sodium stores and may cause water intoxication. The estimated volume of water from ice chips must be recorded as fluid intake. Orange juice or other potassium-containing liquids are not allowed until about the third to fourth postburn day, when renal function is established. Oral fluids are not given until bowel sounds are heard and intestinal atony is definitely not present, or until the presence of gastric dilatation or frequent vomiting is ruled out.

Dietary Progression

By the end of the first postburn week, intensive feedings are given to meet additional nutritional requirements caused by increased cell metabolism, red blood cell regeneration, and tissue repair. Although there is a weight gain in the first 48 hours, there is a loss of up to a pound a day through the first month. This stems from a negative nitrogen balance. More protein is used than is taken into the body. High-protein supplements such as Nutrament or Sustagen may be given to provide for this protein deficit. The high-protein, high-calorie diet, begun about seven to ten days after the burn, includes 2 to 3 gm protein per kilogram body weight, 50 to 70 calories per kilogram body weight, and 1,000 mg of vitamin C to encourage healing. Additional multivitamin capsules are frequently given. The patient may be tube-fed. In this case, no more than 500 ml should be given at one time. The feeding is preceded and followed by an ounce of warm water (105° F.) to clear the tubing. Often, the patient must be hand-fed, and the nurse's willing, patient attitude is vital.

Oral hygiene is essential to decrease development of mucus plugs, which could obstruct an airway, especially if burns involve the mouth. If burns of the mouth are not severe, a soft toothbrush and mouthwash can be used. Glycerin and lemon juice can be swabbed on the dry lips. Frequent gentle suction of the trachea is important, as are humidifiers to help keep the secretions moist and loose.

Vaporizational Heat Loss

One of the main problems is to reduce vaporizational heat loss from large burned areas. The temperature-regulating mechanisms in the skin are destroyed, and the patient feels cold; there is increased evaporation of water from the wound. Interestingly, water is lost to an even greater extent through the dead, dry burn eschar.[20] The room should be kept at 75° to 80° F. and 45 to 70 per cent humidity. Air conditioning should not be used. Warmed sterile sheets may be used to decrease heat loss. The physician may order continuous immersion in baths of controlled temperature or thick dressings wet with chemical bacteriostatic agents such as 0.5 per cent silver nitrate solution to help decrease vaporizational heat loss. (See pp. 161–62.)

Positioning

In the early burn phase, elevation of involved areas aids in reabsorption of edema. The patient is turned and exercised to provide maximal exposure to the burned area. Cradles are used to keep the linen off the affected parts and to provide some degree of warmth. Heating lights are not used because they provide too optimum a temperature for microorganism growth. Splints made of various materials are used on the arms and legs to prevent flexion with contractures. Footboards are used to prevent shortening of the Achilles tendon. The trunk and hips are maintained in anatomic position, and the knees are extended. The elbow is kept extended with rolled towels, bath blankets, or small pillows. The wrist is extended and the fingers flexed with hand rolls. The shoulders are kept in anatomic position, except in burns of the axilla, where the shoulders should be abducted to 90 degrees.[21]

Relief of Pain

Although third-degree burns are painless because the nerve endings are damaged, a person usually sustains a mixture of first-, second- and third-degree burns, and pain is present. Oral or parenteral analgesics are used. Morphine is not given if there are burns of the respiratory tract because it is a respiratory depressant. If it is used, the nurse must count respirations first and withhold the drug if they are 12 or less per minute. Because of the cumulative effects of analgesics that collect in subcutaneous areas with poor circulation, drugs are usually not given subcutaneously.

The Postshock Phase

Stage of Fluid Remobilization

During this period, edema fluid shifts from the tissue phase back into the intravascular phase. It is excreted, along with sodium and potassium, through the kidneys. If the diuresis is too rapid, the patient will experience symptoms of water-loss syndrome with thirst, dry mucous membranes, sudden drop in weight, apathy, and faintness. He must be observed for signs of sodium or potassium depletion (apprehension, anorexia, abdominal distention, cramps, diarrhea, soft muscles, difficulty in breathing, and so forth). Both serum sodium and serum potassium must be maintained during this period, usually by ingestion of oral electrolyte solutions. Intravenous fluids are curtailed because the combined increase in volume from shift of fluids back to the plasma and from an infusion might seriously overload the circulation. As edema fluid is reabsorbed, pulmonary edema becomes a possibility. Symptoms include feeling of chest constriction, moist sound to the respirations, increased restlessness, cyanosis of the nail beds, shortness of breath, coughing of frothy fluid, and venous distention. As the fluid shift takes place, the blood becomes diluted (hemodilution), and this hemodilution, coupled with a decreased number of red cells because of thermal damage, causes anemia.

Infection

The most life-threatening problem to plague the burned patient during this period, and for months after, is infection. The body's great barrier to infection, an intact skin, is broken. Bacteria gain entrance to the body easily and then find excellent growth media in denuded areas. Bacteria survive and grow in sweat glands, and in hair follicles, even if the entire thickness of skin is nonviable. During the postshock phase septicemia is the killer! For this reason, prophylactic doses of antibiotics are often initiated during the period of burn shock and are continued for up to two months after. Prophylactic antibiotics control the spread of beta-hemolytic streptococcus, but *Staphylococcus aureus* and *Pseudomonas* organisms beneath the burn eschar proliferate despite antibiotics. Swab wipings of various parts of the body for culture help in the selection of appropriate antibiotics and determine their probable effectiveness. When catheters are removed, their tips are snipped off and cultured.

The symptoms of infection may develop acutely or insidiously. The nurse must pay special attention to increases in temperature and pulse rate.

Débridement

Débridement means removal of loose, dead skin, crusts, and debris. It is always an ordeal for the patient. It is painful and it "looks unsightedly." It is hard for the patient to understand why this apparently healed area, covered with the thick eschar of tissue and hardened exudate, must be disturbed. Just as soon as the eschar begins to separate, it is gently lifted from the underlying tissues and loose crusts are removed. Débridement is done to decrease the growth of microorganisms favored in the dead tissue and to allow for earlier and more successful "take" of skin grafts. If extensive débridement is required, the patient is taken to the operating room and is anesthetized. Otherwise, débridement is done in the burn unit. Twenty-minute temperature-controlled baths (100° F.) with or without added salts or pHisoHex facilitate the procedure. Then, the nurse or physician gently removes loose crusts with sterile dental forceps and scissors, trying to cause as little bleeding as possible. Blisters are sometimes broken because they harbor infection-causing microorganisms, or they may be left intact and watched carefully. Epithelization may progress better under the covering of the blisters.[22]

Silver Nitrate Treatment

In many burn units 0.5 per cent silver nitrate-saturated dressings are emerging as the treatment of choice. The solution causes bacteriostasis and decreases heat loss through otherwise copious leakage of water vapor from the burn site.[23] This treatment appears to decrease pain, infection, odor, insensible water loss, and the need for blood replacement. It helps to prevent the conversion of second-degree burns to third-degree burns by bacteria. It enhances the "take" of skin grafts and allows débridement without anesthesia. A coarse mesh gauze made without cotton, lint, or paper filling is used. It comes commercially prepared, four layers thick, and is then fan-folded ten times to a 40-layer thickness. It is saturated with 0.5 per cent silver nitrate ($AgNO_3$) solution. A solution greater than 1 per cent is damaging to the tissues. Holes can be cut into the dressings to aid in moistening procedures. If larger areas are to be covered, catheters can be incorporated within the layers to facilitate subsequent moistening. The dressing must be kept continuously wet so that the bacteriostatic solution is in continuous contact with the burn. This "thick pad" should be moistened every two to four hours. The patient should be turned often as this adds pressure to the dressing and helps maintain the wet contact. The entire area is covered with two layers of sterile stockinette sheeting. The edges can be sealed with waterproof tape or with safety pins. A dry blanket covers the whole area. Plastic or other water-impervious materials are not used because some evaporation is necessary to help keep body temperature within reasonable limits. The entire dressing is changed every 12 to 24 hours. At each dressing change, dead skin is gently removed and specimens are taken for culture.

When silver nitrate is used, salt solutions should not be used for débridement because they cause precipitation of the silver salts with a decrease, then, in the silver nitrate's bacteriostatic effectiveness. Only water-soluble solutions should be used. Non-water-soluble solutions act as barriers to the surface action of silver nitrate.[24] The silver nitrate solution is kept at tepid temperature (80° to 95° F.). It is destroyed if submitted to temperatures over 95° F. It is stored in a colored container to prevent exposure to light.

When solutions are used on the face, care must be taken to avoid contact with eyes or with any mucous membranes, e.g., mouth or nose. Prolonged contact causes a bluish discoloration of the skin.

When silver nitrate is used, rigid isolation techniques are not employed. Sterile gloves and instruments are used for débriding and for applying the dressings. Masking and gowning are not routine. Frequent hand washing and restriction of personnel with respiratory infections are precautions taken.

Silver nitrate solution is used directly on grafted areas and on the donor sites, too. The main disadvantage is its dilution of serum electrolytes. It is hypotonic to the plasma. Sodium and chloride diffuse to this area of lesser concentration and are lost in the dressings. Frequent plasma electrolyte analyses allow for adequate oral or intravenous replacement of these electrolytes. The solution stains.

Occlusive Dressings Versus Exposure of Burn Area

Burns of the face, neck, perineum, and trunk are usually cleansed and left exposed to the air. This hastens drying. If the "exposure method" is used, the patient is usually placed on reverse-isolation precautions. Sterile linen and garments are used. The nurse dons sterile gown, mask, and gloves to give care. A burn pack containing all essential items for care is packaged and is autoclaved. If the exposure method is used, the patient feels cold until the eschar forms. Covers are used, but are kept off the body with cradles. Drafts should be avoided. Bath blankets can be used to line the window areas. The temperature of the room should be kept at about 76° F., with a humidity of 40 to 50 per cent. Portable electric humidifiers can be used for this purpose.

Occlusive dressings (pressure dressings) consist of a layer of lightly impregnated petrolatum or sterile, dry fine-mesh gauze on the wound covered with a bulky layer of absorptive gauze and followed by several abdominal pads. This may be covered with an elastic bandage or stockinette. Occlusive dressings are used primarily for burns of the hands or for burns that encircle a part forcing the patient to lie on it. They encourage crust formation; however, the procedure is time-consuming, the materials are expensive, and the mechanical pressure serves to divert burn exudate to surrounding areas rather than decrease its production. Other disadvantages include increased temperature to the dressed part and provision of a warm, moist environment for bacterial growth.

Occlusive dressings *do* protect the wound during transportation, are more comfortable in early burn phases, and seem to allow for earlier grafting. Dressings are changed every four to ten days until skin grafting is done. The part to be dressed must be placed in proper alignment. The position should be changed, if possible, when the dressings are changed. No two skin surfaces should be in contact or they will "heal together." Petroleum gauze can be used to separate parts, e.g., fingers and toes, ears and scalp, genital folds. The nurse must watch for signs of impaired circulation (numbness, pain, tingling) and infection (odor, increased temperature and pulse rate). The part is elevated to encourage absorption of fluid.

Skin Grafting

Grafting is done as soon as the wounds have clean surfaces devoid of necrotic tissue. It is done as early as possible because it speeds healing, decreases the chance of infection, and prevents contractures, especially in full-thickness burns where extensive scar tissue is laid down. Most grafting is done between the fifth and twenty-first day after injury. Partial-thickness autografts are taken from any unburned skin area of the patient, with the Brown electric dermatome. This very thin piece of skin does not prevent regeneration of skin at the donor site. It is placed on the burned site, where it rapidly adheres to granulating surfaces. The serum beneath the graft acts like glue. Grafting may be done on the burn unit with the patient awake and the donor site anesthetized locally, or it may be done in the operating room with general anesthesia used. The graft can be held in place with dressings, liquid adhesive, clips, or sutures. The donor site oozes and is painful. It is covered with a fine-mesh sterile dressing. This can be covered with a pressure dressing or left exposed to facilitate drying.

The pain abates within two days. Grafting is repeated at one- to two-week intervals. Grafts taken from other people (homografts) are used only as an emergency covering. They slough within a few months.

Prevention of Contractures

Early grafting mobilizes the patient much earlier than was possible when grafting was withheld until much later in treatment. However, contractures are still a major problem, and astute nursing attention to frequent planned position changes does much to decrease this sequela. Exercises should be ordered by the physician and supervised by the physical therapist. Here are some points to remember:

1. Maintain joint range of motion by daily passive and/or active, supervised exercise. This should be done at least three times a day and is particularly important to prevent contracture of the hand.

2. Have the patient lie in the prone and supine positions for periods each day. This can be facilitated with use of a Stryker frame or Circ-O-Lectric bed.

3. Do not let the patient remain in one position for extended periods of time "because he says it is comfortable." Be empathic, but firm!

4. If burns involve the face, have the patient exercise by chewing gum or blowing balloons to prevent scars from tightening as they form.

5. If burns involve the face, chin, or neck, have the patient lie with the neck hyperextended (look at the ceiling) for a period each day.

For further discussion of rehabilitation methods see Chapter 37.

21

MULTIPLE WATER AND ELECTROLYTE PROBLEMS: UROLOGIC DYSFUNCTION

The Kidneys

The kidneys are essential to life. Because of their multiple discriminatory functions end products of metabolism are excreted, normal electrolyte levels and a slightly alkaline body pH are maintained, and water volume is regulated. Interference with the functioning capacity of the kidneys or with the free passage of urine out of the body can cause irreparable tissue damage and life-threatening electrolyte imbalance.

What Structures Are Involved in the Production and Excretion of Urine?

The two kidneys formulate urine from the blood. To do this, they receive 25 per cent (1,200 ml) of the heart's output per minute. The blood is delivered to the kidneys through renal arteries that branch directly off the abdominal aorta. The urine is transported to the bladder by a ureter from each kidney. It is stored in the bladder until 300 to 500 ml is collected, at which time it is voided out of the body through a single urethra. The urethra of the male is 7 to 9 in. long; the urethra of the female about 1½ in. long.

The kidneys are encapsulated in tough fibrous connective tissue. They lie behind the peritoneum on either side of the vertebral column at the level of the lower thoracic to the upper lumbar vertebrae. They are shaped like kidney beans and are about the size of a man's fist. They are not anchored in place by ligaments but rest on muscles of the posterior abdominal wall (including the diaphragm) and are held in place by blood vessels, fat, and the pressure of the abdominal organs. A sudden loss of weight can upset the anchoring function of perirenal fat and result in an overly mobile, "free-floating" kidney (nephroptosis). This condition must be repaired surgically. A shift in normal position of the abdominal organs that support the kidneys can also cause displacement.

Parts of the Kidney

The functioning tissue of the kidney, called renal parenchyma, is located in the outer cortex and the inner medulla. Each kidney contains about 1 million "functioning units" called nephrons. A nephron contains a tuft of capillaries (glomerulus) encased in a capsule (Bowman's capsule) that contains an entering vessel called an afferent arteriole and an exiting vessel called an efferent arteriole. This is the only area in the body where capillaries are squeezed between two arterioles! The efferent arteriole courses between the tubules in the cortex and medulla and drains into collecting venules. The glomerulus produces an ultrafiltrate from blood. The nephron also contains a variety of tubules that selectively reabsorb

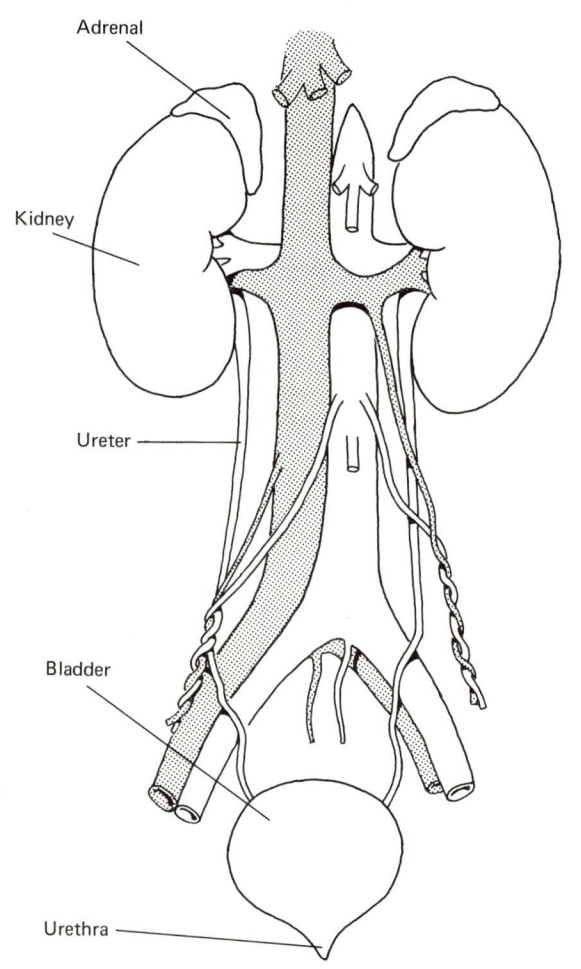

Figure 21-1. The urinary system.

water and electrolytes. Once processed, urine collected in collecting tubules is transported to the renal pelvis, a funnel-shaped extension of the ureter, for its trip out of the body. (See Figs. 21–1, 21–2, 21–3, and 21–4.)

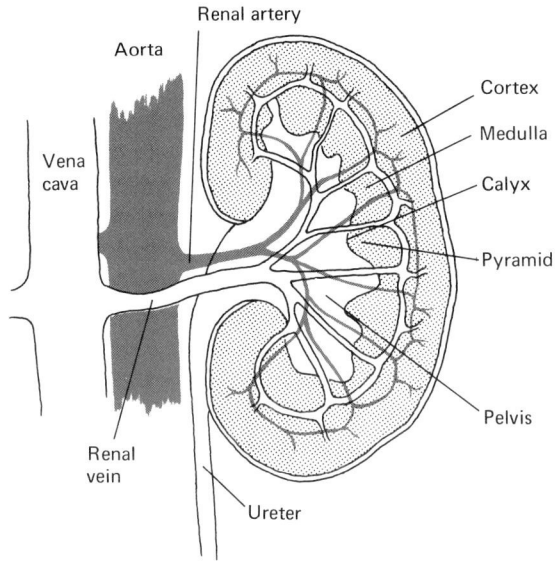

FIGURE 21–2. The internal structure of the kidney.

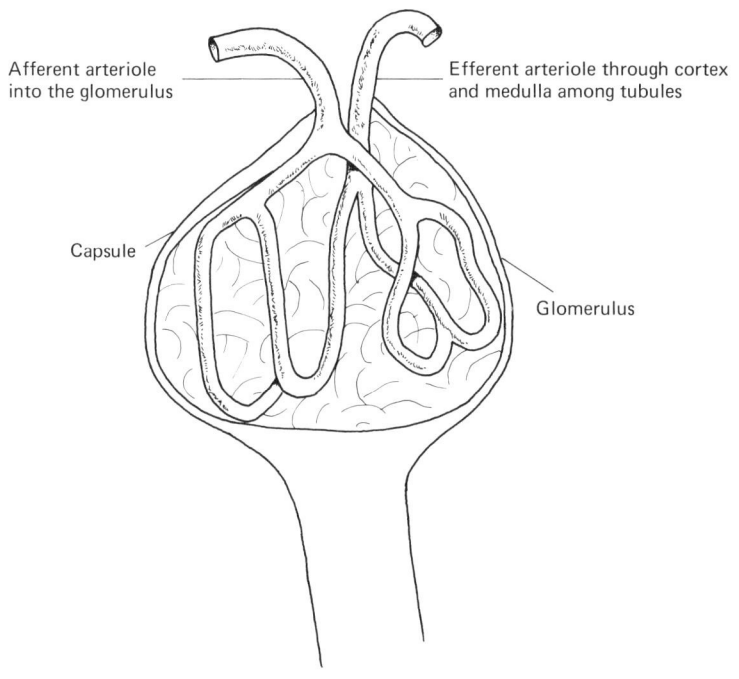

FIGURE 21–3. The glomerulus.

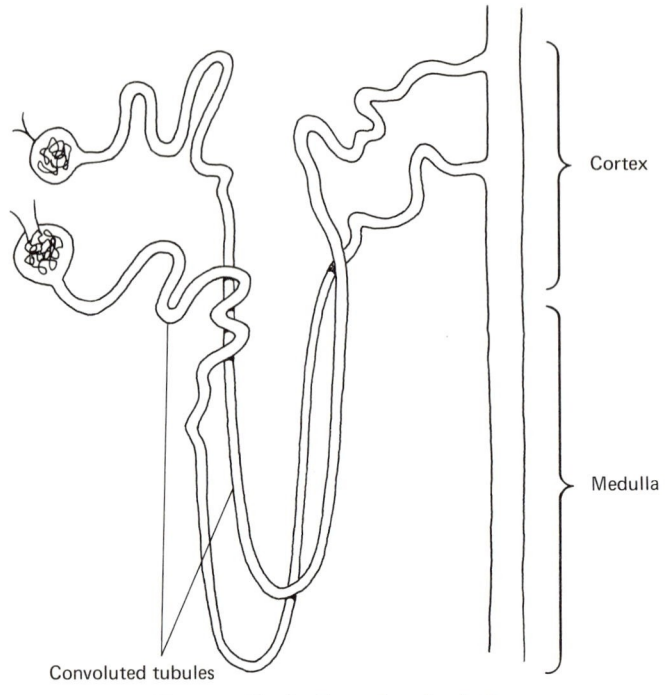

FIGURE 21–4. Convoluted tubules.

How Is Urine Formed?

The major processes involved in the formation of urine are glomerular filtration, tubular reabsorption, tubular secretion, and tubular excretion. Water and solutes are filtered from the blood in the tuft of capillaries at the glomerulus. The filtrates thus formed is protein-free. The blood pressure in the glomerular capillaries drives water and crystalloids through the glomerular membrane. The rate of this filtration varies with the arterial blood pressure. If the systolic blood pressure falls to 75 mm Hg (as in circulatory shock), urine formation is arrested. Interestingly, urine formation is also arrested if the pressure within the ureter is raised 30 mm Hg above atmospheric pressure.[25] This can happen if a ureteral obstruction develops.

Tubular reabsorption involves a very selective, discriminatory process in which excess substances are eliminated, but needed substances are conserved. High-threshold substances such as glucose, protein, vitamin C, potassium, and sodium are reabsorbed; low-threshold substances such as urea, uric acid, phosphates, and sulfates are not reabsorbed. Ninety-nine per cent of the body water, too, is reabsorbed. From the 125 ml of glomerular filtrate passing into the renal tubules every minute, all but 1 ml of water content is reabsorbed.[26]

Tubular secretion is the process through which unfiltered or partly filtered substances are secreted directly from the capillaries around the tubules.[27] In this way, unfiltered materials are transported from areas of low concentration in the plasma surrounding the tubules to areas of high concentration in the glomerular filtrate, quickly. For example, harmful substances in the plasma can quickly be exchanged for desirable ones in the glomerular filtrate.

In tubular excretion the cells of the tubules actually function in an excretory capacity. This type of excretion is of relatively little importance to man, but is involved in the excretion of certain dyes used in testing. If these dyes are maintained at high plasma levels, the tubular cells remove them from the plasma and excrete them into the lumens of the tubules. If the glomeruli are severely diseased, this excretory function of the tubules may be invoked.

Schematically, urine is manufactured and transported this way:

Urinary ultrafiltrate produced in glomerulus → to proximal convoluted tubules —reabsorption water and elec.→ down descending tubules —in medulla→ around loop of Henle → up through ascending tubules —again in medulla→ to distal convoluted tubules again in cortex → back through cortex and medulla → to collecting tubule → through renal pelvis → ureter → bladder → urethra → out

Some Commonly Occurring Observations Necessitated by Interference in the Manufacture or Transportation of Urine

The production and transportation of urine occur in a relatively "closed system." This means that dysfunction in one part of the system can ultimately affect other parts and can lead to irreversible kidney damage.

Here are some of the symptoms that indicate urologic dysfunction:

1. Changes in voiding habits, volume, and voluntary control. The average adult voids when his bladder collects 300 to 500 ml of urine. The quantity voided in 24 hours is roughly equal to the amount of fluid ingested in that same period of time. The average adult voids 1,500 ml a day and empties his bladder four or five times a day. Voiding more often than four or five times a day is called *frequency*. Voiding more than once during the night (once is considered physiologic) is called *nocturia*. If there is pain when voiding (before, during, or immediately after the stream of urine), it is called *dysuria*. An intense, painful need to void is called *urgency*. The patient may say he has a *burning* sensation when he voids. Voiding less than 400 to 500 ml in 24 hours is called *oliguria*. If the patient does not void at all, or voids only minute quantities, it is called *anuria*.

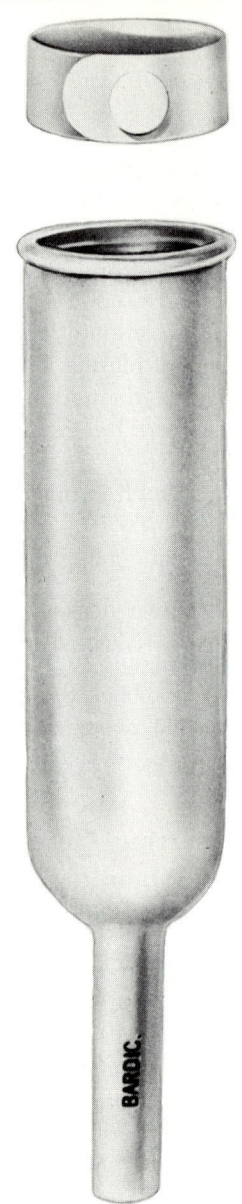

FIGURE 21-5. Urosheath to be slipped over the penis. (Courtesy, C. R. Bard, Inc., Murray Hill, N.J.)

Voiding greater than the average amount, depending on the situation, is called *polyuria*.

The internal bladder sphincter is controlled by the nervous system. When the internal sphincter is open, the external sphincter, voluntarily

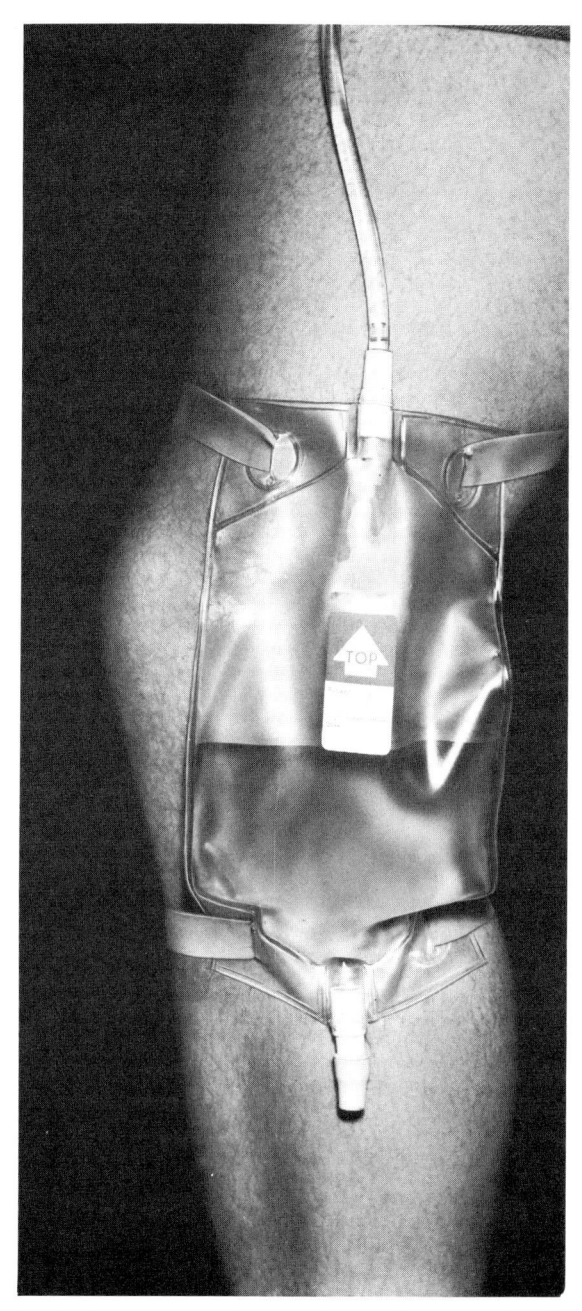

FIGURE 21-6. Leg urine collection bag. (Courtesy, Sterilon Corp., Braintree, Mass.)

controlled by the person, can be opened and voiding takes place. *Incontinence* indicates the loss of the voluntary aspect of voiding. For detailed discussion of incontinence see page 409. The male patient may be protected from urine by use of a urosheath attached to a leg collection bag. (See Figs. 21–5 and 21–6.) The female patient is best protected with sanitary pads and rubber pants.

2. Changes in the appearance of urine. Normal urine is clear and ranges in color from light to dark amber. *Pyuria* indicates pus in the urine. It becomes cloudy to look at. *Hematuria* indicates blood in the urine. Any changes in the usual color of the urine may indicate dysfunction somewhere in the urinary system.

3. Pain. Along with dysuria, the patient may experience pain in the exact area of the dysfunction, e.g., flank pain if the kidneys are implicated, and lower abdomen, midline, if an overdistended bladder is implicated; or the pain may begin in the area of the dysfunction and travel; e.g., a male patient with a ureteral stone may experience pain beginning in the flank area and traveling all the way down to the end of the penis. The pain may be in the low back area. It may be excruciating. It may be continuous (e.g., a continuous dull ache) or intermittent.

4. Chills and fever. This suggests infection with invasion of the blood by bacteria or toxins.

5. Severe imbalances in water and electrolyte levels, e.g., dehydration and/or edema, metabolic acidosis, sodium and potassium excesses and deficits.

Uremia (Azotemia)

Uremia is the most severe syndrome of urologic symptoms. It occurs when the functioning tissue within the kidney is damaged and cannot carry out its normal activity. There is a life-threatening accumulation of waste products circulating throughout the body. The gross accumulation of nitrogenous material is called azotemia. Uremia can occur suddenly as the result of severe trauma to the kidneys, e.g., from a crushing injury or ingestion of poison, or it can occur after long-term kidney disease with decreased functioning capacity of kidney parenchyma. The patient may void less than 150 ml of urine in 24 hours. This is considered the "oliguric phase," of uremia. If the kidney heals, the patient may later void 1,000 ml or more of dilute urine. This is called the diuretic phase of uremia and indicates the early healing within the tubules.

The uremic patient is very sick. His skin and mucous membranes are dry, and he suffers from cell dehydration. He tends to bleed and may have bleeding from the nose (epistaxis), gums, and gastrointestinal tract. Gastrointestinal ulcers may develop. The exact cause of this increased bleeding tendency is not known, though it is believed to be related to the blood-platelet factor. The patient vomits and has diarrhea. His breath and his body have the odor of urine. His skin excretes greater amounts of waste products, and a white "frost" develops. It is called uremic frost. His tongue also becomes coated. His skin itches (pruritus). His respirations become deep and increased to "blow off" excess CO_2. As the imbalances progress, central nervous system symptoms develop. The patient may have muscle twitching. He becomes drowsy and may become stuporous or comatose. Convulsions sometimes occur.

Management of the Patient with Uremia

USE OF ARTIFICIAL DIALYSIS

Dialysis means the transfer of water and electrolytes across a semipermeable membrane. It is a process that normally takes place in the glomeruli and the tubules of the kidneys. If the kidneys are not working, this transfer of water and electrolytes can be attained artificially. Artificial dialysis is used to remove the end products of protein metabolism, maintain safe levels of electrolytes, correct hydrogen ion imbalance (acidosis), and remove excess water.[28] It can be done as an emergency treatment to rid the body of life-threatening excess products and give the kidneys a chance to heal, or it can be done on a more permanent basis for chronically diseased kidneys that no longer function adequately. Artificial dialysis is used to maintain the patient who is waiting for a transplant from a suitable kidney donor.

Artificial dialysis is based on the laws of osmosis and diffusion. The patient's blood flows on one side of a semipermeable membrane, and a prepared electrolyte solution (a dialysate) flows on the other. Electrolytes that are more highly concentrated on the patient's side of the membrane move toward their less concentrated counterpart in the dialysate by diffusion. Excess water, on the other hand, moves by osmosis toward highly concentrated solutes; e.g., dextrose may be added to the dialysate to pull water out of the patient's blood. By regulation of the concentrations of electrolytes in the dialysate, excess electrolytes are removed from the patient's blood.

HEMODIALYSIS: THE ARTIFICIAL KIDNEY

In hemodialysis, the patient's arterial blood is shunted, by cannula, through a machine (the artificial kidney.) The machine contains a synthetic semipermeable membrane. Waste products are removed and the purified blood is returned to the patient's venous circulation. The cannulas are connected to each other with silastic tubing between treatments so that repeated cutdowns are not necessary.

A more recent method of connecting the patient to the machine is called "fistulation" or internal shunting. A fistula is created surgically between the radial artery and the cephalic vein. The opening is only 2 mm wide, but it enables arterial blood to enter and engorge the veins. The deep arteries, then, do not have to be cannulated with each treatment, and a permanent external device is not needed. Two needles are used in the fistula, one a bit higher than the other, and both facing in the same direction. One takes blood through the kidney; the other returns purified blood to the patient. "Arterialization" of the vein increases the diameter and pressure within it. This eliminates the problem of vein collapse with frequent venipuncture. The needles must be reinserted with each treatment. Patients seem to prefer internal shunting because they do not have to worry about the external cannulas becoming dislodged or being knocked or caught on something. No "equipment" shows, and clotting and infection are less of a problem. Because the pressure within this vein is elevated, blood tends to spurt out when the vein is punctured and pressure must be used. The involved arm should not be used for blood pressure readings or for any other treatments. The patency of the system is determined by listening to the sound of the flow of blood with a stethoscope. Only the Kiil negative-pressure artificial kidney can be used with internal shunting.

Both methods are closed. Dialysis takes place by diffusion of molecules from an area where they are greatly concentrated to an area where they are less concentrated. Transfer of water takes place by osmosis (water moves where the particles are) and by alteration of pressure between the cellophane compartment and the dialysate compartment. Water tends to move where there is lower pressure. This can be attained artificially by increasing the pressure in the blood compartment, or by decreasing the pressure in the dialysate compartment.[29]

There are two major types of artificial kidneys in use. The Kolff machine is a coil-type device with a pump. Once in the machine, the pump increases the pressure of the patient's blood, and excess water is removed by "positive pressure." The Kiil Parallel Plates type of device does not use a pump. It removes water by decreased (negative) pressure in the dialysate compartment. The machines are primed with normal saline.

Each dialysis treatment lasts about six to eight hours, depending on the type of machine used. The patient may be dialyzed three times a week. He stays in his bed, or rests on a reclining chair for the period of dialysis. He should be weighed accurately immediately prior to and after the dialysis to determine the exact amount of water removed. This may vary from 0.5 to 7 lb with an average of 4 lb in a six-hour dialysis.[30] A 2-4-lb weight gain is expected between dialysis. Vital signs are noted on arrival in the kidney laboratory, and observations are made and recorded pertaining to the mental status of the patient. Blood pressure determinations (serial blood pressures) are made before the patient is connected to the machine, are taken continuously during the initial treatment period, and are taken every 15 minutes for the remainder of the treatment. Because heparin is used to decrease the chance of clotting, blood studies are done routinely. Correlation of blood pressure and weight is a useful indicator of fluid status. A hypovolemic patient is usually hypotensive, and signs of circulatory shock must be watched for. The nurse must pay particular attention to decrease in blood pressure, nausea, vomiting, and faintness. A decreased flow of blood through the cannula could cause clotting. Between treatments, diet is individualized. Most patients receive some sodium restriction; however, this is flexible. If weight suddenly drops below a desired base level, sodium and water are increased.

Points to Watch for When Patients Are Being Dialyzed.
1. Bleeding due to repeated heparinization, particularly at cannulization sites
2. Symptoms of shock
3. Changes in mental status
4. Tremors
5. Convulsions
6. Vomiting
7. Restlessness
8. Cyanosis

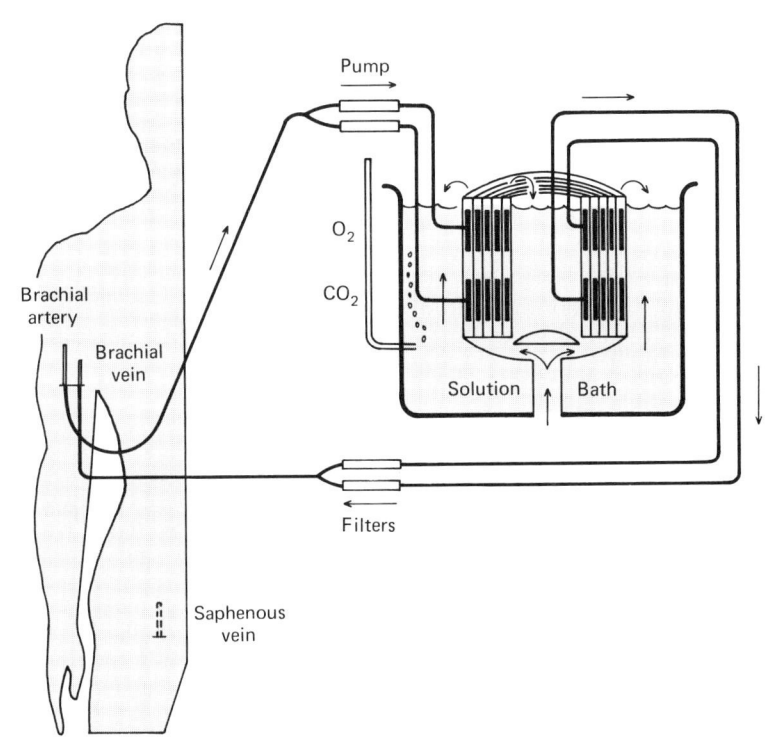

FIGURE 21-7. Diagram of Travenol Twin-Coil Kidney attached to patient. (Courtesy, Baxter Laboratories, Inc., Morton Grove, Ill.)

Nurses working in a hemodialysis unit receive special intensive instruction in the care of the patient and in working with the machine. A nurse is always in attendance when a patient is being dialyzed. In some large kidney centers several patients are dialyzed at one time, and a central dialysate source is used.

Use of the artificial kidney is very expensive. It costs between $10,000 and $20,000 a year to maintain a patient on hemodialysis. The equipment is extremely costly. Many patients are now being taught to use portable machinery in the home to decrease the expense.

PERITONEAL DIALYSIS

In peritoneal dialysis the large surface area of the peritoneal cavity is used as the dialyzing membrane. Although only one sixth to one tenth as efficient as hemodialysis, it does not involve expensive equipment or complex technique and can be utilized easily in the general hospital. Once the procedure is started, it becomes a nursing responsibility.

Baseline vital signs and weight are recorded, and the patient empties his bladder. The physician anesthetizes a small area in the lower left quadrant of the abdomen. A small incision is made and a metal trocar and cannula are inserted. The cannula is replaced by a semirigid, many-eyed catheter, and the trocar is withdrawn.

Two liters of dialysate similar in composition to blood minus protein and formed elements are allowed to run into the peritoneal cavity rapidly, in about ten minutes. Commercial dialysates such as Impersol and Dianeal are available. The solution is warmed to body temperature before infusion. The tubing from the bottles of dialysate is clamped just before the bottles are completely empty. The dialysate remains in the peritoneal cavity (for one or two hours) until ionic equilibrium between the patient's blood and the dialysate is reached. Then, the two bottles are lowered to the floor and the peritoneal fluid is allowed to drain out. There should be a steady stream of fluid drainage. The return takes 20 minutes to one hour. If there is more than a 500-ml difference between what went in and what comes out, the physician is notified, and the second dialysate infusion is not begun. (See Fig. 21–8.) The procedure of infusing dialysate, allowing dialysis (transfer of electrolytes) to occur in the peritoneal cavity, and then lowering the bottles to allow the fluid to drain out is repeated several times, according to the physician's order. Total treatment time is 12 to 36 hours. Electrolyte status is determined by frequent blood studies.

The patient is kept in a supine position with the head slightly elevated to decrease the discomfort of the abdominal organs pushing up against the diaphragm. He may turn toward his side for back care after the end of the fluid return and before the beginning of the next infusion. Vital signs must be taken every 15 minutes during the first exchange and then once each hour for successive exchanges. Weight is checked every 24

Step one

Fluid into peritoneal cavity

Step two

Same bottles are lowered and fluid is allowed to drain out

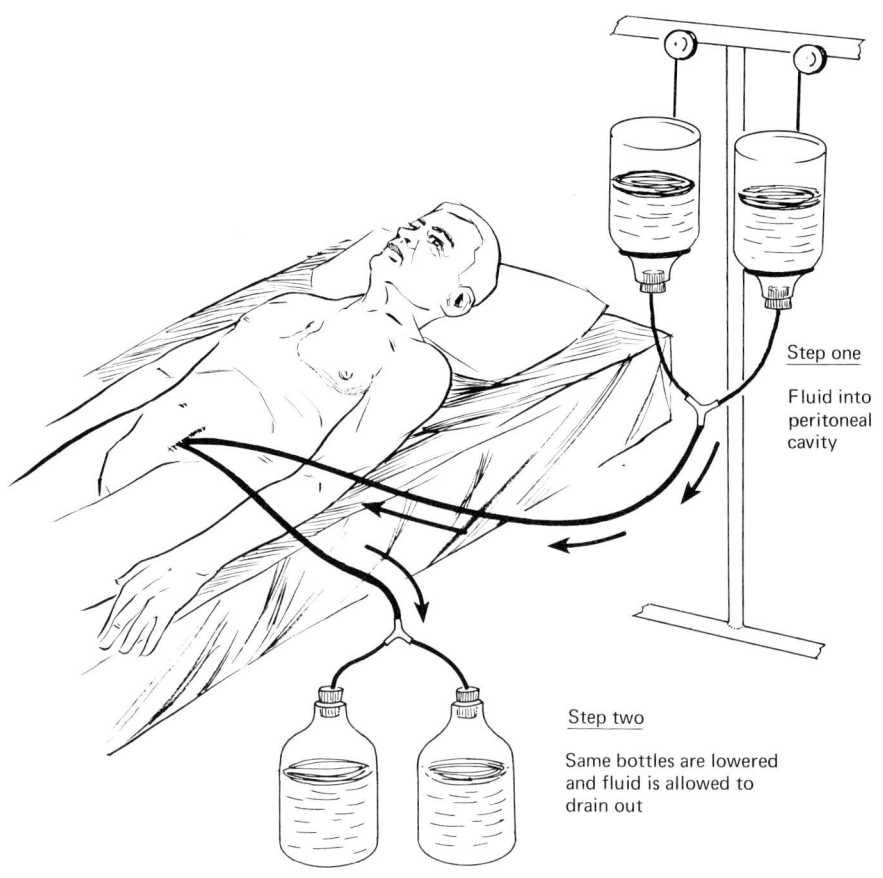

FIGURE 21–8. Peritoneal dialysis.

hours and compared to baseline weights; 0.5 to 1 per cent of the total body weight should be lost each day to prevent overhydration.[31] The nurse must observe carefully for signs of dehydration or overhydration. Pulmonary edema from overhydration may occur, and is life-threatening. Infusions are stopped if there is a moist, bubbly sound to the patient's breathing. The physician may instill an anesthetic agent into the catheter if the patient has abdominal pain.

The risk of infection with peritoneal dialysis is high, and paralytic ileus may result. Peritoneal dialysis cannot be used if there has been a recent abdominal operation.

General Principles in the Management of the Patient with Uremic Syndrome

1. *Specific observations and intervention related to water and electrolyte imbalance and anemia.* Observations are discussed in detail on page

169. The patient with uremia has increased levels of circulating electrolytes, especially during the initial (10 to 20 days) oliguric phase. The patient should be observed for elevations in serum potassium: cardiac arrhythmias, pulse changes, intestinal cramping and diarrhea; elevations in hydrogen ion content (acidosis); shortness of breath on exertion, disorientation, dehydration; deficit in serum calcium levels: tetany; with hyperirritable nerve-muscle response, tingling in the fingers, convulsion. Cation-exchange resins may be used either orally or in a retention enema to help eliminate excess electrolytes through the bowels. These drugs are insoluble, nonabsorbable, synthetic substances that "take up" sodium, potassium, and other cations and excrete them through the bowel. If these resins are used for more than a few days, excess cations lost must be replaced. Sodium polystyrene sulfanate (Kayexalate) is an example.

During the oliguric phase the nurse must watch for signs of sodium and water excess with pitting-type edema and a "swollen" look to the face. During this phase, the physician will limit fluid intake to 800 to 1,000 ml per day and restrict sodium to that amount that is lost each day. Diuretics will be used intermittently to help excrete sodium and water. Toxic effecs of the diuretics are minimized by not giving them every day and/or by altering the diuretic used.

The patient will probably be fed by vein. In this case, the drops per minute should be regulated carefully according to the amount of time the solution should take to run in, per the physician's order. If the patient is allowed oral fluids, they must be spaced judiciously through the day to help appease extreme thirst. *All intake and output must be recorded.* This includes drainage from all catheters, from gastrointestinal suction, from wounds (weigh wet dressings), and so forth. An intake-and-output sign should be posted in an obvious place at the bedside so that all personnel will be aware of the need to record "even the small sip of water." If the urinary output falls below 500 ml per day this should be reported emphatically. The patient should be weighed daily.

During the diuretic phase, which begins when the urine volume approaches 1,000 ml in 24 hours, the patient reacts to the rapid contraction of fluid phases (loss of fluid) from the body. He may bleed internally, vomit blood, and convulse. Fluids are replaced even if symptoms of edema occur.[32]

For chronic renal disease, the physician may order 2,000 to 3,000 ml of water each day to aid in the elimination of wastes, if the patient is able to excrete the large volumes. What goes in must come out!

The cause of the normochromic, normocytic anemia that the uremic patient develops is not known. It seems to be related to the degree of circulating nitrogenous wastes and to the platelet factor.[33] It can contribute to the development of congestive heart failure because the heart must work harder to supply the needs of the body when the blood is "anemic." If the hematocrit falls below 20 per cent or the hemoglobin below 7 gm, packed red cells are administered. The anemia, coupled with the symptoms of electrolyte imbalance, make the patient feel tired, anorexic, and sapped of energy. Mild bleeding, e.g., bruising and bleeding from the gums may occur, or more severe bleeding into the lungs or brain may occur. The nurse must be alerted to a fall in blood pressure (compare with prior readings), an increase in pulse rate or a change in pulse rhythm, increasing lethargy, or a decreasing orientation to surroundings. All body discharges should be inspected for bleeding.

2. *Eating and mouth care.* The physician will make dietary changes according to daily electrolyte findings, the condition of the kidneys, and his own philosophy. His major goal is to decrease the breakdown of body protein because this burdens the kidneys with nitrogen to be excreted and increases the level of circulating potassium. To spare protein breakdown, sufficient calories plus a diet containing at least 100 gm of carbohydrate and moderate amounts of fat is ordered. Carbohydrate can be administered intravenously as glucose solutions or ingested as high-carbohydrate foods (bread, rice, potatoes) in the meal plan. Protein intake is usually restricted to less than 0.5 gm per kilogram body weight per day because every 4 gm of protein furnishes 1 gm of urea that must be excreted by the kidneys. The diet contains moderate to high amounts of fat. Fat provides less water of oxidation than protein or carbohydrate, and would be less likely to cause excess fluid volume. It is also a good source of calories. The patient may be offered a "butter-sugar ball" to eat. If he is fed through a nasogastric tube, high-fat solutions such as Lipomul may be used.

If edema is present, sodium restriction will be ordered; however, it is not an across-the-board rule to restrict sodium for all patients who have kidney failure. If serum potassium is elevated, foods containing large amounts of potassium are restricted, e.g., fruit juices, coffee, tea, meats.

Mouth care is essential. The patient may have soreness, bleeding gums, a sweet, greasy sensation, and a heavily coated tongue, all of which decrease his appetite and interfere with maintenance of adequate balance. Caked blood can be gently removed with hydrogen peroxide. Cotton applicators moistened with glycerin and lemon juice should be used to cleanse the mouth. A stiff bristled toothbrush should not be used because of the patient's bleeding tendency. A ready supply of sourballs at the bedside helps decrease the unpleasant taste in the patient's mouth. Offering foods he is fond of is more logical than stressing foods he is not fond of. The nurse should check his tray after he is finished eating to see what he has actually eaten.

3. *Physical Activity and Comfort.* The nurse must have a clear understanding of the amount of physical activity the patient may have. Usually, it is minimal in order to decrease the rate of metabolism. This requires

that the nurse gives complete care. The patient should be turned, rubbed, reminded to "deep-breathe," and positioned carefully. Between these activity periods, he should be allowed optimum rest. Bathing is extremely important because the skin provides a route for excretion of waste products. If uremic frost or itching develops, a soothing lotion may be applied, or a weak vinegar solution (2 tablespoons of vinegar to 1 pt of warm water) can be used to dissolve deposited crystals.

4. *Maintain a free route for passage of urine.* Make sure catheters are draining freely and are not kinked or compressed. Never leave a catheter clamped unless specifically ordered to do so by the physician. Anchor catheters with tape so that there is no tension or pulling on them.

5. *Protect the patient from hospital-acquired infection.* The urinary drainage system should remain a relatively "closed system." Do not allow drainage tubing to become immersed in urine. Empty the drainage bag only when necessary (usually once each shift) so that the system is not frequently exposed to environmental microorganisms.

Aids in Making the Diagnosis of Urinary Tract Disease

Examination of the Urine

If urine is properly collected, stored, and examined, it can yield a wealth of clinical information.[34] Disease processes may increase urinary constituents or introduce abnormal components, e.g., protein, sugar, bile pigments, casts, or bacteria. A single first-voided morning specimen is often used for analysis because the urine is most concentrated at that time and would, more than likely, contain any atypical substances. Sometimes the physician will request "timed" specimens. For instance, he may want to collect all the urine voided in a 24-hour period (8 A.M. to 8 A.M.). In this case, the patient voids and discards the initial 8 A.M. voiding, and then voids and collects all urine from that point to and including the 8 A.M. voiding on the second day. Or, a multiple-glass test may be indicated. This provides separate specimens from a single voiding. The patient voids 100 ml into the first bottle. This contains urethral washings. Then he voids 100 ml into a second bottle. This provides bladder and kidney washings. If prostatic washings are desired from the male patient, the physician gently massages the prostate gland through the rectum immediately after the second part of the voiding, and the third specimen contains prostatic secretions.

All urine specimens are collected in clean containers unless a sterile specimen is specifically ordered. The urine should be refrigerated until examined. Standing at room temperature causes the formed elements to deteriorate, increases the bacterial growth, and causes chemical changes.

Specimens may be plain-voided directly into a specimen bottle. This is usually the way a routine specimen is collected when the patient is first admitted to the hospital. The physician may want a "clean-catch" specimen. In this case the genitalia of male or female are cleansed with soap and water, and the urethral meatus is gently cleansed with an antiseptic solution, as for a catheterization. The female patient is instructed to hold the labia apart as she voids into the specimen bottle. Some hospitals require nurse and patient to don sterile gloves to collect a "clean-catch" specimen. If a "midstream" specimen is requested, the first 50 ml voided is discarded, and the remaining urine is collected.

Catheterized specimens are being requested less frequently because of serious increases in urinary infection associated with the technique. Bacteria normally found in the urethra (e.g., *Escherichia coli*) cannot be eliminated by cleansing, and are "pushed up" the urinary tract with the catheter. The gram-negative bacilli (*Escherichia coli, Proteus* species, and *Klebsiella aerobacter*) normally found in the intestinal tract or on the skin in the perineal region have a peculiar affinity for damaged urinary tract tissue.[35] Trauma of forceful catheterization damages tissues. Along with *Pseudomonas aeruginosa*, chiefly found in the hospital environment on faucets, sinks, bedpans, water pitchers, and soap dishes, these microorganisms account for 80 to 90 per cent of all urinary tract infection. The remaining 10 to 20 per cent comes from *Streptococcus faecalis, Staphylococcus aureus*, and the tubercle bacilli.[36] The longer a catheter is left in the urinary tract, the greater the bacterial count. The patient is said to have *bacteriuria* if there are more than 100,000 colonies per milliliter of urine of one pathogenic microorganism.

COLOR

Routine urinalysis includes a description of color: normally pale yellow to amber. If the urine is red, there may be blood in it or the patient may have eaten beets or may have taken medication that causes redness. If it is brown to black, it may contain bilirubin or melanin.

ODOR

Urine is faintly aromatic when fresh but develops a strong ammonia odor from bacterial decomposition; a foul odor from infection; a fruity odor from acetone bodies.

pH

Urine is normally acid (pH 4.5 to 7.5).

SPECIFIC GRAVITY

Specific gravity, the weight of dissolved substances in urine, is normally 1.010 to 1.025. An elevated specific gravity may be caused by increased dissolved protein as in kidney disease.

TURBIDITY

Average urine is clear. If the specimen is cloudy, it may indicate the presence of precipitated crystals, pus, or red blood cells, and a microscopic examination should be ordered.

Microscopic examination of the urine indicates the presence of epithelial cells, white blood cells, red blood cells, casts (casts are protein that has coagulated around tubules and has taken the shape of the tubules), crystals, and miscellaneous formed elements. In the Addis count all the urine excreted in 12 or 24 hours is collected and examined microscopically. The patient is not allowed any fluids during the test period.

Urine is analyzed chemically for protein (albumin, globulin, fibrinogen), glucose, ketone bodies, bile, and so forth. Protein is of utmost importance. It is normally not found in the urine. Its presence may result from "leaking" of plasma protein in the glomerulus, damage of the functioning tissue of the kidneys, and inflammatory processes anywhere in the urinary system. Sometimes, protein may be deposited in the urine from the labia. In this case, it is not indicative of disease. A catheterized specimen is often taken to make sure the protein does not come from within the urinary system. A simple dip-stick test may be done by the nurse. (See Fig. 21–9.)

Tests of Renal Function [37,38]

These tests measure the ability of the kidneys to excrete foreign substances (dyes), to concentrate the urine, to maintain water and electrolyte balance, and to excrete products such as urea that are normally removed from the body in the urine.

PHENOLSULFONPHTHALEIN TEST (P.S.P.)

Rather marked kidney damage must be present before this test gives significantly abnormal results; however, it is still used frequently. The patient is allowed a light breakfast but no coffee or tea. One milliliter of dye (phenolsulfonphthalein) is injected, usually intravenously, and the time is noted. The patient is then given one glass of water to drink and a urine specimen is collected 15 minutes after injection of the dye. The patient drinks another glass of water, and urine is collected one and two hours after the injection of the dye. Normally, 40 to 60 per cent of the dye is excreted in the first hour, and an additional 20 to 25 per cent is excreted in the second hour. The dye colors the urine red. Therefore, blood in the urine or use of other drugs that redden urine (e.g., pyridium) makes the test invalid.

NONPROTEIN NITROGEN (N.P.N.) AND BLOOD UREA NITROGEN (B.U.N.)

These are tests of the blood. All proteins contain nitrogen, but many body substances that contain nitrogen are not proteins.[39] A venous speci-

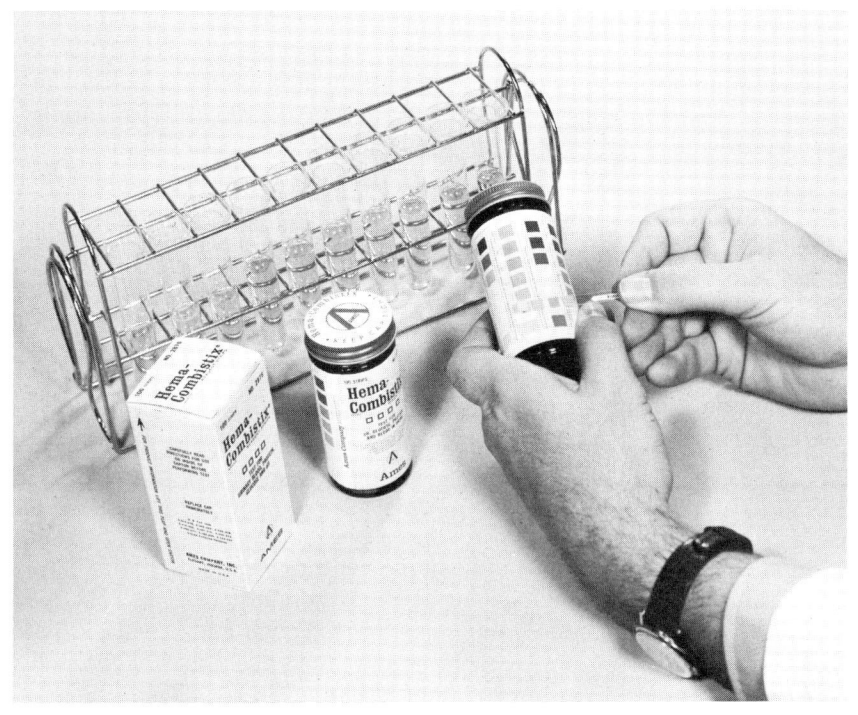

FIGURE 21-9. Urinary dip-stick test of urine for presence of blood, protein, glucose, and pH. (Courtesy, Ames Company, Elkhart, Ind.)

men is used to determine the level of these nonprotein nitrogenous substances. The usual range of nonprotein nitrogen is 15 to 30 mg per cent. Urea is one of the major nonprotein nitrogenous substances and is a major excretory product of the kidneys. Normal blood urea nitrogen is 8 to 28 mg per cent.

FISHBERG'S CONCENTRATION TEST

When renal damage has occurred one of the first functions to be lost is the ability of the renal tubules to concentrate and dilute urine. In this test, the patient is not permitted anything from the evening meal the night before the test until completion of the test at 11 A.M. the following day. Urine is collected at 10 and 11 the second day and checked for specific gravity. This indicates the ability of the kidneys to concentrate urine. Normal specimens have a specific gravity of 1.020 or greater.

UREA CLEARANCE TEST

Normally, 60 to 90 ml of plasma is cleared of urea by the kidneys each minute. The patient is given his usual breakfast at 7 A.M. with sufficient fluid included. At 7:30 he is given two glasses of water to drink to keep urine flow at 2 ml per minute. This is required for accurate laboratory results. At 8 A.M. he empties his bladder and discards the urine. At 9 A.M. he again empties his bladder and saves all the urine. This is labeled "first specimen" with the exact time. A blood specimen is drawn for urea nitrogen determination. One hour later a second urine specimen is voided and labeled "specimen two" with the exact time and is saved. Another blood specimen may be drawn.

With poor renal function, urea in the blood is elevated; urea in the urine is decreased. Creatinine clearance may also be done.

TUBULAR FUNCTION

Substances known to be excreted by the renal tubules are injected. Examples include para-aminohippuric acid and iodopyracet (Diodrast). By determination of blood and urinary levels at specified times after injection, tubular excretory capacity is determined.

RADIORENOGRAPHY

In this test, an intravenous radiopaque contrast medium (dye) such as Hippuran tagged with radioiodine (I^{131}) is administered. Specimens of urine are collected 20 and 90 minutes after injection and are tested with the Geiger counter or similar device for radioiodine content. Normally, 75 per cent is excreted within 30 minutes. Urine can be collected from individual ureteral catheters to test the function of each kidney separately, or tracings may be made over each kidney with a scanning machine.

INTRAVENOUS PYELOGRAPHY (EXCRETORY UROGRAPHY)

In this test, the physician injects an iodide containing dye (Urokon, Diodrast), which the kidneys concentrate, and a series of x-rays are taken at intervals thereafter. The dye makes visible the inner silhouette of the urinary excretory passages. The pelves, calyces, ureters, and bladder are delineated. If the patient has a history of allergy, a test dose of the dye may be given intravenously, or a skin test may be done, to determine the presence of sensitivity. Symptoms of an untoward reaction include urticaria, respiratory difficulty, diaphoresis, clamminess, tingling sensation, and palpitation. Emergency antihistamine drugs (Benadryl, Adrenaline) should be ready. The dye is not used if the patient has serious kidney or liver disease.

The patient is allowed nothing by mouth for 12 hours before the test. This fasting dehydrates his body, the dye is better concentrated, and a clearer picture is obtained. The bowel must be free of feces and gas because these would cause shadows on the picture. A cathartic such as 20 mg of bisacodyl (Dulcolax) is often given at 6 P.M. the evening before the test. A cleansing enema may be ordered the morning of the pyelogram. Results should be observed by the nurse and reported to the physician. A low-residue diet (no whole-grain products, raw fruits or vegetables, and so on) may be ordered the day before the test.

A flat plate of the abdomen is taken first. This shows the presence of any radiopaque stones and can be used as a standard for which later comparisons can be made. Then, the intravenous dye is injected. The patient may feel warm, may flush, and may have a salty taste in his mouth as the dye is injected. Films are taken at 5-, 10-, 15- and 30-minute intervals. If poor kidney function is suspected, another x-ray may be taken two hours after the injection. The patient lies on the x-ray table in lithotomy position, or flat on a full-length table. A large plastic ball [40] may be strapped firmly on the abdomen to prevent the radiopaque dye from passing freely down the ureters until after the picture of the kidneys is taken. Fluids should be encouraged for 24 hours following the test to help eliminate any remaining dye and to help rehydrate the patient.

CYSTOGRAM

This is an x-ray of the bladder. It is done by inserting a catheter into the bladder, removing urine, and instilling a radiopaque dye. An x-ray of the bladder is taken. As the patient voids the dye, an x-ray of the urethra may be taken. This is called a voiding urethrogram.

CYSTOSCOPY

In this test the physician visualizes the inside of the bladder by means of a periscope-like instrument called a cystoscope. The cystoscope contains a series of mirrors to reflect the image viewed and a miniature light bulb at the tip to illuminate the inside of the urethra and bladder.[41] At the other end are a viewing window and inflow and outflow valve to allow for irrigation. The bladder is filled with clear sterile distilled water (normal saline is an electrolyte solution and would interfere with electric current) to distend its wall. This allows better visualization and protects the bladder wall from accidental perforation. The sterile water is drained through the outflow valve.

Cystoscopy is done to inspect the prostate, bladder, and ureteral orifices; to obtain specimens for tissue biopsy; and as a treatment device when cutting, crushing, or cauterizing is required. Special instruments (electrodes, crushing devices) are passed through the cystoscope. The doctor has foot pedals to control cutting or cauterizing. Cystoscopy is done anytime the patient has hematuria, so that a point of hemorrhage can be located. Hematuria is one of the earliest signs of malignant growth.

A signed permit is required for cystoscopy. The patient should be in a hydrated state to ensure continuous flow of urine. If local anesthesia is used, oral fluids are encouraged for several hours before the test, and 400 ml is given about one hour before the test. The patient is not permitted solid foods from midnight the evening before the test. If a general anesthetic is to be used, fluids can be given by vein to ensure adequate hydration. A sedative and narcotic may be given about 30 minutes before the test.

The patient is placed in lithotomy position on the table. A local anesthetic (procaine 4 per cent) may be instilled in the urethra. The cystoscope (20 to 24 French) is passed, and the doctor begins his examination. Ureteral catheters (4 to 14 French) may be passed through the cystoscope and inserted into the ureteral openings in the bladder. In this way, individual kidney specimens may be obtained. Or, a contrast medium may be instilled into each ureteral catheter and an x-ray taken. This procedure is called retrograde (against the usual direction of flow) pyelography. It is done when the information gleaned from an intravenous pyelography is insufficient.

After cystoscopy, the patient is returned to his own room. He may feel dizzy because the blood suddenly drains back into his legs when they are removed from the stirrups, and he must be protected from falls. Urine may be pink-tinged after cystoscopy, but there should be no extensive bleeding. If a contrast medium was used, the urine may be an odd color. This should be reported if it lasts more than 24 hours. A warm tub bath or sitz bath relieves the discomfort. Fluids are encouraged to lessen the irritation of concentrated urine on the lining of the urinary tract. Analgesics (e.g., codeine) may be ordered to relieve discomfort; however, the nurse should report the following symptoms immediately:

1. Sharp abdominal pain: it may mean perforation of an organ.
2. Frank bleeding: it may mean hemorrhage.
3. Anuria.
4. Chills and marked elevation of temperature: although thought to be a general systemic reaction to introduction of foreign substance and pain, it may herald infection and should be reported.

Specific Dysfunction in the Urinary System

Kidney Disease

When the kidneys are diseased, the body's natural inflammatory response is invoked. This response leads to areas of healed but nonfunctioning scar tissue. If there are repeated calls for the inflammatory response, scarred areas may become extensive, and the kidneys may be unable to perform their function adequately. The symptoms of water and electrolyte imbalance previously discussed develop. The patient may become uremic.

Kidney disease can be classified in the following way:[42]

1. Immunologic (e.g., glomerulonephritis)
2. Degenerative (e.g., ischemic nephrosclerosis)
3. Infectious (e.g., pyelonephritis)

The disease is considered acute during the initial period when symptoms are severe; subacute if complete recovery has not occurred within six to eight weeks; chronic if symptoms continue beyond one year; and latent when no symptoms are present but albumin and casts continue to be spilled in the urine.

Glomerulonephritis (Bright's Disease)

Glomerulonephritis is a nonbacterial, diffuse inflammatory disease of the kidneys. They become somewhat enlarged, congested, and tense. There is impaired blood flow through the glomerules. Glomerulonephritis always affects both kidneys. It can be acute, subacute, or chronic. If it becomes chronic, the kidney appears small, atrophied, and full of scar tissue. The disease usually affects preschool children, males more frequently than females; however, people of any age are susceptible.

Glomerulonephritis is now believed to be the result of an antigen-antibody response to infection by Group A, beta-type hemolytic *Streptococcus*. In some way, the streptococci stimulate the cells of the glomeruli to form antibodies against themselves.[43] The patient reports having had a "sore throat," or "flu" one to three weeks before the onset of renal symptoms. The streptococci themselves have never been recovered from glomerulonephritic kidneys. On examination, the patient may have puffiness about the eyes (periorbital), some ankle swelling, headaches and visual disturbances, retinal edema, breathlessness, costovertebral angle pain, and hypertension. He complains of anorexia and may have a low-grade fever. His urine may be smoky-colored and decreased in quantity. Microscopically it contains protein, red blood cells, and casts.

Some patients are totally asymptomatic, and the disease is accidentally discovered when urine is checked during a routine physical examination.

Management is primarily supportive with the goal being rest for the kidneys to give them a chance to heal and control of individual symptoms as they present themselves. For instance, fluid is restricted to less than 600 ml above urinary output if edema is present. Hypertension is treated vigorously with antihypertensive drugs such as reserpine (Serpasil). If symptoms of uremia are present, hemo- or peritoneal dialysis is done. Sometimes infection develops because there is stasis of urine behind scar tissue, and bacterial invasion occurs. If infection develops, antibiotics are administered. The patient remains in bed during the acute phase, until renal tests indicate that function has returned to normal. Diet restrictions depend on symptoms. If edema is present, sodium is restricted. Protein is usually restricted to 40 to 60 gm of complete protein a day to decrease the work load of the kidneys in excreting their metabolic end products. During the acute phase, the nurse must watch for complications that may occur if the kidneys are not quickly repaired.[44] These include cardiac failure, pulmonary edema, and increased intracranial pressure with convulsions.

As healing progresses, gradual ambulation is allowed. The patient is encouraged to rest often, avoid strenuous exercise, and keep away from people who have upper respiratory infections. No other specific limitations are prescribed. An annual physical examination with kidney function tests is stressed.

The vast majority of patients with acute glomerular nephritis (80 per cent) heal completely. About 5 per cent die of complications during the acute phase. Only 10 per cent progress to the chronic form of the disease.[45] Although chronic glomerulonephritis may follow the acute disease, most patients with the disease give no history of having had the acute form. In chronic glomerulonephritis the kidneys gradually lose their ability to concentrate urine. Fibrotic tissue increases, and both the glomeruli and the tubules eventually degenerate. The progress of chronic glomerulonephritis is unpredictable, and many patients lead normal lives for years. Ultimately, though, uremia develops.

Nephrotic Syndrome

Half the patients who have glomerulonephritis develop a severe generalized edema with puffiness about the eyes and swelling in the abdominal region.[46] There is probably an increased glomerular permeability with albuminuria, hypoalbuminemia, and hyperlipemia. With loss of protein from the blood there is a decreased osmotic pressure in the capillaries. Fluid tends to remain in the tissue spaces rather than being pulled back into the circulation, and the patient becomes generally edematous. During the nephrotic stage the physician will make judicious use of diuretics and will restrict sodium intake. The nephrotic syndrome may disappear spontaneously or may progress to uremia.

The nephrotic syndrome may develop in a "pure" form, without any history of glomerulonephritis.

Degenerative Ischemic Conditions

RENAL HYPERTENSION

Hypertension may develop as a result of a lesion in the renal blood vessels, as a result of renal disease or obstruction, or from a nonrenal cause. In any case, unchecked hypertension causes renal artery sclerosis and decreases the supply of blood to the kidneys. This is called ischemic nephrosclerosis.

THE GOLDBLATT PHENOMENON

Hypertension and kidney disease go hand in hand. The Goldblatt phenomenon attempts to explain this in this sequence: [47]

1. Occlusion of renal artery or its branches.
2. Decreased blood supply to kidneys (ischemia).

3. Ischemia triggers the release of renin (a hormone that causes protein lysis).

4. Renin hydrolyzes a blood protein to form vasopressor principle (angiotensin; hypertensin).

5. Hypertension develops.

Because a kidney may have relatively good function but still have significant stenosis, renal arteriography is done. A contrast medium is injected intravenously into the renal arteries just above their take-off point from the aorta. Rapid-sequence roentgenograms outline the vascularity of both kidneys simultaneously.[48] Medical management includes rest, sodium restriction, and the use of antihypertensive drugs such as *Rauwolfia* derivatives; however, if the hypertension is of the malignant type, developing suddenly with extremely high elevations, and is extremely difficult to control, surgical intervention is required. Stenosed arteries may be repaired, or a kidney may have to be removed to save the patient's life.

PYELONEPHRITIS

Pyelonephritis is an infectious disease of the kidneys. It occurs at any age. The bacteria gain a stronghold in the kidneys from the lower urinary tract, via the lymph, or via the blood. The kidneys respond with an inflammatory process in the glomeruli and tubules. Abscesses develop and fibrous tissue forms to wall them off. As healing occurs, scar tissue remains. If only a small area is involved, there is little loss of kidney function; however, a severe infection or repeated bouts of infection cause so much abscess formation and leave so much scar tissue that the functioning areas of kidney tissue are depleted. Pyelonephritis can be acute or chronic. In its chronic form, pyelonephritis causes a slow, insidious decrease in the functioning ability of the kidneys, with ultimate renal failure and death. It is the renal lesion that is most frequently associated with uremia.[49] There is a spontaneous cure of chronic pyelonephritis in 20 per cent of the cases.[50]

Pyelonephritis is extremely common clinically. It is second only to respiratory disease in frequency.[51] It is seen four times more frequently in women than in men because of the short female urethra and the ease with which microorganisms gain access to it from the vagina and rectum. *Escherichia coli* and *Streptococcus faecalis* are usually the culprits. One or both kidneys may be involved. Although the patient may be asymptomatic, he usually experiences some urologic difficulty. There may be a dull pain and tenderness in the area of the involved kidney (flank pain) from inflammatory swelling. The patient may state that he has "a backache." If the disease is blood-borne, there may be chills and a spiking fever. There may be frequency, dysuria, and/or nocturia. Pus and pathogenic microorganisms are found in the urine. An increase in leukocytes is found in the blood.

Management of Pyelonephritis. The patient is put to bed to rest. Liberal fluid intake is ordered to keep the urine dilute. A urine culture is done to identify the causative organism, and a sensitivity test is done to determine which antimicrobial agent will be most effective. Antibiotics must be used for at least ten days, sometimes up to six weeks, to bring the infection under control. If untreated or treated for too short a time, acute pyelonephritis may become chronic pyelonephritis! Follow-up cultures are done to determine the effectiveness of the drug. Sometimes the antibiotic does not come into contact with the pathogenic microorganisms because of the presence of lesions and scar tissue. In this case, the symptoms of infection may subside, only to "flare up" again at a later date. Polymyxin, neomycin, and bacitracin are toxic to the kidneys and are not used.[52] If sulfa drugs are used, intake and output must be checked carefully. Even the most soluble sulfa products cause crystalluria and hematuria if urinary output is not adequate. The nurse must make sure the patient is drinking adequate quantities of fluid.

Because most common bacteria are killed at a pH of less than 5.0 (acid), an acidifying agent may be given. Mandelic acid is an example. The acidity of the urine can be easily checked with nitrazine paper strips.

As soon as possible, x-ray studies must be made to determine whether an obstruction is causing stasis of urine and infection. Pending removal of an obstruction, catheter drainage is essential. The catheter must "bypass" the obstruction so that urine has a way out.

When pyelonephritis is chronic, the goal is to arrest the infection and try to slow down the progress of the disease. The patient's resistance becomes severely decreased, and he must be protected from further infection. Vitamins are often given. A course of antibiotic treatment that lasts for one week out of every month may be tried.

OBSTRUCTIONS IN THE URINARY SYSTEM: OBSTRUCTIVE UROPATHY

Any obstruction to the free flow of urine out of the body can ultimately cause irreversible damage to the kidneys. The areas behind the obstruction are affected. First, there is stasis of urine behind the obstruction. The static fluid provides an optimum environment for bacterial growth, and infection develops. Second, the increase in fluid behind the obstruction causes an increased "back pressure" and there is distention. A distended ureter with increased fluid and pressure is called *hydroureter*. A distended kidney is called *hydronephrosis*. There is pain from the "stretch" on the organ. If the obstruction is not removed, or temporary bypass drainage established with a catheter or tube, there can be permanent damage to the functioning tissue of the kidneys. Strictures, stones, tumors, and encroachment on the urethra by an enlarged prostate gland are all examples of obstruction.

PROSTATIC HYPERTROPHY (PROSTATISM)

The most common cause of obstruction within the urinary system is an enlarged prostate gland that impinges on the urethra and the bladder outlet and prevents the free passage of urine out of the body. Sixty-five per cent of all men over 50 have some prostatic enlargement.[53] Of those seeking medical help for the symptoms of prostatism 80 to 88 per cent have a benign enlargement, and 12 to 20 per cent have malignant hypertrophy.[54] The cause of hyperplasia is not always known, though decreased hormone levels associated with the aging process are believed to be implicated.

The prostate gland is one of the accessory structures in the male reproductive system. It is made up of glandular and muscular tissue and surrounds the proximal part of the male urethra. The urethra enters the base of the prostate gland and descends through it. In the adult, about 2 ml of prostatic secretion is produced every day (more during sexual activity). This secretion is found in the early fraction of the male ejaculate and is beneficial to sperm motility. The total ejaculate, called semen, is made up of sperm and the secretions that are added along the way to assist the sperm. Secretions from the epididymis help ripen sperm; from the seminal vesicles stimulate motility and aid in nutrition of sperm; from the bulbourethral glands provide an alkaline medium for the sperm; and from the prostate gland aid in motility of sperm.

Symptoms of Prostatic Hypertrophy. The symptoms are caused by gradual impingement of the enlarged gland on the neck of the bladder. The man first realizes that he must void more often (frequency) and that there is a smaller urinary stream with each voiding. He may have difficulty starting the stream. He finds that the desire to void becomes painfully necessary (urgency) and may be accompanied by a burning sensation and bleeding (hematuria). He is often awakened more than once during the night to void (nocturia). As the impingement increases there is stasis of urine in the bladder, and he may develop a bladder infection (cystitis) with systemic symptoms (chills, fever, and so on). If prostatic enlargement is not diagnosed and treated early, acute urinary retention with ultimate destruction to kidney tissue may ensue.

How Is the Diagnosis Made? How Is the Patient Prepared for Surgery? Every man should have an annual physical examination. A rectal examination is a part of this physical. By inserting a gloved, lubricated finger into the rectum the physician can palpate the prostate gland. The patient is draped and placed in the knee-chest position. The female nurse usually leaves the room after the patient is draped and positioned. If an enlarged gland is suspected, the physician orders other confirming tests. He will catheterize the bladder to see if there is residual urine. He may order a blood urea nitrogen or nonprotein nitrogen test to determine adequacy of kidney function. A cystoscopy is done to determine the extent of prostate impingement on the bladder neck. Renal function tests, cystoscopy, and presence of residual urine help the physician determine the need for preoperative catheterization to provide an outlet for trapped urine, and help him determine how immediate the need for surgery is. *The physician is always concerned about the possible damage to the kidneys from the obstruction to the free flow of urine.*

A way out must be provided for trapped urine. If retention of urine is of short duration (the physician learns this from a careful history), straight catheter drainage of the bladder is usually instituted. If, however, the retention has been chronic, and a residual amount of 1,000 to 1,500 ml is suspected, decompression catheter drainage will be ordered. Gradual removal of urine, against gravity, helps prevent bleeding from rupture of capillaries in the bladder lining, helps the bladder muscles retain their tone, and decreases the chance of shock caused by the sudden decrease of the mechanical pressure of a filled bladder on blood vessels. If this "long-term" mechanical pressure is suddenly released, the abdominal vessels and bladder mucosal vessels fill with blood, decrease the blood to the brain, and fainting results.[55] A Y tube is attached to a standard at a level prescribed by the physician (high 5 to 8 in. above bladder level; medium 3 to 5 in. above bladder level; low at bladder level).[56] One arm of the Y tube is attached to the catheter tubing and one arm to the drainage bottle. The center arm of the Y is left open as an air outlet. The catheter is usually attached to the high decompression drainage first, and then the level is lowered an inch at a time (usually every hour), until the catheter is ultimately connected to straight drainage. (See Fig. 21–10.) The patient is made ready for surgical removal of the prostate gland by elimination of infection, adequate intake of fluids, a well-balanced diet, and rest. Unless surgical intervention is of an emergency nature, an attempt is made to have the patient in optimum condition before the surgery is done.

Surgical Intervention for an Enlarged Prostate. Unless radical surgery is indicated for cancer, the procedures are all subcapsular. The gland is "shelled out" and the capsule is left behind.[57] Goals of surgery include relief of symptoms and the ability to hold urine from three to five hours.

Transurethral Resection (T.U.R.). Transurethral resection is a closed procedure that usually takes place in the cystoscopy room of the operating suite. Although an incision is not made, aseptic technique is adhered to. The procedure takes about one hour. The patient is anesthetized with a general or a local anesthetic and is placed in lithotomy position. He is grounded against shock with a lubricated plate placed under his hips. A resectoscope is passed through the urethra. It is similar to a cystoscope but is a bit larger and contains a loop for cutting and cauterization. The

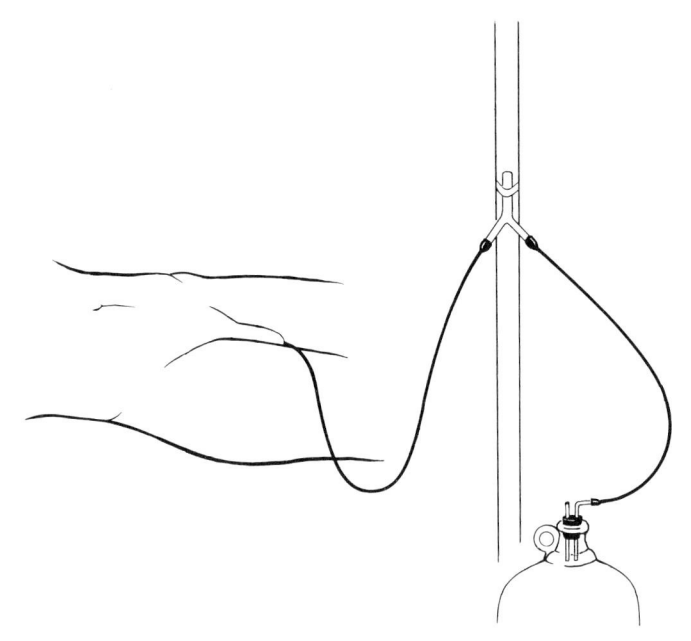

FIGURE 21–10. Decompression drainage. (From K. Shafer, J. Sawyer, A. McCluskey, and E. Beck, *Medical Surgical Nursing*, 4th ed., 1967. Reprinted with the permission of the C. V. Mosby Co., St. Louis, p. 448.)

electric current to the loop is controlled with a foot pedal. The bladder is filled with an irrigating solution through an opening in the resectoscope. A non electrolyte solution such as sterile water may be used because it is less likely to interfere with the electric current used for cauterization in the procedure. Filling the bladder decreases the risk of perforation of its walls. Pieces of enlarged gland are sliced away in bits, fall into the bladder, and are washed out with the irrigating solution. Bleeding is controlled with electric fulguration (cautery).

Transurethral resection is selected when prostatic enlargement is to the lobe directly surrounding the urethra. It is most frequently used for elderly men who would not withstand an "open" procedure. It can be used only as a palliative procedure when malignancy is present because there is uncertain removal of all of the hypertrophied tissue. It is not suitable as a curative procedure for early cancer. The procedure is technically difficult and requires special skill on the part of the surgeon. There is always the chance that the bladder may be accidentally perforated. Mortality with T.U.R. is low, and the patient usually has a mild convalescence.

The patient goes to the recovery room with a straight catheter connected to drainage, or with a "three-way catheter" that provides continuous gentle irrigation of the bladder with an antiseptic solution, e.g., neosporin genitourinary irrigant in 1,000 ml normal saline. Never irrigate a retention catheter unless specifically ordered, because the pressure of the irrigant may cause hemorrhage. Sometimes a Foley-type catheter with a large (30-ml) inflation bag is inserted. The inflated bag is pulled down so that it rests in the prostatic fossa and its pressure provides a means of controlling bleeding (hemostasis). The bag puts pressure on the internal urinary sphincter and may make the patient feel as though he has to void, even though the catheter is draining urine for him. Explaining the reason to him helps decrease his concern about it. He should not try to "void around the catheter" as this increases the discomfort. The catheter must be checked frequently for patency; it may become blocked by blood clots and would then obstruct the flow of urine. The catheter is removed as soon as the urine is clear of blood, usually between the third and seventh postoperative day. If antispasmodic drugs are used to control bladder spasms, e.g., methantheline (Banthine), they are discontinued a day before the catheter is removed so that the bladder resumes its muscle tonus. A bladder spasm is the painful contraction of the detrusor muscle. Some spasms accompany T.U.R. They should decrease in intensity by the end of the first or second postoperative day.

Some hematuria will be present in the early postoperative period; however, copious amounts of bright red blood mean hemorrhage, and the physician should be called immediately. To decrease the risk of postoperative hemorrhage the patient may be given a laxative for three days after surgery so that he does not strain at stool. Straining may start bleeding from the fossa. Enemas and rectal thermometers are discouraged during the first postoperative week.

Because large amounts of irrigating solutions are used and may be absorbed there is always the possibility of hemodilution. The patient may show signs of increased blood volume (elevated blood pressure; moist bubbly sound to breathing) and hyponatremia (restlessness, apprehension, weakness, faintness, muscle fatigue), and this should be reported to the physician. If these symptoms do not present themselves, a large intake of fluid is usually ordered. The fluid ensures a constant passage of fluid over the bladder mucosa and helps lessen irritation and resultant discomfort.

If the patient should suddenly develop severe abdominal or pelvic pain, it may mean the bladder has been perforated and its vessels are leaking blood into the peritoneal cavity. This should be reported immediately!

The patient is discharged about one week after surgery with instructions not to do any heavy lifting or vigorous exercise for about three weeks. He is also told to call the physician if he notices any bleeding. Secondary hemorrhage sometimes occurs during the second to fourth postoperative week as coagulated vessels slough.

Open Surgical Techniques for Removing Enlarged Prostate Glands. The three open techniques are suprapubic prostatectomy, perineal prostatectomy, and retropubic prostatectomy. All allow complete removal of hypertrophied tissue. Perineal prostatectomy allows total removal of the gland and its capsule and is suited for early cancer cure.

Suprapubic Prostatectomy. This technique allows wide exposure of the bladder and is used when a large gland extends into the bladder or when stones or other conditions complicate the picture. A low midline incision is made directly over the bladder, the bladder is opened, and through an incision into the urethral mucosa the prostate tissue is enucleated (scooped out). The technique is relatively simple for the surgeon. It is not suitable for malignancy.[58] To control bleeding, the physician may use a hemostatic device in the prostatic fossa, e.g., a retention catheter with a 30-ml inflation bag pulled down into the fossa, or gauze packing. Postoperative hemorrhage is often difficult to control (the bladder is very vascular), and the mortality risk to the patient is increased because of this. Because the bladder is incised, there is a surgical urinary fistula that drains urine for a few days to a month. This suprapubic wound is drained with a tissue drain or with a cystostomy tube. The amount of drainage should be recorded and the patient's skin should be protected. The suprapubic wound is a potential site for bacterial invasion. Infection would further delay an already lengthy (about a month) healing time. The causative organism of infection is often *Bacillus pyocyaneus.* If infection occurs, drainage appears a light bluish-green. Special wound irrigations with antiseptic solutions will more than likely be ordered.

The suprapubic catheter is removed about five days after surgery and the urethral catheter about ten days after surgery.[59] Some urologists do not use packing or catheters to provide hemostasis because they feel these devices increase bleeding by preventing normal contraction of the fossa.[60] Or, they may use these devices but remove them in 24 to 72 hours.

Analgesics and antispasmodics are used to control pain. The total convalescent period is longer than that for T.U.R.

Retropubic Prostatectomy. A low abdominal incision similar to that used for a suprapubic prostatectomy is made. The bladder is retracted (it is not incised!), and the hypertrophied prostate is removed through an incision into the anterior prostatic capsule. There is a relative absence of postoperative pain with this technique because bladder spasms do not occur. Bleeding is not severe, and the indwelling catheter does not get clogged. There is no urinary fistula, and the convalescent period is short and mild. The patient usually has a Penrose drain in the tissues of the operative site. It is removed when all drainage has stopped. The urethral catheter is usually removed about five days after surgery.

Perineal Prostatectomy. A perineal incision is made (between the scrotum and the rectum) with the patient in lithotomy or jackknife position. The posterior capsule of the prostate gland is incised, and the hypertrophied tissue is removed. This technique is often selected for elderly men with very large glands who are considered poor operative risks for suprapubic prostatectomy. The position on the table, though, may cause circulatory embarrassment. A frozen section biopsy of suspicious tissue is done while the patient is on the table. If cells are malignant, a radical procedure can be done at the same time. This technique allows total removal of the gland for early cancer.[61] It is a technically difficult procedure with the ever-present danger of damage to the rectum and to the external sphincter. Mortality is low, and convalescence mild. The patient returns with a urethral catheter and a tissue drain in the perineal area.

RADICAL PROCEDURE FOR MALIGNANCY [62]

Most cancerous lesions are adjacent to the rectal wall and can be detected prior to symptoms by a rectal examination. A biopsy may be done by needle aspiration. A long needle is inserted through the perineum. A syringe is attached and material is aspirated. Or, a biopsy may be done through a surgical incision into the perineum. If malignant cells are found, a radical perineal resection follows. This involves removal of the prostate gland and its capsule, the seminal vesicles, and adjacent tissue. The remaining urethra is anastomosed to the bladder neck. The patient may be incontinent, impotent, and sterile after the procedure. If the cancer is inoperable, a bilateral orchiectomy may be done. This is the removal of both testicles (castration) to eliminate male hormones (androgens). The procedure is palliative. It seems to slow down the progress of the malignancy and decrease pain.

For all the open surgical procedures, catheter and tube drainage is used. (See pp. 200–201.)

OBSTRUCTION OF THE URINARY SYSTEM BY CALCULI (UROLITHIASIS)

Calculi, commonly called "stones," are hardened deposits of inorganic salts. The salts often settle around tiny particles of pus, blood, tumor, or bacteria. Or, they may precipitate about a catheter. Oddly enough, stones may form in a sterile as well as a nonsterile medium.

Calculi are identified according to their chemical composition. Most calculi contain either calcium, e.g., calcium oxalate and calcium phosphate, or a protein derivative, e.g., cystine and uric acid. Those stones containing calcium usually precipitate in an alkaline urine. Those derived from protein precipitate in acid urine.

Stones form in the renal pelvis, the ureters, and the bladder. They may be minute (about the size of the head of a pin) or large. If they are 0.5 cm or larger, the usually do not pass out of the body spontaneously. No chemical has been found to successfully dissolve stones while they are in the body.[63]

Laboratory analysis of the stones is done to determine their mineral composition.

Factors Implicated in Cause of Calculi. Although a single cause has not been established, calculi are usually related to inborn errors in metabolism (excess uric acid excretion in gout); to hormonal imbalance (e.g., excess calcium excretion in hyperparathyroidism); to severe vitamin A deficiency; to changes in urinary pH toward the alkaline side; to infection (infection and calculi coexist); and to immobility. Immobility causes stasis of urine in the lower renal calyces. The human organism is designed to function in the upright rather than the supine position. Stasis provides an optimum medium for bacterial growth. Some bacteria are "urea splitters." They break up urea and form ammonia, and this converts the urinary pH toward the alkaline side. Salts precipitate, and stones develop.

Symptoms of Calculi. Some stones are "silent." They produce no pain at all. Others produce varying degrees of ache and pain in the flank area. The patient may have urinary frequency, difficulty voiding in the usual position, retention, pyuria, and hematuria if the stone irritates or tears the urinary mucosa. As the body attempts to excrete the stone spontaneously (90 per cent are excreted this way,[64]) the patient has attacks of severe colic-like pain in the flank and abdominal area. This comes from violent contractions of the ureter as it attempts to dislodge a stone that is temporarily "stuck" and push it along its way. The pain is excruciating and the patient "doubles up." He cannot lie still and usually must get up and walk around. The walking actually helps pass the stone. It should be saved for chemical analysis. Analgesics such as Demerol and morphine are used for the pain; smooth-muscle depressants such as methantheline (Banthine) relieve the spasms. The patient should be encouraged to rest after the attack. It sometimes takes two or three attacks before the stone is passed.

The diagnosis of calculi is made by a combination of history, flat plate of the abdomen (calcium-containing stones show up this way), intravenous pyelography, and sometimes cystoscopy. Cystoscopy is done if the kidney cannot concentrate the contrast medium because of disease and the physician wishes to instill the dye retrograde fashion through a ureteral catheter, or if he wishes to leave a ureteral catheter in place for 24 hours to dilate the ureter and facilitate passage of the stone. Or, the catheter may "bypass" the stone and remain in the renal pelvis to ensure a nonobstructed exit for the urine. This makes the patient a better surgical risk because there is no urinary stasis with infection. The ureteral catheter(s) is marked "left" or "right" with adhesive tape. It exits through the urethra and is attached to a drainage bag. It must be observed frequently for patency because it is so narrow and may easily be blocked with pus, and so forth. The patient is kept in a low Fowler position to prevent dislodgment of the catheter. It is irrigated only by order and is never irrigated with more than 5 ml of sterile solution. That is all the kidney pelvis can hold safely.

Some small, soft bladder stones may actually be removed through the cystoscope. If these procedures are anticipated, the patient receives a general anesthetic and must realize that open surgery will be done immediately if the cystoscopic procedure is not successful. An instrument called a *lithotrite* may be used to crush bladder stones (litholapaxy), through the transurethral approach. Or, specially designed catheters wtih expanding baskets or loops may be passed to snare the stones. These procedures always carry the danger of rupture with them. Larger stones are removed through open surgical procedures, e.g., ureterolithotomy. The word describes the area of the incision and the removal of stones, e.g., pyelolithomy: into the renal pelvis; nephrolithotomy: into the kidney tissue; cystolitotomy: into the bladder. Occasionally the kidney must be split to remove a stone that fills the entire renal pelvis (staghorn calculus).

Medical and Nursing Management. After the physician has determined the presence of stones in a particular area, he must find out what they are made of. *All urine must be strained.* The nurse may do this through two opened 4-by-8 gauze squares. The stones are sent to the laboratory for chemical analysis. The physician may want to alter the urinary pH if he finds that the inorganic salts are precipitating in either an acid or alkaline urine. He can do this with medication, e.g., sodium acid phosphate to acidify the urine or sodium bicarbonate to alkalinize it; or he may modify the diet. For a calcium-containing stone he may give a drug that binds calcium, e.g., sodium phytate (Rencal) or aluminum hydroxide gel (Amphogel), and restrict dietary intake of calcium to 250 mg per day. For a phosphate-containing stone he may give the patient sodium acid phosphate or methionine and a diet that leaves an acid ash, e.g., one high in meat, fish, eggs; low in certain fruits and vegetables. For uric acid stones he may use a uricosuric agent, e.g., probenecid (Benemid), and an alkaline ash diet, e.g., one high in vegetables and fruits. A simple exclusion of some foods often does the trick. Citrus fruits and carbonated beverages may be eliminated to acidify the urine; large quantities of orange juice may be ordered to alkalinize it. In any case, the patient's nutritional needs must be balanced. Exclusion of one type of food must be replaced with another similar in essential nutrients.

Encourage the patient to drink 2,500 to 3,000 ml of fluid each day. Adequate fluids decrease the precipitation of salts and the chance of stone formation.

Ensure adequate mobility so that stasis of urine does not develop. If the patient cannot get out of bed, make sure he changes his position frequently. Schedule a visit to his room every one or two hours to guide this. Frequent range-of-motion exercises should be done. The physician may order the use of a tilt table or a Circ-O-Lectric bed for long-term immobilization.

The patient must be observed for any signs of infection. Urinary tract infections and stones often coexist. Check the temperatures carefully; count the pulse for one full minute.

Even if the patient has had his calculi removed surgically, the basic cause of their formation may still be in operation. He may still be "a stone former." He should leave the hospital understanding the need for medical supervision, adequate daily fluid intake, exercise, and knowledge of any dietary restrictions.

Pre- and Postoperative Management of Any Patient Having Surgery upon the Urinary System

The patient is made the best possible surgical risk preoperatively. Infection is controlled. Water and electrolyte levels are studied and balanced. Temporary urinary drainage may be established to ensure the free flow of urine out of the body. The preoperative preparation is similar to surgical preparation for any major procedure. With the exception of cystoscopy, the bladder should be empty.

An operative permit must be signed, and if a sterilization procedure is contemplated, e.g., bilateral oophorectomy or orchiectomy, an additional permit for sterilization must be signed.

Surgical Approach and Shave

The patient is shaved according to the approach to be utilized. Most hospital procedure books diagram the specific areas to shave. The usual approaches and areas to be shaved are: a flank incision just under the diaphragm for surgery of the kidney or upper ureter: shave skin on affected side from spine to beyond midline anteriorly and from nipple line to pubic area; a suprapubic incision in the lower abdomen above the symphysis pubis for bladder surgery or lower urethral surgery: shave from below breasts to and including pubic area in female; from nipple line to and including pubic area in male; for perineal, urethral, penile, or scrotal incision: shave from the umbilicus to and including the pubic area, perineum, and adjacent thighs in female; include the penis and scrotum in the male.

The patient is allowed nothing by mouth from the evening meal the day before surgery. He is medicated one-half hour before surgery usually with a sedative and atropine.

Naming the Urologic Procedure

As previously mentioned, the name of the surgery designates the organ or area to be operated upon, e.g., *nephrectomy:* removal of a kidney; *heminephrectomy:* removal of half a kidney; *calycectomy:* removal of calyces, e.g., to eradicate stone-forming areas; *ureterotomy:* incision into the ureter; *cystectomy:* removal of the bladder; *prostatectomy:* removal of the prostate tissue; and so forth.

Major Points in the Care of the Patient Following Urologic Surgery

1. Know which body cavity is being intubated with a catheter, tube, or drain. Know what drainage should come from each catheter. Make sure it is open (patent). Record drainage from each catheter separately.

FOR URINARY DRAINAGE

A variety of catheter tips are used to drain urine. They ensure free flow of urine out of the body. The catheter may bypass the operative area until healing occurs. It may be inserted through a suprapubic incision, e.g., a nephrostomy tube inserted into the kidney. A catheter may not only drain urine, it may also "splint" the wound, e.g., a ureterostomy tube. As soon as the patient returns from the operating room, the catheter should be connected to its drainage collection system. Do not leave it clamped. The end of the drainage tubing should never be immersed in urine. The catheter should be clamped temporarily and the drainage tubing "milked" away from the patient, toward the collection device, to rid it of any sediment that might block it. The catheter should be anchored to the patient to prevent pull and tension on it. If tape is used

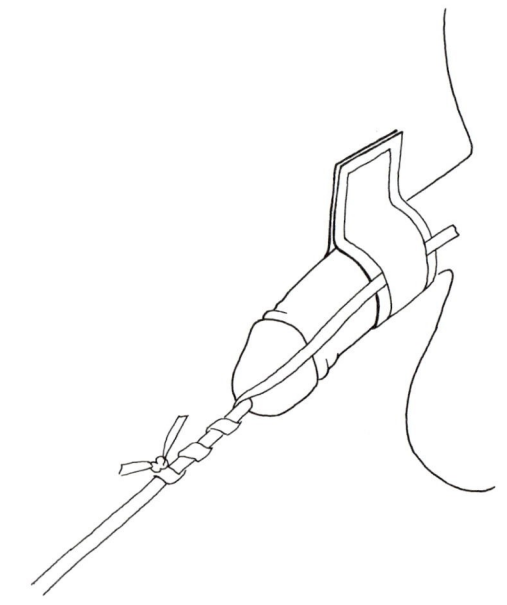

FIGURE 21–11. Straight catheter anchored in male urethra.

on the penis, the area should be shaved and benzoin tincture applied. The edges of the tape should be brought together beyond the penis to allow for an erection.[65] (See Fig. 21–11.) The drainage tubing should be pinned to the sheet.

Do not allow tubing to become kinked, compressed, or bent at right angles.

Do not irrigate unless there is a written order; do not instill more than the cavity can hold. Instill no more than 8 to 10 ml in a ureteral catheter, no more than 5 to 100 ml in a urethral catheter.

Do not force fluid through the catheter; allow it to flow in by gravity.

Record output for each catheter separately.

FOR SEROUS DRAINAGE

Drains may be inserted into a tissue space to help draw out serous secretions. They should not drain urine. A Penrose drain is usually positioned in the empty space left following nephrectomy. Tissue drains may be easily lost into the wound. Pin a sterile safety pin to the exposed portion.

FOR EXTERNAL WOUND DRAINAGE: PROTECT THE SKIN

If drainage is expected from the wound site, a catheter may be placed in the superficial wound tissues and incorporated in the dressings, or it may simply be incorporated in the dressing. The dressing, then, does not have to be disturbed for changing as frequently. Some urinary drainage may come from the wound. It should be minimal if a nephrostomy or pyelostomy tube is in place. The physician should be notified if the drainage is copious, if it contains blood or pus (any sediment), or if it has an odor. The skin should be protected by keeping dressings dry and by using protective ointments such as zinc oxide, specifically ordered.

2. *Watch for postoperative hemorrhage from the catheters or from the wound site.* The kidney parenchyma is highly vascular; hemorrhage is always a possibility. The urine is usually dark red immediately after surgery. It gradually lightens to a pink color and by the end of the second postoperative day will be amber to yellow. It should not be bright red or viscid or contain clots. It should not suddenly change from a light color to a darker red. The dressing should not be bloody. There are two danger periods when hemorrhage may occur. The first, and most serious is immediately after surgery. The second is between the eighth and tenth postoperative days when tissue and coagulated blood vessels slough. The ambulatory patient may be returned to bed for those three days.

3. *Feeding.* Usually the patient is not permitted anything by mouth during the operative day. He may have a nasogastric tube inserted to decrease vomiting and distention. The abdominal distention may be the

result of paralytic ileus following pain of surgery. Oral fluids are begun gradually. They should not be iced because iced fluids may produce flatus. The patient should be observed for distention. Foods are added gradually, and the patient is usually eating a full diet by the third postoperative day.

4. *Make sure the patient turns and deep-breathes at least every two hours.* This is likely to be painful if a flank incision was made because of its proximity to the thoracic cavity and diaphragm. Splint the incision with your hands or with a draw sheet and encourage the deep breathing. Hypostatic pneumonia and atelectasis are potential hazards if these precautions are not taken. Most patients have no restrictions concerning their position and should be encouraged to move about frequently. The exception is the patient who has a nephrostomy tube in place. To prevent kinks or compression of this tube, the patient can be "tilted" toward his side. Be sure all catheters are patent and are not accidentally kinked or compressed while the patient is turning.

5. *Control of pain.* Most patients will have some pain, and analgesics are ordered for about 48 hours postsurgery. If the side-lying hyperextended position was used, as for renal procedures, the patient will feel "achy." Supporting the back with pillows helps to relieve the ache.

6. *Keep the patient comfortably warm and check his temperature.* Large volumes of irrigating solutions may have been used and the patient is likely to be chilled.

7. *Encourage walking rather than sitting in a chair.* Most patients will be out of bed within 24 hours after the surgery. Sitting in a chair encourages stasis of blood in the venous system and should be discouraged.

8. *If a nephrectomy was performed, the pleura may have been accidentally perforated. Observe for signs of pneumothorax: sudden, sharp chest pain; dyspnea; diaphoresis; shock.*

Urinary Diversion Procedures

When the bladder is removed (cystectomy), another route out must be found for the urinary drainage. The ureters can be transplanted into several areas.

ILEAL CONDUIT (ILEAL BLADDER)

The most frequently used procedure at this time is the formation of an ileal conduit through which urine is excreted. A segment of the ileum is resected from the intestine, leaving its blood and nerve supply intact. This segment is sutured closed at one end, and the other end is brought to the skin. A pouch is thus formed. Both ureters are transplanted into this new conduit. Urine is not stored in it, but is passed through it. The remaining intestine is reanastomosed. It is not in any way connected to the ileal conduit. Urine is excreted through the ileal conduit; stool is excreted by the regular route. The bowel is prepared for surgery by use of enemas, cathartics, and usually sulfonamide preparations. The patient is given a clear liquid diet for three days before surgery. Vitamins may be given.

After Surgery. When the patient returns from surgery he has a long vertical or transverse abdominal incision. The male patient will also have a perineal incision because a radical perineal prostatectomy is performed simultaneously. There may be a catheter inserted through the ileostomy opening to provide for urinary drainage. The physician may dilate the stoma with this catheter or with a sterile, well-lubricated finger cot daily in the initial postoperative period, and then weekly, to ensure an open passageway free of strictures. The patient learns to do this himself. Because the ileum secretes mucus, there may be an order for gentle irrigation of the catheter. Or, instead of a catheter, a temporary plastic ileostomy bag may be placed over the stoma immediately after surgery to collect and drain urine. It is like a colostomy bag. (See Fig. 21–12.) The nurse measures the stoma size and cuts the opening in the bag a bit larger than the stoma so that it is not irritated by the adhesive backing. The protective covering is peeled off to expose the sticky surface, and the bag is sealed in position around the stoma. It is connected to a usual urinary collection device attached to the bottom of the bed. These temporary bags are used until the stoma shrinks to a normal size, about three to six weeks later. At that time the patient can be fitted with a permanent-style appliance with an opening that is custom-cut for him. There are rubber models available or semidisposable vinyl bags. The patient will develop a distinct preference for one type of bag depending on the ease with which it can be handled and put on independently. Strap-on models using a strap around the waist give an added sense of security. The permanent bag requires use of a cement, e.g., Skin-Bond Cement, on the skin and on the appliance. When they are pressed together, a leakproof seal is formed. A solvent such as Uni-Solve must be used to remove the appliance. The appliance is left on the body (though emptied regularly!) for several days without change. The patient should have two appliances so that one can be in use while the other is being aired. A twisted hanger-like device fits in the bag and keeps its rubber sides separated. The bag must also be deodorized. It is soaked in a deodorant-detergent solution such as Uri-Kleen or a homemade deodorant solution such as 4 tablespoons of vinegar in 1 pt of water, for ten minutes. A few drops of a concentrated liquid deodorant, e.g., Banish, is placed in the tail spout of the appliance to help stop odor between changes and emptyings and to help dissolve caked salt deposits around the outlet. Spray-on tincture of benzoin can be used on the skin surrounding the stoma to protect it and create a base for the cement substance. The skin around the stoma should be gently but thoroughly washed when the appliance is changed. The patient should

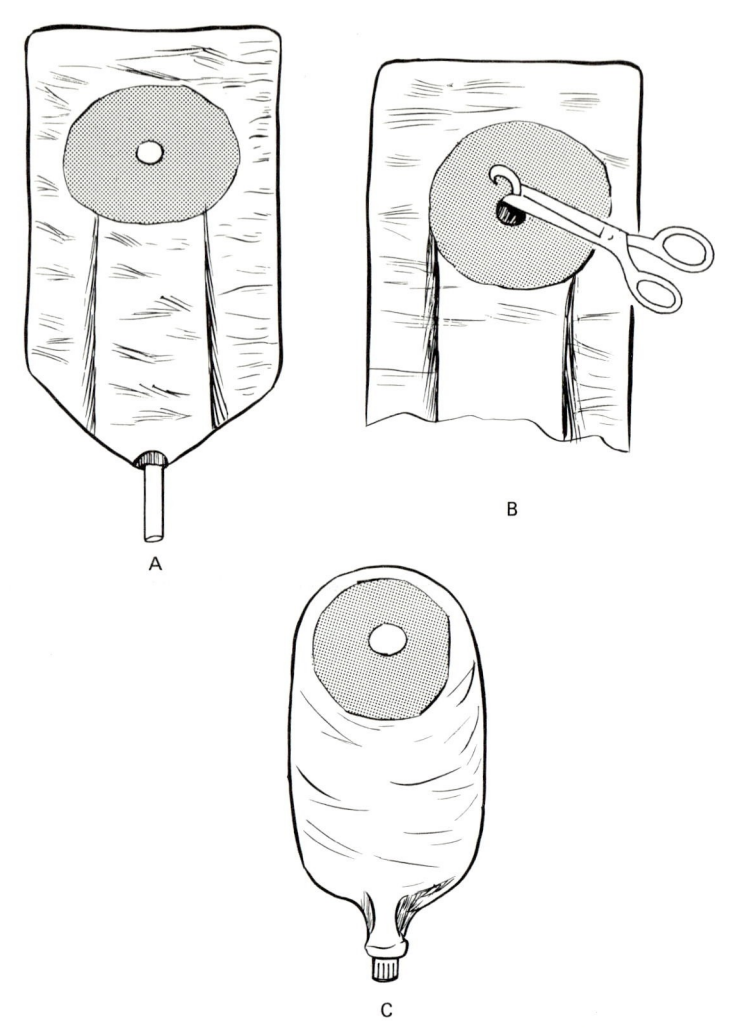

FIGURE 21–12. A. Temporary urinary drainage bag for ileal conduit. B. Protective backing is cut to fit stoma size. Backing is peeled off. Exposed adhesive surface is then placed on skin around stoma. C. Permanent urinary drainage bag designed to fit healed stoma. (Courtesy, United Surgical Corp., Largo, Fla.)

sit in a tub of water to cleanse and soothe the bud. A liquid hexachlorophene-containing substance, e.g., Liquid Ostomy soap, can be used. The bag is emptied by turning the screw at the bottom of it. The physician may want the bag unscrewed, attached to tubing, and allowed to drain into a bottle during sleep.

The female patient may cut a hole in her girdle for the stoma. The nurse must sense the patient's readiness to learn about his appliance and its care and begin teaching at this point.

Unless specifically limited by the physician, the patient with an ileal conduit can participate in sports, including swimming.

Points to remember in the Postoperative Period.

1. The bag should always be emptied before it is completely full so that backup pressure does not develop.

2. The nurse must observe for signs of distention of the ileal conduit. Distention might cause the suture line to rupture. She watches for decreased urinary output, abdominal pain, and so on.

3. The nurse must observe for signs of peritonitis from leakage of urine or fecal material into the peritoneal cavity (fever, abdominal pain, and boardlike rigidity). This is an emergency that requires further surgical intervention.

4. When allowed, the patient should be encouraged to drink adequate amounts of fluid (e.g., 2,500 to 3,000 ml per day) and to walk about. Activity favors fecal and urinary evacuation.

OTHER URINARY DIVERSION PROCEDURES

Cutaneous Transplant. In this procedure the ureters are transplanted directly into the skin of the abdomen, leaving two permanently draining fistulas, on either side of the abdomen or both on the same side. The ends of the ureters are rolled and attached to the skin in such a way that a circle of mucosal lining is exposed to the air. These are called ureteral buds.[66] The ureters are initially drained with catheters. Later, they are covered with special cups or, more recently, with a rubber flange that is cemented around the ureteral stoma and can remain in place for several days, and a detachable cap that is removed as frequently as necessary for cleaning the stoma and the inside of the cap. (See Fig. 21–13.)

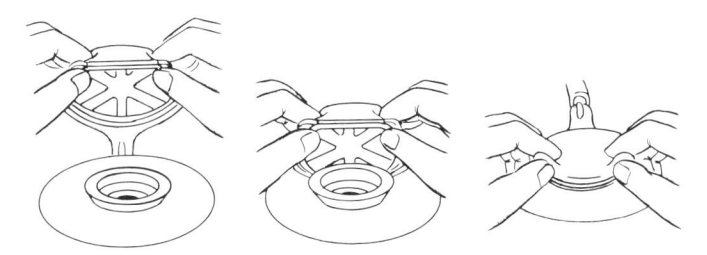

FIGURE 21–13. Cutaneous ureterostomy appliance. The flange is cemented around the stoma. The cap can be removed to cleanse stoma. (Courtesy, United Surgical Corp., Largo, Fla.)

Ureteral Intestinal Anastomosis. In these procedures, the ureters are transplanted somewhere in the intestinal tract. For example, they can be transplanted into the sigmoid colon (ureterosigmoidoscopy) or into the terminal end of the ileum (ureteroileostomy). The patient voids and defecates through the anus. As the bowel begins to adjust to being a reservoir for urine, the patient begins to be able to tell when he has to void.

These procedures may result in ascending infection of the urinary system with fecal content or a backup of urine because the rectum has a normally higher pressure than the bladder and the kidney is poorly emptied. There is also an electrolyte problem because the bowel reabsorbs electrolytes that would have normally been excreted by the kidney. The patient may develop metabolic acidosis. He may lose potassium through diarrheal stool or through the need to have chloride re-excreted after it is wrongly absorbed by the intestine. The chloride latches on to cations like potassium for this re-excretion, and there is a resultant potassium depletion. People with normal renal function can withstand the absorption of electrolytes without significant changes.[67] However, they should be encouraged to void every two to three hours to limit absorption time.

KIDNEY TRANSPLANTATION

Since the 1960's kidney transplantation has become a therapeutic alternative for the patient who has chronic, near-fatal renal insufficiency. Because the surgery involves the kidney of another person (a homograft), it is recognized by the patient's body as a "nonself," [68] and a rejection crisis is always expected, unless the donor and the recipient are fortunate enough to be identical twins. To be a candidate for this type of surgery the patient should have irreversible renal disease with a life expectancy limited to a few weeks or months. He should have no major element of infection at the time of transplantation and should have a normal lower urinary tract. Diseases secondary to the renal failure (e.g., cardiac and vascular diseases) should be deemed reversible. Although best results seem to occur if the patient is under 35, many older people have had successful transplantation.

A suitable donor should be "genetically favorable" to the recipient. Identical twins are ideal. The least number of rejection problems in nonidentical donor-recipient combinations occur when the donor is the parent or the sibling of the recipient. (Parent to child seems best.) The greatest number of problems occur when the donor is unrelated to the recipient; however, tissue typing helps predetermine compatibility by establishing which white blood cell antigens present in the donor might invoke a strong antibody response in the recipient. This is critically important when the donor and recipient are unrelated.

Close relatives under 45 have priority as donors. They are told of the risks to themselves and the possibility of early failure for the recipient. They are given a thorough physical examination to see if they can undergo the nephrectomy safely, to see if their kidneys are functioning optimumly, and to see if the renal-vascular anatomy of the potential donor kidney is suitable for anastomosis in the recipient. It must have a single renal artery that is long enough and wide enough.[69]

Much experimentation is being done on the use of compatible cadaver kidneys. The principal deterrent is the ischemic injury that occurs in the kidney. This can be deterred if hypothermia can be established soon after death. It is accomplished by use of temperature-controlled solutions injected through catheters inserted in the femoral vessels. Then, the kidneys can be surgically removed in a slower manner. Sometimes, it is extremely time-consuming to obtain permission to remove the kidneys after death because of a lack of understanding on the part of the relatives of the deceased and a repulsion that they feel at the thought of "cutting into" the body and desecrating it. Much public education is needed regarding use of all cadaver organs.

The Surgery. The patient must be put in the best possible condition for surgery; therefore, the hemodialysis unit is an essential part of the transplant program. Uremia must be reversed, excess body fluid removed, and serum electrolyte abnormalities corrected. Preoperative conservative management decreases the total number of dialyses required. Water intake is restricted to the previous day's output, plus 400 to 1,000 ml for insensible loss. Protein may be limited to 20 to 40 gm a day, although it may actually be increased in badly debilitated patients, and a greater number of dialyses performed.

A regimen of immunosuppressive drugs may be started eight to ten days before surgery. White blood counts are done every day to determine a dosage range that does not cause bone marrow depression with a decrease in white blood cells and concomitant increase in susceptibility to infection. Azathioprine (Imuran) is the most important single drug in the management of possible rejection. It is believed to interfere with nucleic acid synthesis, and is continued on a long-term basis. ALG (antilymphocytic globulin) is given three to five days before the transplant. Prophylactic doses of prednisone may also be used in the preoperative period. (See p. 209.)

Donor and recipient surgery takes place in separate operating rooms, at the same time. The donor kidney is removed and is carried into the recipient operating room where it is perfused with a cold solution. The recipient's kidneys and spleen are removed through an upper midline incision. The spleen is removed because of its role in antibody formation. Great care is taken to avoid any breaches in aseptic technique, and to ensure absolute hemostasis (control of bleeding), so that hematomas do not provide a focus of infection later. Because the bladder is a potential source of contamination, a separate ten-minute perineal preparation is done, and 50 ml of saline with 1 gm of neomycin and 50,000 units bacitracin is inserted into the bladder through a Foley catheter. Then, when the bladder is opened to insert the ureters, contamination does not occur. Cystostomy tubes and drains are not used, because they may cause retrograde (backup) contamination of the wounds.

A homograft bed is prepared in the extraperitoneal space of the iliac fossa. If the donor's left kidney is used, it is implanted in the recipient's right side; if the right kidney is used, it is implanted to the left side. Once positioned, the ureter is anastomosed to the bladder. The donor renal artery is anastomosed to the recipient's hypogastric artery, the donor renal vein to the recipient's external iliac vein.

Massive diuresis begins while the patient is still on the operating table and reaches a peak four hours postoperatively. Built-up waste products and tissue fluids are excreted. There is a weight loss of 5 to 35 lb in the first few days.[70] The patient's mental responsiveness improves almost immediately. He "feels well" and becomes euphoric.

The bed is kept flat for 24 hours despite tension on the lower abdominal incision, to protect ureteral and vascular anastomosis. The head of the bed is elevated about 20 degrees after the first day.[71] Vital signs are taken every 15 minutes, temperature every hour. The Foley catheter is irrigated only by the physician and is removed on the first postoperative day. Urine is measured every hour, and all urine is collected for study. Intravenous replacement is calculated on an hourly basis, according to urinary excretion, and "spot checks" of serum and electrolyte levels are made every four to eight hours. The patient is initially fed a liquid diet through a nasogastric tube. This is gradually increased to a solid, bland diet, and then to a regular, high-caloric diet. There are no fluid or salt restrictions until the onset of a rejection crisis. If steroids are used, a bland diet is continued because it lessens the chance of steroid-induced ulcers.

If blood pressure increases, antihypertensive drugs are used. The patient is weighed daily. Intake and output is measured on an eight-hour basis after the first 48 hours and on a 24-hour basis once the patient is home. Biweekly nose, throat, skin, and urine cultures are done throughout hospitalization.

In the recent past, elaborate reverse-isolation techniques were always carried out; however, it was learned that most infections were endogenous (from the patient himself) and occurred as a result of lowered resistance associated with vigorous use of immunosuppressive drugs. Now, precautionary measures include donning masks, gowns, and gloves before entering the patient's room. Nurses with colds or with any signs of infection do not care for kidney transplant patients. If a severe rejection crisis occurs, reverse isolation may be enforced.

The patient is encouraged to ambulate after 48 hours and leaves his room after three to four days. He may leave the hospital after the second week. He is treated as an outpatient, even when the almost inevitable rejection crisis occurs.

Rejection Crisis. A rejection crisis occurs in 80 to 90 percent of patients with homograft kidneys.[72] It is a reaction by the patient's body to the implantation of a foreign tissue. Symptoms are systemic and are from acute renal failure. Early rejection crisis occurs from 1 to 42 days after surgery with an average between the second and sixteenth day.[73] The critical postoperative period is one to three months. Late rejection crisis may occur four months or more after surgery. The nurse first notes psychologic changes in the patient. He may be anxious, lethargic, and apathetic. His appetite decreases. His urinary output decreases. There are tenderness over the transplant site, fever, and an elevated blood pressure. There may be alternating periods of diarrhea and constipation. Laboratory study indicates an elevated B.U.N., leukocytosis, lymphocytosis, casts, and increased white blood cells in the urine. When a late crisis occurs, there is gross deterioration of renal function.

Control of Rejection Crisis. Most rejection crises can be reversed with proper use of immunosuppressive drugs. The regimen [74] includes use of azathioprine (Imuran), a cytotoxic agent believed to interfere with nucleic acid synthesis; prednisone, a steroid that serves as an adjunct to the cytotoxic agent and reduces the inflammatory reaction; actinomycin C, a mixture of three antibiotics that has cytostatic or cytocidal action on lymphoid tissue (it is used for an established reaction, often in conjunction with irradiation of the kidney); and the newest agent, antilymphocytic globulin (ALG). With use of this drug, doses of steroids can be reduced. ALG has significantly decreased the death rate. More than 90 per cent of the recipients of intrafamilial homografts can be expected to live beyond the first postoperative year;[75] many are living after five years. To prepare ALG, lymphocytes are collected, washed, and injected into horses. The horse reacts against this foreign protein. The globulin fraction of the horse serum is given, intramuscularly, to the patient. With use of ALG, large doses of prednisone can be reduced in the postoperative period. Twenty percent of the patients getting ALG develop anaphylactic reactions to the horse serum with shortness of breath, flushing or cyanosis, drop in blood pressure, weak rapid pulse, increased respirations, chest pain, and nausea and vomiting.

The major complications of renal homotransplantation come from rejection crisis and from reaction to the immunosuppressive agents. By causing a serious drop in white blood cells, they increase the patient's susceptibility to infection. The most frequent septic complications are pneumonia, wound infections, pyelonephritis, and septicemia. Once leukopenia is evidenced, reverse-isolation precautions are enforced to protect the patient from microorganisms of others. A Life-Island isolator might be used. It provides a sterile unit, all enclosed, for the patient and all materials used for his care.

The moral question involved in the area of transplantation is a piercing one.[76] Some questions that must be answered are: Who should get the transplant? Is the unknown life extension of the recipient worth the possible reduction in life-span to the donor? Who should decide when artificial dialysis should be stopped when a transplant fails? Is there a violation of the patient's right to die after the disease has run its natural course?

REFERENCES

1. Metheny, N. M. and Snively, W. D., Jr., *Nurse's Handbook of Fluid Balance.* J. B. Lippincott Co., Philadelphia, 1967, pp. 9, 10.
2. *Ibid.*, p. 29.
3. Dutcher, I., and Fielo, S., *Water and Electrolytes: Implication for Nursing Practice.* The Macmillan Co., New York, 1967, p. 46.
4. *Ibid.*, pp. 70–71.
5. Metheny, *op. cit.*, p. 248.
6. *Ibid.*, pp. 70–71.
7. Bennett, H., "Burns: First Aid and Emergency Care," *Amer. J. Nurs.,* 62:96, 1967.
8. Beland, I.: *Clinical Nursing: Pathophysiological and Psychosocial Approaches.* The Macmillan Co., New York, 1965, p. 1340.
9. Shulman, A., "Ice Water as Primary Treatment of Burns," *J.A.M.A.,* 173:1916, 1960.
10. Larsen, D., and Gaston, R., "Current Trends in the Care of Burned Patients," *Amer. J. Nurs.,* 67:319, Feb. 1967.
11. *Ibid.*, p. 320.
12. Metheny, *op. cit.*, p. 163.
13. Wood, M., Kenny, H. A., and Price, W., "Silver Nitrate Treatment of Burns: Technique and Controlling Principles," *Amer. J. Nurs.,* 66:518, Mar. 1966.
14. Goldberger, E., *A Primer of Water, Electrolyte, and Acid-Base Syndromes.* Lea and Febiger, Philadelphia, 1965, p. 115.
15. Larsen, *op. cit.*, p. 322.
16. Metheny, *op. cit.*, p. 164.
17. Shafer, K. N., Sawyer, J. R., McCluskey, A. M., and Beck, E. L., *Medical Surgical Nursing.* The C. V. Mosby Co., St. Louis, 1967, p. 60.
18. Dutcher, *op. cit.*, p. 133.
19. Maxwell, P., Linss, M., McDonnough, P., and Kinder, J., "Routines on the Burn Ward," *Amer. J. Nurs.,* 66:522, Mar. 1966.
20. Larson, *op. cit.*, p. 322.
21. Beland, *op. cit.*, p. 1350.
22. Larson, *op. cit.*, p. 325.
23. Wood, *op. cit.*, p. 518.
24. Price, W., and Wood, M., "Operating Room Care of Burned Patients Treated with Silver Nitrate," *Amer. J. Nurs.,* 68:1706, Aug. 1968.
25. Colby, F., *Essential Urology.* The Williams and Wilkins Co., Baltimore, 1961, p. 24.
26. Sawyer, J., *Nursing Care of Patients with Urologic Diseases.* The C. V. Mosby Co., St. Louis, 1963, p. 20.
27. *Ibid.*, p. 20.
28. Albers, J., "Evaluation of Blood Volume in Patients on Hemodialysis," *Amer. J. Nurs.,* 68:1678, Aug. 1968.
29. *Ibid.*, p. 1678.
30. Dutcher, *op. cit.*, p. 107.
31. Shafer, *op. cit.*, p. 436.
32. Metheny, *op cit.*, p. 188.
33. *Ibid.*, p. 190.
34. Mohammed, M., "Urinalysis," *Amer. J. Nurs.,* 64:7, June 1964.
35. Santora, D., "Preventing Hospital Acquired Urinary Infection," *Amer. J. Nurs.,* 66:791, Apr. 1966.
36. *Ibid.*, p. 791.
37. French, R. M., *Nurse's Guide to Diagnostic Procedures.* McGraw-Hill Book Co., New York, 1967, pp. 136–42.
38. Sawyer, *op. cit.*, pp. 179–80.
39. French, *op. cit.*, p. 104.
40. Sawyer, *op. cit.*, p. 188.

41. Smith, D. W., and Gipps, C. D., *Care of the Adult Patient*. J. B. Lippincott Co., Philadelphia, 1966, p. 888.
42. White, A. G., *Clinical Disturbances of Renal Function*. W. B. Saunders Co., Philadelphia, 1961, p. 31.
43. Baltzan, R. B., "Glomerulonephritis," *Canad. Nurse*, 62:45, Aug. 1966.
44. Shafer, *op. cit.*, p. 439.
45. White, *op. cit.*, p. 41.
46. *Ibid.*, p. 46.
47. Avery, D., "Hypertension Secondary to Renal Artery Stenosis," *Amer J. Nurs.*, 66:2685, Dec. 1966.
48. *Ibid.*, p. 2686.
49. Hamm, F. C., and Weinberg, S. R.: *Urology in Medical Practice*. J. B. Lippincott Co., Philadelphia, 1962, p. 93.
50. Colby, *op. cit.*, p. 144.
51. White, *op. cit.*, p. 66.
52. Colby, *op. cit.*, p. 140.
53. Sawyer, *op. cit.*, p. 239.
54. Hamm, *op cit.*, p. 54.
55. Sawyer, *op. cit.*, p. 241.
56. Shafer, *op. cit.*, p. 462.
57. Rubin, E., "Type of Prostatectomy Discussed; Good Nursing Service Essential," *Hosp. Topics*, 43:110, Apr. 1965.
58. Colby, *op. cit.*, p. 407.
59. Smith, *op. cit.*, p. 930.
60. Sawyer, *op cit.*, p. 246.
61. Colby, *op. cit.*, p. 407.
62. Sawyer, *op. cit.*, p. 290.
63. Colby, *op. cit.*, p. 173.
64. Sawyer, *op. cit.*, p. 258.
65. *Ibid.*, p. 60.
66. Smith, *op. cit.*, p. 903.
67. Metheny, *op. cit.*, p. 193.
68. Starzl, T. E., *Experience in Renal Transplantation*. W. B. Saunders Co., Philadelphia, 1964, p. 2.
69. *Ibid.*, p. 35.
70. *Ibid.*, p. 113.
71. Bois, M., Barfield, N., Taylor, C., and Ross, C., "Nursing Care of Patients Having Kidney Transplants," *Amer. J. Nurs.*, 68:1238, June 1968.
72. Starzl, *op. cit.*, p. 143.
73. Frankson, C., *Kidney Transplantation*. Almquist and Wiksell, Stockholm, Sweden, 1968, p. 24.
74. Bois, *op. cit.*, p. 1245.
75. Martin, A., "Renal Transplantation: Surgical Technique and Complications," *Amer. J. Nurs.*, 68:1241, June 1968.
76. Starzl, *op. cit.*, p. 357.

ADDITIONAL READINGS

BETSON, C., "Blood Gases," *Amer. J. Nurs.*, 68:1010, May 1968.
BONINE, G., "Burn Treatment with Silver Nitrate," *RN*, 29:47, Aug. 1966.
BURROWS, K., "Treatment of Acute Renal Failure," *Nurs. Times*, 63:8, Jan. 6, 1967.
CLAUSS, R. H., "Monitoring Blood Gases and pH During Open Heart Operations." Paper presented at the American Society of Extracorporeal Circulation Technicians, Washington, D.C., May 1966.
CRAIG, I.; "Collecting Specimens of Urine," *Nurs. Times*, 62:531, Apr. 22, 1966.
DAVIS, J., "Drugs for Urologic Disorders," *Amer. J. Nurs.*, 65:107, Aug. 1965.
DE VEBER, G., "Fluid and Electrolyte Problems in the Postoperative Period," *Nurs. Clin. N. Amer.*, 1:275, June 1966.
GANDEE, N. C., and LAYMAN, J. D., "Cyanosis in Burn Patients," *J. Amer. Ass. Nurs. Anes.*, 35:105, Apr. 1967.
HEARN, A., "Wilms Tumour," *Nurs. Times*, 63:1167, Sept. 1, 1967.

Noonan, J., and Noonan, L., "Two Burned Patients on Flotation Therapy," *Amer. J. Nurs.*, **68**:316, Feb. 1968.
Pearson, J., "Water and Electrolyte Balance," *Nurs. Times*, **63**:415, Mar. 31, 1967.
Schlegel, J. U., "Pyelonephritis," *J. Urol.*, **86**:12–16, July 1961.
Seidler, F. M. "The Nurse and the Isolator," *Nurs. Clin. N. Amer.*, **1**:587, Dec. 1966
Spector, A., "Effect of Postburn Serum on in Vitro Respiration of Normal Myocardium," *J. Appl. Physiol.*, **18**:821, 1963.

UNIT V

THE PATIENT WITH A PROBLEM TRANSPORTING MATERIAL TO AND FROM CELLS

22

THE CARDIOPULMONARY EMERGENCY

An adequately pumping heart, sufficiently oxygenated blood, and a patent roadbed of blood vessels are essential to the transportation of materials to and from cells. Transfer of materials takes place at the capillaries where oxygen and essential nutrients are supplied to the cells, and carbon dioxide and waste products are removed from them. Impairment in the smooth functioning of any part of this supply-and-removal system can deprive vital organs of life-giving blood.

Shock

Shock is a condition in which inadequate blood is supplied to the capillaries for transfer of materials. In any circumstance in which there is insufficient cardiac output to adequately perfuse the capillaries, shock may develop. When enough adequately oxygenated blood is brought to the cells, a series of complex chemical reactions take place that lead to the synthesis of adenosine triphosphate (ATP),[1*] the ultimate source of cell energy; but when insufficient oxygenated blood is supplied to the cells, metabolism takes place in a less-than-effective way. It is called anaerobic (without oxygen) metabolism and causes the accumulation of acid end products in the tissues. Metabolic acidosis develops. It is life-threatening to the cells and tends to perpetuate any pathology. Shock can lead to metabolic acidosis and death.

The sequence of events leading to metabolic acidosis from shock looks like this:

Insufficient blood → decrease in cardiac output → decrease in circulation to vital tissues → hypoxia → anaerobic metabolism → metabolic acidosis → cell injury and death

Shock may stem from a single cause or from a combination of several causes. Examples include blood loss (hematogenic), trauma to the nervous system with reflex inhibition to the heart (neurogenic), interference of heart function (cardiogenic), and massive infection (septic shock).

* References for Unit V are on pages 299–302.

Assessment of the Patient in Shock

Signs of shock vary with the individual and the cause. They are most meaningful to the physician if they can be compared with previous reactions. Usually there is a drop in systolic and diastolic blood pressure with the degree of drop proportionate to the severity of the shock. In a person with an average systolic reading of 110 to 130 mm Hg a drop to 90 to 100 mm Hg would indicate impending shock, below 80 mm Hg would indicate shock.[2] Pulse becomes rapid and thready. Sympathetic nervous system stimulation causes the skin to feel cold and sweaty, and it is pale. The hands are valuable indicators of circulatory status. In shock, the nail beds frequently become cyanotic, and capillary filling time is increased. If the nail bed is compressed, it will normally fill within a fraction of a second after the pressure is released. In shock, capillary filling time is longer. The decrease in blood volume causes the patient to be thirsty, and there is usually a drop in urine volume. The patient becomes apprehensive and agitated. Frequently agitation is the forerunner of cardiac difficulty and will appear before any other telltale signs. If the shock progresses, the patient becomes unconscious.

What to Do for Shock

If there is no evident cessation of respiratory or cardiac function, the patient is placed in a flat position, or in a position in which his thorax is lower than his pelvis. His legs are elevated to a 45-degree angle, with the knees straight. The trunk is horizontal or very slightly inclined. This is *not* the traditional head-down Trendelenburg position. The head is level with or slightly higher than the chest. The Trendelenburg position should be used only if specifically ordered by the physician because it can increase intracranial pressure in a patient who may already be suffering from this neurologic problem. Elevating the legs may help to increase venous return by gravity, if the decreased blood supply is only moderate.[3] A bath blanket can be placed over the patient; but use of many blankets further increases the metabolic rate and heightens the hypoxia.

Oxygen, 100 per cent concentration, is administered. Although it does not increase the saturation in hemoglobin, it does substantially increase the amount of oxygen dissolved in plasma. In this way, the oxygen tension in the venous end of the capillary is increased and this helps to correct the hypoxia.

In hypovolemic (decreased blood volume) shock, intravenous replacement solutions are utilized according to need. If whole blood has been lost, it will probably be replaced with whole blood or dextran; if the shock is from uncontrolled vomiting or diarrhea, physiologic solutions matching the electrolytes lost will be used. (See Chap. 19.)

The physician may also elect to use drugs that cause vasoconstriction and elevate the blood pressure. Examples are Levarterenol bitartrate (Levophed) and metaraminol bitartrate (Aramine). When they are administered in an intravenous solution, the rate must be watched carefully. It is slowed or stopped completely if the blood pressure reaches a high point, specified by the physician; it is increased if the blood pressure reaches a low point, specified by the physician. These drugs cause sloughing of tissues if they infiltrate.

The physician will determine the cause of the shock, and then will treat the patient according to his findings.

Cardiac and Respiratory Arrest

If the heart or respirations suddenly stop, the patient is in danger of death. This can happen at any hour of the day or night, and from a wide variety of causes. The patient may have reacted adversely to a central nervous system depressant such as Dilaudid or an anesthetic; he may have been submerged in water; he may have had electric shock; he may have had a myocardial infarction. His life is in jeopardy unless resuscitation is instituted promptly, accurately, and continuously. When the heart stops pumping, the vital organs are not supplied with oxygen and they become hypoxic. The brain utilizes what oxygen is left in the stagnant blood, but it can survive without irreversible damage for only four to six minutes. Closed-chest cardiac massage with mouth-to-mouth breathing is often successful in restarting the pumping action of the heart, and re-establishing exchange of gases by the lung. The nurse must first evaluate the situation to see whether breathing or heartbeat has stopped. Apnea, cyanosis, dilated pupils, and absence of pulse and blood pressure are indicators of the need for immediate resuscitative measures. If the patient is unconscious, this means his heart has been arrested at least six seconds; if his pupils are dilated, he has been in arrest 30 to 60 seconds.[4] Cardiopulmonary resuscitation is usually not started when it is known definitely that cardiac arrest has persisted for more than six minutes, or in patients known to be in the terminal stages of an incurable disease.[5]

The ABC's of the technique include:[6]

1. Airway
2. Breathing
3. Circulation
4. Definitive treatment

Steps in Emergency Resuscitation

1. Place the person on a hard surface such as the floor or ground or use a specially designed board placed on the bed under the chest or entire body.

2. *Establish a clear airway.* This is by far the most important single factor contributing to successful resuscitation. Tilt the head backward as far as it will go by placing one hand under the patient's neck and lifting it, the other on the patient's forehead with gentle pressure down. The mandible is, thus, pulled forward and the tongue is lifted away from the back of the throat. Remove any obstruction in the throat or nasal passages. Make sure dentures are out!

3. *Ventilate the lungs.* The operator takes deep breaths and places his wide-open mouth over the patient's mouth, with the patient's nostrils pinched, or over the patient's mouth and nose. A tight seal should be made. The operator inspires atmospheric air and then blows this into the patient's mouth. He then removes his mouth to allow the patient to expire the air passively. He watches to see if the patient's chest expands. This tells whether the airway is, in fact, clear. If ventilation is not effective after proper positioning, the patient is rolled onto his side, and firm blows are delivered over his spine between the shoulder blades to dislodge the obstruction. The cycle of blowing air into the patient and then letting the patient blow it out is repeated 12 times per minute. If there is only one operator doing cardiac massage and mouth-to-mouth breathing, he must ventilate the lungs with three-to-five breaths initially, then massage the heart for 15 seconds, stop, and give two or three breaths of air, and then massage again with a 15:2 ratio of massage to ventilation. If the mouth cannot be used because of injury or because the operator prefers to use the mouth-to-nose route, the operator tilts the patient's head back with one hand and uses the other hand to push the lower jaw closed. If the operator cannot, esthetically, place his mouth directly over the mouth of the patient, a gauze square or clean handkerchief can be used. Many hospitals have emergency S-shaped airways that can be placed in the mouth over the tongue for mouth-to-mouth breathing, or a breathing bag may be used. It fits over the patient's nose and mouth and is squeezed to aerate the lungs. It can be connected to an oxygen source or atmospheric air can be used.

If the patient vomits he should be turned on his side to decrease the chance of aspiration.

If infants and small children are to be ventilated, the same position is used though the tilt should not be exaggerated. Less volume of air is blown in and the rate of inflation should be 20 to 30 times per minute.

4. *Re-establish circulation.* The operator positions himself at the side of the patient and places the heel of one hand over the lower half of the sternum, not over the tip of the sternum (xiphoid process of the sternum, which extends down over the abdomen). He places his other hand on top of the first and then rocks forward, keeping his arms straight. He must exert enough pressure (80 to 120 lb) to depress the lower sternum 1½ to 2 in. in an adult, once a second. Sixty compressions per minute maintains blood flow, and still allows the heart to refill. The operator must release

all pressure to allow this refill. The compressions should be continuous, and under no circumstances should they be interrupted for more than five seconds. This requires practice. Nurses should use adult-like manikins for periodic practice.

When there are two operators, optimum ventilation and circulation are achieved with five chest compressions to every one inflation, without any pause in compressions. Resuscitation measures should be continued until cerebral and cardiovascular status can be assessed by the physician. He checks for carotid or femoral pulse, blood pressure, and pupillary reaction. A pupil that constricts when exposed to light indicates adequate oxygenation and blood flow to the brain. The decision to stop resuscitation is a medical one.

The method of cardiac compression is basically the same for children; however, the heel of only one hand is used for children up to about ten years of age, and only the tips of the index and middle fingers are used for infants. Of course, less pressure is exerted.

If the procedure is done properly, complications resulting from cardiopulmonary resuscitation are minimized. For instance, keeping the fingers off the ribs decreases the chance of rib fracture; keeping the heel of the hand off the xiphoid process at the lower end of the sternum decreases the chance of laceration of the liver; compressing the chest, not the abdomen, decreases the chance of rupture of the liver. Fat emboli remain a potential problem.

In the Hospital

Most hospitals have a trained emergency team and a "crash cart" of specialized equipment that is wheeled to the bedside of the patient. The team has periodic practice drills to maintain their speed, knowledge of the equipment, and supplies to be used. The machinery is checked for operating efficiency. In the event of an emergency, the telephone operator is called. She uses the hospital page system to announce, by a predetermined code name, the existence and location of the emergency. "Dr. Pacemaker—Dr. Pacemaker— 359" and "Code 6—Code 6—Emergency Room" are examples of coded phrases in use. Members of the emergency team, including physicians, anesthetist, inhalation therapist, and nurses, immediately rush to the area. All other elevator traffic stops. How important it is to explain this fact to *all* hospital personnel! A planned sequence of activities, with each member knowing exactly what his job is, helps decrease the confusion and ineffectiveness of many curious bystanders with no one really sure of what his job is.

A possible activity sequence might be:

Nurse # 1. Examines the patient for signs of cardiorespiratory embarrassment. Finds apnea, pupil dilatation, and no blood pressure. She calls code # 6, begins mouth-to-mouth respiration (an Ambu breathing bag may be used) and closed-chest massage.

Nurse # 2. Places board under patient's chest; connects oxygen and takes over closed-chest massage. She will prepare and replace solutions used by the emergency team, e.g., epinephrine, sodium bicarbonate, Isuprel, intravenous solutions.

When the crash cart and emergency personnel arrive, the monitor is plugged in, the ECG electrodes are applied, and the ECG is recorded. The defibrillator is charged and ready for use. The anesthetist establishes an open airway. He may insert a cuffed endotracheal tube. It has a balloon-like attachment that, when inflated, creates a seal between the tube and the trachea and prevents leakage of oxygen or aspiration of fluid through the trachea. He may use an automatically cycled controlled ventilation respirator to establish and maintain gas exchange. This machine does the work of breathing for the patient. He does this in conjunction with a physician or member of the inhalation therapy department who continues closed-chest massage. He times the inspiratory cycle of the respirator to fit between compressions of the heart.[7] The person performing the massage must allow lung expansion to take place between cardiac compressions. While cardiac and ventilatory resuscitation is being performed, a physician studies the admitting diagnosis, checks blood pressure and pulse, watches the heart rhythm through the ECG tape, and administers medications and intravenous solutions. He judges the efficacy of the resuscitative measures. He may elect to use the defibrillator and/or the external pacemaker. He determines the point at which artificial respiration and circulation should be discontinued.

Emergency Equipment and Its Use
WHAT IS AN ARRHYTHMIA?

The use of specialized emergency equipment is based on an understanding of the heart as an electrical conduction system and on the nature of this rhythm system.

AUTONOMIC CONTROL

The heart is innervated by the autonomic nervous system. Its normal rate is the result of balance between the slowing affect of parasympathetic (vagal nerve) stimulation and the speeding effect of the sympathetic stimulation. The autonomic system, in turn, responds to innervation by pressure receptors in the carotid sinus that inhibit heart rate when distended and by chemoreceptors in the carotid body that increase heart rate in the presence of elevated carbon dioxide.

THE COMMUNICATION SYSTEM OF THE HEART

Even if all of its nerve fibers were cut, the heart would continue to beat[8] because of its own innate electrical system. The electrical impulse starts in the sinoatrial node in the right atrium between the venae cavae. It is transmitted through the atria, causing them to contract together. It travels to the atrioventricular node, down both sides of the bundle of His, and through the Purkinje fibers to cause contraction of both ventricles together. All the cardiac tissue is capable of originating rhythmic contractions if the normal communication system is faulty.

DISTURBANCES IN RHYTHM

ARRHYTHMIA. A disturbance in rhythm: from "a," meaning without, and rhythmia, rhythm.

N.S.R. Normal sinus rhythm.

SINUS TACHYCARDIA. Increase in heart rate.

SINUS BRADYCARDIA. Decrease in heart rate.

ECTOPIC BEAT. One that originates in a place other than the SA node.

If normal sinus impulses are too slow or irregular, other areas of the heart may take over initiating the beat. These are called ectopic beats. They may be occasional, as when an ectopic beat escapes and causes a single premature contraction of the atria or ventricles; or they may be permanent, as when the beat originates in the atrioventricular node on a regular basis, causing a decreased heart rate (40 to 60 beats per minute). If the ectopic beat originates in the ventricles (idioventricular beat), it may cause an excessively slow rate, especially if impulses from the atria are not getting to the ventricles at all. Idioventricular beats may lead to a Stokes-Adams attack in which there are a temporary absence of pulse, cerebral ischemia with loss of consciousness, and convulsion.

Delays in transmission are called "blocks." A delay between the atria and ventricles is called an atrioventricular block. This is often caused by use of digitalis. A delay in the impulse through the bundle of His is called bundle branch block. It can be right-sided or left-sided. Complete heart block indicates total ineffectiveness in the cardiac conduction system.

ATRIAL FIBRILLATION

In this most commonly seen arrhythmia, the atria "shake" ineffectively, at fantastically high rates. They do not contract. The ventricles do contract and maintain adequate body circulation. Ventricular rate is usually increased. The pulse is irregular and frequently slower than the ventricular rate would indicate because all the ventricular contractions are not strong enough to cause radial pulsation. A difference between the apical and radial rates (pulse deficit) is often evident. This arrhythmia is most amenable to therapy by drugs, e.g., digitalis, quinidine sulfate, procaine-amide hydrochloride, or by insertion of an implantable pacemaker. It is the most frequently seen arrhythmia.

VENTRICULAR TACHYCARDIA AND FIBRILLATION

In these most serious arrhythmias the action of the ventricles is controlled by an abnormal source of impulse in the ventricular muscle.[9]

Ventricular rate is rapid (120 to 200 per minute), the QRS complex is bizarre, and cardiac arrest may ensue. If the ventricles actually begin fibrillating (shaking with ineffective contractions), they are no longer capable of supplying the body's blood needs, and shock follows. There is complete electrical disorganization. Cardioversion is often the emergency method of choice. (See pp. 223–24.)

Emergency Machinery and Its Use

ELECTROCARDIOGRAPHY

The electrocardiogram is a pictorial record of the electrical current passing through the heart. The human body, by virtue of the chemical nature of its fluids (they conduct current), is essentially a volume conductor through which current generated in any part of the body can reach any other part.[10] So, the electric impulses of the heart are conducted through the body and are picked up and recorded in the galvanometer (ECG machine). Metal is also a conductor of electricity; therefore, metal electrodes, with conductive jelly applied to the skin under them, are placed in a variety of predetermined body areas. They conduct the electrical current that comes from the heart. In a complete ECG recording, 10 or 12 leads are used. Lead simply designates the direction of flow of electricity from one predetermined area of the body to another. For example, lead 1 involves the flow of current from the right and left arms just above the wrists. If the flow from the right arm is relatively negative and from the left arm is relatively positive, an upward curve is recorded on the graph paper.[11] An upright wave indicates depolarization toward a positive electrode; a downward wave indicates depolarization away from a positive electrode toward a negative electrode.

Two electrodes are needed to pick up and record patterns. They are usually placed on each limb, with the right limb at "O" potential. This is called the "indifferent" electrode and serves as the second lead for several exploring or moving electrodes. There are at least six precordial (chest) leads that use this "indifferent" lead to make a pair. A dial on the machine is labeled with the lead connections, e.g., 1, 2, 3, aVR, aVL, aVF, V, and the technician turns the dial to the designated setting to record the electrical reading from that particular pair of electrodes.

MEANINGS OF THE LETTERS USED

V, potential (used in frontal plane and chest leads)
R, right arm
L, left arm
F, left leg
a, augmented

The graph paper on which the electrical picture is recorded contains many tiny boxes that indicate time and amplitude. Time is determined by measuring the width between the vertical lines. The distance between each vertical line is equal to 0.04 second. Amplitude is the distance between the horizontal lines. A normal ECG recording consists of a repetitive series of P, Q, R, S, T waves that conform to established standards for size, shape, and time. (See Fig. 22–1.) These time and amplitude averages are derived from lead 2 and are for adults.

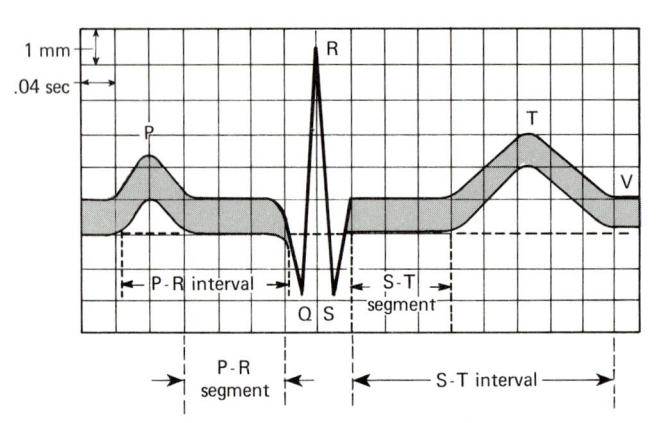

FIGURE 22–1. Normal electrocardiogram.

MEANING OF ECG SEGMENTS [12]

P WAVE. Depolarization (electrical excitement and activity) of atria. 0.06 to 0.11 second; 0.3 to 2.5 mm high. If P wave is present and precedes the QRS complex, the impulse has originated in SA node; otherwise, another area of heart is working as pacemaker.

PR SEGMENT. The time it takes for the impulse to travel from the atria to the ventricles.

PR INTERVAL. The time required to depolarize the atria, plus the delay in transmission of the impulse through AV node to beginning of ventricular excitement. 0.20 second with cardiac rate of 70 to 90. Prolongation or reduction indicates defect in conduction system.

QRS COMPLEX. Depolarization in ventricles. 0.06 to 0.10 second with cardiac rate of 70 to 90. Increase in seconds indicates slowing in conduction through ventricles, e.g., bundle branch block. Decrease in seconds indicates a more rapid rate. Amplitude 4.0 to 23.0 mm at R wave.

S–T SEGMENT. Between the end of the QRS complex and the beginning of the T wave. The interval of time between completion of ventricular depolarization and beginning of repolarization (re-establishment of electrical balance). Time varies with cardiac rate and sex of individual. In men with rate of 70, 0.135 second. Women with rate of 70, 0.150 second.

S–T INTERVAL. Duration in seconds from end of QRS complex to end of T wave. Represents time from completion of depolarization to completion of repolarization.

T WAVE. Ventricular repolarization. Average amplitude 0 to 8.0 mm.

V WAVE. An "after-potential" wave which follows the T wave and is low in amplitude. May first become apparent in potassium depletion.[13]

The interpretation of the ECG is left to the physician; however, nurses are now being prepared to recognize anything "that does not look right." More specifically, she recognizes [14]

1. Abrupt speeding or slowing of heart rate. Rate of appearance of R waves.
2. Appearance of irregularity of heart beat. R waves.
3. Change in the form of QRS complex.
4. Disappearance or marked change in form of P waves (atrial depolarization).
5. Failure of the normal sequence of P wave followed by QRS complex.

Nurses working in highly specialized areas, such as intensive or coronary care units, are taught to recognize specific arrhythmias and to take emergency action depending on their findings.

The ECG recording is a valuable adjunct to making the diagnosis. It helps in determining effectiveness of the electrical conduction through the heart, indicating myocardial change, injury, and ischemia, showing the effect of drugs on the heart, and so forth. The patient, however, may have a normal ECG and still have serious cardiac disease. The ECG is used along with other diagnostic tools, not by itself.

THE DEFIBRILLATOR

The defibrillator is an electric-shock machine. It momentarily shocks the heart into total electrical activity so that the sinus node, the body's natural pacemaker, can effectively take over. It's like erasing a messy chalkboard and beginning all over again on a clean slate with a better chance of doing it properly. The procedure can be utilized in an emergency when atrial or ventricular fibrillation (shaking, ineffectual contractions) is present, or can be used as an elective measure for the patient who experiences long-term, uncomfortable palpitation. Cardioversion, the electric-shock method of reverting the heart to a normal rhythm, enhances ventricular filling in these patients, and they feel much better.

Lown [15] describes two major phases in cardioversion. The first is electrical and external. It involves the actual mechanical delivery of energy to depolarize the heart. This is usually successful. The second phase is physiologic and internal. It involves take-over of pacemaking by the heart and herein lies the difficulty. The original factors that caused the abnormal sinus rhythm are still operative, and although an effective rhythm can be established by cardioversion, it cannot always be maintained by the heart. Several factors decrease the capacity of the heart to sustain long-lasting sinus rhythm. Among these are atria that have been injured or are inflamed or infarcted or that are depressed by drugs. Large maintenance doses of digitalis decrease the chance of successful cardioversion. If an elective procedure is contemplated, digitalis is withheld for one or more days prior to the treatment.

The Defibrillation Procedure (See Figs. 22–2 and 22–3). Two paddles, 3½ to 5 in. in diameter (about the size of small grapefruits) with heavily insulated handles are coated with conductive paste and are applied to two areas of the chest. In the anterolateral positions one paddle is placed on the lower end of the sternum and the other is placed to the side of the apex of the heart.[16] In the anteroposterior method the patient lies flat on the posterior paddle, which is placed in the left infrascapular region (below the shoulder blade), while the anterior paddle is placed at the lower end of the sternum. This anteroposterior position seems to shorten the pathway between the electrodes, augments the density of the electrical field, and decreases the amount of electricity required for reversion.[17] The nurse holds the paddles in position over the chest and stands away from

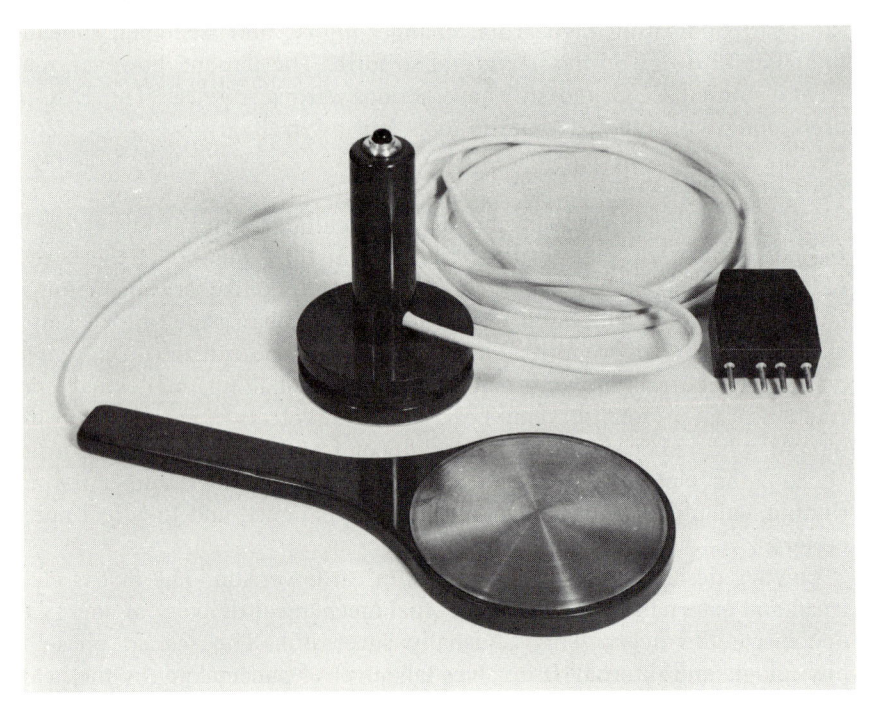

FIGURE 22–2. Defibrillation paddles. (Courtesy, Air-Shields, Inc., Hatboro, Pa.)

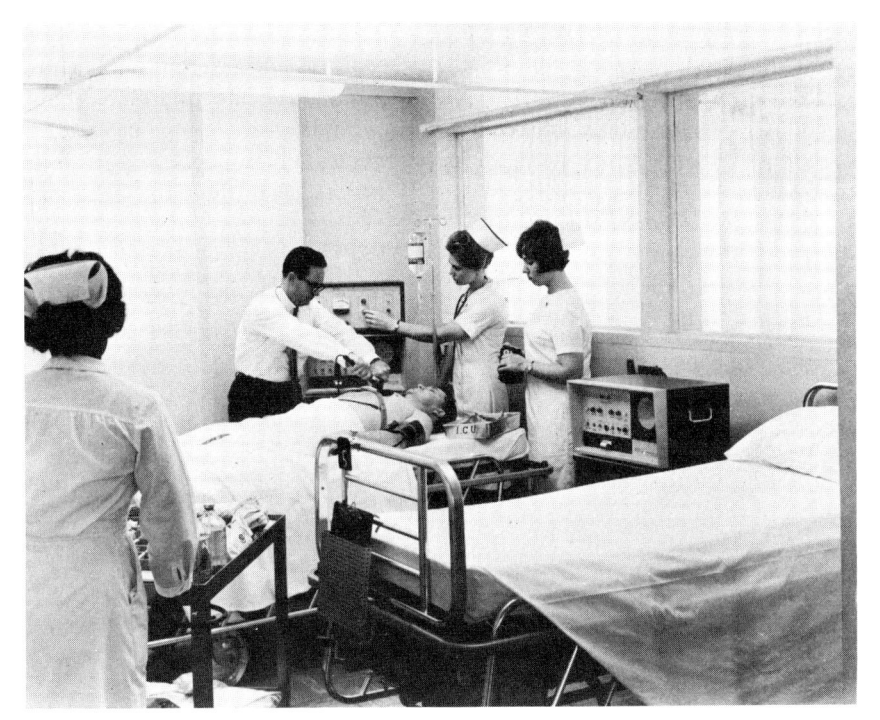

FIGURE 22-3. Emergency defibrillation. (Courtesy, Electrodyne, Westwood, Mass.)

the bed so that no part of her body touches a metal conductor. The physician sets the amount of current to be administered and actually pushes the button that discharges the current. In some hospitals, nurses are taught to recognize ECG abnormalities that can be corrected with electric shock (atrial and ventricular fibrillation are examples) and are given the prerogative to institute the treatment. The patient will respond with a twitch of the thoracic muscles and a jerk of the arms. If several shocks have to be administered a red ring outlining the circumference of the paddles will develop and the area will be tender for 24 hours. The procedure is painless. Shocks of 75 to 100 watt-seconds are given initially. If this fails to restore sinus rhythm, successively larger shocks are given to a maximum of 400 watt-seconds.[18] Defibrillation can be initiated with the maximum.

Some complications of cardioversion include technical errors of procedure, release of the shock during the vulnerable "T"-wave period in older equipment (this can cause ventricular fibrillation in a patient being cardioverted for atrial fibrillation), failure to explain the elective procedure to the patient (this causes increased anxiety, increased circulating catecholamines, which increase the susceptibility of the heart to arrhythmias), and systemic or pulmonary embolism. The incidence of embolism is increased immediately following reversion to sinus rhythm.[19] Some patients are not suitable candidates for cardioversion. They include those who have been reverted with quinidine and, despite adequate maintenance doses, had the arrhythmia recur; patients with very enlarged atria; elderly patients with very advanced atrioventricular block; and patients immediately before or during valvular surgery. Handling the atria precipitates fibrillation.

Until 1960, cardioversion by electricity was employed only for terminating ventricular fibrillation. However, it has been found to be successful in terminating many arrhythmias, especially chronic atrial fibrillation, the most frequently occurring arrhythmia.[20]

THE PACEMAKER

In the normal heart, rhythm is controlled through an electrical stimulus originating in the sinoatrial node (the physiologic pacemaker) and traveling through the atria to the atrioventricular node, down the bundle of His and out through the Purkinje fibers to the ventricles. This occurs rhythmically and controls the heart rate. In some instances this rhythm is interrupted and short- or long-term electronic control of the rate is indicated. The pacemaker is a mechanical device that controls this rhythm by continuously stimulating ventricular contractions. It provides short- or long-term electrical stimuli that the physiologic pacemaker is incapable of doing effectively.

Pacing at the Bedside. In an emergency, electrodes can be strapped directly over the skin on the chest and can be connected to a pacemaker machine. Since 1957, however,[12] electrodes placed directly into the myocardium have proved more effective, especially for long-term pacing. If the patient is too sick to be moved to a fluoroscopy room, a cutdown can be made into the antecubital vein, and a Teflon-coated stainless steel wire, with electrode, can be guided into the right atrium using electrocardiograph monitoring to determine its proper position.[22] When the heart rate is stable, the pacemaker can be disconnected.

For Long-Term Pacing. Until 1960 patients were treated with implanted electrodes attached to rather cumbersome pacemaker units, sort of a half-in–half-out operation. The patient carried the machine with him when he moved about. Since 1960 the unit has been miniaturized, given battery power, and transistorized, and is capable of total implantation.[23]

Types of Units. (See Figs. 22–4, 22–5.) The two basic types of implantable pacemaker units are the asynchronous unit, which is regulated prior to implantation at a rate set by the physician, and the synchronous unit, which is physiologically controlled. At present, the asynchronous, fixed-rate models are the units of choice because of their simplicity of design, dependability, and lower cost. Their major drawbacks are their inability to accelerate or decelerate rate according to metabolic need or activity, and the fact that atrial and ventricular activity are not synchronized. The efficiency of the atrium as a booster pump is lost.[24]

The synchronous pacemaker is physiologically controlled. The atrial and ventricular activity are synchronized so that the ventricles contract at a preset interval after the atria contract. This is a more natural sequence. A device is implanted in or on the atrium. It "senses" a P wave, amplifies it, and conducts it to the ventricles by an electronic circuit.[25] It causes a device implanted in the ventricle to stimulate ventricular contraction. It "bypasses" the ineffectively working electrical communication system of the AV node and Purkinje fibers.

Newest pacemakers are powered by atomic energy. They contain a half-gram of plutonium 238 and are about two thirds the size of a pack of cigarettes. They are designed to operate for ten years. There is no radiation risk.

HOW ARE PACEMAKERS AND ELECTRODES INSERTED?

Intravenous Route. A radiopaque electrode catheter is passed through the external jugular, femoral, or subclavian vein into the right ventricle. The method is similar to that of cardiac catheterization in which the

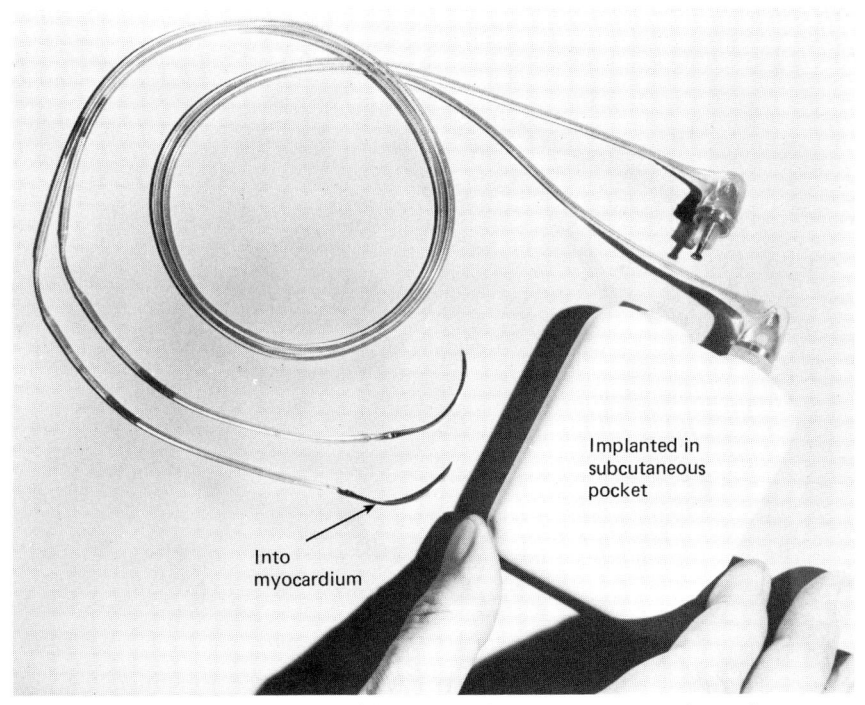

FIGURE 22–4. An implantable pacemaker. (Courtesy, Electrodyne, Westwood, Mass.)

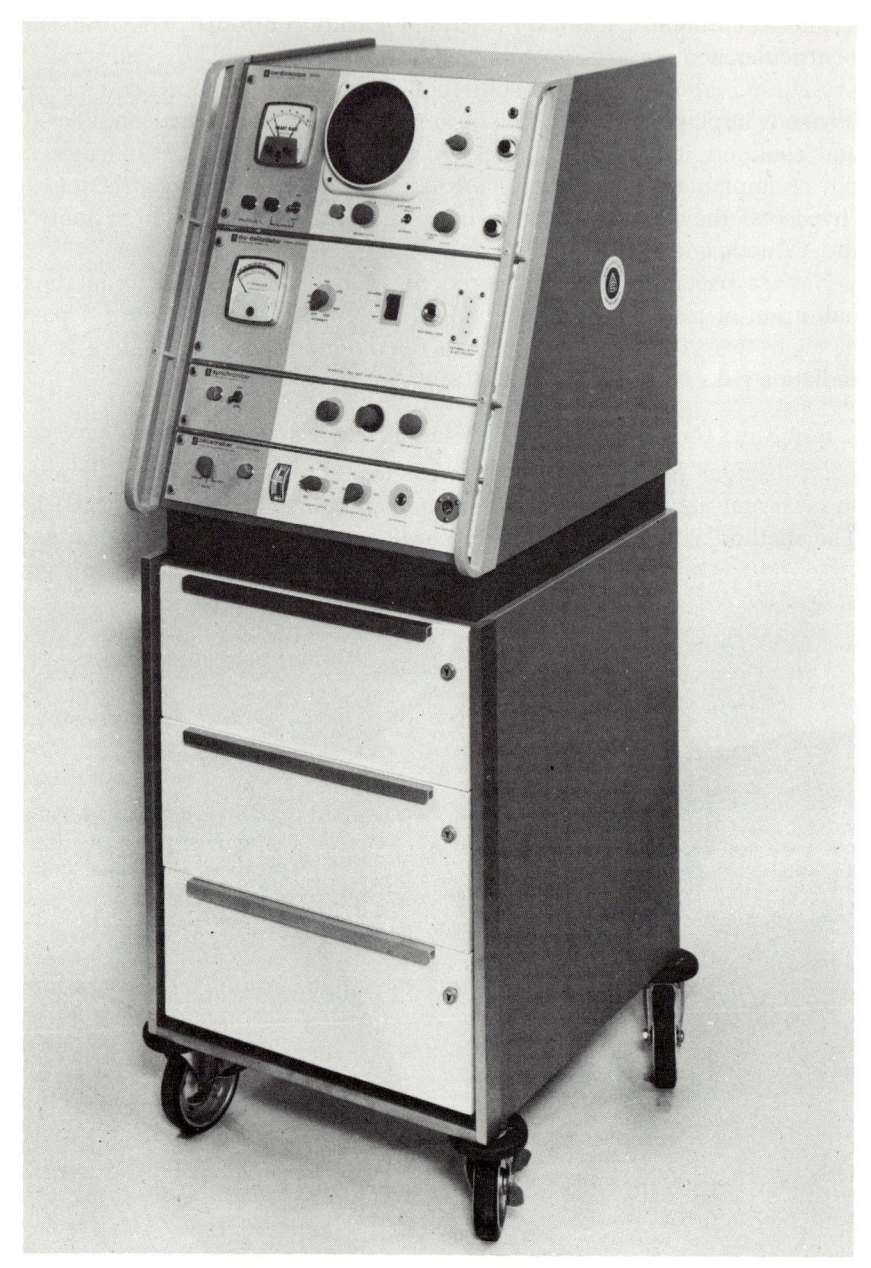

FIGURE 22–5. This machine is a combination defibrillator, monitor, pacemaker. Other equipment is stored in the drawers. (Courtesy, Air-Shields, Inc., Hatboro, Pa.)

catheter is observed as it is passed through the veins and vena cava into the heart by means of the fluoroscope machine. The electrodes are placed against the ventricular endocardium. A subcutaneous pocket is then made for the pacemaker unit in the axilla or abdominal wall. The latter site poses some problems because bending puts a strain on the wire leading to the electrodes and may cause wire breakage. The abdominal site is used in tall, thin people who have inadequate chest musculature.[26] A wire or group of wires extend freely from the pacemaker unit in the subcutaneous tissue around the implantation site. They are emergency wires that are easily located, can be exposed under local anesthesia, and can be used for pacemaker failure, for connection to an external unit, to charge batteries, and for ease of accessibility to the implanted unit. The life of the batteries differs according to the type of battery, and, interestingly, according to the particular patient.[27] Batteries last anywhere from one to five years. Periodic x-ray studies show the state of battery depletion. The patient, too, can note changes in effectiveness of the unit. Theoretically, the pacemaker increases 5 to 8 beats per minute as the batteries near exhaustion, but other variables, such as temperature, confuse the issue.[28] The patient may be told to take his pulse daily and report a 10 per cent increase or decrease in rate to the physician. Change in rate usually indicates impending battery failure and the physician has a seven-to-ten day safety period for replacement.[29]

Surgical Route. The main deterrent to use of the intravenous route is the fact that the catheter tip may flip back into the right atrium, or move out into the pulmonary artery. There is, then, a return to the arrhythmic state that necessitated the pacemaker implantation. Placement of the catheter must be checked under fluoroscope examination and repositioned.

When the surgical route is used, two incisions are made, the first to give access to the myocardium, either over the left or right ventricle, and the second to give access to a suitable bed of subcutaneous tissue for implantation of the unit. A vertical incision is made into the pericardium for placement of the electrodes in as bloodless an area as possible. They are placed parallel to the long axis of the heart so that there will be a minimum of flexion of electrodes with each heartbeat.[30] They are inserted deep into the myocardium. The electrodes may be tied on top of electrode platforms.[31]

The physician selects a second site in which to form a subcutaneous pocket for the pacemaker unit. If the axillary area is selected, an incision is made that curves beneath the left breast toward the axilla. If an abdominal pocket is to be used, an incision is made in the left lower quadrant at the level of the umbilicus. The pocket is formed under the external oblique muscle and the unit is inserted. It rests against the inguinal ligament where it cannot drift downward and put tension on the electrodes.[32] The electrodes are brought up into the chest in the free space behind the rectus muscle. They are passed through a large chest tube to decrease possible damage to the tissues and/or delicate electrodes, and are sutured in place.

The most common complication arising from pacing is fracturing of the wires. If the broken wire touches the left diaphragm, the patient may have persistent hiccuping; there may be muscular twitching from current leakage; or there may be intermittent pacing if the wires touch, become separated during activity, and then touch again. Multiple spot x-rays of suspected sites prove or disprove the wire break.

Another complication is ventricular fibrillation if improperly grounded hospital equipment is used near the patient who has a line-powered (from the electric outlet) pacer. The electrodes in the myocardium allow small currents to bypass skin and other tissue barriers and pass directly into the heart. This is not a hazard with battery-operated pacers.[33] "Grounding" simply means carrying the current to earth by means of some kind of conductor, where it is safely dissipated. Metal objects that are not covered by dust or thick paint may be used. The three-pronged plug is a coded plug containing a ground wire and is a reliable method of grounding line-powered equipment. Proximity to certain radiofrequency-emitting apparatus, such as diathermy units, should be avoided as they may interfere with the pacemaker's transistors and cause arrhythmias. Long-term, elective insertion of pacemakers is used in a variety of arrhythmic conditions including surgical damage to the AV conduction system, in elderly patients with arteriosclerosis and AV block, carotid-sinus syndrome in which the chemo- and pressure receptor is hypersensitive and the slightest pressure to the carotid sinus in the neck causes shocklike symptoms, and for people with Stokes-Adams disease in which there is unpredictable disturbance in ventricular rhythm with AV block leading to cerebral ischemia (lack of oxygen). Once the pacemaker is inserted the person senses a marvelous change, a "calm in the chest," and a sense of well-being. His cardiac output is improved.

The Coronary Care Unit

The concept of progressive patient care involves placement of the patient in an area determined by his medical and nursing needs; thus, a patient in serious cardiopulmonary distress will, more than likely, be cared for initially in an intensive care unit or, more specifically, in a coronary care unit. These are either open-ward, multibed units with pull curtains around each bed or individual one- or two-bed rooms. The common denominators, in either case, are specially prepared nurses (one nurse to every three patients) around the clock, the use of a cardiac monitor, and the ready availability of a defibrillator and external pacemaker. Many monitors are "three-in-one" devices, with the monitor, pacer, and defibrillator combined in one unit. (See Fig. 22–5.)

The cardiac monitor provides a continuous record of the body-function status of the patient and indicates the first clues of impending arrhythmias. It has an automatic audio and/or visual alarm system that is triggered by changes in heart rate and pulse range; however, the alarms are so sensitive that they are also triggered by patient movement in bed, such as using a bedpan and touching a metal bedframe. The alarm does, however, produce an "instant nurse," who assesses the situation and can take appropriate action. Some models have visible lights with remote audible sounds. The "beep" sound of each ventricular contraction is not heard by the patient, nor is the alarm sound. There is cardiac monitor equipment provided for each patient, with the oscilloscope either at the bedside, outside the room, and/or centrally located at the nurses' station. Most monitors allow for electrocardiograph recordings, with write-out strips that can be run electively or that are synchronized to print rhythm strips automatically during and preceding alarm situations. They have pulse-rate meters with a preset range (e.g., if the pulse falls below 50 beats per minute, an alarm sounds); temperature gauges (a special rectal thermometer is left in place in the patient); and a blood pressure gauge that measures blood pressure by means of the familiar cuff left in place on the arm. If the patient is conscious the nurse tells him she is taking his blood pressure so that he is not surprised by the sudden inflation of the cuff as if by magic. The nurse inflates the cuff by turning a dial on the monitor unit.

The patient is "connected" to the oscilloscope in much the same way that he is connected to a galvanometer for an electrocardiogram. At least two electrodes must be used; usually electrodes are placed on all four limbs, and sometimes on the chest. Before placement, the skin must be washed and dried. Perspiration and skin oils interfere with conduction. The search still goes on for a perfect electrode. They come in all sizes and shapes from a flat plate to a top hat; are disposable or reusable; are made of metal, plastic, rubber, or a combination of these materials; and are attached to the skin with powdered straps, adhesive or hypoallergenic tape, transparent tape, and contact cement. The effectiveness of the contact electrodes depends on the adequate use of conductive jelly (it contains an electrolyte solution) and remaining in place. The permanent types are usually removed, the skin washed and observed for redness, and their placement rotated daily. New contact jelly is applied. The disposable types are inspected daily but are usually changed every two days. Needle electrodes, implanted in subcutaneous tissue, serve as very effective electrodes and need rarely be changed; however, nurses are reluctant to use them though they cause no discomfort once they are inserted.

Many hospitals prefer to use direct measurement of arterial blood pressure [34] by means of arterial cannulation. This is done by inserting a catheter 3 in. into an artery, often the radial artery, and connecting it to a special pressure gauge that responds to blood pressure (a strain gauge). This, in turn, is connected to an arterial blood pressure monitor. Stopcocks attached to the strain gauge allow blood samples to be collected easily, and at any time, for blood gas measurement. This is an excellent means of estimating cell hypoxia and of evaluating adequacy of ongoing therapy. With arterial cannulation air embolism is a potential problem. All tubing and connections must be inspected regularly to prevent them from loosening. There are no standard arterial blood pressure values; a normal range must be developed for a given patient by recording several readings and determining an average for him.

Direct venous pressure can be obtained by inserting of a catheter 12 to 24 in. into a central vein (venae cavae; innominate, subclavian, or iliac veins). This gives direct estimate of hypo- or hypervolemia (blood volume). It measures the amount of pressure exerted against the venous wall. A low pressure might indicate blood loss or reaction to some drugs; a high pressure might mean congestion of the systemic veins from heart failure. Normal venous pressure is 0 to 4 cm water in the right atrium and 6 to 12 cm water in the venae cavae. All catheters inserted for monitoring purposes are inserted using sterile technique. The tubing should be positioned so that there is no tension on the catheter. Under no conditions should fluid be forced into a venous catheter to clear an obstruction. It may dislodge a large clot and cause an embolus!

Care is planned for the patient so that he will have maximum undisturbed time for sleep. During the first 24 hours in intensive care his blood pressure, pulse, and respirations are checked once an hour while he is awake, and every four hours while he is asleep. He is given complete care by the nurse, who encourages him to lie as still as possible.

The Environment of Coronary Care

There is a continuous, all-pervading sense of urgency in the unit. The constant attendance by staff and frequent check of patient condition often prevent the patient from sleeping. Lights and movement go on around the clock. Day becomes night and night becomes day for him. He loses all sense of time and date. He experiences an extreme lack of privacy. He is frequently bedded down next to a patient of the opposite sex. He is aware of emergencies happening around him. The threat of death and of nonbeing looms over him continuously. He experiences overabundant sensory input into the form of pain, light, noise, and activity around him, but he experiences sensory deprivation in the form of familiar communication with people. There is physical overstimulation and emotional deprivation.[35] He may become totally dependent on the monitor and the people caring for him, and may lose his autonomy as an individual and an adult. He may be in a state of emotional shock and amnesia and may not remember that he has had visitors or that equipment was explained to him. His conversation may be superficial and "cheerful," or he may not want to talk at all. In any case, the nurse must support him and must by her attitude convey the feeling of "I am with you. I will not push you but I will listen to you when you are ready to share your thoughts with me."

Major Alarms [36]

The following changes in patient condition warrant immediate action by the nurse:

Loss of consciousness for more than 15 seconds
Change in heart rate of 40 beats per minute or more
Drop in heart rate of 20 beats per minute if the rate was less than 70
Convulsions
Respiratory distress: mouth breathing, use of accessory muscles, apnea of 15 seconds' duration
Ventricular fibrillation

Hospitals vary in their routines for handling major alarm situations; however, in most instances the nurse would:

Ensure adequate airway: begin artificial respiration if patient is apneic or very cyanotic: use respirator or mouth-to-mouth breathing
Record ECG on strip recorder
Take blood pressure
Begin or be ready to have the physician begin intravenous fluids if pressure is less than 80 mm Hg systolic
Begin external cardiac massage if systolic reading is less than 30 mm Hg
Turn on the defibrillator and have paddles ready
If hospital policy allows, defibrillate if ventricular tachycardia or fibrillation is evidenced on oscilloscope
Prepare emergency drugs: lidocaine, sodium bicarbonate, epinephrine, procaine amide, and so on

The physician is called for any major alarm. He is also called if the patient should suddenly experience nausea, visual disturbances, dizziness or faintness, chest pain, pain in the left arm, jaw, or substernal area, respiratory difficulty, or change in the respiratory rate of plus or minus 5 breaths per minute lasting more than three consecutive minutes,[37] and change in the level of consciousness.

23

CORONARY DISEASE—CORONARY PRONENESS

CARDIOVASCULAR disease is the leading cause of death in the United States. Fourteen hundred Americans are killed by it each day.[38] Through the activities of the United States Public Health Service, a federal publicly supported agency, and the American Heart Association, a voluntary privately supported agency, much information is being compiled that points a menacing finger at several high-risk factors. Much of the information that now implicates these factors has been collected over a 20-year period in a study of over 5,000 adults living in Framingham, Massachusetts. The adults chosen for the study were between 30 and 62 years of age, and were free of heart disease at the inception of the study. They came from all walks of life. Each received a thorough examination that included blood tests, x-rays, blood pressure readings, and electrocardiograms. Detailed histories that included specific living habits were obtained. The same examination was repeated every two years. Each illness, no matter how small, was recorded in the interim periods. If the person died, an autopsy was performed to establish the specific cause of death.

These risks, if present, tend to increase the chances of a person's developing heart disease before he is 65 years of age. The risk is 1 in 20 to 50 if none of the factors is present, but 1 in 2 if two or three of the factors are present.[39] None of the factors is absolutely proved to be a cause of heart disease; however, all are proved to be associated with the increased incidence and prevalence of it.[40] All can be corrected! The high-risk factors are:

1. Diet
2. Obesity
3. Hypercholesteremia
4. Cigarette smoking
5. Hypertension
6. Lack of exercise with decreased lung vital capacity
7. Tension and stress
8. Heredity

We are definitely the products of modern Western socioeconomics. Our way of life is such that we gorge ourselves on high-status foods that tend to be very rich, that are high in fats, and that contain many "empty" calories. They make us put on weight but do not provide essential nutrients. We eat a diet extremely high in meat, eggs, and dairy products. These contain a great percentage of saturated fats (those loaded with hydrogen), which require cholesterol for their transport. (See p. 263.) The greater the quantity of saturated fat, the greater the amount of circulating cholesterol derived from synthesis in the liver and from ingested sources. In the famous Framingham study,[41] begun in 1948, data obtained through biennial examinations of a sample of the adult population in the 30-to-62-year-old showed that a high serum cholesterol level of 260 mg per cent (normal in United States is 200 to 210 mg per cent) predisposed to development of new heart disease. Interestingly, it is man's current level of cholesterol, rather than his past levels, that seems to affect development of new disease.[42] Of the total calories in the American diet, 40 to 45 per cent come from fats. It is suggested that this percentage be reduced to 30 per cent, and that half of this be in the form of polyunsaturated fats.

Physical fitness through regular activity seems to decrease the level of circulating cholesterol regardless of ingestion of saturated fats. In a study conducted by Mann et al.[43] it was found that, though the Masai people of Tanzania consume a diet rich in dairy fat and animal products, their high physical fitness level seems to preclude their developing coronary artery disease. Yet, we are geared to a physically inactive existence in the United States. We ride to work rather than walk; we clean our houses with a menagerie of electric devices that "save energy"; we enjoy our leisure passively in front of the television set. We gain weight insidiously over the years. We develop the chronic diseases of Western society: diabetes with its ultimate damaging effect on blood vessels, obesity, and coronary artery disease.[44] We develop hypertension with systolic readings over 140 mm Hg and diastolic readings over 100 mm Hg. Diastolic "minor" elevations over 90 mm Hg over a long period of time increase the risk of heart disease.

We support a multimillion-dollar cigarette industry though there is ominous statistical evidence that those who smoke a pack a day or more increase their risk of premature heart disease by three to six times that of the noncigarette smoker. On autopsy there is extensive deterioration in the arteries and arterioles of heavy smokers.[45] The exact mechanism of this change is poorly understood, though it is believed that the nicotine causes arterial vasoconstriction.

Underlying all these high-risk factors is the stress of modern-day living, especially in highly populated metropolitan areas. When emotional tension is high, we eat and smoke compulsively, our blood pressure is elevated, we tend to fatigue more readily, and then we are disinclined to exercise. In a study of Benedictine monks who ate a high-saturated-fat diet but who were isolated from the stresses of everyday living, there was little coronary disease. On the other hand, a high-saturated-fat diet, combined with the stresses of modern living, seemed to predispose to coronary artery disease. Russek [46] calls this the "atherogenicity of emotional stress."

A coronary-prone behavior type has been suggested through many studies.[47] This hypothetical person probably has a drive for upward social mobility, is aggressive and ambitious, is involved in competitive activities, has an enhanced sense of time urgency with vocational deadlines and pressure for vocational productivity, has a history of past social and vocational achievement and job status, takes a leadership role, seems to be unable to delegate responsibility, and is admittedly irritated at delays. He is restless and his verbal style is quick and staccato. He may house much hidden hostility.

On the other hand, the low-coronary-risk behavior type is more relaxed and easygoing, seldom becomes impatient, and takes more time to enjoy avocational pursuits. He is not easily irritated and works steadily but without a feeling of being driven by a lack of time. He is less competitive and does not seem preoccupied with social achievement. He moves and speaks in a slow and more smoothly modulated style.

A family history of premature heart disease gives a 2 to 1 increase in the chance of developing the disease.[48]

Each high-risk factor seems to be related to every other factor. Though premenopausal women seem to have a greater degree of protection than men, they approximate the male rate later in life.

Making the Diagnosis

The physician uses many tools to make the diagnosis of heart disease. His approach includes (1) the history, thought by some to be the most important factor in the examination; (2) the physical examination; (3) one or a series of electrocardiograms; (4) a chest x-ray; and (5) laboratory studies and other specialized diagnostic procedures that are indicated. Hurst [49] likens the making of a diagnosis to the five open fingers of a hand with each finger representing one part of the total procedure and the clenched fist suggesting that the best diagnostic tool is developed when all techniques are welded together.

The History

The history gives many important clues to the possible physiologic disturbance. By subtle questioning, the physician elicits the symptoms and the patient's response to them. He is particularly interested in some specific symptoms; for instance: When, where and what kind of pain does the patient have? Does he experience palpitation (a disagreeable awareness of the heartbeat described as "pounding," "jumping," or "stopping")? Is there dyspnea, and if so, when does it occur? Does the patient faint? This may indicate a transient loss of consciousness from inadequate cerebral blood flow. Does he cough? Have bloody sputum? This may indicate an increased pulmonary vascular resistance. Is he excessively fatigued? Fatigue may indicate the presence of hypoxia. The physician assesses the patient's personality and finds out what high-risk factors are present in his life, e.g., what is his diet like? Does he smoke? What familial diseases is he aware of?

The Physical Examination

In the physical examination the physician utilizes all of his special senses (touch, sight, sound, smell). He observes the vital signs, especially the blood pressure, and compares them with previous vital sign recordings. He inspects and palpates the organs to determine enlargement or ascites. These may be present in congestive heart disease. He listens to the sound of the heart and lungs. This gives him clues to the effectiveness of passage of blood through the heart chambers, the presence of edema, and so on. He compares electrocardiograph recordings and, if necessary, does an ECG after the patient exercises. He may do a phonocardiograph, in which the heart sounds are translated into electrical energy and are recorded on paper,[50] or a ballistocardiogram, in which the patient is placed on a table so delicately balanced that any vibration of the body caused by systolic ejection of blood into the aorta can be recorded.[51] The physician is particularly interested in the ophthalmoscopic examination of the retinal fundi, for this is a spot in the body where he can actually see small blood vessels. He can see arterosclerotic vessels, retinal hemorrhages, swelling of the head of the optic nerve (papilledema), and so on.

RADIOLOGIC EXAMINATION OF THE HEART

The physician utilizes fluoroscopy to actually visualize motility of the heart and lungs, and he may use cineradiography [52] to take moving pictures of fluoroscopic observations with specialized equipment. This provides a permanent record of fluoroscopic observations. He does a standard chest x-ray to gain information about the size of the heart and the presence or absence of enlargement of particular chambers.

ANGIOCARDIOGRAPHY

Angiocardiography is the method utilized to render cardiac chambers, heart valves, and blood vessels visible by use of a contrast medium (dye). The medium, usually an iodinated substance, can be injected intravenously and thereby outline all the structures; or it can be injected more selectively into specific vessels or chambers through a catheter. (See below.) Selective coronary arteriography reveals decreases in the internal diameter of the vessels, as in occlusion by atherosclerosis. Sometimes angiocardiography is misleading. Arteries appear perfectly patent on x-ray when coronary heart disease is surely present because of other findings.[53]

CARDIAC CATHETERIZATION

Using surgical aseptic technique, a catheter may be placed in either side of the heart to collect blood samples for blood-oxygen determinations, to obtain measurement of pressures in each of the heart's chambers (see Fig. 23–1), to outline cardiac cavities in an effort to detect abnormal pathways, to confirm clinically suspected lesions, to evaluate the effect of surgery, to allow for selective injection of contrast media for angiocar-

```
                    Right atrium        Left atrium
                    5 mm Hg             8 mm Hg

                    Right ventricle     Left ventricle    Aorta 130 mm Hg
                    25 mm Hg            130 mm Hg

Pulmonary artery
to lungs
25 mm Hg
```

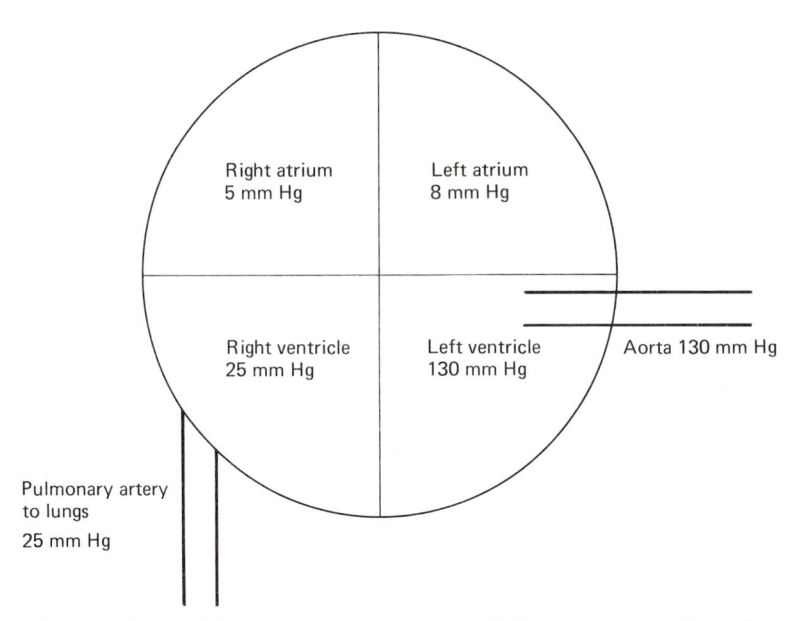

FIGURE 23–1. Schematic representation of the pressures within the heart chambers and major vessels.

diography, and so on. Many hospitals now have facilities for cardiac catheterization. It is carried out in a room that has fluoroscopy equipment so that passage and placement of the catheter can be visualized. For right-sided catheterization a catheter is inserted into a peripheral vein, usually an arm vein, to the vena cava, the right atrium, right ventricle, and pulmonary artery. For left-sided catheterization a venous cutdown is done and a long needle with a curved tip is advanced through a thin-walled catheter into the right side of the heart and then across the septum. It is then advanced until it is free in the left atrium. The needle is withdrawn, and the catheter can be advanced through the mitral valve into the left ventricle.[54] Retrograde (against the flow of blood) catheterization through the aorta and percutaneous catheterization (through the skin) into the left ventricle are sometimes selected for left-sided catheterization.

The patient is admitted the day before the catheterization. The procedure is explained to him by a member of the cardiovascular team, and he signs the permit for the test. An area 4 in. in diameter is shaved around the artery or vein to be used. If abdominal or renal aortography is scheduled, the patient is given a cathartic. He is allowed nothing by mouth for six hours before the test and is given a prophylactic antibiotic about two hours before and a sedative about a half-hour before. The patient lies on a fluoroscope table and is given a local anesthetic. He is asked to assume a variety of positions for different x-ray views and is frequently asked to deep-breathe and to perform the Valsalva maneuver in which he momentarily contracts his thorax and holds his breath.

Kelly [55] suggests the following ways of describing the sensations the patient will experience: "stinging" from injection of anesthetic; "tingling" in fingers from blunt dissection of brachial artery in antecubital area because of its proximity to nerves; "coldness-numbnesss" distal to the area of arterial incision until the artery is resutured; "low-back discomfort" from lying on the hard fluoroscope table for up to three hours; "warmth" if more than a few milliliters of contrast media is used.

Complications stemming from cardiac catheterization are not frequent; however, the nurse must observe for signs of local infection (redness, swelling, heat, elevated temperature); signs of phlebitis (swelling, pain, coldness in the limb, pallor, redness along the line of the vein); signs of pulmonary thrombosis from flushing a small clot in the pulmonary artery (sudden thoracic or abdominal pain, dyspnea, cough, hemoptysis); pyrogenic reaction (shivering, coldness); shock from loss of blood or perforation of atrium, ventricle, and so on (drop in blood pressure, increased pulse); and toxicity from the contrast media (headache, nausea, vomiting, urticaria). There will be cerebral symptoms if the brain supply of oxygen was decreased from the catheter insertion in a stenotic pulmonary valve, and so on. The nurse should watch for confusion, twitching, slurred speech, aphasia, amnesia, vertigo, visual disturbances, convulsions, and agitation.

CIRCULATION TIME

The time it takes for an intravascular substance to get to a sampling site and be subjectively experienced by the patient is the circulation time. Indicators may use color, vasodilator effect, radioactivity, effect on respirations, neuromuscular stimulation, smell, or taste.[56] Most frequently, taste is utilized. A substance, like sucrose, is injected intravenously with the patient in a supine position, and his arm abducted at midchest level. He is instructed to say "now" when he first tastes the indicator. A stop watch is used. Circulation time varies with age (it is longer in people over 40), sex (it is longer in men than in women), with position of the arm, and in certain diseases in which there is increased blood volume and therefore increased circulation time. Congestive heart disease is an example. The normal arm-to-tongue time is 15 seconds or less. The patient need not be fasting.

VENOUS PRESSURE TIME (See Fig. 23–2)

An increase in pressure in the venous circulation indicates inefficient pumping of the heart. The test is done at the bedside. The patient's right arm is positioned on a pillow so that the vein is level with the right atrium. A stopcock is attached between the syringe and needle. The needle

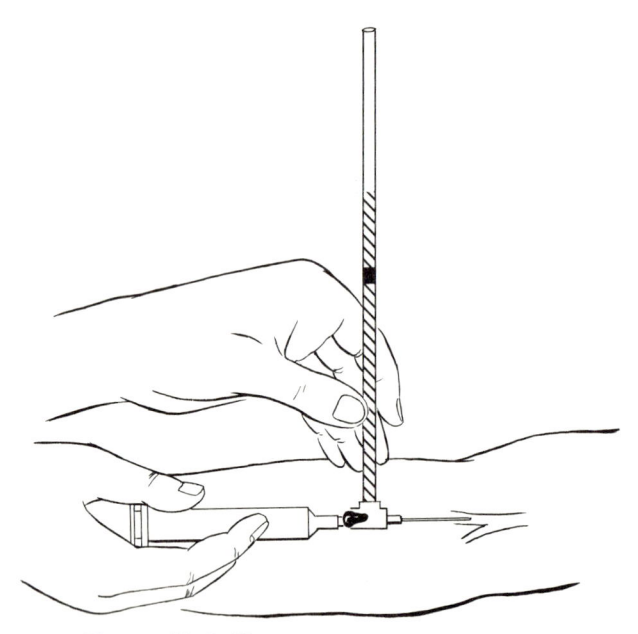

FIGURE 23–2. Venous pressure measurement.

with syringe is attached to one side of the stopcock, and a glass manometer calibrated in millimeters or centimeters is attached to the other side of it. The physician draws 5 ml of sterile normal saline or 3 per cent sodium citrate solution into the syringe, does a venepuncture, draws 2 to 3 ml of blood into the solution containing saline, attaches a glass manometer to the stopcock, and the blood and saline are then injected into the manometer. The stopcock is opened, and the mixture is allowed to run into the vein. The fluid level falls to the point at which the venous pressure supports it, and is then read. Normal venous pressure is 6 to 12 cm of saline or 40 to 100 mm of saline. It is elevated in diseases such as congestive heart failure.

General Laboratory Tests

A complete blood count, hemoglobin or hematocrit, and urinalysis are standard procedures for patients with suspected heart disease. Abnormalities indicate presence of infection, necrosis, degree of blood oxygenation, kidney involvement, and so on. Blood and throat cultures isolate specific microorganisms. An antistreptolysin titer may be done if rheumatic heart disease is suspected. Beta-hemolytic *Streptococcus* is implicated in the disease. Antistreptolysin titer of 400 Todd units occurs four to six weeks following infection with beta-hemolytic *Streptococcus* and may return to normal levels in four months. Serum cholesterol levels are studied. Normal United States levels are 160 to 270 mg per cent.

PROTHROMBIN TIME

This test indicates the ability of the blood to form clots. It may be done routinely on all patients with heart disease or daily for patients receiving anticoagulant drugs. The daily prothrombin time is used to evaluate the effectiveness of the amount of anticoagulant used. This is important. Too much of the drug can cause hemorrhage. Normal prothrombin time is 14 to 18 seconds.

ENZYME TESTS

The serum levels of certain enzymes normally found in heart, liver muscle, kidney, and pancreas are elevated following tissue damage. Levels of glutamic oxaloacetic transaminase (GOT or SGOT) are elevated within 6 to 12 hours following a myocardial infarct (death to the heart muscle from lack of blood supply). The normal SGOT serum level is 10 to 40 units; this is elevated to 160 to 400 units after an infarct. The greater the elevation, the grimmer the prognosis.[58] The lactic dehydrogenase enzyme (LDH) is elevated in almost all patients within a few hours following an infarction. Normal level is approximately 79 units.[59] Creatine phosphokinase (CPK) is also elevated following infarction. Normal range is 0 to 200 sigma units. Monoamine oxidase [60] is also elevated following infarction. Clinical study is currently being done to determine the effectiveness of inhibiting these enzymes with medication. When they are inhibited, there is an increased level of catecholamines (l-epinephrine and norepinephrine) and the vasopressor serotonin. These substances seem to increase the tone of heart contractions and, by doing this, decrease the deleterious effect of anoxia on the heart. On the other hand, they may produce increased myocardial oxygen consumption and increased arterial pressure.

Vessel Deterioration

Changes in the arteries and veins predispose to many kinds of disease. (See Fig. 23–3.) In arteriosclerosis, the vessels become hard, stiff, and brittle. There is atrophy of the muscle and elastic tissue. In atherosclerosis, stemming from the Greek word for "gruel or porridge," fatty lesions develop in the arterial wall. There is thickening in the intima with lipid deposition (laying down of fat) in the intimal and subintimal layers. The elastic

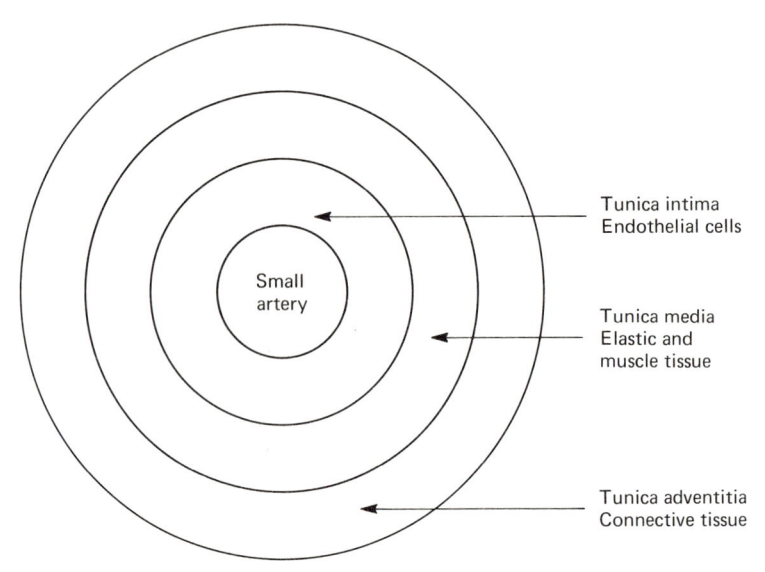

FIGURE 23–3. Schematic representation of a normal artery.

membranes become deformed and fragmented, with fibrosis and calcification. The fatty deposits cause lesions that appear yellow and are called fatty plaques; the increase in fibrous material causes lesions that appear whitish and are called pearly plaques. Both tend to block up the artery, causing occlusion and decrease in free flow of blood. Pieces of the plaque may break off and cause fatal embolus or perforate a vessel and cause ulceration and hemorrhage.[61] Most lesions develop in "high-stress" areas of the circulation. Because of the continuous contraction-relaxation of the myocardium, vessels supplying this area are prone to lesion formation. This disintegrative process also weakens the arterial walls and predisposes them to aneurysm formation. An aneurysm is an arterial dilatation or "outpouching" that is extremely prone to rupture.

The degenerative process occurs in this sequence:

1. Accumulation of lipid-laden cells.
2. Fibrous material surrounds fatty substance with thickened intima.
3. Capillaries form in the fibrous wall of the lesion to nourish this new tissue; prone to bleeding.
4. Crystallization and calcification of fatty material occurs.
5. Vessel is gradually occluded.

Arterial degeneration apparently is the result of a host-environment interaction (see discussion of high-risk factors, p. 234) and begins, in many Americans, very early in life. During the Korean War autopsies were performed on men in the 20-to-30-year age group. Forty per cent were found to show some coronary artery degeneration;[62] 70 to 80 per cent of men reaching 70 years of age show arterial degeneration.

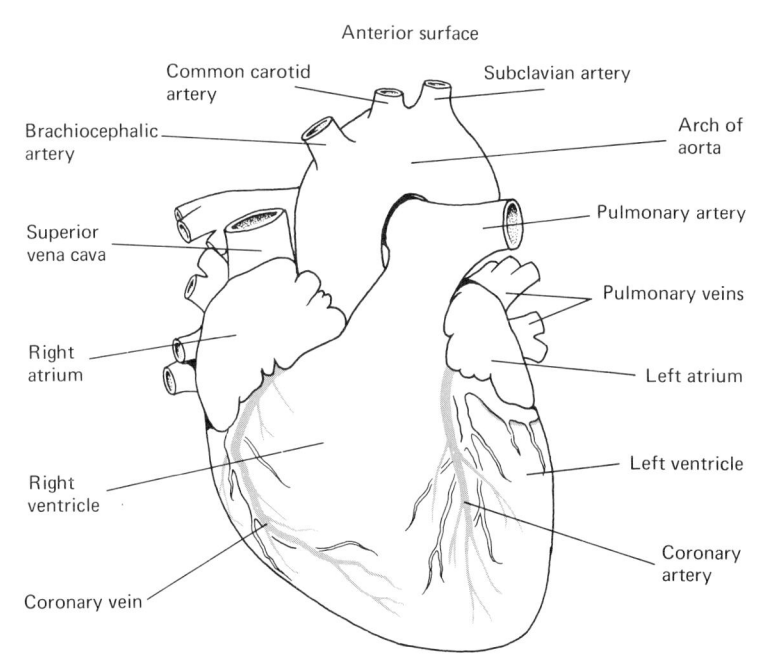

FIGURE 23-4. The heart and blood supply to the myocardium.

As the occlusion progresses there is a decrease in oxygen to the myocardium (heart muscle). This is called ischemia. Ischemia is responsible for a composite of clinical syndromes jointly referred to as coronary artery disease. They are the greatest single health problem in the United States [63] with a peak incidence in men between the ages of 50 and 60, in women between the ages of 60 to 70, after menopause.[64] The disease seems to be accelerated by the high-risk factors already discussed, and by the presence of other diseases such as hypertension and thyrotoxicosis (overactive thyroid gland). The two major syndromes associated with myocardial ischemia are angina pectoris, in which the myocardium remains alive, and infarction, in which the myocardium dies. This is called necrosis.[65] Midway between the severity of angina pectoris and absolute myocardial infarction is a "catchall" group of diagnostic titles, sometimes called coronary insufficiency, coronary failure, or intermediate coronary syndrome. The pain is not associated with the precipitating factors of angina pectoris, nor does it last as long (usually no longer than one hour) as the pain of acute infarction. Friedberg[66] suggests that careful diagnosis would probably place the patient in either of the two major categories of coronary artery disease. (See Fig. 23-4.)

Angina Pectoris

Angina comes from the Greek word meaning "strangle" and pectoris from pectus, meaning "breastbone." Angina pectoris has come to mean a sense of strangling or suffocation. Stemming from myocardial ischemia, it has two very distinctive features that help distinguish it from other coronray diseases: It is always precipitated by physical or emotional stress, and it is always relieved by nitroglycerin.

The pain of angina pectoris is characteristic, too. It usually radiates from the sternum in broad, horizontal bands over the left pectoral region and the left shoulder, to the inner aspect of the left arm, and through the forearm to the hand along the ulnar nerve.[67] It can, however, radiate to the left and right side, or to the right side alone, and occasionally it extends upward to the throat, face, jaws, and teeth.[68] Sometimes it begins over the scapular region and moves to the anterior chest. The pain is described by the patient in a very characteristic way, too. He says he experiences pressure, tightness, squeezing, choking, heaviness, a load on the chest, a desire to belch, or a feeling of a band tightening around his chest. There is extreme anxiety with the pain that seems to be more severe than the distress would warrant. The patient may break out in a sweat.

Severe emotion, pleasant or unpleasant, is one of the precipitating factors. Anger, fear, sudden tenseness or expectancy, loud or enthusiastic speech, an exciting book, television show, or movie, or a telephone call can precipitate an attack, as can passion and sexual intercourse. At times, an attack occurs during the night, probably the result of a nightmare.

Physical stress can precipitate an attack, too. Walking out of doors on a cold day, especially against the wind, is very significant. Pain may be induced by climbing stairs, by eating a large, heavy meal, or, in very severe cases, by performing usual activities of daily living, e.g., shaving, dressing, or washing. The distress is not always precipitated by the same amount of activity. Sometimes, a person can walk a block carrying a heavy bundle with no distress at all, and at other times, just carrying a bundle will cause pain in the same person.

Anginal pain comes during the stress, not afterward. It usually lasts only a short time, e.g., one to ten minutes, unless the stress factor continues. Patients experiencing the pain will be seen stopping in the middle of what they are doing and placing a nitroglycerin tablet, gr 1/400 (0.16 mg) or gr 1/200 (0.32 mg), under their tongue where it dissolves and is absorbed through the mucous membranes. It cannot be swallowed because it is inactivated by the gastrointestinal secretions. Relief comes in two to four minutes. The patient is advised to carry the drug with him at all times. It is one of the few medications he is allowed to keep at his hospital bedside. It is a good idea to have the nurse count the number he has at regular intervals during the day, e.g., when she gives other medications. In persons with normal coronary arteries, the nitroglycerin seems to increase blood flow by dilating the vessels; however, the mechanism by which nitroglycerin helps the person with angina pectoris appears to be a bit different.[69] In the person with angina, the arteries are rigid and narrowed and do not respond by dilating. The drug, though, seems to reduce blood pressure or venous return by temporary venous pooling of blood, and in this way temporarily decreases the work load of the heart. Sometimes the patient develops headaches from the nitroglycerin, but he develops a tolerance to the headaches after he uses the drug for awhile. He is instructed that he may take as many tablets as needed, sometimes up to 20 a day, *as long as the anginal pain is relieved by them*. If there is no relief within five minutes after taking one tablet, he takes another. If there is still no relief, the pain was not from angina pectoris![70]

Activities need not be greatly restricted if the angina pectoris is stable. They are adjusted to a level below that which causes pain. The patient comes to recognize those situations, physical or emotional, that cause him difficulty. He avoids them; or if stress activity is anticipated and essential, he is advised to take a prophylactic tablet of nitroglycerin prior to the activity.

The patient finds that wearing warmer clothes in the cold weather helps, and, of necessity, he tends to remain indoors on particularly cold and windy days.

Some patients must alter their eating habits. If large meals cause pain, they eat several small meals at more frequent intervals.

Collateral Circulation

Often, the heart muscle develops new arterial channels. This is called collateral circulation. It is believed that moderate, regular exercise encourages this developing circulation.

Patients with angina pectoris are able to live near-normal lives. Many have normal life-spans. However, angina pectoris has a significantly greater mortality for a given age.[71] Sudden death may be caused by myocardial infarction or coronary insufficiency.

Patients in whom angina pectoris appears for the first time, without other clinical abnormality, require a two-to-three-week rest period at home, while collateral circulation is being established. Hospitalization for one to two weeks is necessary for the management of intractable angina pectoris in an attempt to exclude the stresses precipitating the attacks. The patient is not allowed newspapers, television, and so forth until he is free from pain. The nurse observes the attacks especially to note changes in the pain. If the pain is "different," it may mean another cardiac problem. A small percentage of people with angina pectoris develop angina decubitus. This is a life-threatening advanced state of the disease that causes agony for one to three months.[72] It occurs in recumbency and seems to be relieved in the upright position.[73]

For those patients who do not respond to conventional medical treatment, surgery is contemplated. Coronary arteriography is done to determine the extent of the lesions. If they are localized, and if there is a significant decrease in blood supply to the anterior or lateral wall of the myocardium, endarterectomy or the Vineberg or Sewell procedures are done. Direct-vision coronary endarterectomy involves opening the artery and removing its thickened intima. The Vineberg procedure involves implanting the mammary artery into a tunnel made in the myocardium to increase circulation to that area. The Sewell procedure is a modification of the above. A pedicle containing artery, vein, muscle, and connective tissue is implanted into the myocardium. Sometimes a physician will elect to make a euthyroid (normal thyroid) person hypothyroid with the use of I^{131}. It is known that too much thyroid hormone aggravates angina pectoris. Use of irritant substances placed in the pericardial sac (cardiopericardiopexy) to encourage inflammation and revascularization is not done very often any more.[74]

Sympathectomy, the severance of the upper dorsal sympathetic nerves, completely denervates the heart, coronary vessels, head, neck, and upper extremities.[75] It is sometimes elected for stubborn angina complicated by hypertension.

Myocardial Infarction

Infarction means death to the tissues. A myocardial infarction is death to a portion of the myocardium as a result of ischemia. The ischemia may come from distinct occlusion of the coronary artery, as from thrombus, hemorrhage, embolus, or atheromatous plaque; or from unusual demands made upon a coronary circulation unfit, because of the degenerative processes, to contend with them. The most common site of myocardial infarction is in the anterior wall of the left ventricle near the apex. It results from occlusion of the descending branch of the left coronary artery. The second most common site of infarction is in the posterior wall of the left ventricle near the base, behind the posterior cusp of the mitral valve. It results from occlusion of the right coronary artery or circumflex branch of the left coronary artery.[76] If the infarction involves the entire thickness of muscle it is called a transmural infarction and is usually associated with coronary artery occlusion. If the infarct is not full-thickness, and is confined to the endocardium, occlusion is usually not present.[77]

Myocardial infarction is the leading cause of death as well as a major cause of disability among those between the ages of 40 and 70.

SYMPTOMS OF MYOCARDIAL INFARCTION

The symptoms can occur during the day or night, and are not necessarily precipitated by physical or emotional stress. Myocardial infarction is commonly known as a "heart attack" or "coronary." The pain is sudden, severe, horribly frightening, and long-lasting. Unlike the pain of angina pectoris, it is not relieved by nitroglycerin, and lasts an hour or more. The patient describes the pain as being crushing, compressing, viselike, like a red-hot poker, like someone sitting on his chest, or like an elephant stepped on him. It begins spontaneously and is constant, not intermittent. It frequently starts in the substernal area and radiates to the left or right arm and down through the arm to the wrist and hand. It can, however, begin anywhere in the anterior chest, the back, epigastrium, jaw, neck, shoulder, or arm. Because of the interrelated nature of the nerve supply to the gastrointestinal and coronary systems, the patient often is nauseated, has diarrhea, and feels like "he is having indigestion." The act of defecation may precipitate an attack because of vagal (vagus nerve) stimulation. The vagus nerve slows the heart.

PAIN IN MYOCARDIAL INFARCTION

The pain is triggered by extreme tissue hypoxia and by accumulation of by-products of tissue necrosis. The patient becomes gravely frightened. His fear stimulates the parasympathetic nervous system, which causes reflex vasoconstriction with pallor, severe perspiration (he "breaks out" in a cold sweat), nausea, vomiting, faintness, and vertigo.[78] He has difficulty breathing. His pulse may be irregular from tachycardia, and he may be in severe cardiogenic shock. (See p. 214.)

Infrequently, the patient has a "silent coronary." It happens so gradually, or so rapidly, that metabolism stops in the totally anoxic muscle. There is no product to trigger the pain response, and the patient is unaware that he has had an infarction.[79]

STAGES IN INFARCTION AND HEALING

Stage One. Inflammation and leukocyte infiltration. Lasts about three days. The inflammatory response to body injury causes dilatation of blood vessels; leukocytes converge around the periphery of the infarct; area is deep red if infarct was hemorrhagic, clay-colored if ischemic.

Stage Two.

1. Muscle fiber removal
2. Development of collateral circulation

From the end of the third day; dominates second week; may last days or weeks. All necrotic tissue is removed beginning at the periphery and progressing to the inner parts of the infarct. There is a depressed, reddish-purple band close to the center of the infarct; a yellowish band between its periphery and viable tissue. The border between viable and non-viable tissue is uneven. Some "borderline" muscle lives; some dies. Regardless of the size of the infarct, most necrotic tissue is removed by the end of the fourth week. Removal of muscle fiber causes thinned cardiac wall.

Collateral circulation develops and nourishes the areas adjacent to the infarct.

About the twelfth day collagen begins to form in preparation for scar formation.

Stage Three. Scar formation.

Third week to second to third month. Increased laying down of collagen bundles causes change in the color of the depressed red ring to a "ground-glass" gray hue. Scar tissue completely replaces necrosed muscle. Area is now firm, shrunken, and white.

LABORATORY STUDIES IN MYOCARDIAL INFARCTION

There will be an increase in blood sedimentation rate and an increase in leukocyte count about the second to third day. This results from the inflammatory response to the trauma. Glycosuria may develop in a diabetic or a nondiabetic patient. In the former it is a result of sugar imbalance caused by the stress of the infarction; in the latter it results from stress stimulating the adrenal cortices to produce more glucocorticoids, one function of which is insulin antagonism.

Serum Enzymes. An elevation in certain serum enzymes may help in making the diagnosis. These enzymes are produced by organs of the body and are spilled into the blood when necrosis occurs. An increase in serum glutamic oxaloacetic transaminase (SGOT; GOT) from the normal range of 10 to 40 units is usually present 6 to 12 hours after an infarction. Lactic dehydrogenase (LDH) is elevated above the normal 79 units a few hours after the infarction. This is also true of monoamine oxidase (MAO). These enzymes are also elevated in other kinds of diseases and cannot be used as the sole diagnostic tool. (See p. 241.)

ECG IN MYOCARDIAL INFARCTION

Very definite changes occur in the electrocardiograph tracings following myocardial infarction;[80] however, changes frequently do not become apparent for 24 hours or more following the infarction. An early ECG recording may be deceptive in its normal appearance! Soon after the infarction, there are changes in the S-T segment. It is either elevated above or depressed below the baseline depending on whether the tracing comes from a lead facing toward or away from the infarcted area. The S-T change is thought to be caused by injured but living tissue, and it regains its normal tracing as the tissue either becomes ischemic, dies, or returns to normal. There is an inversion of the T wave that persists if the area of ischemia is large, and the Q wave takes on a deep, broad, conspicuous appearance representative of electrically dead tissue and scar tissue. These unusual Q waves often persist after the infarction is healed.

COMPLICATIONS OF MYOCARDIAL INFARCTION

Nine per cent of all patients experiencing infarction develop one of the complications arising from it.[81] The first week is the most critical period, with many deaths occurring during the first 48 hours. However, complications continue to be a problem throughout the total healing process.

Pericarditis

This results from extension of the infarct to the epicardium, the outer coat of the heart muscle. It can appear within 24 hours after the infarct, or several days later, and disappears spontaneously. Sometimes it becomes more extensive, with effusion, changes in the ECG, and severe pain.

RUPTURE OF HEART MUSCLE

As the heart muscle degenerates and muscle fibers are removed, the muscle wall becomes thinner. There is a paradoxical cutting-like movement between the involved and noninvolved areas during contraction,[82] and the myocardium tears. Blood pours into the pericardial sac and prevents the heart from filling. Death follows. Danger of rupture, present from the fourth to fourteenth day,[82,83] is more common among women than among men. It seems to be precipitated by a sudden increase in intracardiac pressure or excessive effort.

THROMBOEMBOLI

If the infarct spreads to the endocardium, or if the infarcted wall dilates, a thrombus may result. This may break off, become an embolus, and cause death.

Congestive Heart Failure

This condition occurs in many patients during the second to sixth week. It develops when the left ventricle decreases in efficiency as a pump and there is an acute buildup of fluid in the pulmonary circulation. The older the patient is, the more likely he is to experience this complication. The condition is grave if it lasts a length of time. (See below.)

Other complications are rupture of the papillary muscle, arrhythmias, aneurysms, and spread of the infarction, especially from excessive exertion by the patient.

Congestive Heart Failure

This is a syndrome of symptoms produced when the heart loses its effectiveness as a pump and causes circulatory congestion throughout the body. Although it is frequently seen as an acute complication of myocardial infarction, it usually is a chronic disease, seen in adults over 40, and developing gradually over a period of months and years. The pumping impairment often originates in the left ventricle; however, because the heart and blood vessels make up a closed-circuit system, the right side responds to left-sided impairment. It cannot continue to pump out more blood into the pulmonary artery than the left side is pumping through the aorta. The output of the right side, then, is secondarily decreased when the left side is deficient. Often, both ventricles fail simultaneously.[84] The two major precursors [85] to all the symptoms are decreased cardiac output with inadequate oxygenation of the tissues and an elevated venous pressure with backup or congestion of fluids in the left and right side of the heart, the lungs, and throughout the body. With the decreased cardiac output there are a decreased renal blood flow and glomerular filtration rate. This results in an increase in renal reabsorption of sodium and edema. The elevated venous pressure pushes water out of the capillaries and into the tissue spaces. This, too, causes edema. Blood volume is decreased and probably stimulates the secretion of aldosterone by the adrenal glands. Aldosterone also causes sodium retention. Liver congestion interferes with the normal breakdown of aldosterone in that organ, further increasing its level in the circulation with additional retention of sodium.

Sequence of Events Causing Symptoms of Congestive Heart Failure

1. Failure of left ventricle to pump enough blood through the aorta → decrease in blood and oxygen to body tissues → forward failure

2. Failure of left ventricle to pump enough blood through the aorta → failure of left ventricle to empty completely → buildup of blood in pulmonary veins and capillaries → increased pressure and congestion in lungs → lymph drainage unable to keep up with excess fluid formation → backward failure with pulmonary edema

3. Response of right ventricle to impaired left ventricle pumping → decreased pumping activity of right side of the heart → congestion of fluids

in the pulmonary artery and the venae cavae → tissue edema throughout the body

Congestive heart failure is considered "latent" when symptoms do not occur at rest but are precipitated by increased stress. It is considered "compensated" when normal physiologic mechanisms, medical intervention with drugs, and so forth cause a decrease in or control of the symptoms. Hypertrophy of the left ventricle in an attempt to pump with adequate effectiveness is a compensatory mechanism. Increased sympathetic stimulation in response to increased carotid pressure and so forth is a compensatory mechanism. It causes increased contractility of the heart and helps to maintain the blood pressure by increased stimulation to the arteries and veins.

Symptoms of Congestive Heart Failure

For ease of discussion, the symptoms are separated into those resulting from right-sided failure and those resulting from left-sided failure. Most symptoms, however, are seen simultaneously.

SYMPTOMS FROM LEFT-SIDED FAILURE

These symptoms stem primarily from increased lung congestion. Fluid is backed up in the pulmonary vein. There is cough, which is often dry and nonproductive and occurs most frequently at night. There is dyspnea (shortness of breath), which is often relieved in the upright position and tends to decrease venous return and, by doing this, increases vital capacity. The dyspnea frequently awakens the person during the night (paroxysmal nocturnal dyspnea) probably when a full bladder or a nightmare suddenly causes an increased need for oxygen and an increased pumping action of the left ventricle. The patient frequently has difficulty sleeping, and may have Cheyne-Stokes respirations (periods of apnea and periods of hyperpnea). He may have cardiac asthma in which pulmonary edema causes bronchospasm and wheezing during expiration. An attack of acute pulmonary edema is life-threatening. The patient can "drown in his own lung fluid." He suddenly sits up or stands upright and becomes very anxious, pale, and drenched in sweat; his skin may be cyanotic and cold and clammy. Respirations are rapid with very dramatic use of the accessory muscles of respiration. There may be prolonged respiratory wheezing, rattling sensations in the trachea, and profuse watery or blood-tinged sputum. Shock may follow.[86]

THERAPEUTIC INTERVENTION FOR PULMONARY EDEMA

Specific therapeutic measures include treatment with diuretics, rotating tourniquets, and phlebotomy.

Rotating Tourniquets.[87] With the production of stasis of blood in the veins, about 1,000 ml less is transported to the heart and lungs. Rubber-tube tourniquets can be used. They are tightened sufficiently to cause venous congestion without obliterating the arterial pulse. Sphygmoman-

A. 10:00 A.M. Apply tourniquets to three limbs.

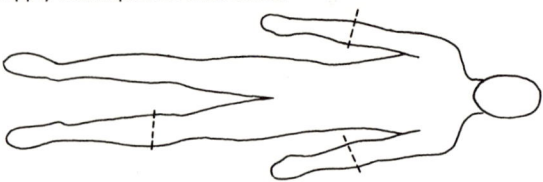

B. 10:15 A.M. Remove tourniquet from left leg and place on right leg.

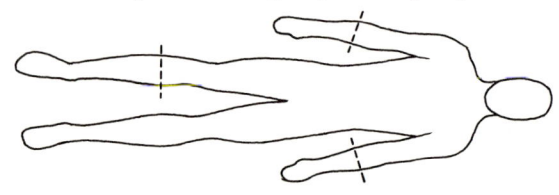

C. 10:30 A.M. Remove tourniquet from left arm and apply to left leg.

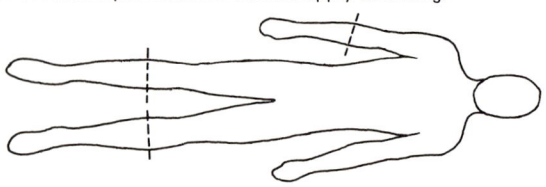

D. 10:45 A.M. Remove tourniquet from right arm and apply to left arm.

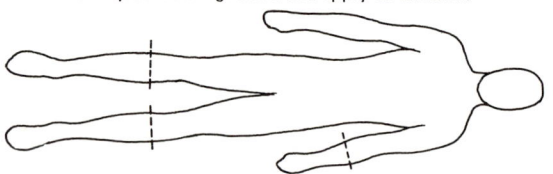

E. 11:00 A.M. Remove tourniquet from right leg and apply to right arm.

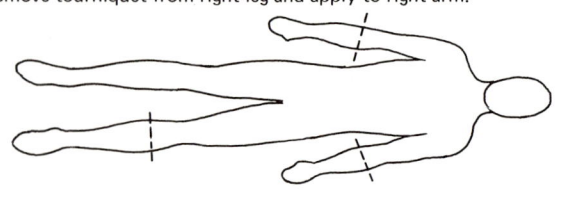

FIGURE 23–5. Rotating tourniquets. (From I. Dutcher and S. Fielo, *Water and Electrolytes: Implications for Nursing Practice*, 1967. Reprinted with permission of The Macmillan Co., New York.)

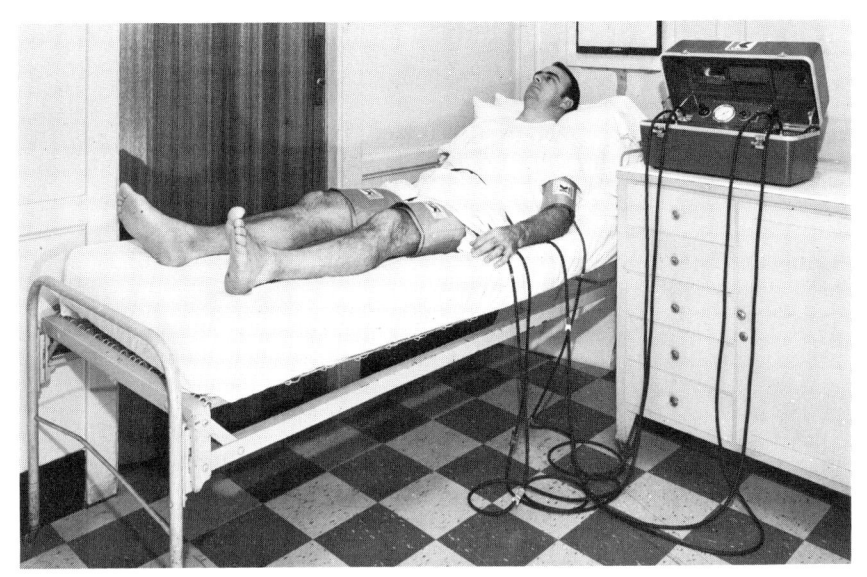

FIGURE 23-6. Automatic rotating tourniquets. (Courtesy, Walter Kidde & Co., Belleville, N.J.)

ometer cuffs, if available, are more accurate. They are inflated to a point slightly above the level of the diastolic pressure.[88] The tourniquets are left on three of the four limbs for no more than 45 minutes each limb. Using a counterclockwise schedule, one tourniquet is removed every 15 minutes and is applied to the unbound limb. The congested extremities will appear blue. Automatic rotating tourniquets are preset to change every 11 minutes. (See Figs. 23-5 and 23-6.)

Phlebotomy (Venesection). This procedure is used only if rotating tourniquets fail to produce the desired effect. With a standard blood donor set, 350 to 1,000 ml of blood is removed from a vein, thereby reducing circulating blood volume.

Paracentesis. In this procedure, fluid is removed from a body cavity, usually the abdominal cavity, for ascites. (See a fundamentals-of-nursing textbook for procedure.) The pericardial sac may also be "tapped" for fluid.

SYMPTOMS OF RIGHT-SIDED FAILURE

These stem, primarily, from backup of fluid and increase in pressure in the venous systemic circulation causing edema throughout the body. There is an initial weight gain from the retention of sodium and water. Frequently there is a reversal in urinary excretion. Instead of voiding during the day, the patient finds himself up during the night to void. Edema develops in the course of the illness and is first seem in the periphcral areas of the body. Fingers swell and rings become too tight. There is edema in the ankles, and this travels up the entire leg. It is the "pitting" type: when a finger is pressed on the skin a pitlike indentation remains even after the pressure is removed. The legs become very heavy, and it is difficult for the patient to move them. The skin is stretched taut and thin from the buildup of interstitial fluid. The skin is poorly nourished and likely to break down.

Congestion in the abdominal organs and in the liver causes anorexia, nausea, vomiting, distention, and pain. The liver is enlarged and tender.

One of the earliest warning signs of congestive heart failure, frequently not heeded by the patient, is profound fatigue. It is out of proportion to the activity that precipitates it. It is caused by hypoxia of the tissues. Not enough blood is pumped to them to supply additional oxygen when metabolism is increased.

The trilogy of symptoms seen with congestive heart failure is dyspnea, edema, and fatigue.

24

MANAGEMENT OF PATIENTS WITH CARDIOVASCULAR DISEASE

MAJOR goals in the medical-nursing management of the patient with cardiovascular disease include all measures designed to provide the patient with a "physiologic environment" conducive to healing. Specific measures include:

1. Decrease of the oxygen requirements of the heart muscle
   a. Relief of pain
   b. Physical and emotional rest; decreased stress factors
   c. Relief of dyspnea
   d. Decrease of edema
   e. Modification in activities of daily living
   f. Modification in diet
2. Control or modification of cardiovascular function
   a. Use of cardiotonic glycosides, antiarrhythmic drugs, anticoagulants
   b. Use of surgery
3. Prevention of complications associated with immobility
4. Awareness of and speed in handling concomitant emergencies
5. Long-term modification of high-risk factors
6. Rehabilitation (transcends each goal)

The Experience

The heart symbolizes life. It is a profoundly devastating experience to have an attack upon it. The patient responds to the crisis in much the same way he responds to grief, first with shock, then with denial ("this did not happen to me, the doctors are all wrong"), and gradually, through an uneven course, to accepting his changed health image and adjusting or not adjusting to what has happened. The end effectiveness of adjustment depends on the patient's own philosophy as a human being, on the way that he has learned to cope with crises in the past, and on the support he gets in the hospital, at home, and in the community. His family experiences grief, too. If they are supported effectively, feedback to the patient is beneficial rather than harmful. *Rehabilitation begins the day the patient comes to the hospital.* The major goal is to help him attain his maximum potential according to his own medical status. Although he must go through a period of almost total dependence on people and machines, he is weaned as soon as it is deemed safe. After an initial period of absolute rest, he is allowed as much sharing in decisions concerning his daily care as is possible. If he is permitted only limited activity, he helps to decide which activities he can tolerate having others do and which he feels he must do himself. It is understood that this is an adult who has had a monumental interruption in his developmental tasks, and the fact that he is in the hospital does not magically remove his responsibilities. A nurse who has developed an attitude that conveys, "I care; I am with you; I understand your reaction" supports him as he progresses through the stages of grief and toward understanding and adjustment. There will be changes in his life that he will discuss with his doctor; the decisions made during these discussions will more likely be fruitful if the patient is given ample and frequent time to explore his feelings with the nurse.

Providing Rest

The major goal of care during the first three to six weeks after a myocardial infarction is to decrease the oxygen requirements of the heart so that it has the chance to heal and so that extension of the infarct does not occur. The length of time required for complete rest following congestive heart failure depends on the extent of coronary insufficiency. How difficult it is to achieve rest! The word implies freedom from undue anxiety as well as decrease in physical activity. A calm but decisive nurse helps to attain this. She controls environmental stimuli by reminding people to lower their voices, by not being afraid to turn off the television set, and by limiting the number of visitors allowed in the patient's room at one time and observing the patient's reaction to them. Those who are very upsetting to the patient must have their visits restricted. The nurse plans care to allow for maximum periods of undisturbed quiet time.

Control of Pain

During the first week following a myocardial infarction and for varying lengths of time following congestive heart failure, there is pain. This continues in varying degrees during the postacute phase of the illness. When there is pain, the patient cannot rest; therefore, he is usually sedated and given analgesics during the first 48 hours, and then given analgesics according to need thereafter. The nurse must pay particular attention to the number of respirations per minute and question the administration of an opiate if they fall below 12 to 14. She must also keep the side rails up if the patient is sedated. After the initial period of severe pain, the nurse begins to help the patient differentiate between types of pain he experiences so that he does not leave the hospital believing every commonly occurring ache means he is "having a heart attack"! If he has angina pectoris, he should be aware of the specific nature of and relief for the pain.

Activity

The actual amount of activity allowed depends on the degree of the involvement and the philosophy of the physician. *It must be clarified explicitly.* During the first 48 hours no activity is allowed. The patient then progresses through gradual addition of activities. He is observed before, during, and after any new addition. If pain, dyspnea, or extreme fatigue follows, the activity is excluded for the time being. The pulse, too, should be felt and counted by the nurse for a full minute before and after the activity. If it becomes thready, irregular, or greatly increased in rate, the activity is terminated. Many physicians introduce activity early because of its thrombolytic effect.[89]

Armchair Therapy

In this treatment the patient is lifted from his bed to a comfortable chair so that there is no expenditure of energy on his part. This sitting position decreases the work load of the heart by decreasing venous return from the limbs. Gravity tends to mobilize fluid in the legs, and pulmonary congestion is decreased.[90]

Control of Dyspnea

If the patient has difficulty breathing, he will not be able to rest. Frequently, he breathes easiest in nonrecumbent positions. If he is "orthopneic," his dyspnea is decreased in the sitting position. He often sleeps in this position. Oxygen is administered by mask, nasal catheter, or cannula, or by tent if an air-conditioning effect is desired or if the oxygen is to be used for periods longer than 48 hours to decrease irritation to the nasal passages. Intermittent positive-pressure breathing may be used for pulmonary edema. It tends to decrease the transudation of fluid from the pulmonary capillaries.

Control of Edema

Edema increases the work load of the heart, makes breathing more difficult, is extremely frightening to the patient, and does not allow him to rest. The physician may prescribe diuretics to control this, or he may prescribe use of rotating tourniquets.

Bathing

During the first 48 hours the patient is usually not bathed, though his face can be gently sponged to make him more comfortable. He is then gradually allowed a partial bath, then a full bath, and ultimately assists the nurse with the bath. By the end of the sixth week he is usually participating in complete self-care. After the first 48 hours the physician will probably allow passive limb exercise, four to five times every day. Bathtime is one appropriate time for taking the limbs through full range of motion. Later, active limb exercise will be allowed, and the nurse must ensure scheduling of this activity. Keeping the pressure of covers off the patient's feet and use of a footboard help maintain proper body alignment.

Feeding

Feeding often begins with intravenous fluids and progresses to liquid, soft, and regular diets. Calories are usually restricted to 1,200 or less a day because of decreased metabolic needs. Low-caffeine beverages usually replace coffee and tea, and gas-forming foods are eliminated. Special therapeutic diets are utilized if warranted by the patient's condition. Sodium restriction is prescribed when edema is a problem. (See p. 261.) It may not be required following a myocardial infarction. Fat restriction may be indicated for coronary artery disease. In any case, therapeutic regimes are usually continued when the patient returns home, and instruction of the patient and his family should begin early. Feeding is an important facet in the patient's care. It should be done in a leisurely manner. It is a good idea to actually sit when feeding a patient and say to him, "I have time; I'm in no hurry." Foods should not be too cold because cold produces a reflex vasoconstriction. Ice water should not be "automatically" placed on the bedside stand. Very hot foods cause distention, and they should be avoided, too.

Elimination

During the first 48 hours most physicians require the patient to use the bedpan and the urinal in bed. The nurse's attitude in this area makes the use of this equipment easier for the patient. Ensuring privacy is important, though not always easy. Odor and sound cannot be made "private" in a multibed room. If the patient's roommate(s) is ambulatory, it might help to have him spend some time in the solarium while the patient is attempting to use the bedpan. There are some dangers associated with bowel evacuation. The great wandering vagus nerve has branches that supply the heart as well as the intestines. Vagal stimulation slows the heart. Defecation frequently causes enough vagal stimulation to actually slow the heart to a serious level. For this reason, stool is kept soft with stool softeners, the patient is encouraged to drink sufficient quantities of water and fruit juices, and he is observed carefully before and after defecation. Enemas, if they must be given, should be given from a height no greater than 12 in. above the buttocks, and should be given with an 18 to 20 French catheter. Rectal thermometers should be well lubricated and inserted gently if they must be used. Any procedures involving the rectum should be done with caution.

Many physicians allow use of a bedside commode and allow male patients to stand at the side of the bed and use the urinal. They find that this activity involves less expenditure of energy than attempting to void or defecate in the unnatural in-bed position.

Ambulation

When the patient is finally allowed out of bed, he feels he has crossed a major landmark. His enthusiasm, however, must not cause him to do too much at once. Ambulation is often introduced at the end of the third week, and should take seven to ten days to accomplish.[91] It is a gradual process. The patient is observed for pulse change, dyspnea, pain, and extreme fatigue before and after the activity. A schedule should be mapped out, with the nurse signing her name when a particular phase of ambulation is accomplished. Ambulation begins with balancing on the edge of the bed and progresses through sitting in a chair, walking to the bathroom and using it for elimination purposes only, using the bathroom for longer periods of time, taking short walks in the halls, and so on.

COMPLICATIONS ASSOCIATED WITH IMMOBILITY

After the initial period of absolute bed rest, all efforts must be made to decrease complications associated with immobility. The patient should be encouraged to take frequent deep breaths and to turn from side to side, to decrease the possibility of stasis of secretion in the lungs. His joints should be passively and then actively exercised. They should be taken through complete range of motion at least four or five times each day. The patient should be encouraged to periodically dorsiflex his feet and move his knees and hips. These activities help prevent muscle atrophy and contractures and decrease the chance of phlebitis. Often, elastic bandages, with equal pressure applied from the ankle to the knee, are used. The knee gatch is not used as it puts pressure in the popliteal space.

Shoulder-Hand Syndrome

In this syndrome there are pain, tenderness, and limitation of motion at the shoulder girdle. The hand on the affected side may be discolored, and the fingers stiff. This may occur anytime between the second week and fourteenth month following a myocardial infarction;[92] although the pain and swelling subside, flexion deformity of the fingers often remains.

Anterior Chest Wall Syndrome

This is a painful affection of the structures of the chest wall. When the chest is touched, there is exquisite tenderness. This may be the result of inadequate chest expansion and improper body alignment.

Diversion

Diversional activity is a must after the initial acute phase is over. Once the pain subsides the patient feels remarkably well, and it is very difficult for him to remain inactive and in bed for what seems like an unbearable length of time. His likes and dislikes are considered in planning diversional activity. Beginning with spectator-type activities, the patient gradually becomes involved in participant activity. He reads, paints, watches television, visits, as long as the activity is not too exciting. Common sense plays an important part here. The patient would probably be upset by the latest detailed report of heart disease in a current magazine for laymen, by a horror show on television, and so on. He might benefit from telephone conversations with family or friends. His personality plays an important role in determining what he should or should not do. Discussing this with him and with his family may help in initial decisions.

At Home

Gradual return to a comparatively active life is possible for most patients who have experienced cardiac problems. After they leave the hospital there is a convalescent period of three to six months at home, with some modifications made in daily routines. For instance, if the patient lives in a two-floor house all of his daily activities should be on one floor so that he does not have to run up and down the steps. A bed or couch should be available for rest periods. If the convalescing person is a woman with young children, some household help may be indicated. Many communities have trained visiting homemakers for this purpose. In any case, a visiting nurse might be very helpful in guiding this transitional phase. The physician can refer the patient to a visiting nurse association before he leaves the hospital.

The patient returns to work a few hours a day three to four months following an infarction, or when his condition permits in congestive heart failure. Sometimes, adjustments must be made in the type of work done, but in many instances the patient can resume his previous occupation. In a study reported by Lewis,[93] it was found that the patient's perception of his own disability was significantly related to his future activity. In patients with the same severity of disease, marked pessimism seemed to accompany failure to return to work, decreased off-job activity, decreased sexual activity, and so on. These patients are rejected or overprotected by their families, are unable to tolerate their cardiac status, and are in constant fear of a new attack. They become "cardiac invalids." On the other hand, those patients who were optimistic about their cardiac status returned to work. In most cases, this group had been working continuously for five years prior to the attack, had a high-school education or better, were "white-collar workers" or, if "blue-collar workers," belonged to unions, and were not known to any welfare agency. Family members did not reject or overprotect them. They resumed adjusted, but relatively normal lives.

Diet Modification

Most changes in diet are prescribed for long periods of time, sometimes for the rest of the patient's life. He and his family must be involved in learning about the diet throughout the hospitalization. The nutritionist does diet teaching; however, the nurse must implement and clarify material for the patient and his family.

SODIUM RESTRICTION

Although sodium attached to chloride is common table salt, sodium can also be attached to a variety of other chemicals used for many purposes. The person on a restricted-sodium diet limits sodium chloride as well as other sodium-containing chemicals, according to the amount of restriction prescribed by the physician. This is an integral part of the total therapeutic regime. Just as the physician orders a precise amount of a drug (you would not administer "just a little" morphine sulfate), he also orders the amount of sodium allowed. Terms like "low-sodium diet," "salt-poor diet," and "salt-free diet" are not explicit enough, nor is it enough to tell a patient to "cut down on his salt." Unless specific levels of restriction are ordered, the term may be misleading. The average American diet contains 3 to 6 gm of sodium. The American Heart Association has compiled several booklets pertaining to specific restriction levels, with food-exchange lists and number of servings allowed according to calories for the day. The lists include milk and milk products, vegetables, fruit, bread, meat, fat, and free choice. Booklets can be obtained from the American Heart Association, 44 East 23rd Street, New York, New York 10010.

The following levels of restriction with specific instructions follow:

MILD RESTRICTION (2,400–4,500 mg per day)

A limited amount of sodium may be used in cooking. Decrease the amount used to one half that normally used. Use no sodium at the table. Omit obviously "salty" foods (see p. 262).

MODERATE RESTRICTION (1,000 mg per day)

Use no sodium in cooking or at the table, with the exception of ¼ teaspoon (1 teaspoon equals 2,300 mg sodium) a day either at the table or combined in such foods as regular bakery bread (1 slice equals 200 mg sodium) and salted butter (2 teaspoons equal 100 mg sodium). Omit obviously "salty" foods.

STRICT RESTRICTION (500 mg per day)

Use no sodium in cooking or at the table. Avoid "salty" foods.

SEVERE RESRICTION (250 mg per day)

Diet is the same as strict restriction, but substitute appropriate amounts of low-sodium whole or nonfat milk (8 mg sodium per pint) for the milk allowance. Liquid "low-sodium" milk is not available in all parts of the country. Many patients use the powdered form and find it more palatable if flavored with honey, liquid flavorings, and so on, according to calories allowed. Severe restriction is usually prescribed for in-hospital use. The patient is observed carefully for signs of sodium depletion (see p. 126).

Regardless of the level of restriction, all sodium-restricted diets contain limited amounts of foods with high natural sodium content, e.g., milk and meats, because they are rich sources of essential nutrients. In general, meat, poultry, fish, and eggs are high in natural sodium; fruits contain little natural sodium; and vegetables range from little content to large amounts, with beets, beet greens, celery, kale, dandelion greens, carrots, chard, white turnips, and spinach containing large quantities.

Omit these "salty" foods: [94]

1. Smoked, processed, cured meats and fish, e.g., ham, bacon, frankfurters, smoked salmon, sausage, salt pork, anchovies, cold cuts
2. Meat extracts and sauces, e.g., bouillon cubes
3. Obviously salted foods, e.g., pretzels, saltine crackers, potato chips
4. Prepared condiments, e.g. catsup, pickles, olives, prepared mustard
5. Vegetable salts and flakes, e.g., onion and garlic salt, parsley flakes, monosodium glutamate (Accent)
6. Sodium in any form, e.g., preservatives, some medicines
7. Bread or bakery products unless prepared without salt; baking powder and baking soda contain sodium
8. Frozen fish fillets and shellfish, except oysters
9. Prepared flours, flour mixes, baking powder, and baking soda
10. Frozen peas and Lima beans; sauerkraut
11. All canned meats and vegetables unless prepared without salt, called "dietetic pack"
12. Canned pears, figs, applesauce unless prepared without salt, "dietetic pack"

13. Butter, cheese, peanut butter unless prepared without salt, "dietetic pack"

Low-sodium milk, unsalted canned meats, low-sodium cottage and cheddar cheese, butter and margarine, bakery goods, and baking powder are now available. Most spices can be used safely, with the exception of allspice, dehydrated parsley flakes, whole mace, and celery seed.[95] Particular attention must be placed on reading labels for their sodium content. Many foods, medicines and dentifrices contain sodium, though not necessarily sodium chloride. For instance, sodium sulfite is used to bleach dried fruits; sodium benzoate is a food preservative; disodium phosphate and sodium alginate are used in processing some quick-cooking cereals, cheese, ice cream, and chocolate milk; sodium propionate is used to inhibit growth of mold. Patients must be alerted to sodium found in many patent medicines, e.g., laxatives, alkalizers, cough preparations, and analgesics, and should discuss their use with the physician. If the local water supply is high in its sodium content, distilled water may have to be used.

No salt substitute should be used unless specifically prescribed by the physician. Commercially prepared salt substitutes contain potassium or ammonium chloride and, if used in large amounts, may be detrimental to patients with liver or kidney impairment.

FAT RESTRICTION

The significant classes of lipids in the body are fats, glycolipids (triglycerides), sterols (cholesterol and its esters), and the phospholipids.[96,97] Many of these lipids combine with protein and circulate as "lipoproteins" to give them solubility in water.

The quantity of circulating lipids, especially serum cholesterol, seems to be implicated in development of atherosclerosis. Although the ultimate therapeutic role of diets intended to retard atherosclerosis has yet to be proved, changes in the total calories derived from fats and an increase in the proportion of polyunsaturated to saturated fats seems to lower the level of circulating cholesterol.

Body cholesterol comes from two sources. It is ingested in certain foods (brains, kidney, liver, oysters, fish oils, egg yolk, and so on) and it is manufactured by the liver in response to levels of saturated fatty acids in the blood. Cholesterol is involved in the transport and the digestion of fats and is a precursor to vitamin D.[98]

Chemically, the fats are made up of carbon, hydrogen, and oxygen. If each carbon atom contains all the hydrogen possible, it is called *saturated*. It is "full of hydrogen." Saturated fats are usually solid at room temperature. They come primarily from animal and dairy products (animal fat, butter, cream, lard, mutton tallow, coconut oil, cocoa butter, hydrogenated shortenings, and so on).

Polyunsaturated fatty acids, comprising a preponderance of body fat depots, are not "loaded with hydrogen." They contain more than one double bond in the carbon chain. Of the three polyunsaturated triglycerides, two are essential. Linoleic and arachidonic acids must be ingested to maintain health because they are not synthesized in significant amounts in the body. Usually liquid at room temperature, they include corn oil, cottonseed oil, peanut oil, fish oil, and "special margarines" that contain no more than 25 per cent saturated fatty acid and a minimum of 25 per cent linoleic (polyunsaturated, essential) fatty acid. These percentages are indicated on the labels.

Modified fat diets have one common denominator: the total percentage of fat is decreased from 40 to 45 per cent found in the average American diet, to 30 per cent; and the ratio of polyunsaturated to saturated fatty acids is altered so that at least half the total fat is made up of polyunsaturated fatty acids. The proportion of saturated fat is lowered by reducing the animal, dairy, and hydrogenated fats ingested. Polyunsaturated fats are increased by introducing liquid vegetable oils, "special margarines," fish, and foods containing linoleic and other polyunsaturated fatty acids.[99] It must be stressed that all the polyunsaturated fatty acids must be utilized every day in order to maintain this ratio. Dietary cholesterol may be restricted to 300 to 400 mg a day in contrast to 700 mg a day found in the average American male diet. If cholesterol is to be restricted, the patient is instructed to avoid shellfish, caviar, and organ meats, and is allowed no more than four eggs each week.

SOME HINTS FOR THE PATIENT ON A FAT-RESTRICTED DIET

1. The 14 main meals (lunches and dinners) should contain a good quality protein: poultry, fish, eggs, but limit the use of lean beef, lamb, and pork to a total of three to four meals each week.

2. Trim all visible fat. Even after trimming, meats contain 7 to 11 per cent fat by weight.[100]

3. Remove poultry skin. The skin contains fat.

4. Avoid "marbled" meat.

5. Broil foods. If they are baked or roasted, use a rack to collect the fat drippings. If they are potted, refrigerate overnight and remove fat from surface next day.

6. Use vegetable oils for frying.

7. Use desserts made of fruit, tapioca, sherbet, angel-food cake; omit chocolate and caramel-type candies prepared with cocoa butter.

8. Use uncreamed cottage cheese and skim milk.

Most foods contain both saturated and polyunsaturated fatty acids. It is the proportion of one to the other that is regulated.

Food-exchange lists for fat-restricted diets are available from the Council on Foods and Nutrition of the American Medical Association. They are planned for diets of 1,200, 1,800, and 2,400 calories. Booklets can also be obtained from the American Heart Association.

Many drugs are being tested to determine their lipid-lowering effects. There has been some success with aluminum nicotinate, with thyroid therapy, and with gonadal hormone therapy.[101]

Table 24–1. Drugs Used in Treating Myocardial Infarction [*]

Indication or Expected Action	Drug	Dosage and Route	Precautions
ANALGESICS Relieve pain and anxiety	meperidine (Demerol)	25-100 mg I.M. May be given I.V. initially if pain is severe, then 25 mg increments q30 min. in I.V. tubing	May cause dizziness, visual disturbances, sweating, dry mouth, weakness, nausea and vomiting, euphoria, dysphoria, hypotension, peripheral vasodilation, respiratory depression. I.V. use may cause tachycardia
Given to relieve dyspnea of congestive heart failure or for persistent pain	morphine	gr. 1/6-1/4 I.V. or I.M.	Suppresses AV conduction. Respiratory depressant. May cause constipation, nausea, vomiting, itching, sweating, flushing and warmth of face, neck, and upper chest
SEDATIVES Used routinely to keep patient in resting mental state and to reduce heart work	chloral hydrate	0.5 gm q4h p.o.	Chloral hydrate is used for older patients who may not tolerate barbiturates, tranquilizers, and antiemetics. Should not be given if B.P. is unstable
	phenobarbital	gr. 1/4-1 q4h p.o. while awake	
	various tranquilizers used to control severe anxiety or nausea and vomiting		

[*] From M. S. Rawlings, "Inside the Coronary Care Unit: Trends in Therapeutic Management," *Amer. J. Nurse.*, **67**:2323, 1967. Reprinted with permission of the American Journal of Nursing Company, New York.

TABLE 24–1. [*Continued*]

Indication or Expected Action	Drug	Dosage and Route	Precautions
DIGITALIS Increases force of myocardial contraction; slows rate in atrial fibrillation Most important use is in congestive heart failure May be used for cardiogenic shock; atrial flutter or fibrillation; atrial and AV nodal paroxysmal tachycardia	*Fastest acting* ouabain (Strophanthin G) digoxin (Lanoxin) lanatoside C (Cedilanid) digitoxin (Crystodigin) ↓ *Slowest acting*	0.25 mg I.M. or I.V., repeated in 1 or 2 hr Initially, 0.25 to 1.0 mg p.o., I.M., or I.V. Initially, 0.8-1.6 mg I.M. or I.V. Initially, 1.0-1.5 mg p.o., I.M., or I.V.	Any form of digitalis may cause partial or complete AV block and almost any arrhythmia, including paroxysmal tachycardia, atrial tachycardia, fibrillation, or standstill, and ventricular tachycardia or standstill. First ECG signs of toxicity are ST segment sagging, PR prolongation, and possible bigeminal rhythm. Clinical signs of toxicity are mostly gastrointestinal and visual: excessive salivation, anorexia, nausea, vomiting, diarrhea, abdominal discomfort or pain, headache, weakness, confusion, blurred vision, and disturbed color vision (objects may appear haloed or frosted)
DRUGS USED IN CARDIOGENIC SHOCK **Vasopressors and cardiotonics** Combined alpha and beta adrenergic stimulating drugs, used to stimulate the myocardium and cause peripheral vasoconstriction for the support of coronary perfusion in the first hour or so	levarterenol (Levophed) metaraminol (Aramine)	5-15 mg per liter given in I.V. infusion with drip regulated to control B.P. 100-300 mg in an I.V. infusion; up to 50 mg by direct I.V. injection	All vasopressors can themselves cause arrhythmias. Levophed causes sloughs if it infiltrates. Use 5 mg phentolamine (Regitine) in infusion or inject directly into extravasated area to help prevent sloughing. Levophed rapidly increases B.P. Should be infused at a rate to maintain B.P. at 90-100 mm Hg systolic. Peripheral vasoconstriction should not be permitted to continue for long

Indication or Expected Action	Drug	Dosage and Route	Precautions
Primarily beta adrenergic stimulating drugs, used to stimulate the myocardium and improve blood flow to the body for improved tissue perfusion (cardiotonics)	mephentermine (Wyamine) isoproterenol (Isuprel)	15 mg I.M. or I.V. q1h P.R.N. 2 mg in 500 ml dextrose in water as a regulated drip	If B.P. is below 90 systolic
Primarily alpha adrenergic blocking drugs, used to prevent inappropriate and persistent peripheral vasoconstriction that usually perpetuates shock	phenoxybenzamine (Dibenzyline) hydralazine (Apresoline)	1 mg per kg I.V. 20 mg I.V. q2h as needed	May cause nasal congestion, miosis, postural hypotension, tachycardia. Dibenzyline should not be used in patients with congestive heart failure. Apresoline may cause tachycardia, headaches, dizziness, numbness, nausea, urticaria
Steroids Effective in treatment of shock; exact mechanism unknown	dexamethasone (Decadron) or betamethasone (Celestone)	2ml 8 mg I.M. q6h	May cause sodium retention, aggravating any edema or heart failure. May aggravate preexisting diabetes, uremia, or peptic ulcer
Alkali To combat metabolic acidosis due to lactic acid accumulation in the poorly perfused tissues	sodium bicarbonate	3.75 gm I.V. May be repeated in a few minutes if necessary	
Volume expanders	dextran	Average amount is 500 ml, I.V. drip	Requires central venous pressure monitoring to regulate quantity
ANTICOAGULANTS To prevent thrombophlebitis, mural thrombi, and pulmonary embolism			

TABLE 24-1. [*Continued*]

Indication or Expected Action	Drug	Dosage and Route	Precautions
Rapid acting To start anticoagulation before coumarin takes effect	heparin	150 mg deeply S.C.	Given as long as Lee-White coagulation time (taken before each dose) is less than 20 minutes. Watch for ecchymoses, G.I. bleeding, nosebleeds. Antidote: Protamine 100 mg I.V.
Slower acting For maintenance anticoagulation, usually for 3 months to 1 year	coumarin (Warfarin)	Initially, 30-40 mg p.o.	Prothrombin level should be kept at approximately twice normal in seconds or at about the 20 per cent control level. Antidote for coumarin and phenindione: Vitamin K (AquaMephyton) 2 ml I.V.
	sodium warfarin (Coumadin)	Initially, 25 mg p.o., then usually 5 mg daily	
	phenindione (Hedulin)	Initially, 150 mg p.o., then usually 75 mg. daily	
CATHARTICS **Stool softeners** To prevent straining at stool and fecal impactions	calcium bis-dioctyl sulfosuccinate (Doxidan)	1 b.i.d. p.o.	Potassium salts, digitalis, procainamide, and quinidine may all cause diarrhea
	dioctyl sodium sulfosuccinate with casanthranol (Peri-Colace)	1 b.i.d. p.o.	Caution patient not to strain at stool, as this is one of the most common causes of extension of heart damage and sudden death
Other mild laxatives	Milk of magnesia, mineral oil Dulcolax suppositories	1 oz p.o.	

Drugs That Affect Cardiovascular Function

The cardiotonic glycosides increase tone and strength of myocardial contraction, slow the heart rate by stimulating the vagus nerve, and depress the electrical conduction from the atria to the ventricles.[102] The drugs most frequently used include whole-leaf digitalis, digitoxin, gitalin, digoxin, lanatoside C, and ouabain. They differ in their onset and duration of action from the very slow-to-act whole-leaf digitalis preparations and digitoxin, to the more moderate-acting lanatoside C, digoxin, and gitalin, to the very rapidly acting strophanthin ouabain. In an emergency, the physician may elect to use one of the rapid strophanthins intravenously. They work in a matter of minutes but the effect lasts only one or two hours. The physician follows this with an oral dose of one of the intermediate-acting glycosides that take four to eight hours to work well but continue to exert their action for two or three weeks. The dosage must be individualized for each patient. If he has not been taking a digitalis preparation before, he must be "digitalized" first. This is a gradual process of building up the necessary amount of drug to produce the desired cardiac effect. It is a difficult balancing act because the quantity producing the desired effect and that producing a toxic effect are so close. Full digitalization is best accomplished over a period of days. This is followed by doses sufficient to maintain the desired blood level and cardiac effect. The dosage is "custom-tailored" to meet the needs of the particular individual.

Digitalis cardiotoxicity [101] remains a problem for many reasons. First, there is a wide variation in individual tolerance to the drugs, and a given individual's tolerance is changeable. Second, use of the purified and potent glycosides produces fewer gastrointestinal side effects so that the patient may be unaware of a developing toxic response. Third, many older people are taking the drugs, and they are less tolerant to its effects than young people. They show signs of toxicity with relatively small doses. And fourth, digitalis tends to cause a cellular depletion of potassium. The effects of digitalis are magnified in the presence of low potassium levels. Any factors that further deplete cell potassium, e.g., the use of thiazide diuretics or intravenous feeding without potassium replacement, may cause digitalis cardiotoxicity.

Toxic effects include anorexia, nausea, vomiting, diarrhea, yellow vision, and the more serious cardiac rhythm abnormalities including bradycardia, premature beats, and irregularity. For these reasons, frequent electrocardiograms are done to identify possible cardiac irregularities, and the nurse must take an apical pulse before giving any cardiotonic glycoside. Ideally, this involves simultaneous listening to the apical rate with a stethoscope by one nurse and feeling the radial pulse by another. If the pulse rate is 60 beats per minute or less, the drug is withheld and the physician is notified.

Antiarrhythmic Drugs

POTASSIUM SALTS

Intravenous potassium salts are used to suppress many ectopic beats in emergencies. The therapeutic effect is transient, but effective, in 80 per cent of the patients for which it is used.[102] Quinidine sulfate is the most frequently used antiarrhythmic drug. It is given by mouth in doses of 200 to 600 mg up to six times a day, often with an initial test dose of 200 mg. The drug seems to influence abnormal electrical activity of the myocardium by increasing the refractory period, thereby terminating atrial fibrillation and establishing normal rhythms. Some patients are hypersensitive to the drug. Toxic reactions include visual disturbances, ringing in the ears, vertigo, nausea, vomiting, abdominal cramps, diarrhea, respiratory depression, and vascular collapse. If a toxic reaction occurs, the dosage must be reduced or the drug discontinued.

Procaine amide (Pronestyl), a synthetic antiarrhythmic drug, can be given by mouth or by intramuscular or intravenous injection. It works in much the same way as quinidine sulfate with similar toxic effects. It may cause hypotension, allergic reaction, and agranulocytosis.[103] The oral or intramuscular dose is 500 mg to 2 gm four times a day.

Propranolol (Inderal) is a beta adrenergic blocking agent. It protects the heart against overstimulation by catecholamines (epinephrine) and decreases excessively rapid irregular heartbeats. It is particularly useful in controlling arrhythmias from digitalis intoxication. It is given orally in doses of 10 to 30 mg four times each day before meals and at bedtime, or 1 to 3 mg intravenously, not to exceed 1 mg (1 ml vial) per minute. ECG monitoring is used to check effectiveness. The drug may cause mental depression.

Lidocaine (Xylocaine) is a local anesthetic that has been found successful in reducing cardiac excitability and conductivity. It seems to act like procainamide. It is used by some physicians in treating ventricular arrhythmias.

Diphenylhydantoin (Dilantin) and the antihistamine antazoline are being studied for their antiarrhythmic effects. Dilantin seems particularly useful in treatment of ventricular arrhythmias, especially those caused by digitalis intoxication.

Anticoagulant Drugs

The use of anticoagulant drugs remains a controversial issue. The drugs do not dissolve clots already formed, but by decreasing the coagulability of the blood they decrease the chance of new clot formation. The physician must weigh the advantage of decreased chance of clot formation against the disadvantage of often serious bleeding. Most physicians utilize anticoagulants while the patient is in the hospital. They check clotting time daily and have vitamin K and whole blood available in case of bleeding. There is controversy as to which one of the laboratory tests is most suitable to measure effectiveness of a particular type of anticoagulant. Many physicians do a daily prothrombin time when the patient is on a coumarin or indanedion derivative. The Quick one-stage method involves adding a mixture of thromboplastin and calcium to a serum specimen. The patient does not have to be fasting for this test. The time of formation of fibrin threads is measured with a stop watch.[104] Normal range is 11 to 18 seconds; with use of an anticoagulant, it is kept at two to two and one-half times normal, or 27 to 45 seconds. The test is done daily. Drug dosage is regulated according to the results and given after the laboratory test. When heparin is used, the Lee-White test is often selected. Its accuracy depends on collection of a "clean" blood specimen, one free from tissue juice. Normal values are below 20 minutes. The goal of anticoagulation is to keep the value at twice that amount.

The anticoagulant drugs interfere with various stages in the clotting response. Coumarin derivatives reduce the levels of clotting factors. Heparin has an antithromboplastin and antithrombin effect. It apparently blocks several enzymatic reactions in the clotting mechanism.

STAGES IN COAGULATION OF BLOOD

At least eight known factors are responsible for the formation of intrinsic thromboplastin.

Stage I: thromboplastin formation

Stage II: prothrombin $\xrightarrow{\text{thromboplastin}}$ thrombin

Stage III: fibrinogen $\xrightarrow{\text{thrombin}}$ fibrin clot

Heparin most nearly approaches the ideal anticoagulant. Best used for immediate and short-term hypocoagulability, it is rapidly absorbed, readily excreted, and practically nontoxic. It does cause a local reaction at the site of injection. It is not, however, practical for long-term use because it must be given by injection and must be given every 12 to 24 hours to maintain its effect. Five to thirty thousand units are given intravenously, 20,000 to 40,000 units intramuscularly every 12 to 24 hours.

The coumarin and indanedione derivatives are more practical for long-term use. They can be administered by mouth, are less expensive, and have a longer-lasting effect; however, their action builds up more slowly, and there is a latent period of 24 to 48 hours before their peak effectiveness is reached.[106] Usual initial dose is 200 to 300 mg daily, with 100 to 200 mg daily thereafter according to prothrombin determinations.

SOME COUMARIN DERIVATIVES

Bishydroxycoumarin (Dicumarol)
Warfarin (Coumadin, Panwarfin)
Acenocoumarol (Sintrom)
Ethyl biscoumacetate (Tromexan)
Phenprocoumon (Liquemar)

SOME INDANEDIONE DERIVATIVES (WORK LIKE COUMARIN)

Phenindione (Hedulin; Danilone)
Anisindione (Miradon)
Diphenadione (Dipaxin)

If anticoagulants are to be continued when the patient returns home, he should be given a written dosage schedule, and he should have an appointment scheduled with his physician. He should be advised of the importance of keeping the visit with his physician and should be told that he has a greater tendency to bleed while on the anticoagulant and should report to the physician bruises, nosebleeds, dark urine, dark or bloody stools, weakness or feeling faint, and so on. He can carry an American Heart Association card that says he is on anticoagulant therapy.

Studies of drugs to dissolve clots once they are formed are underway. Streptokinase, a protein produced by hemolytic streptococci, apparently activates the body's fibrinolytic system. The problem of its use focuses on the patient's own antibody response. He most often has developed antibodies for the streptococci, and an extremely large dose of the medicine, marketed as Actase or Thrombolysin, is required to counteract this effect. Urokinase, taken from human urine, contains naturally occurring fibrinolytic activators. It, too, is being studied.

25

CARDIAC SURGERY

The Pump Oxygenator

With the perfection of a machine to pump and oxygenate blood, open techniques of cardiac surgery have been made possible. This machine allows the blood to bypass the heart and lungs; it does the work of these two organs so that the surgeon can work directly inside the heart in a relatively bloodless field, for one to three hours. The technique of cardiopulmonary bypass is called "extracorporeal circulation." The machine is called a heart-lung machine or pump oxygenator. It is primed with matched whole blood or a glucose-dextran solution. The patient is anesthetized, and a bilateral incision through the thorax into the pericardium is made. Intravenous heparin is administered to decrease the chance of clotting. Blood normally returned to the heart by way of the superior and inferior venae cavae is routed through two catheters to the pump oxygenator. Once oxygenated, it is pumped through a heat exchanger and a filter and back to the aorta by means of a cannula or catheter in the femoral artery. Flow through the aorta is reversed, retrograde fashion. This tends to keep the aortic valve closed and supplies the coronary arteries with blood. Other measures of supplying the coronary vessels must be instituted if repair of the aortic valve is to be done. (See Fig. 25–1.)

Profound Hypothermia

This is a technique often used along with extracorporeal circulation when an immobile heart is needed for complicated repair. The temperature of the body is lowered, through the blood, to 80 to 10° C. (46 to 50° F.), at which point the body metabolism is so low that the rate through the heart-lung machine can be slowed or can be stopped completely for up to 45 minutes.[107] The heart is virtually in a state of "suspended" animation.

Surface Hypothermia

This technique is used for very short cardiac surgery, without use of the pump oxygenator. Body temperature is lowered by "surface cooling" with

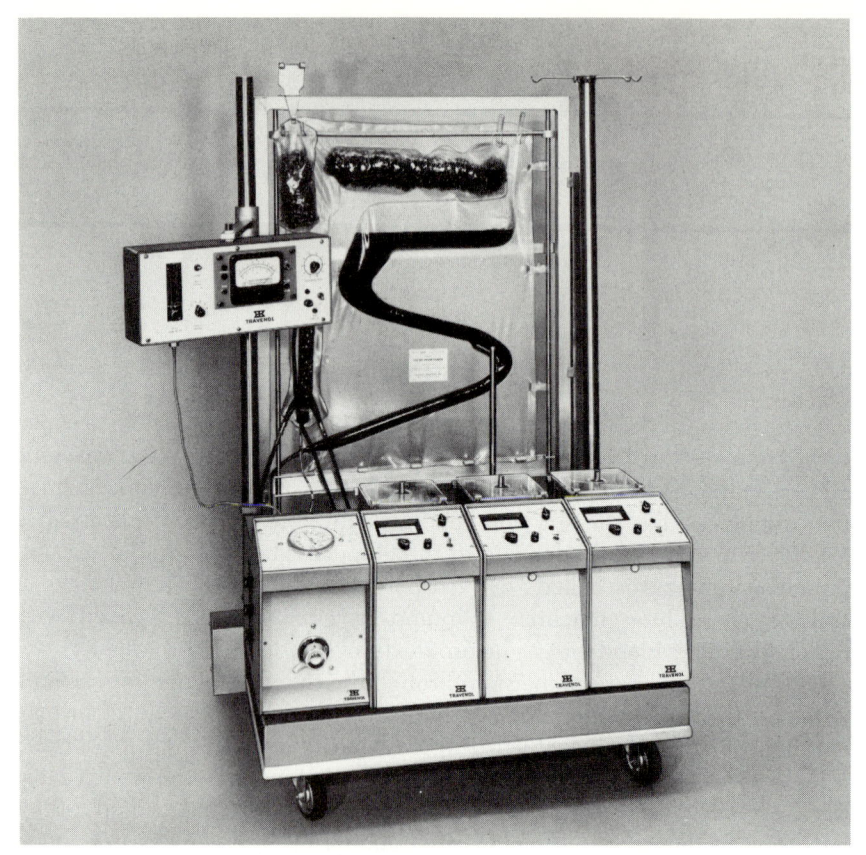

FIGURE 25-1. The pump-oxygenator console. (Courtesy, Travenol Laboratories, Inc., Morton Grove, Ill.)

a hypothermia machine and water-circulation blanket. The patient is anesthetized. This stops shivering, which would only defeat the purpose of cooling because it increases body metabolism. The cooling is stopped as the surgery begins. The temperature drifts down to 28° to 30° C. The superior and inferior venae cavae are tied, and the field is "bloodless." The tolerance of the brain to cardiac standstill at this temperature in only eight to ten minutes.[108]

Much intricate surgery of the heart is now being accomplished by trained teams. Cardiac transplantation, the use of someone else's heart, is a newly developing area.

The patient having surgery of his heart will certainly wonder if he will live or die. The nurse must be sensitive to the cues he gives her to determine at what point he is ready to participate in learning about the surgery, the equipment around him, and what activities he will be asked to do post-

CARDIAC SURGERY   [275

operatively. For instance, he will be asked to "cough" postoperatively and should practice the technique preoperatively.

To cough productively [109]

1. Deep-breathe five times.
2. Sip water to help loosen secretions.
3. Take a deep breath, hold it, slowly blow it all the way out.
4. On the next breath hold it and cough from the chest.

The nurse must also confer with the physician for some specific information, e.g., what time will the surgery be performed, where will the incision be made, how much information may she give the patient, should anything be withheld? Then she plans definite teaching periods with the patient. Visual aids or actual equipment may make the teaching more meaningful. A picture of the heart and lungs may clarify information. Actually seeing bottles and tubing used for closed-chest drainage and being told very specifically that they will probably remain in for 24 to 72 hours helps. Practicing deep-breathing, coughing, and other prescribed exercises helps.

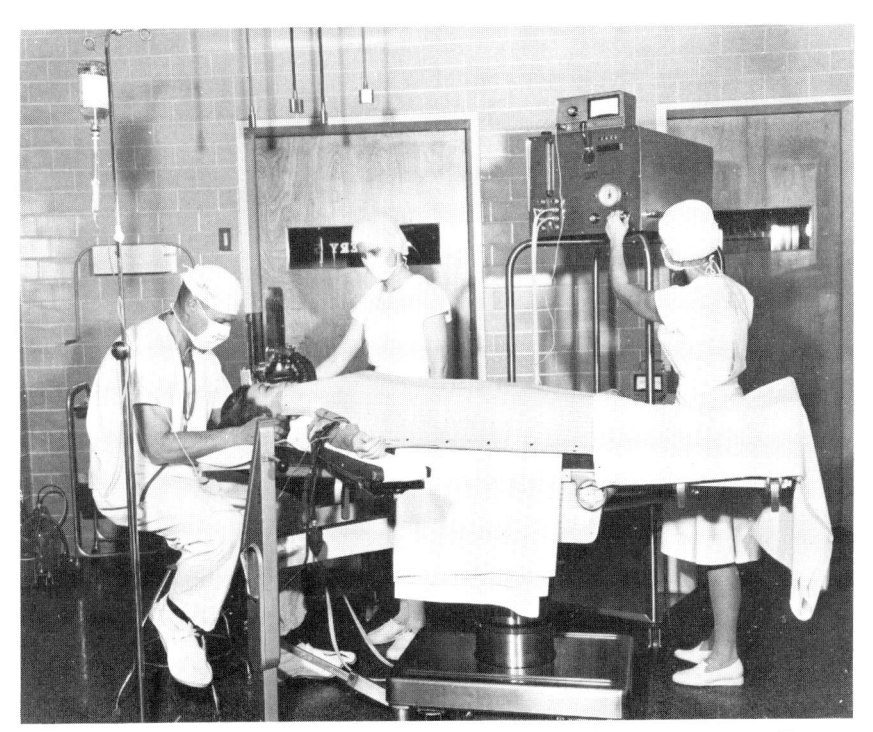

FIGURE 25-2. Hypothermia unit in use. (Courtesy, Gorman-Rupp Industries, Inc., Bellville, Ohio.)

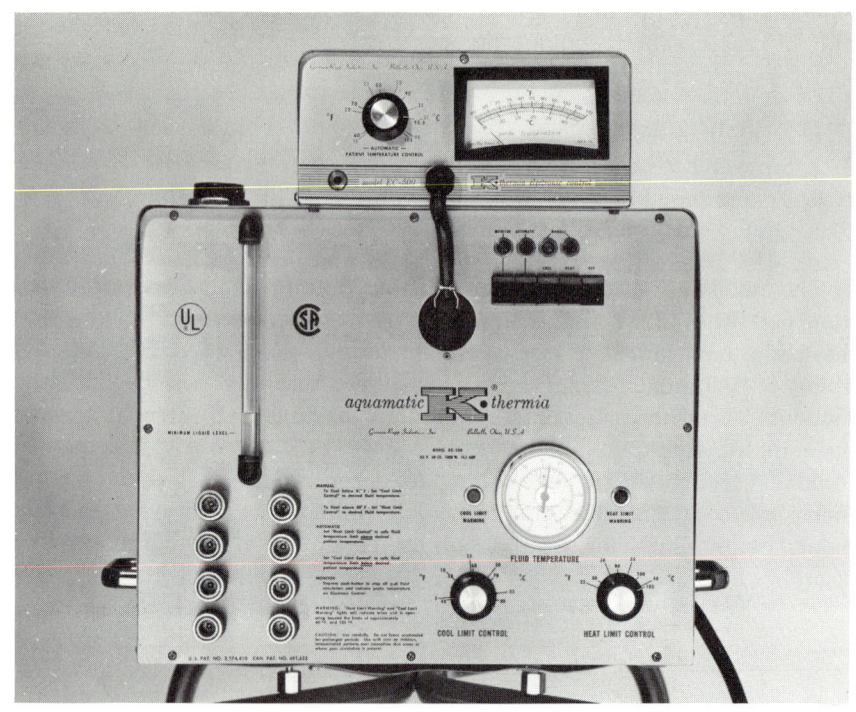

FIGURE 25-3. Hypothermia unit. (Courtesy, Gorman-Rupp Industries, Inc., Bellville, Ohio.)

Replacing Failing Hearts

Homotransplantation; Mechanical Pumps

The first human heart transplant was performed on December 3, 1967, by Dr. Christian Barnard in Cape Town, South Africa. Dr. Barnard, with the help of a specially trained team, replaced the heart of 55-year-old Louis Washkansky with that of a 25-year-old girl mortally injured in a road accident. Mr. Washkansky died of pneumonia 18 days later; however, his surgery initiated a new era in the treatment of advanced, long-standing heart disease for which there was no cure.

Up to this time, heart surgery concentrated on correction of congenital, pericardial, and valvular defects, excision of cardiac aneurysms, and revascularization procedures. These techniques, though, did not correct "pump" failures caused by heart muscle disease or impaired myocardial blood supply. Homotransplantation, using the heart of a deceased person anastomosed in the chest of a living person, seemed the answer.

Homotransplantation has been performed by surgeons in large medical centers all over the world. The original technique involved removal of the recipient's whole heart and placement and anastomosis of the donor heart in the pericardial cavity. In later techniques portions of either atria and the atrial septum were left in the host, making the surgery less complicated and requiring fewer vessels to suture. The sinus node of the donor heart takes over. The donor heart is kept alive by extracorporeal circulation (cardiopulmonary bypass). It is cooled, excised, and transferred to the recipient's operating room in an isotonic salt solution cooled to 4° to 10° C. It is connected to the recipient heart-lung machine until it is implanted. The recipient, too, is connected to the heart-lung machine while parts of his diseased heart are excised. His blood is cooled. The donor right atrium, atrial septum, left atrium, aorta, and pulmonary artery are sutured in place, in that sequence. Blood is gradually rewarmed, and the new heart is defibrillated with an electric shock. It begins to beat on its own. Total cardiopulmonary bypass lasts about three hours.

The patient is transferred from the operating room to the intensive coronary care unit where one or two nurses and at least one physician are present at all times. Goals during the postoperative period are to maintain satisfactory cardiac output, prevent infection, and control immunologic rejection crisis.

The chest cavity is drained with catheters. A tracheostomy may be done to ensure adequate ventilation. It is connected to a Bennett pressure cycled respirator for mechanical ventilation. A warmed, humidified mist is provided through this respirator. Saline is instilled in the tracheostomy tube to liquefy secretions, and the tube is suctioned frequently. The patient is turned every 30 to 60 minutes. Vital signs are taken every 15 minutes for the first 12 postoperative hours. Temperature, venous pressure, and cardiac function are monitored. Apical radial pulses are taken simultaneously by the same person. Bedside chest x-rays are taken. Urinary output is measured. Blood and electrolyte replacement solutions are administered as needed. The head of the bed is elevated 20 degrees for patient comfort.

To control infection, swabbings of the skin, nose, throat, and rectum are taken from the patient and from staff caring for him, for culture.

Steroids, azathioprine, actinomycin C, antilymphocytic globulin, and local irradiation to the heart are methods employed to lessen the effect of expected immunologic crisis. (See p. 209.)

The moral-ethical question of what constitutes death is a puzzling one. Four criteria used to determine death are absence of natural heartbeat, absence of respiration, absence of reflexes, and absence of brain waves as seen on an electroencephalogram. For further discussion refer to kidney transplantation (p. 206).

Mechanical pumps to replace diseased hearts are being developed and tested. They are designed to support the circulation indefinitely with some form of indefatigable power source.

26

PERIPHERAL VASCULAR DISEASE

PERIPHERAL vascular disease is a group of diseases that affect the arteries and veins in the peripheral areas of the body. The hands and feet are most frequently involved though the nose and ears are sometimes affected. The common denominator in all these diseases is decrease in flow of blood to the involved areas, causing ischemia, or decrease in the return of blood from the area, causing stasis. Symptoms may be mild and cause little more than inconvenience to the patient, as seen in many cases of Raynaud's disease; or they may be severe with ischemia leading to necrosis, as in some cases of arteriosclerosis obliterans.

The pathology involved may be degenerative (arteriosclerosis obliterans), arteriospastic (Raynaud's disease), inflammatory (thromboangiitis obliterans), or the result of anatomic imperfections (varicose veins). A patient may have a single disorder or a combination of disorders. In any case, the most common sites of occlusive disease (except Raynaud's disease in which the hands are involved) are the aortoiliac vessels below the renal vessels and the large arteries leading to and in the lower extremities, such as the femoral or popliteal artery. Prognosis is most favorable when the occlusion is "higher up" because collateral circulation develops effectively; prognosis is less favorable when the more distal vessels are involved.

Atherosclerosis is now believed to be the major underlying cause of peripheral occlusive disease.[110] It involves the deposition of fat and fibrous tissue in the inner layer of the vessels and causes the gradual occlusion of the vessel lumen.

Description of Some Peripheral Vascular Diseases

Arteriosclerosis Obliterans

This is a generalized degenerative disorder in which there is hardening of the arteries, primarily the middle layer of the vessel. Decrease in elasticity renders the vessel less flexible. Calcium deposits gradually block the lumen. Arteriosclerosis obliterans is the most prevalent of the peripheral vascular diseases. It affects men in the 45-to-70-year age group

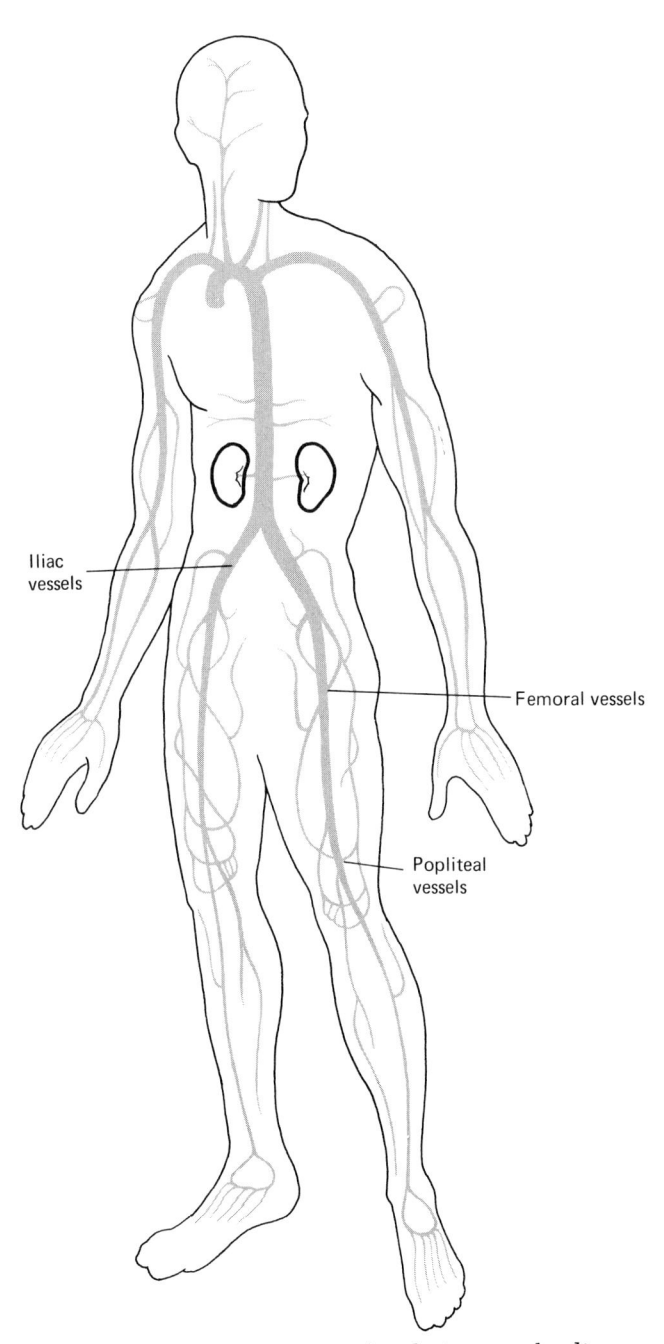

FIGURE 26–1. Common sites of occlusive vascular disease.

more than women. Women seem to be protected by circulating estrogen levels. The patient experiences symptoms when the blood supply is no longer adequate to meet the needs of the limbs. The disease is usually present in both limbs, although symptoms may be apparent in only one.

Thromboangiitis Obliterans (Buerger's Disease)

This is a sclerosing, inflammatory disease of arteries and veins in which arteries, veins, and even nerves become bound in a mass.[111] Thrombus formation is frequent. Small-to-medium-sized vessels in the feet are involved initially. Later, the hands, too, may be involved. The disease runs a progressive course beginning in the peripheral vessels of the fingers and toes (usually the toes first) and traveling to more central sites in the hand and foot. The patient experiences persistent coldness in one or both lower extremities and aching pain in the fingers, instep, ankle, calf, wrist, or forearm following exercise of those corresponding muscles. There may be migratory phlebitis with tender, red, patchy areas along the veins. The disease is associated with the use of tobacco. Abstinence causes gradual remission of symptoms. The disease strikes young men in the 20-to-35-year age group more frequently than women. Although seen in all nationalities, it is most commonly seen in Jews.

Raynaud's Disease

In this disease, spasm in the arteries of the extremities develops in response to cold and to emotion. The hands are more frequently affected than the feet, with spasm and cyanosis appearing in one to four fingers of one or both hands. The thumb is usually not involved. As the vasospasm disappears, vasodilation occurs and the finger becomes hyperemic; it is red in color. If the attack is severe, the fingers ache, and there is awkwardness in fine movement.[112] In many instances the attacks disappear spontaneously or remain stationary for several years. Gangrene is rare. The disease is seen in women more than men, with underweight, emotionally labile women most frequently affected. Nationality does not seem to play a part. The disease occurs at any age, though it is less common before puberty and after 40. Its incidence is most frequent between the ages of 17 and 35.

If the symptoms are secondary and can be traced to a specific underlying cause, e.g., trauma or arteriosclerosis obliterans, the condition is called Raynaud's phenomenon rather than Raynaud's disease. Raynaud's phenomenon may occur unilaterally and is usually associated with systemic symptoms, e.g., fever, anemia, elevated sedimentation rate. There is a greater likelihood of lesions developing from Raynaud's phenomenon.

Thrombophlebitis and Phlebothrombosis

Both of these conditions involve clot formation in the veins. In thrombophlebitis local and systemic inflammatory symptoms are present. The veins may be hard, thready, and sensitive to pressure. The area along their length is red, warm to touch, and swollen. The remaining part of the limb may be pale and cold. In thrombophlebitis, the inflammatory process tends to hold the clot firmly in place, and it is less likely to dislodge and become an embolus. Phlebothrombosis is the more serious condition. The inflammatory process is not involved, and clots often break loose, travel in the bloodstream, and lodge in a vital organ such as the lung or brain. This may cause sudden death. Initial symptoms are not as obvious as those of thrombophlebitis. Edema and cyanosis are present, but may be overlooked until more drastic signs of embolus occur. There may be a sudden increase in the circumference of the limb, pain in the calf and/or popliteal space, or dorsiflexion of the foot (Homan's sign). There may be decreased pulsation in the femoral artery. Stasis of venous blood, as from immobility, local trauma to the vessel, and systemic hypercoagulability, seems to be implicated in the cause of thrombus formation.[113]

Varicose Veins

These are dilated, elongated, tortuous veins usually associated with the saphenous system of the lower limbs and trunk. Ten per cent of all adults over 35 have some degree of varicosity,[114] though women in the third,

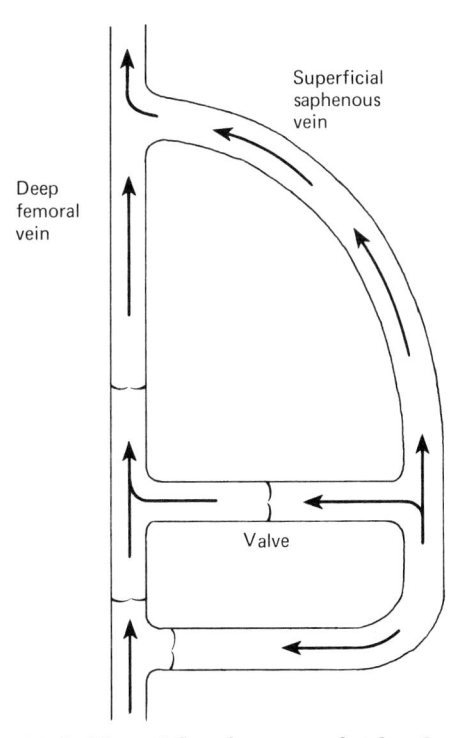

FIGURE 26–2. Normal flow from superficial to deep vein.

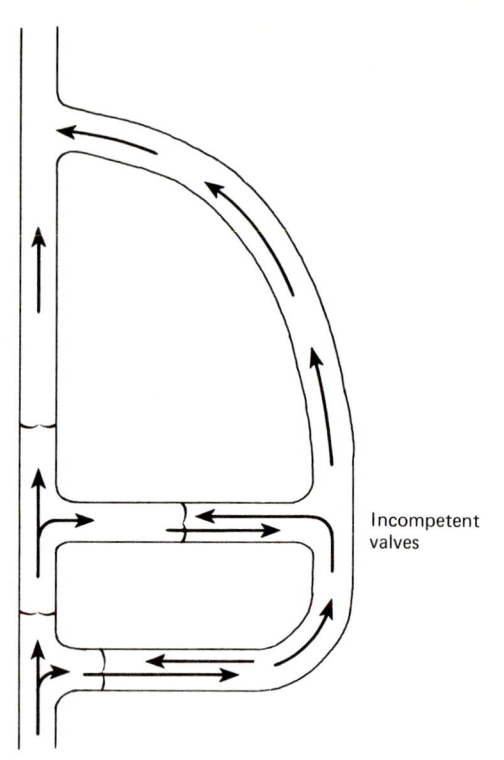

FIGURE 26-3. Incompetent valves in connecting veins cause flow from deep veins into superficial veins with increased pressure in superficial veins.

fourth, and fifth decades of life are most commonly affected. The disease is associated with a hereditary weakness in the vein walls and valves. Incompetent valves, especially those in the connecting veins between the deep and the superficial systems, allow blood with a greater than normal pressure to fill the superficial venous system. The superficial venous system is less able to cope with the stress of the increased pressure than the deep system because it lies relatively unsupported in the subcutaneous tissue.[115] (See Figs. 26-2 and 26-3.) Venous flow in the deep system often remains normal because flow is aided by contractions of strong muscle and by fascia. Any circumstance that places additional pressure on the venous system in a susceptible individual may predispose to varicosities. Examples are pelvic tumors, pregnancy, immobile upright posture for long periods of time, and constricting round garters and tight panty leg girdles.

The patient experiences a feeling of heaviness and fullness in the involved limb and a stinging sensation along the course of the veins after standing for some time.[116] Superficial varicosities are unsightly, but usually not incapacitating. Deep varicosities are of a more serious nature. They may cause ulcerations in the skin, loss of blood through rupture, and so on. The most severe symptoms are from complications of varicose veins. They include dermatitis with the skin scaly and discolored, or red and itchy; "varicose ulcers" stemming from a decreased blood supply in the area around inflamed veins; and superficial thrombophlebitis with a tender, red area overlying a firm segment of vein.

Conservative treatment includes use of elastic stockings from toes to groin or injection of a sclerosing solution directly into the vein. This offers temporary relief, but is contraindicated in uncontrolled diabetes, when local ulcers or inflammation are present, in some cardiovascular diseases, and in advanced arterial disease of the legs.[117] Incidents of death from emboli following injection are recorded. Vein ligation and stripping is the treatment of choice. (See p. 289.)

Symptoms and Diagnostic Tools in Vascular Disease

The severity of the symptoms is related to the amount of obstruction, the extent of the lesion, and the status of collateral circulation.

Intermittent Claudication and Pain

Claudication means lameness. When the blood-oxygen needs of muscles are not met, the patient experiences lameness, soreness, and pain. For instance, the great calf muscles respond to inadequate blood flow through the femoral arteries; the patient often experiences pain in the legs after a certain amount of walking, or, if the occlusion is in the iliac vessels, the patient will experience pain in the muscles of the buttocks and thighs. The pain is described as burning, boring, throbbing, sharp, and shooting. It may be continuous or paroxysmal. For instance, a sudden occlusion from a thrombus might cause severe, sudden pain. The pain may occur at rest. It often wakes the patient up at night, and he must walk or hang his legs over the side of the bed for relief.

Appearance

The appearance of the skin in the involved area changes. It becomes thick and hairless. Nails become hard, brittle, thickened, and ridged, and their growth is impaired. There may be excessive dryness, sweating, or edema. Ulcers often appear.

Color and Temperature

Color of the skin will appear pale if there is acute obstruction or spasm of the arteries. It will be red if there is arterial dilation or inflammation. It will be cyanotic if there is pooling of blood in the vessels. Color is also indicative of approaching gangrene. Changes from red and blotchy areas to dark-brown-black "mummified" areas are characteristic of necrosis. If

284] TRANSPORTING MATERIAL TO AND FROM CELLS

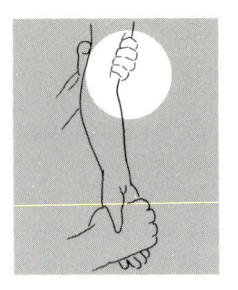

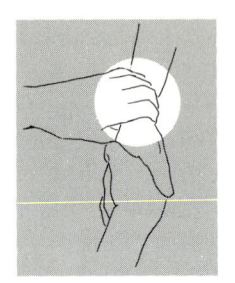

Brachial artery   Radial artery

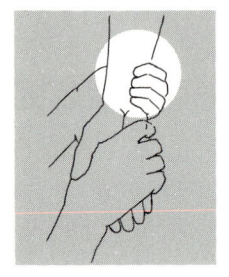

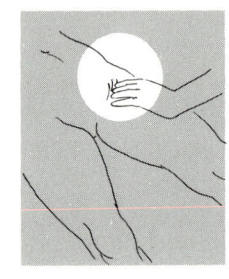

Ulnar artery   Femoral artery   Popliteal artery

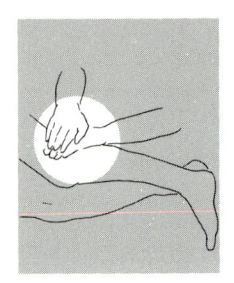

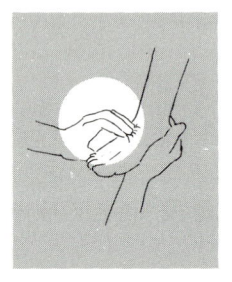

Dorsalis pedis artery   Posterior tibial artery

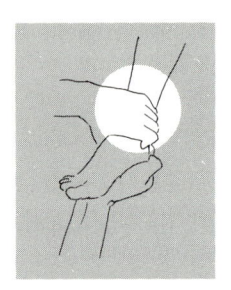

FIGURE 26–4. Palpation for peripheral arterial pulsations. (Courtesy, Mead Johnson & Co., Evansville, Ind.)

the flow of blood is seriously obstructed, minor trauma to the limb may cause spontaneous gangrene.

Color tests are used to judge the status of circulation. In the *position test* the limb is elevated and will blanch. Then it is lowered, and color normally returns within five seconds in the arms, ten seconds in the legs. The speed at which color returns indicates circulatory status.

In the *histamine test*, histamine is injected under the skin and will normally produce a wheal surrounded by a flare within five minutes. In obstructive disease, the wheal takes longer to develop.

In the *reactive-hyperemia test* a blood pressure cuff is used to produce temporary occlusion. Sudden release of the pressure normally produces a flush in less than five seconds,[118] longer if obstruction is present.

The temperature of the extremity depends on environmental temperature, availability of blood flow, and vasomotor activity governed by the autonomic nervous system. In general, stimulation of the sympathetic system is a response to stress. There is vasoconstriction in the peripheral blood vessels in an effort to divert blood to more crucial areas. The limb feels cold. Parasympathetic stimulation generally causes vasodilation; however, regardless of parasympathetic stimulation, the limb will continue to feel cold if its blood flow is impeded because of vascular pathology. At 77° F. (25° C.), the fingers are about 99° F. (33° C.) and the toes 78° F. (26° C.).[119] The nurse can compare temperatures in both sides of the body as clues to peripheral vascular disease.

Pulses are palpated in involved body areas, and their volume is "graded" by the physician. The nurse is frequently asked to palpate the pedal or popliteal pulse for changes in tone, absence or presence of pulse, and so on. (See Fig. 26–4.) Measurements of pulse volume can be quickly attained through use of an oscillometer. Oscillometric studies reveal the effectiveness of the larger arteries. An inflatable cuff is wrapped around the limb, usually at the lower thigh or upper calf. It is connected to a delicate diaphragm that transmits arterial pressure to a needle moving across a dial. Values are listed as units.[120] For instance, the normal reading at the calf is 3 to 10 units at a cuff pressure midway between diastolic and systolic pressure.[121] Values are slightly lower in the thigh. The readings are lower than normal in affected limbs. Pulse wave can be interpreted by observing the needle of the oscillometer. Quick, sharp swings of good magnitude usually indicate patent vascular tree.

Arteriography has become the definitive diagnostic technique in evaluating occlusive vascular disease. It is essential when reconstructive vascular surgery is contemplated.

Management of the Patient with Peripheral Vascular Disease

The major goals [122] include protection of the tissues from injury, prevention and relief of symptoms, and promotion of effective collateral circulation. Measures include those that produce systemic effects, such as the use of vasodilator drugs, and those that produce local effects, such as specific exercises and surgical reconstruction.

Tissue Protection

The key words here are gentle handling and avoidance of extremes of heat and cold. Treatment is long-term and very tedious for the patient.

Measures instituted in the hospital must be continued at home. Teaching is an important aspect of every technique utilized.

Decreased blood supply to involved areas seriously jeopardizes the nutritional health of the involved tissue. It becomes extremely susceptible to trauma of any kind. A "minor" bump can increase the ischemia and cause gangrene. Eighty per cent of the cases of gangrene begin with a preventable injury.[123]

Foot Care

Limbs must be handled carefully, with meticulous attention to foot care. Feet should be kept clean, well lubricated, and free from fungous infection. Nails should be trimmed carefully, straight across, to prevent incidental trauma and ingrown toenails. The toes are very vulnerable. Minor trauma may lead to deep abscess formation. Weight of bedcovers should be kept off the limbs with a bed cradle, and particular attention should be paid to prevention of decubiti, at the heel and ankle. Mild soap may be used in bathing, but antiseptics and other medications should be used only at the specific request of the physician. Temperature of the bath water should be checked with a thermometer. Limbs should be patted dry, not rubbed. Lanolin or petrolatum can be applied to keep the feet adequately lubricated and prevent cracking. Limbs should not be massaged as this may dislodge a clot. Shoes should be properly fitted and not too tight.

Encourage Collateral Circulation

Warmth promotes vasodilation and relieves pain, but heat increases skin metabolism and may cause burns. Because of peripheral nerve degeneration the limbs become insensitive to heat; therefore, direct heat to the area must be avoided. Treatments providing warmth rather than heat are utilized. Contrast baths in which the patient alternately immerses his feet in warm and cold water one minute at a time over a 15-minute period tend to improve circulation. Contrast baths may be used only if the physician specifies temperatures. Maximum vessel dilation occurs between 86° F. and 95° F.[124] This can be attained with a thermostatically controlled heat cradle. Use of an electric pad or blanket might increase area metabolism and cause burns and is generally contraindicated.

The patient is advised to avoid extremes in temperature both indoors and out. If he must go out on a particularly cold day, warm clothing helps protect the limbs from the vasoconstrictor effect of chilling.

Tobacco is also implicated as a vasoconstrictor. Each patient must work out a personal program to decrease cigarette smoking.

A well-balanced diet containing adequate protein to prevent tissue breakdown is suggested.

Position and Posture

The general rule for any patient with peripheral vascular disease is that he should not remain in any one position too long. If the physician wishes to have the patient's legs elevated or in a dependent position, he will specify this. The nurse should know whether the disease involves the arteries, the veins, or both. If there is arterial insufficiency, elevating the legs for lengthy periods of time may actually damage the vessels because they are further drained of their meager supply of blood. If the veins alone are involved, elevating the limbs above the level of the heart actually helps in venous return and prevents stasis of blood. If the patient has a combination of arterial and venous disease, the legs may be elevated, but for only a few minutes. Some general rules for the patient with artery or venous involvement are:

1. Avoid standing for long periods of time.
2. Alternate short periods of standing with exercise such as rapid walking.
3. Do not remain in one position for long periods of time.

Exercise

Passive, continuous exercise can be attained by use of electrically operated beds, e.g., an oscillating bed, which tilts at regular intervals and intermittently fills and then empties the arterioles, capillaries, and venules, thus improving circulation. It is difficult for the patient to get used to. Active exercise also improves collateral circulation. The physician may prescribe walking for specific lengths of time. The nurse then must allow walking only for this specified period. Or, he may order walking to the point of claudication: the point at which pain and lameness begin. The patient must understand that walking beyond this point may be harmful.

Buerger's Exercises

In these exercises the patient elevates his legs at a 45-degree angle so that all venous blood is emptied. He maintains this position for one minute. (See Fig. 26–5.) The capillaries become hypoxic, and this hypoxia serves as a maximum stimulant to vasodilation. The patient then lowers his legs and exercises the feet for two or three minutes. Arterial blood, assisted by gravity, fills the capillary tree. The legs are then kept at rest in a horizontal position for five to seven minutes. Slight, but definite benefit accrues from repeated use of the Buerger cycle, three times each day. The exercise can be done with a chair placed on the bed, or it can be done on the floor at home.

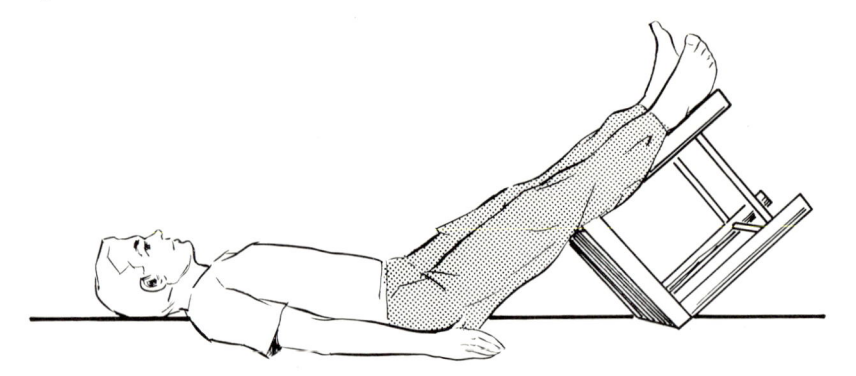

A. Legs elevated at a 45° angle for one minute

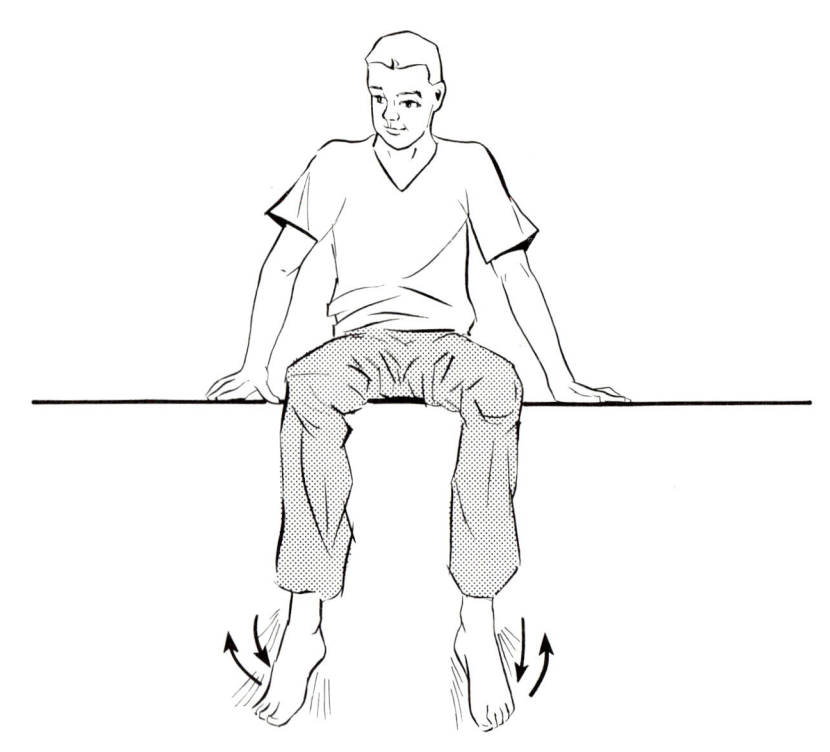

B. Legs lowered, feet exercised for 2-3 minutes

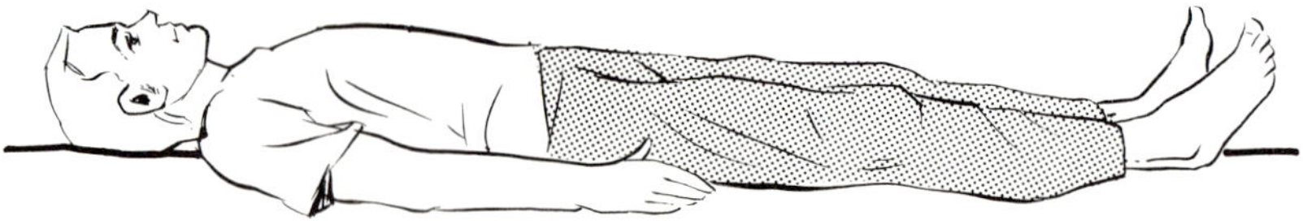

C. Legs in horizontal resting position for 5-7 minutes

FIGURE 26–5. Buerger's exercises.

Surgical Intervention for Peripheral Vascular Disease

Lumbar Sympathectomy

In this surgical procedure a lower lateral abdominal incision is made, and the ganglionic fibers supplying the legs are cut. The technique is used as an adjunct to reconstructive therapy, or alone when the patient is not a suitable candidate for vascular surgery. The vessels of the legs are ordinarily under tonic contraction in response to sympathetic motor stimulation. By severance of the fibers supplying the lumbar region, blood vessels tend to remain dilated, and there is an increase in blood flow to the limbs. The major advantageous effect seems to be improved skin nutrition. When these nerves are severed, the patient no longer responds to emotion, heat, cold, shock, and so on with reflex vasoconstriction. Sometimes, vasomotor activity returns after sympathectomy.[125] Postoperatively, the patient may have a feeling of warmth and fullness in the feet and legs and abdominal distention from decreased peristalsis. Neuralgia is sometimes felt in the tissues of the inner aspect of the thigh, beginning on the tenth postoperative day and lasting for a few weeks.[126] Sympathectomized patients are extremely sensitive to ether; it is not used for the surgery.

Vein Ligation

In this procedure the entire length of saphenous vein is removed, from the groin to the ankle. The great saphenous vein is ligated and separated at the saphenofemoral junction in the groin. It is separated from all the branches arising from this area, and the entire length is "stripped." Separate incisions may be made to remove clusters of veins that are only indirectly connected with the main stream. The incisions are covered with sterile dressings in the operating room, and elastic bandages are applied firmly from the foot to the groin. The foot of the bed is elevated immediately postoperatively (see Fig. 26–6). The patient is often asked to take a short walk as soon as he recovers from anesthesia. This is a painful time, and analgesics are utilized. He returns home in two or three days with instructions to elevate his legs when sitting, avoid standing for long periods of time, and refrain from wearing any garment that would cause constriction. If varicose ulcers have developed, the physician may order elevation of the leg and "Unna's paste boot." This is a circular gauze bandage [127] and a gelatin paste that dries and "sets" after about 20 minutes. It provides a firm support that compresses the superficial varicose veins, aids the return of venous blood, and protects the area. Bandage already impregnated with the paste is available commercially. The patient rests for 30 minutes before application of the bandage with his leg elevated. Then, the leg is shaved and the boot is applied. It is covered with a sock or stocking and is changed about every ten days.

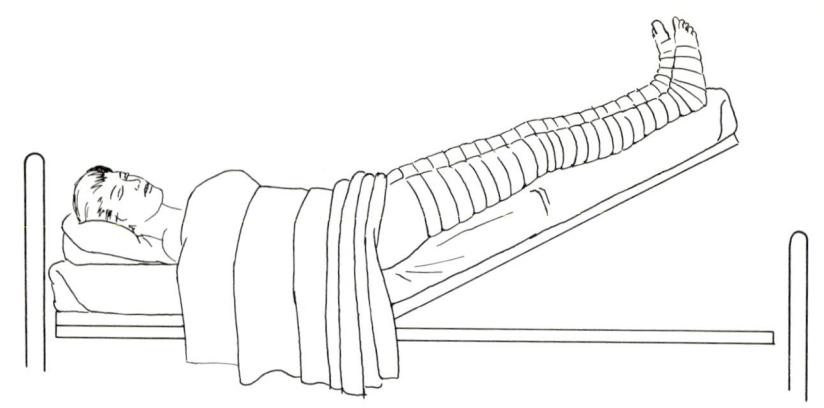

FIGURE 26-6. The foot of the bed is elevated immediately after vein ligation.

Reconstructive Vascular Surgery

ENDARTERECTOMY

In this surgical procedure the occluded vessel layers are dissected free and the atheroma lifted out. One long incision (open endarterectomy) extending the entire length of the vessel can be used, or two or more arteritomies (incisions) can be used to get to and remove the lesion (see Fig. 26-7). The vessel is clamped at the upper and lower end of the obstruction, and heparin is instilled into the distal patent tree (the part that is free of occlusion). Mattress sutures are used to hold the loose intima against the media after the obstruction is removed. The most favorable endarterectomies are performed on large vessels with high blood flow, the least favorable on small vessels with restricted flow. Aortoiliac and femoropopliteal repairs are common.

Reconstructive procedures utilize several kinds of graft materials either to bolster weakened vessels in the form of patches and "sleeves," to actually replace segments of vessels that have been removed in an end-to-end anastomosis (joining), or to "bypass" involved areas when endarterectomy is not feasible. The most acceptable graft substance for its long-term effectiveness is a venous autograft taken from the patient's own femoral or saphenous vein. If the saphenous vein is used, it is removed from the knee to the saphenofemoral junction. It is then reversed to place its valves in the proper direction and is attached to patent vessels at either end of the obstructed area by end-to-side anastomosis.[128]

If an autograft cannot be used, a synthetic graft is used. Synthetic grafts are made of Ivalon, nylon, orlon, dacron, teflon, and so on. The most popular and effective material is woven dacron. Ultimate healing of the graft depends on its ability to become "endothelized." It becomes an integral part of the patient's body when it is penetrated by granulation

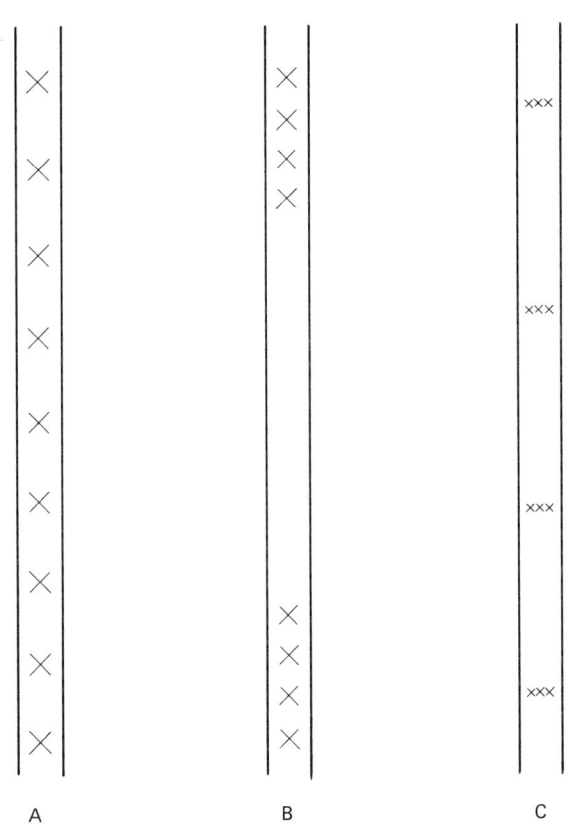

FIGURE 26–7. Incisions for endarterectomy. A. Full-length open endarterectomy. B. Endarterectomy through two arteriotomies. C. Endarterectomy through many transverse arteriotomies.

tissue, and a firmly adherent lining similar to endothelium is established. Failure of a synthetic graft stems from the fragility of its new lining and the tendency for it to stiffen, kink, and crack when flexed. Grafts are also employed in treating aneurysms. These are dilated vessel outpouchings that are very prone to rupture. They are resected and replaced by grafts.

The major complications of vascular surgery are hemorrhage, especially at the anastomosis site, and thrombosis in the reconstructed segment. The nurse must observe keenly for any untoward changes, especially pertaining to circulation in the involved limb. Hypotension, if persistent, slows the rate of flow through the vessels and increases the chance of thrombus formation, cerebral ischemia, and impaired renal function. The nurse palpates peripheral pulses and compares skin color in involved and non-involved limbs. A warmer feel, pink color, and palpable pulse in the involved limb indicate increased circulation, but a colder feel with paler tones and absent pulse is indicative of complication. Acute pain distal to the graft site may be from a thrombus.

POSTOPERATIVE CARE IN RECONSTRUCTIVE SURGERY

On the first postoperative day the patient lies flat on his back with no flexion at the operative site. By the second postoperative day he is usually allowed out of bed and walking a short distance. He is instructed to walk or lie down, but not to sit with the legs in a dependent position. If the graft crosses the knee, he will be restricted to lying down or standing up for two to four weeks postoperatively. If the graft does not cross the knee, he is encouraged to avoid sitting with his hip or knee flexed for long periods of time. He is discharged within ten days of the surgery.

27

INADEQUATE COMPOSITION OF MATERIAL TO CELLS: THE PATIENT WITH A BLOOD DYSCRASIA

Anemia

Anemia is a disease in which there is a decrease in red blood cells either from faulty formation in the bone marrow or from excess loss as in hemorrhage. There is normally 6,000 ml of circulating blood in an adult of average size. He can lose 500 ml of blood without developing symptoms. There are normally 4½ to 5 million red cells per cubic millimeter of blood, with 14½ to 15 gm of oxygen-carrying hemoglobin per 100 ml. The red cells live about four months and are destroyed in the bone marrow, liver, and spleen. In order to continuously maintain the supply of red blood cells, the body requires intrinsic factor produced by the stomach mucosa and extrinsic factor (vitamin B_{12} and iron) derived from ingested food. If these substances are inadequate, the classic symptoms of anemia may develop. They include fatigue, pallor, and asthenia (lack of strength).

Nutritional Anemia

Otherwise called "iron-deficiency anemia" this is common during infancy and pregnancy, during adolescence when onset of menstruation and spurts in growth are often associated with teen-age eating patterns deficient in iron- and protein-containing foods, and in diseases in which low gastric acidity interferes with absorption of iron. Iron remains in solution only in an acid medium.[129] Sometimes, lack of understanding of essential nutrients and lack of enough money to buy essential foods are causative factors.

Foods high in iron, protein, and vitamin B_{12} promote blood regeneration and should be included daily, e.g., lean meat, eggs, whole-grain and enriched bread and cereal, potatoes, kidneys, heart, green leafy vegetables, dried fruits, legumes, and molasses. Liver should be eaten once each week.

Once anemia is present, extra amounts of protein, minerals, and vitamins are required. Oral iron preparations are usually prescribed. Ferrous sulfate, 0.3 gm three times a day, is an example. Iron preparations may be given after meals when food is in the stomach, to decrease their irritant effect; however, most physicians now feel that better absorption occurs when the drug is given on an empty stomach before or between meals. This should be clarified before administration. Iron preparations cause the stools to turn black, and the patient should be told that this is a normal effect. If iron is not tolerated by mouth, a parenteral preparation such as iron-dextran (Imferon) may be used. This is given with a long needle, deep into the muscle. It is extremely irritant to subcutaneous tissue and should be given only with full understanding of the instructions for use that come in each package of the drug.

Pernicious Anemia

In this type of anemia there is a lack of intrinsic factor produced by the stomach mucosa and found in the gastric juice. Intrinsic factor is necessary for the absorption of vitamin B_{12}. Vitamin B_{12} is necessary in the maturation process of red blood cells. In pernicious anemia the number of red blood cells is decreased; however, their size is increased. They become macrocytic. There may be a change in their color. They are hyperchromic if there is a greater concentration of hemoglobin with greater intensity of color; normochromic if concentration of hemoglobin is normal. There is usually an absence of free hydrochloric acid in the stomach. The anemia affects the patient's nervous system, too. He becomes irritable and depressed. There is personality change. He may experience numbness, tingling, or a burning sensation in his hands or feet. He may become less coordinated. If not treated, symptoms may become irreversible.

Patients with pernicious anemia require an adequate diet; however, they also require regular injections of vitamin B_{12} because it is the vitamin B_{12} that is not being absorbed through the gastrointestinal tract. *Diet alone will not help the patient with pernicious anemia.* He will get injections for the rest of his life, though their frequency will decrease with improvement in the disease condition. Along with the chronic fatigue, pallor, and asthenia, the patient with severe pernicious anemia has a low resistance to infection, is anorexic, and often has diarrhea. His mucous membranes become very tender, and his mouth and tongue very sore. Gentle mouth care should be given before and after meals. Toothbrushes are not used. Teeth and gums should be swabbed with cotton applicators and warm water or a weak solution of hydrogen peroxide, 1 per cent. A softening cream should be applied to the lips.

Highly nutritious foods are offered initially, e.g., eggnogs and creamed foods. If the anemia has progressed for a long period of time without treatment, neurologic symptoms are evidenced. The patient may have tingling in the hands and feet, ataxia (lack of balance), and personality changes. It is difficult to determine how much of the neurologic symptomatology will disappear with treatment, though personality changes usually disappear as the condition improves.[130] Severe mental disturbance is sometimes seen.

Hemolytic Anemia

In this type of anemia cells are destroyed at such a fast rate that bone marrow cannot make up for the loss in a satisfactory manner. The disease can be acquired, as with poisoning from bacterial toxins, drugs, or snake venom; or it can be inherited, such as the inherited, noncurable sickle-cell anemia seen in Negroes.

Diagnostic Measures

Routine tests include red and white blood cell count, hemoglobin and hematocrit determination, and bleeding and clotting time.

Special Tests

CAPILLARY FRAGILITY TEST

In some blood disorders capillaries become fragile and rupture easily. In this test a blood pressure cuff is placed on the patient's arm and inflated to a point midway between systolic and diastolic pressure, and this is maintained for 15 minutes. When the cuff is removed, only one or two petechiae (small hemorrhagic spots) per square inch are normally found. If many petechiae develop, this is called the Rumpel-Leede phenomenon and indicates some abnormality.

BONE MARROW ASPIRATION

In this test a bone marrow sample is taken for biopsy. It can be aspirated from a variety of sites including vertebrae, sternum, and iliac crest. The sternum is most frequently used. The patient lies on his back. A pillow placed under the thorax helps bring the sternum forward. After the site is cleansed and anesthetized, a sternal needle, one that is short and stout with a protecting hub that prevents it from being inserted too far,[131] is inserted and tipped gently with a small mallet until the center of the bone is entered. The stylet is withdrawn, a dry 5-to-10-ml syringe is attached, and the material is aspirated and placed in a specimen bottle containing sodium oxalate. The patient feels discomfort as the specimen is aspirated and soreness over the puncture site for several days.

Hemophilia

This is a hereditary hemorrhagic disease that is usually transmitted to the male by the female through a recessive sex-linked characteristic. The woman carries the disease trait and the man develops the disease. (One form of the disease can affect both sexes.) It is a disease of childhood and is rarely seen in adults over 30.

Coagulation time is prolonged and bleeding can occur at any time. Herein lies the problem! Even the slightest bump can cause internal bleeding into the tissues and joints. Repeated injuries cause bone destruction and deformity.

Treatment revolves around preventing bleeding, stopping the bleeding once it occurs, and replacing lost blood. Hemorrhage is difficult to stop. Extreme care must, therefore, be taken to prevent it. For instance, an injection should be given only with a small needle, and the site should be observed carefully for bleeding afterward. Diet should be high in iron. Local application of fibrin foam and thrombin helps stop external bleeding. Blood transfusions are used for internal bleeding.

Leukemia [132]

This is a disease in which there is widespread proliferation of immature white blood cells in the bone marrow, liver, spleen, and lymph nodes. These cells are reproduced at fantastic rates, at the expense of normal cells. Normal bone marrow is replaced by leukemic cells. These white blood cells (precursors) do not function the way white blood cells are intended to function. The type and name of the leukemia are based on which type of white blood cell is being predominantly overproduced, e.g., lymphocytic, myelocytic, or monocytic leukemia. If the cells are in such a stage of development that they cannot be classified, the leukemia is called "stem-cell leukemia."

The specific cause of leukemia has not been established; however, it is believed to be neoplastic and is often referred to as "cancer of the blood." Some factors that appear to be implicated in cause are exposure to radiation and chemical agents that damage bone marrow (e.g., benzol). Hormonal imbalance, genetic predisposition, and viral origin are being studied.

The disease is uniformly fatal, though life can be prolonged with intensive chemotherapeutic intervention. If the disease is in its acute form, death may occur within a few weeks to one year after onset of symptoms; if it is in its chronic form, the patient may survive three to five years.

In the United States, 40 per cent of patients develop acute forms, 60 per cent chronic forms. The incidence is highest in acute lymphocytic leukemia in people under 25, in chronic myelocytic and lymphocytic leukemia in middle life (especially after 45).

Symptoms develop as abnormal cells proliferate and spread. Proliferating cells press on other body organs. Bleeding occurs as the rate of red blood cell production drops. Anemia develops. Infection is a problem anywhere in the body.

In acute leukemia, symptoms occur abruptly with weakness, anorexia, pallor, fever, sudden increase in the size of the lymph nodes, bone or joint pain, and bleeding from mucous membranes or into the skin (petechiae form). The patient often traces the onset of these symptoms to a respiratory infection that "didn't go away the way it usually does." He may have discovered an upper quadrant abdominal mass (enlarged spleen) while bathing. The total number of leukocytes may rise to 15,000 to 30,000 per cubic millimeter of blood, although the range may be normal at the onset of the disease.

In chronic forms the symptoms appear insidiously. The disease is often discovered "accidentally" during a routine physical examination. There may be a few enlarged lymph nodes, especially in the axilla or groin. Anorexia, weight loss, weakness, and pallor develop gradually. The patient becomes anemic and may develop fever late in the course of the disease. There may be marked enlargement of the liver and spleen. Leukocyte count is high with 30,000 to 100,000 cells per cubic millimeter of blood in chronic lymphocytic leukemia.

The diagnosis is confirmed by examination of peripheral blood and bone marrow. Aspirated bone marrow consists of an almost solid mass of immature white blood cells.

Any patient with leukemia is extremely susceptible to infection because white blood cell function is inadequate. Pain develops from infiltration of abnormal cells into the periosteum. It may be constant or intermittent.

The goal of treatment is to provide the patient with as long and as normal a life as possible.

Oral hygiene is very important because there is bleeding in the gums, often with ulceration and a "spongelike" quality from the infiltration. The teeth seem to submerge. Gentle mouth care with swabs, glycerin, and lemon juice helps. Infection, too, is always a possibility and must be watched for closely.

Drugs used include antimetabolites that interfere with the synthesis of nucleic acids, e.g., 6 mercaptopurine, A-methopterin, and corticosteroids that decrease inflammatory response and induce remissions (successive remissions are progressively shorter). Oral chlorambucil (Leukeran), a nitrogen mustard product that is cytoxic to lymphoid tissue, is beneficial in some patients with chronic lymphocytic leukemia; oral busulfan (Myleran), an alkylating agent that combines with cellular substances and prevents the cells from splitting into more daughter cells, may be used. (See p. 94.)

Transfusions of whole blood and/or platelets are used for anemia and for bleeding episodes.

Irradiation with a radioactive isotope such as oral or intravenous sodium phosphate (P^{32}) is done in an attempt to maintain levels of peripheral blood and bone marrow near normal.

Drugs are used one at a time, so that resistance does not develop to all at once. Remissions may last up to two years. Patients should be examined every one to three months and should be instructed to seek immediate medical attention if symptoms occur.

Hodgkin's Disease

This, too, is considered a neoplastic disease. It involves all lymphatic tissue. There are lymphomas (tumors arising from lymph tissue) throughout lymphatic areas of the body. The disease is uniformly fatal. It affects males twice as frequently as females, and more than one case is often found in a family. There may be painless enlargement of a localized group of nodes initially, often beginning in the cervical area. But the disease spreads to the axillary and inguinal areas and eventually becomes generalized. There is usually spread to the chest, with cough, chest pain, dyspnea, and cyanosis. Other symptoms arise as lymphomas press on surrounding organs.

Treatment involves localized x-ray therapy to involved regions with intravenous nitrogen mustard given on successive days as an adjunct to x-ray therapy. Transfusions and antimicrobial agents may be used as supportive therapy. Care must be used if aspirin is given because it can cause a serious drop in temperature when the patient has Hodgkin's disease.

Infectious Mononucleosis

This is an infectious disease believed to be of viral origin and believed to be spread through secretions of the mouth and throat. The incubation period is not definitely established, but seems to be several weeks. The incidence of the disease is slightly higher in males than in females. The disease is most prevalent in the 15-to-30-year age group.

At the height of the disease the white blood count is elevated to 10,000 to 20,000 cells per cubic millimeter of blood with an absolute lymphocytosis that persists over a period of several days or more. The lymphocytes are abnormal, but, unlike those in leukemia, are chiefly mature cells. Along with the lymphocytosis there are enlarged, tense liver and spleen, sore throat, and fever. The patient may look jaundiced.

The diagnosis is confirmed by a positive heterophil agglutination test in which, for some reason, the patient develops an unusually high level of antibodies that agglutinate erythrocytes of sheep's blood.

The disease may run in spurts or may be of epidemic proportion. High-risk groups seem to be college students and health personnel. This may only be because serology is done in these people when mild symptoms develop.

The disease is usually not serious. It disappears in two weeks but may continue in chronic form for several weeks and even months. Relapses occur. There is always the possibility that the tense spleen may rupture. Treatment includes rest, rest, and more rest! This may be very difficult for college students!

REFERENCES

1. Simeone, F., "Shock: Its Nature and Treatment," *Amer. J. Nurs.*, **66**: 1287, June 1966.
2. Smith, D., and Gipps, C., *Care of the Adult Patient*. J. B. Lippincott Co., Philadelphia, 1966, p. 67.
3. Simeone, *op. cit.*, p. 1287.
4. Modell, W., Schwartz, D., Hazeltine, L., and Kirkham, F., *Handbook of Cardiology for Nurses*. Springer Publishing Co., New York, 1966, p. 122.
5. Statement by Ad Hoc Committee on Cardiopulmonary Resuscitation of the Division of Medical Sciences, National Academy of Sciences-National Research Council, *J.A.M.A.*, **198**:138, Oct. 24, 1966.
6. *Ibid.*, p. 138.
7. Fields, Sister M. L., "The C.P.R. Team in a Medium Sized Hospital," *Amer. J. Nurs.*, **66**:87, Jan. 1966.
8. Berger, A., *Elementary Human Anatomy*. John Wiley and Sons, New York, 1967, p. 126.
9. Modell, *op. cit.*, p. 115.
10. Burch, G., and Winsor, T., *A Primer of Electrocardiography*. Lea and Febiger, Philadelphia, 1960, p. 25.
11. *Ibid.*, p. 29.
12. *Ibid.*, pp. 19–24, 276.
13. Sutton, A., *Bedside Nursing Techniques*. W. B. Saunders Co., 1966, p. 209.
14. Modell, *op. cit.*, p. 108.
15. Lown, B., "Electrical Reversion of Cardiac Arrhythmias," *Brit. Heart J.*, **29**:469, July 1967.
16. Modell, *op. cit.*, p. 154.
17. Lown, *op. cit.*, p. 475.
18. Donoso, E., Cohn, L., and Friedberg, C., "Ventricular Arrhythmias After Precordial Electric Shock," *Amer. Heart J.*, **73**:595, May 1967.
19. Lown, *op. cit.*, p. 483.
20. *Ibid.*, p. 475.
21. Lillehei, C., Sellers, R., Eliot, R., and Shafer, R., "Implanted Cardiac Pacemakers," *Amer. J. Surg.*, **114**: 69, July, 1967.
22. Kastor, J., De Sanctis, R., Harthorne, J., and Schwartz, G., "Transvenous Atrial Pacing in the Treatment of Refractory Ventricular Irritability," *Ann. Intern. Med.*, **66**:939, May 1967.
23. Lillehei, *op. cit.*, p. 69.
24. Hann, V. K., "Cardiac Pacemakers," *Amer. J. Nurs.*, **69**:751, Apr. 1969.
25. *Ibid.*, p. 447.
26. *Ibid.*, p. 448.
27. Lillehei, *op. cit.*, p. 73.
28. *Ibid.*, p. 73.
29. Tabrisky, J., Lobe, W., Newman, M., and Seibert, C., "Internal Cardiac Pacemakers," *Amer. J. Roentgen.*, **100**:446, June 1967.
30. Cunningham, L., *Advanced Medical Surgical Nursing*. Wm. C. Brown Co., Dubuque, Iowa, 1966, p. 46.
31. Lillehei, *op. cit.*, p. 71.
32. *Ibid.*, p. 71.
33. Tabrisky, *op. cit.*, p. 454.
34. Brown, S., Iannarella, F., Menchetti, G., and Tuman, M., "Body Function Monitoring," *Nurs. Clin. N. A.*, **1**: 569, Dec. 1966.
35. De Meyer, J., "The Environment of the Intensive Care Unit," *Nurs. Forum*, **3**:263, Summer 1967.
36. Los Angeles County General Hospital Coronary Care Unit Major Alarms, in Jones, B., "Inside the Coronary Care Unit," *Amer. J. Nurs.*, **67**:2315, Nov. 1967.
37. Jones, B., "Inside the Coronary Care

Unit," *Amer. J. Nurs.*, **67**:2316, Nov. 1967.
38. Blakeslee, A., and Stamler, J., *Your Heart Has Nine Lives*. Prentice-Hall Co., Englewood Cliffs, N.J., 1964, p. 4.
39. *Ibid.*, p. 5.
40. Russek, H., "Emotional Stress in Etiology of Coronary Heart Disease," *Geriatrics*, **22**:84, June 1967.
41. Kahn, H., and Dawber, T., "The Development of Coronary Heart Disease in Relation to Sequential Biennial Measures of Cholesterol in the Framingham Study," *J. Chronic Dis.*, **19**:611, May 1966.
42. *Ibid.*, p. 616.
43. Mann, G., Shaffer, R., and Rich, A., "Physical Fitness and Immunity to Heart Disease in Masai," *Lancet*, **2**:1308, Dec. 25, 1965.
44. *Ibid.*, p. 1310.
45. Blakeslee, *op. cit.*, p. 128.
46. Russek, *op. cit.*, p. 85.
47. Jenkins, C., "Components of the Coronary Prone Behavior Pattern," *J. Chronic Dis.*, **19**:600, May 1966.
48. Blakeslee, *op. cit.*, p. 153.
49. Hurst, J., and Logue, R., *The Heart, Arteries, and Veins*. McGraw-Hill Book Co., New York, 1966, p. 44.
50. *Ibid.*, p. 123.
51. Shafer, K., Sawyer, J., McCluskey, A., and Beck, E., *Medical Surgical Nursing*. C. V. Mosby Co., St. Louis, 1967, p. 317.
52. Hurst, *op. cit.*, p. 148.
53. Likoff, W., Segal, B., and Kasparian, H., "Paradox of Normal Selective Coronary Arteriograms in Patients Considered to Have Unmistakable Coronary Heart Disease," *New Eng. J. Med.*, **276**:1066, May 11, 1967.
54. Hurst, *op. cit.*, p. 167.
55. Kelly, A., "Current Cardiovascular Diagnostic Measures and Associated Nursing Care," *J. Nurs. Educ.*, **5**:13, Nov. 1966.
56. Hurst, *op. cit.*, p. 211.
57. Modell, *op. cit.*, p. 67.
58. Kinlein, M., "Myocardial Infarction: the Critical Hours," *Amer. J. Nurs.*, special supplement, **64**:C11, Nov. 1964.
59. Thompson, R., and King, E., *Biochemical Disorders in Human Disease*. Academic Press, New York, 1964, p. 123.
60. Kinlein, *op. cit.*, p. C11.
61. Hurst, *op. cit.*, p. 622.
62. *Ibid.*, p. 623.
63. Modell, *op. cit.*, p. 76.
64. Hurst, *op. cit.*, p. 66.
65. Beeson, P., and McDermott, W., *Cecil-Loeb Textbook of Medicine*. W. B. Saunders Co., Philadelphia, 1963, p. 703.
66. *Ibid.*, p. 703.
67. Modell, *op. cit.*, p. 76.
68. Friedberg, C., "Angina Pectoris," *Geriatrics*, **22**:144, June 1967.
69. *Ibid.*, p. 147.
70. *Ibid.*, p. 152.
71. Hurst, *op. cit.*, p. 716.
72. *Ibid.*, p. 673.
73. Friedberg, *op. cit.*, 146.
74. Hurst, *op. cit.*, p. 716.
75. Modell, *op. cit.*, p. 83.
76. *Ibid.*, p. 85.
77. Hurst, *op. cit.*, p. 662.
78. Kinlein, *op. cit.*, p. C11.
79. *Ibid.*, p. C11.
80. *Ibid.*, p. C9.
81. Hazeltine, L., "Myocardial Infarction: The Weeks of Healing," *Amer. J. Nurs.*, special supplement, **64**:C15, Nov. 1964.
82. Hurst, *op. cit.*, p. 665.
83. *Ibid.*, p. 665.
84. Hurst, *op. cit.*, p. 251.
85. Dutcher, I., and Fielo, S., *Water and Electrolytes: Implications for Nursing Practice*. The Macmillan Co., New York, 1967, p. 77.
86. Hurst, *op. cit.*, p. 252.
87. Dutcher, *op. cit.*, p. 82.
88. Brunner, L., Emerson, C., Ferguson, L., and Suddarth, D., *Textbook of Medical Surgical Nursing*. J. B. Lippincott Co., Philadelphia, 1964, p. 547.
89. Billimoria, J., Drysdale, J., James, D., and Macagan, N., "Determination of Fibrinolytic Activity of Whole

Blood with Special Reference to the Effects of Exercise and Fat Feeding," *Lancet*, **2**:471, 1969.
90. Modell, *op. cit.*, p. 89.
91. Hazeltine, *op. cit.*, p. C18.
92. Modell, *op. cit.*, p. 96.
93. Lewis, C., "Factors Influencing the Return to Work of Men with Congestive Heart Failure," *J. Chronic Dis.*, **19**:1193, Nov.–Dec. 1966.
94. Krause, M., *Food, Nutrition and Diet Therapy*. W. B. Saunders Co., Philadelphia, 1966, p. 344.
95. *Ibid*.
96. Haskin, S., "The Relation of Diet to Atherosclerosis and Infarction," *Amer. J. Nurs.*, **60**:3, Mar. 1960.
97. Brest, A., and Moyer, J., *Cardiovascular Drug Therapy*. Grune and Stratton, New York, 1965, p. 347.
98. Cooper, L., Barber, E., Mitchel, H., Rynbergen, H., and Greene, J., *Nutrition in Health and Disease*. J. B. Lippincott Co., Philadelphia, 1958, p. 28.
99. Zukel, M., "Fat Controlled Diets," *Amer. J. Clin. Nutr.*, **16**:270, Feb. 1965.
100. *Ibid.*, p. 270.
101. Brest, *op. cit.*, p. 347.
102. *Ibid.*, p. 424.
103. *Ibid.*, p. 455.
104. Garb, S., *Laboratory Tests in Common Use*. Springer Publishing Co., New York, 1963, p. 68.
105. Brest, *op. cit.*, p. 229.
106. *Ibid.*, p. 229.
107. Davis, L., *Christopher's Textbook of Surgery*. W. B. Saunders Co., Philadelphia, 1966, p. 469.
108. Sutton, A., *Bedside Nursing Techniques*. W. B. Saunders Co., Philadelphia, 1966, p. 218.
109. Varvaro, R., "Teaching the Patient About Open Heart Surgery," *Amer. J. Nurs.*, **65**:111, Oct. 1965.
110. Barker, W., *Peripheral Arterial Disease*. W. B. Saunders Co., Philadelphia, 1966, p. 55.
111. *Ibid.*, p. 56.
112. Beeson, *op. cit.*, p. 786.
113. Brest, *op. cit.*, p. 215.
114. Davis, *op. cit.*, p. 1308.
115. *Ibid.*, p. 1308.
116. Beland, I., *Clinical Nursing: Pathophysiological and Psychosocial Approaches*. The Macmillan Co., New York, 1965, p. 654.
117. Davis, *op. cit.*, p. 1310.
118. Sister Mary Elizabeth, "Occlusion of the Peripheral Arteries," *Amer. J. Nurs.*, **67**:562, Mar. 1967.
119. *Ibid.*, p. 568.
120. Ajemian, S., "Bypass Grafting for Femoral Artery Occlusion," *Amer. J. Nurs.*, **67**:565, Mar. 1967.
121. Barker, *op. cit.*, p. 72.
122. Sister Mary Elizabeth, *op. cit.*, p. 562.
123. Barker, *op. cit.*, p. 89.
124. Beeson, *op. cit.*, p. 777.
125. Barker, *op. cit.*, pp. 95.
126. *Ibid*, p. 94.
127. Smith, D., and Gipps, C., *Care of the Adult Patient*. J. B. Lippincott Co., Philadelphia, 1966, p. 649.
128. Ajemian, *op. cit.*, p. 565.
129. Cooper, *op. cit.*, p. 365.
130. Smith, *op. cit.*, p. 508.
131. Shafer, *op. cit.*, p. 402.
132. Beeson, *op. cit.*, p. 1127.

ADDITIONAL READINGS

ANTAR, M. OHLSON, M., and HODGES, E., "Changes in Retail Market Food Supplies in the United States in the Last Seventy Years in Relation to the Incidence of Coronary Heart Disease with Special Reference to Dietary Carbohydrates and Essential Fatty Acids," *Amer. J. Clin. Nutr.*, **14**:169, 1964.

BARNARD, C. N., "A Human Cardiac Transplant: An Interim Report of a Suc-

cessful Operation Performed at Groote Schuur Hospital, Cape Town," S. Afr. Med. J., **41**:1271, Dec. 30, 1967.
BARNARD, M. S., "Heart Transplantation: An Experimental Review and Preliminary Research," S. Afr. Med. J., **41**:1260, Dec. 30, 1967.
BETSON, C., and UDE, L., "Central Venous Pressure," Amer. J. Nurs., **69**:1466, July 1969.
BOSMAN, S. C. W., "Selection of Donor for Cardiac Transplant," S. Afr. Med. J., **41**:1262, Dec. 30, 1967.
BRENNAN, R.: Nutrition: A Book of Readings. William C. Brown Co., Dubuque, Iowa, 1967.
DAVIS, J., and WIESEL, B., "Treatment of Angina Pectoris with a Nitroglycerine Ointment," Amer. J Med. Sci., **230**:259, 1955.
Editorial, Circulation, **31**:641, May 1965.
ELIOT, R. and MARK, J., "Aortic Regurgitation Past Fifty," Geriatrics, **22**:90, June 1967.
GEORGE, J., "Electronic Monitoring of Vital Signs," Amer. J. Nurs., **65**:68, Feb. 1965.
GEORGE, J., "Monitoring the Myocardial Infarction Patient," Nurs. Clin. N. Amer,. **1**:549, Dec. 1966.
GRIFFITH, G., "Home Care of the Aged Patient," Geriatrics, **22**:140, June 1967.
HEAP, B., "Sodium Restricted Diets," Amer. J. Nurs., **60**:206, Feb. 1960.
HELLER, A., "Nursing the Patient with an Artificial Pacemaker," Amer. J. Nurs., **64**:87, Apr. 1964.
JENKINS, A., "Successful Cardiac Monitoring," Nurs. Clin. N. Amer. **1**:537, Dec. 1966.
JORDAAN, P., "The First Human Heart Transplant," Nurs. Times, **64**:956, July 1968.
JUDE, J., KOUWENHOVEN, W., and KNICKERBOCKER, G., "External Cardiac Resuscitation," Monogr. Surg. Sci., **1**:59, 1964.
LEHMAN, E., "Social Class and Coronary Heart Disease: A Sociological Assessment of the Medical Literature," J. Chronic Dis., **20**:381, June 1967.
LITWAK, R., LEV, R., BARON, M., SILVAY, J., and GADBOYS, H., "The Surgical Treatment of Aortic Aneurysms," Geriatrics, **22**:105, June 1967.
MACLEAN, D. M., and FOWLER, E. A., "Heart Transplant—Early Postoperative Care," Amer. J. Nurs., **68**:2124, Oct. 1968.
McCALLUM, H., "The Nurse and the Respirator," Nurs Clin. N. Amer., **1**:597, Dec. 1966.
MELTZER, L., "Coronary Care, Electrocardiography and the Nurse," Amer. J. Nurs., **65**:12, Dec. 1965.
MERKEL, R., and SOVIE, M. D., "Electrocution Hazards with Transvenous Pacemaker Electrodes," Amer. J. Nurs., **68**:2560, Dec. 1968.
PARKER, J., DIGIORGI, S., and WEST, R., "Selective Coronary Arteriography: Arteriographic Patterns in Coronary Heart Disease," Canad. Med. Ass. J., **95**:291, Aug. 13, 1966.
PINNEO, R., "Nursing in a Coronary Care Unit," Cardiovasc. Nurs., **3**:1, Jan.–Feb. 1967.
RAWLINGS, M., "Inside the Coronary Care Unit: Trends in Therapeutic Management," Amer. J. Nurs., **67**:2321, Nov. 1967.

ROBINSON, B., "Relation of Heart Rate and Systolic Blood Pressure to the Onset of Pain in Angina Pectoris," *Circulation,* **35:**1073, June 1967.

RODRIGUEZ, J.: *An Atlas of Cardiac Surgery.* W. B. Saunders Co., Philadelphia, 1957.

SCHWID, S., and GIFFORD, R., "The Use and Abuse of Antihypertensive Drugs in the Aged," *Geriatrics,* **22:**172, June 1967.

SHUMWAY, N. E., ANGELL, W. W., and WUERFLEIN, R. D., "Heart Replacement," *J. Lancet,* **88:**171, July 1968.

SMITH, D., and PETERSDORF, R., "Prevention of Infection in Patients with Cardiovascular Disease," *J. Chronic Dis.,* **19:**587, May 1966.

UNIT VI

THE PATIENT WITH A PROBLEM IN SUPPLY AND REMOVAL OF GASES

28

THE RESPIRATORY SYSTEM

THE respiratory tract serves as a passageway for air. It also conditions the air to protect our internal environment. In addition to the nose and nasopharynx it is composed of the larynx, trachea, bronchi, and lungs. The thorax (chest) is a large cavity that is protected on all sides, except at its broad base, by bones and cartilage. The ribs extend from the vertebral column posteriorly to the sternum in front. The diaphragm, an important muscle of respiration, is broad and flat. It separates the chest and abdominal cavities. (See Fig. 28–1.)

TABLE 28–1. THE RESPIRATORY SYSTEM *

This chart of the respiratory system shows the apparatus for breathing. Breathing is the process by which oxygen in the air is brought into the lungs and into close contact with the blood, which absorbs it and carries it to all parts of the body. At the same time the blood gives up waste matter (carbon dioxide), which is carried out of the lungs with the air breathed out.

1. The *sinuses* (frontal, maxillary, and sphenoidal) are hollow spaces in the bones of the head. Small openings connect them to the nasal cavity. The functions they serve are not clearly understood, but include helping to regulate the temperature and humidity of air breathed in, as well as to lighten the bone structure of the head and to give resonance to the voice.

2. The *nasal cavity* (nose) is the preferred entrance for outside air into the Respiratory System. The hairs that line the inside wall are part of the air-cleansing system.

3. Air also enters through the *oral cavity* (mouth), especially in people who have a mouth-breathing habit or whose nasal passages may be temporarily obstructed, as by a cold.

4. The *adenoids* are overgrown lymph tissue at the top of the throat. When they interfere with breathing, they are generally removed. The lymph system, consisting of nodes (knots of cells) and connecting vessels, carries fluid throughout the body. This system helps to resist body infection by filtering out

* Reprinted from *Introduction to Respiratory Diseases*, copyright National Tuberculosis and Respiratory Disease Association.

306

TABLE 28-1. [*Continued*]

foreign matter, including bacteria, and producing cells (lymphocytes) to fight them.

5. The *tonsils* are lymph nodes in the wall of the pharynx that often become infected. They are a part of the bacteria-fighting system of the body.

6. The *pharynx* (throat) collects incoming air from the nose and mouth and passes it downward to the trachea (windpipe).

7. The *epiglottis* is a flap of tissue that guards the entrance to the trachea, closing when anything is swallowed that should go into the esophagus and stomach.

8. The *larynx* (voice box) contains the vocal cords. It is the place where moving air being breathed in and out creates voice sounds.

9. The *esophagus* is the passage leading from mouth and throat to the stomach.

10. The *trachea* (windpipe) is the passage leading from the pharynx to the lungs.

11. The *lymph nodes* of the lungs are found against the walls of the bronchial tubes and trachea.

12. The *ribs* are bones supporting and protecting the chest cavity. They move to a limited degree, helping the lungs to expand and contract.

13. The trachea divides into the two main *bronchi* (tubes), one for each lung, which subdivide into the lobar bronchi—three on the right and two on the left. These, in turn, subdivide further.

14. The right lung is divided into three *lobes*, or sections. Each lobe is like a balloon filled with sponge-like lung tissue. Air moves in and out through one opening—a branch of the bronchus.

15. The left lung is divided into two *lobes*.

16. The *pleura* are the two membranes, actually one continuous one folded on itself, that surround each lobe of the lungs and separate the lungs from the chest wall.

17. The bronchial tubes are lined with *cilia* (like very small hairs) that have a wave-like motion. This motion carries *mucus* (sticky phlegm or liquid) upward and out into the throat, where it is either coughed up or swallowed. The mucus catches and holds much of the dust, germs, and other unwanted matter that has invaded the lungs and thus gets rid of it.

18. The *diaphragm* is the strong wall of muscle that separates the chest cavity from the abdominal cavity. By moving downward, it creates suction to draw in air and expand the lungs.

19. The smallest subdivisions of the bronchi are called *bronchioles*, at the end of which are the alveoli (plural of alveolus).

20. The *alveoli* are the very small air sacs that are the destination of air breathed in. The *capillaries* are blood vessels that are imbedded in the walls of the alveoli. Blood passes through the capillaries, brought to them by the *pulmonary artery* and taken away by the *pulmonary vein*. While in the capillaries the blood discharges carbon dioxide into the alveoli and takes up oxygen from the air in the alveoli.

308]   SUPPLY AND REMOVAL OF GASES

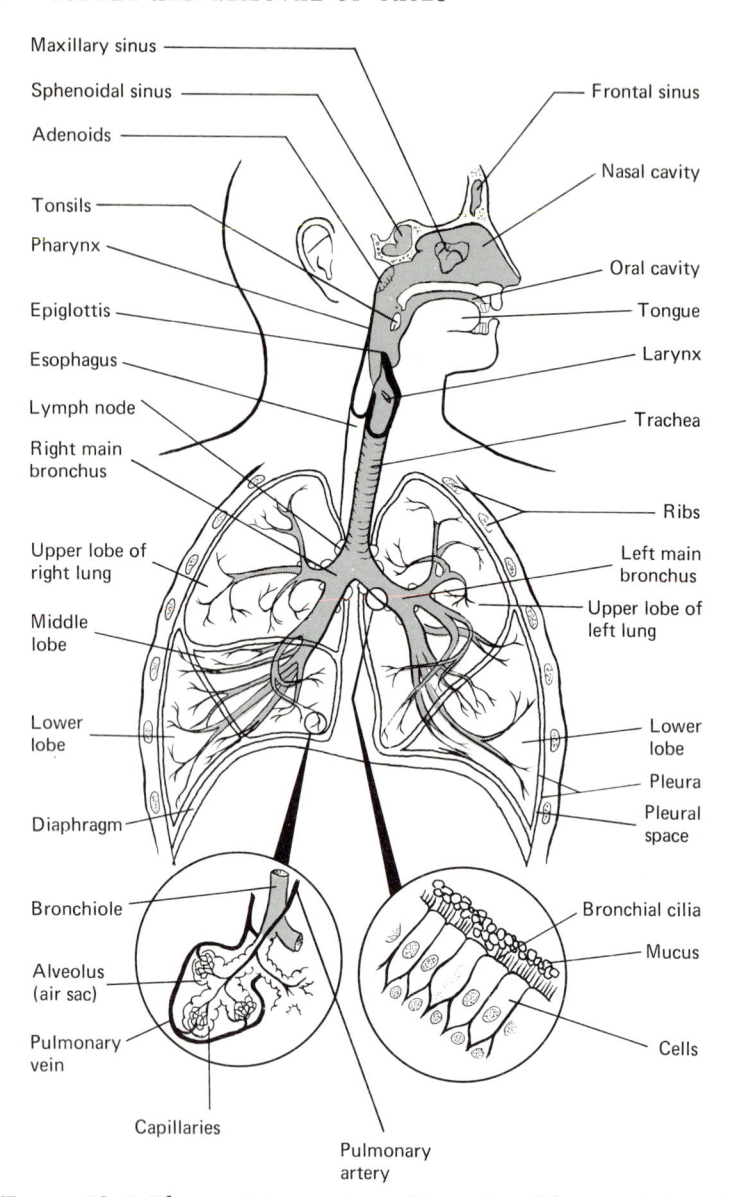

FIGURE 28-1. The respiratory system. (Reproduced by permission of the National Tuberculosis and Respiratory Disease Association, New York.)

The lungs fill both sides of the chest and are separated in the midline by a space called the mediastinum. This space contains the esophagus, the trachea, and the great vessels to and from the heart. The heart is located in the lower part of the mediastinum and extends into the left side of the chest.

Each lung is covered with a thin membrane made up of the visceral pleura, which is continuous with the lung, and the parietal pleura, which lines the surface of the chest.[1*] Thus, a potential space is formed called the pleural cavity. It contains a small amount of fluid that enables the pleurae to glide over each other smoothly. When the pleurae become inflamed, friction develops and there is pain. This is called pleurisy.[2]

The lung contains elastic fibers and will contract and collapse if the normal negative pressure of the pleural space is lost. Each lung is porous and spongy. Owing to the presence of air, they float in water. Each lobe is composed of a number of lobules. In each lobe a bronchiole enters and terminates in one of the alveolar sacs.

Branches of the pulmonary artery, which bring blood from the right ventricle, accompany the bronchial tubes and form a complex of capillaries around the alveoli. The walls of these alveoli are composed of thin elastic tissue and simple squamous epithelium. Here the exchange of gases between the blood in the capillaries and the air in the alveoli takes place. The *pulmonary artery* carries *venous* blood to the lungs. The oxygenated or *arterial blood* is returned to the left atrium by the *pulmonary veins*. Bronchial arteries originating from the thoracic aorta supply arterial blood to the lungs for the nourishment of these organs.

The bronchioles are made up of smooth muscle and elastic tissue. They are thin-walled, and each bronchiole terminates in an alveolar sac. Each sac bears on all parts of its surface small, irregular projections known as *alveoli,* or *air cells*. In these alveoli oxygen is absorbed into the blood and carbon dioxide removed.

The walls of the trachea, bronchi, and larynx are strengthened with cartilage. In the trachea and bronchial tubes these rings are incomplete dorsally, which permits some alteration in their size and shape during various phases of breathing.[3]

Breathing is controlled by the central nervous system and is an autonomic process, although some voluntary control exists.[4] Breathing also helps to equalize the temperature of the body and to get rid of excess water.

Breathing consists of inspiration (breathing in) and expiration (breathing out). *External respiration* consists of the exchange of carbon dioxide and oxygen between the alveoli of the lungs and the blood. *Internal respiration* consists of the exchange of carbon dioxide and oxygen between the blood and body cells. External respiration takes place between the air and the lungs. Internal respiration takes place in the cells that make up the tissues. The respiratory rate (16 to 18) per minute is influenced by emotion, exercise, heartbeat, age, and muscular structure.

* References for Unit VI are on page 339.

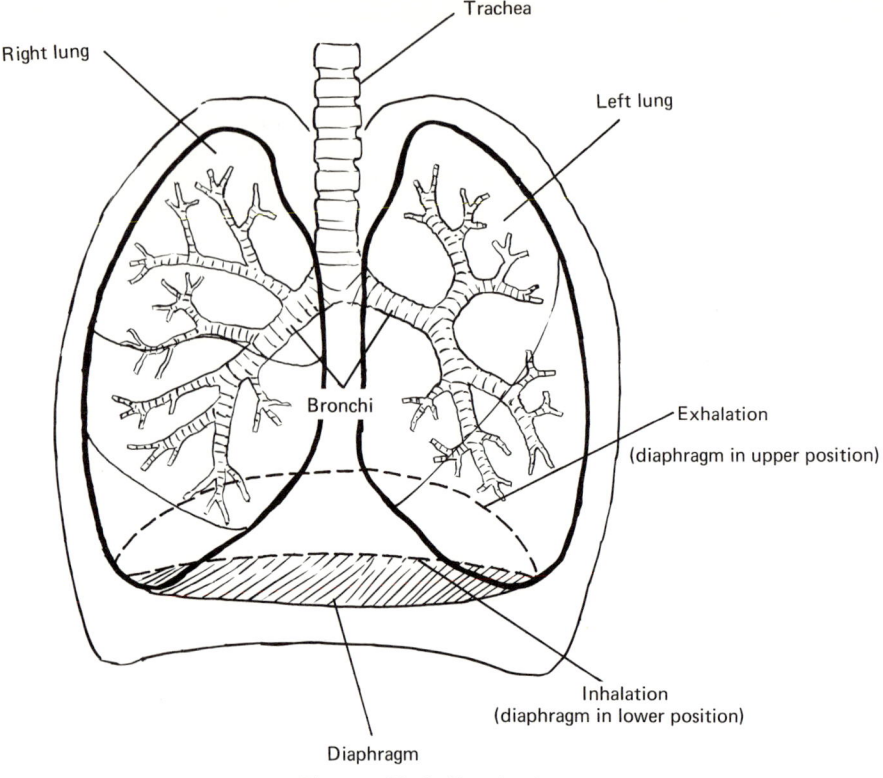

FIGURE 28–2. Respiration.

As mentioned earlier, the act of breathing is controlled by the central nervous system. The respiratory center is located in the medulla oblongata.[5] This is the center for nervous control of the depth and frequency of respiration. From the respiratory center, nerve impulses pass via the spinal cord and spinal nerves to the intercostal muscles, the diaphragm, and the abdominal muscles, adjusting respiratory depth and rhythm to body needs.

Pressure Changes During Respiration

Intrapulmonic pressure is pressure within the air passages and lungs. During the brief interval between inspiration and expiration it is at 760 mm Hg, or atmospheric pressure. During inspiration the diaphragm lowers, the volume of air within the lung increases, and its pressure falls below atmospheric pressure. During expiration the volume of air within the lung decreases, and its pressure rises above atmospheric pressure. (See Fig. 28–3.)

Intrathoracic or intrapleural pressure is that pressure which exists out-

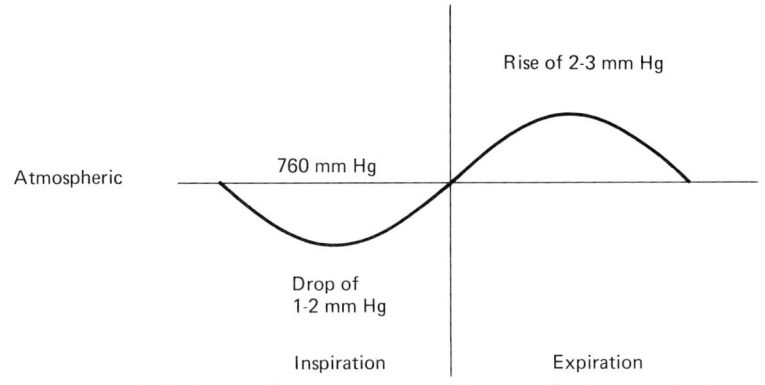

FIGURE 28-3. Intrapulmonic pressure changes during respiration.

side the lungs but within the chest cavity. It exists between the two pleural layers. It is always a negative pressure that is lower than atmospheric pressure. It falls 6 to 8 mm Hg below atmospheric pressure after inspiration and rises to 2 to 4 mm Hg below atmospheric pressure during expiration. If the intrapleural pressure rises above atmospheric pressure, the lungs collapse. This is called spontaneous pneumothorax. It may result from a stab wound to the area. (See Fig. 28-4.)

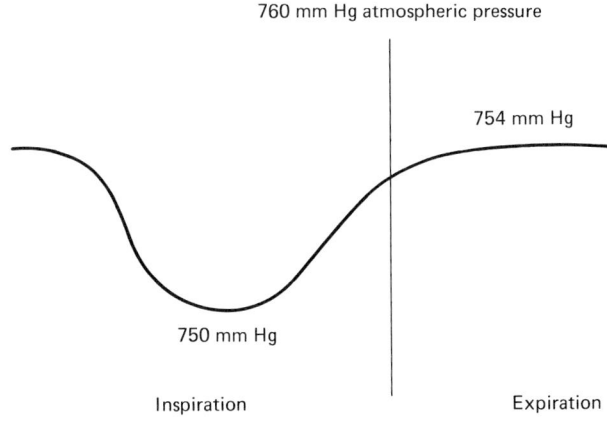

FIGURE 28-4. Intrapleural pressure changes during respiration.

Pressure changes are explained according to the laws of physics: Boyle's law, Charles's law, and the law of solubility of gases.[6] Students are referred to appropriate texts for further discussion.

Adequate ventilation depends on a patent (open) airway. It is jeopardized when a patient is immobilized, unconscious, or taking depressant drugs, and when he has disease within the respiratory tract, an inadequate cough reflex, an obstruction, and so on.

29

DIAGNOSTIC TESTS

DIAGNOSTIC procedures are performed to observe respiratory anatomy, study mucus composition, assess lung function, rule out nonorganic types of dyspnea, and differentiate diseases of the lungs. In addition, they are used to determine the degree of disability caused by disease in the respiratory tract.[7]

X-ray

X-ray of the chest is routinely done on admission. If disease is suspected, several different views may be taken. X-rays may be done at the bedside. Metal objects should be removed. X-rays provide a permanent record of the lungs. Fluoroscopy shows the lungs in motion. The record is not permanent.

Sputum Examination

The patient is instructed to cough deeply and expectorate into a sputum cup (see p. 275). Only specimens obtained from deep within the chest are suitable. First morning specimens are usually the best. The specimens are examined grossly for color, consistency, presence of blood, odor, and so on. They are examined microscopically for specific microorganisms or cancer cells (Papanicolaou test.) Gastric analysis may be done to examine swallowed mucus.

Thoracentesis (Chest Tap)

For this test the patient is in a sitting position, often leaning over an overbed table. Sterile technique is used. Fluid is aspirated by needle through the chest wall for study, biopsy, and so on. The patient should rest after the procedure and should be observed for any respiratory symptoms or bleeding from the injection site. Thoracentesis may also be done to rid the chest cavity of excess fluid. In this case, the patient must be observed for signs of shock.

Measurement of Pulmonary Volumes and Capacities [8,9]

Tidal Volume

This test measures the gas inspired and expired with each normal breath. Average tidal volume is 500 ml.

Residual Volume

This test measures the gas remaining in the lungs after the deepest possible expiration. The patient is usually instructed to breathe through his mouth through a mouthpiece. A noseclip is applied so that he does not breathe through his nose. Time should be allowed for the patient to get used to this clip. A recording device is used. Average volume of residual air is 1.5 L.

Vital Capacity

This test measures the maximal amount of air that can be exhaled after maximal inhalation. This test is timed for 0.5 to 3 seconds. Average vital capacity is 4,500 ml.

Bronchospirometry

This test measures the ventilatory efficiency and the oxygen absorptive function of each lung separately, at the same time. It gives accurate determinations of the degree of respiratory impairment. A double-lumen catheter is introduced into the trachea. A noseclip is applied. Air is inhaled and exhaled through the tracheal catheter, which is attached to a device that measures the amount of air inhaled and exhaled. Samples of arterial blood are taken to determine the arterial oxygen and carbon dioxide tensions.

Bronchoscopy

In this test a long instrument called a bronchoscope is passed through the mouth and pharynx to the bronchi. The area is sprayed with an anesthetic agent. The physician views the area through the bronchoscope. He may obtain tissue for biopsy or remove a foreign agent through it. The procedure is uncomfortable for the patient. It helps if he can practice breathing through his nose and practice relaxing his shoulders and hands while lying on his back. Clenching the fists during the test causes neck muscles to contract and increases the discomfort. Careful mouth care is essential. Dentures must be removed. The physician is gowned, masked, and gloved for bronchoscopy. Following the procedure the patient should be kept quiet. Foods and fluids are withheld until the gag reflex returns. The patient should be observed for bleeding and for laryngeal edema both of which might obstruct the open airway and necessitate emergency tracheotomy.

Bronchogram

A bronchogram is a roentgenographic picture of the bronchial tree. A radiopaque substance is introduced by atomizer or through a catheter passed through a metal laryngeal cannula into the trachea. The patient is tilted into various positions to distribute the radiopaque substance, and roentgenograms are made. Postural drainage may be ordered following a bronchogram to help remove the radiopaque substance. (See p. 317.) The patient is not permitted anything by mouth for eight hours before treatment. He is not given food or fluid until the gag reflex returns.

30

CARE OF ANY PATIENT WITH RESPIRATORY INVOLVEMENT

Changes Seen with Respiratory Interference

1. Change in breathing. Dyspnea, apnea, Cheyne-Stokes respirations. Unusual sounds such as bubbling or rattling.
2. Cough. It can be productive or nonproductive. It interferes with rest.
3. Chest pain.
4. Changes in sputum: appearance, odor, quantity, thickness.
5. Increased body temperature if infection is present.
6. Hypoxia: dizziness, tachycardia, drop in blood pressure, increase in pulse, cyanosis, headache, dyspnea, restlessness, epistaxis.

Major Points in Care of Any Patient with Respiratory Involvement

1. Follow aseptic precautions. Wash hands carefully before and after caring for patient. Provide patient with tissues and with a paper bag for their proper disposal. Turn your head away from him when he sneezes or coughs.
2. Encourage patient to cough if his cough is productive. Splint his chest with hands or with a drawsheet to decrease pain. (See p. 275 for method used to produce adequate cough.)
3. Encourage deep breathing rather than shallow breathing. Encourage frequent turning and movement. This facilitates lung expansion.
4. Encourage the patient to rest. Administer cough medicines before sleep to depress the cough center. Administer expectorants and preparations that increase secretions during the day.
5. Provide frequent oral hygiene to decrease the sour taste and crusting caused by increased mucous secretions.
6. Understand the prescribed inhalation therapy and know how to use the equipment. Oxygen is usually administered by nasal catheter or cannula; it is less frequently administered by tent. Assist the patient with

intermittent positive-pressure breathing and aerosol sprays that help to liquefy secretions and make them easier to expectorate. In intermittent positive-pressure breathing a positive pressure is created by use of compressed air or oxygen. This aids pulmonary ventilation by increasing tidal volume, distribution of inhaled gas, and elimination of carbon dioxide. Some equipment can be regulated according to the patient's own respiratory rate; other equipment has a preset rate and allows the patient no control. The pressure range is ordered by the physician. It is usually 12 to 20 cm water. The treatment lasts 20 minutes and is administered three to four times each day. After initial instruction by the inhalation therapist, the patient may administer the treatment himself with nurses' guidance. *Supervise careful adherence to precautions for the use of oxygen.*

TABLE 30–1. PRECAUTIONARY MEASURES IN USE OF OXYGEN

ADMISSION AND CARE OF PATIENTS FOR OXYGEN THERAPY:

1. Undress patient completely; use hospital gown.
2. Remove matches, cigarettes, hearing aids, radios, battery or electrically-run devices from room.
3. Remove call cord from unit.
4. Check history of patient to ensure patient has no ointments, salves, or other oily substances applied to his skin surfaces.
5. Post "No Smoking" signs conspicuously. Warn visitors.
6. Do not use alcohol, ether, or other flammable liquids, or wool or nylon within tent hood. (Special rubbing lotions are available.)
7. Do not use combs or brushes on patients in oxygen tents. No lighted candles permitted in the area.
8. Do not handle oxygen cylinders or apparatus with oily hands, greasy gloves or rags.
9. Report worn or frayed cords or malfunctioning equipment immediately.

7. Encourage fluid intake to decrease dehydration.

8. Suction adequately whenever necessary. Insert catheter with the tubing pinched to protect mucous membranes; release tubing to provide suction and remove mucus. Hold catheter in the direction of natural drop. Do not suction more than ten seconds. Slowly withdraw catheter by gently rotating it. Cleanse it by soaking in suitable disinfectant, as ordered. Do not let it become clogged!

9. Postural drainage exercises are frequently ordered to help rid the patient of excess secretions. (See Figs. 30–1 through 30–11.)

The patient is placed in a position in which his head and chest are lower than his trunk so that gravity drainage takes place. Time the treatment and gradually work up to a 20-minute period. Never use postural drainage for a longer period of time, and never after meals. Make sure

[*Text continued on page 320.*]

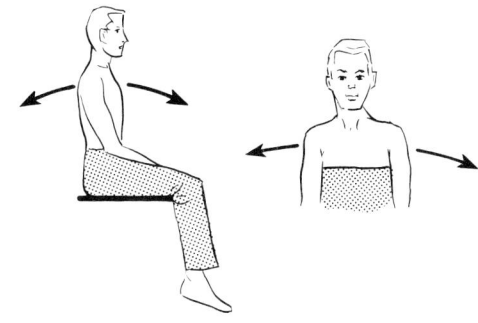

CARE OF RESPIRATORY PATIENTS [317

FIGURE 30-1.

Sit upright on edge of bed or chair, lean slightly back, forward, left and right. Hold each position half a minute.

FIGURE 30-2.

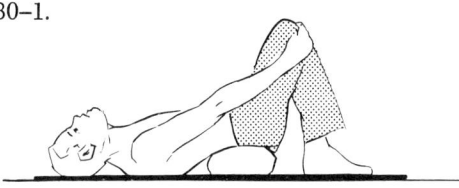

Lie on back, with small rolled blanket or cushion (6 inches thick) under hips. Bend knees, pull thighs toward chest. Keep feet on bed. Hold position for half a minute.

Note: Foot of bed may be elevated 18 inches for greater effectiveness.

FIGURE 30-3.

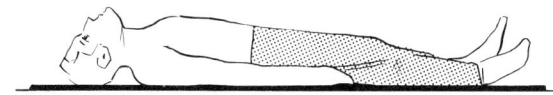

Lie flat on back without pillow, arms at side. Hold position half a minute.

FIGURE 30-4.

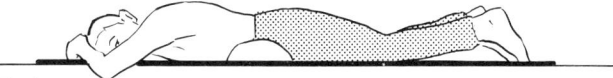

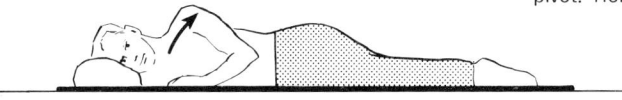

Lie face downward, head on arms, with small rolled blanket or cushion (6 inches thick) under lower abdomen. Hold position half a minute.

FIGURE 30-5.

Lie on right side with pillow supporting head, as shown. Hold half a minute. Then swing left shoulder forward, using right shoulder as a pivot. Hold half a minute.

FIGURE 30-6. Lie on left side with pillow supporting head, as shown. Hold half a minute. Then swing right shoulder forward, using left shoulder as a pivot. Hold half a minute.

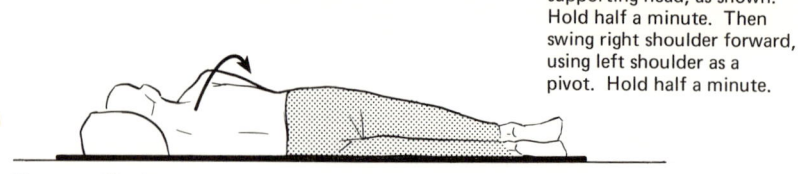

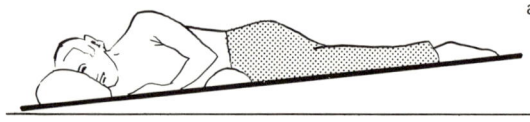

FIGURE 30-7. With foot of bed elevated 18 inches, lie on right side. Place small rolled blanket or cushion (6 inches thick) between hip bone and bottom rib. Hold position half a minute.

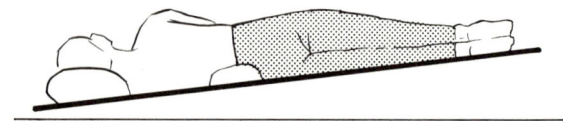

FIGURE 30-8. With foot of bed elevated 18 inches, lie on left side. Place small rolled blanket or cushion (6 inches thick) between hip bone and bottom rib. Hold position half a minute.

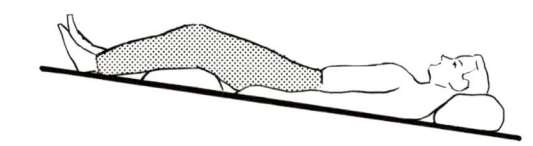

FIGURE 30-9. With foot of bed elevated 18 inches, lie on back, with pillow under knees. Hold position half a minute.

FIGURE 30-10. With foot of bed elevated 18 inches, lie on back, with body turned slightly onto left side, pillow under knees. Hold half a minute. Then turn body slightly onto right side. Hold half a minute.

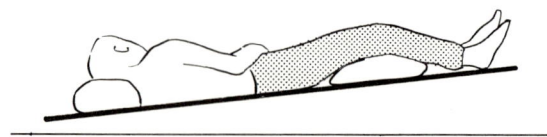

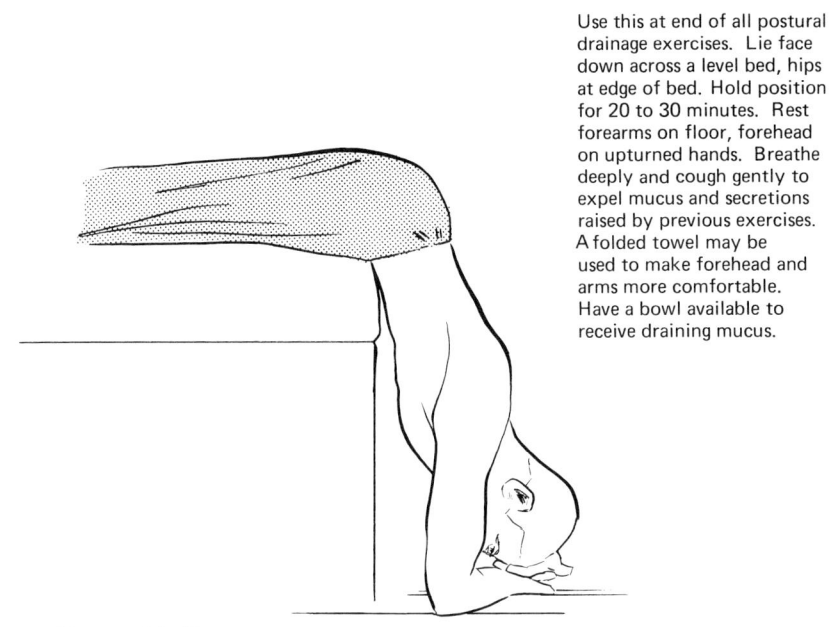

Use this at end of all postural drainage exercises. Lie face down across a level bed, hips at edge of bed. Hold position for 20 to 30 minutes. Rest forearms on floor, forehead on upturned hands. Breathe deeply and cough gently to expel mucus and secretions raised by previous exercises. A folded towel may be used to make forehead and arms more comfortable. Have a bowl available to receive draining mucus.

FIGURE 30-11.

FIGURES 30–1 through 30–11. Postural drainage exercises. Begin exercise session with aerosol medication if ordered. When mucus accumulates in the lungs, it thickens and forms "plugs" that block the alveoli and make breathing difficult. Postural drainage is a way of letting gravity help clear out these plugs and mucus and get them to the mouth where they can be expectorated. The doctor orders the exercises that are best for the patient. The benefit the patient gets from these exercises depends on the regularity and care with which they are carried out.

Preparation: Postural drainage exercises are usually performed four times a day—on arising, before lunch and dinner, and before bedtime. Before beginning the exercises, remove tight or restrictive clothing. If prescribed by the physician, inhale an aerosol medication according to his directions. This will relax and open the airways in the lungs and loosen tenacious mucus and plugs so they will drain more easily. In addition, a chest-tapping procedure can be used to help dislodge mucus. In exercises where it is recommended that the foot of the bed be elevated, it may be found most practical to use shock blocks or to adjust the foot lift of the bed, thus adjusting the bed to the desired height. Do the exercises in sequence. Keep a container available for the draining mucus. Cover the pillow with a towel to prevent soiling. Do not hurry—hold each position as long as required. In all cases, finish the exercises with the basic position, that is, Figure 30–11. (Adapted, by courtesy of Breon Laboratories, Inc., New York.)

the patient gets mouth care afterward. Many patients tend to forgo this treatment because the position is uncomfortable, the foul sputum that is raised leaves an unpleasant taste in the mouth, and nausea and vomiting frequently occur. Stay with the patient. Make sure he is adequately supported so that he feels secure.

10. Use depressant drugs such as morphine with extreme care: count respirations frequently. Do not administer if less than 12 per minute.

11. Tracheotomy. Maintenance of a patent airway is a concern whenever respiratory illnesses are discussed. When there is interference with the free passage of air through the larynx or pharynx, a tracheotomy may be necessary. A tracheotomy is the creation of an artificial airway through the neck by incision.

With the neck extended an incision is made in the midline over the upper part of the trachea. After the trachea is exposed, an incision is made through two or three of the cartilaginous rings, and the tracheotomy tubes are inserted. When a temporary tracheotomy is performed, the tube itself is the only thing that holds the air passage open. When a permanent tracheotomy is done, the trachea is sutured to an opening in the skin, and closure of the opening is not a problem. Each tracheotomy set contains an outer and an inner tube that fit, one into the other. Responsibility for removing and replacing the outer tube rests with the physician; responsibility for removing, cleaning, and replacing the inner tube rests with the nurse. The outer tube is held firmly in place by tapes around the neck. Tapes should not be knotted because knots cause irritation. The tapes can be pulled through slits made at the ends of each tie. Bronchial secretions are profuse initially and should be gently wiped away with cellulose tissues or with gauze squares. Facial tissues should not be used because they contain lint that might be aspirated. Care must be taken to prevent gauze threads from catching on the protruding parts of the tubes. The tube is suctioned of mucus whenever necessary. The catheter is inserted 5 to 6 in. into the tube with the Y connecting tube open. This protects the delicate mucous membranes from too much suction. The open end of the Y tube is covered with the thumb to produce suction. The catheter is gradually removed by rotating it. Suction should not last more than ten seconds. The air in the room should be humidified so that the air reaching the lungs is warm and moist. Sometimes the physician will request use of a moistened gauze square draped over the tracheotomy tube. A tray should be set up with all needed equipment. It should include sterile water or saline to clear the catheter and keep it patent. Three to five drops of sterile water can also be instilled through the tracheotomy tube to loosen dried secretions. A second tracheotomy set must also be available. Each set contains an inner and an outer tube of the same size (0–10), an obturator, and any other emergency equipment that might be needed. (See Figs. 30–12, 30–13, and 30–14.)

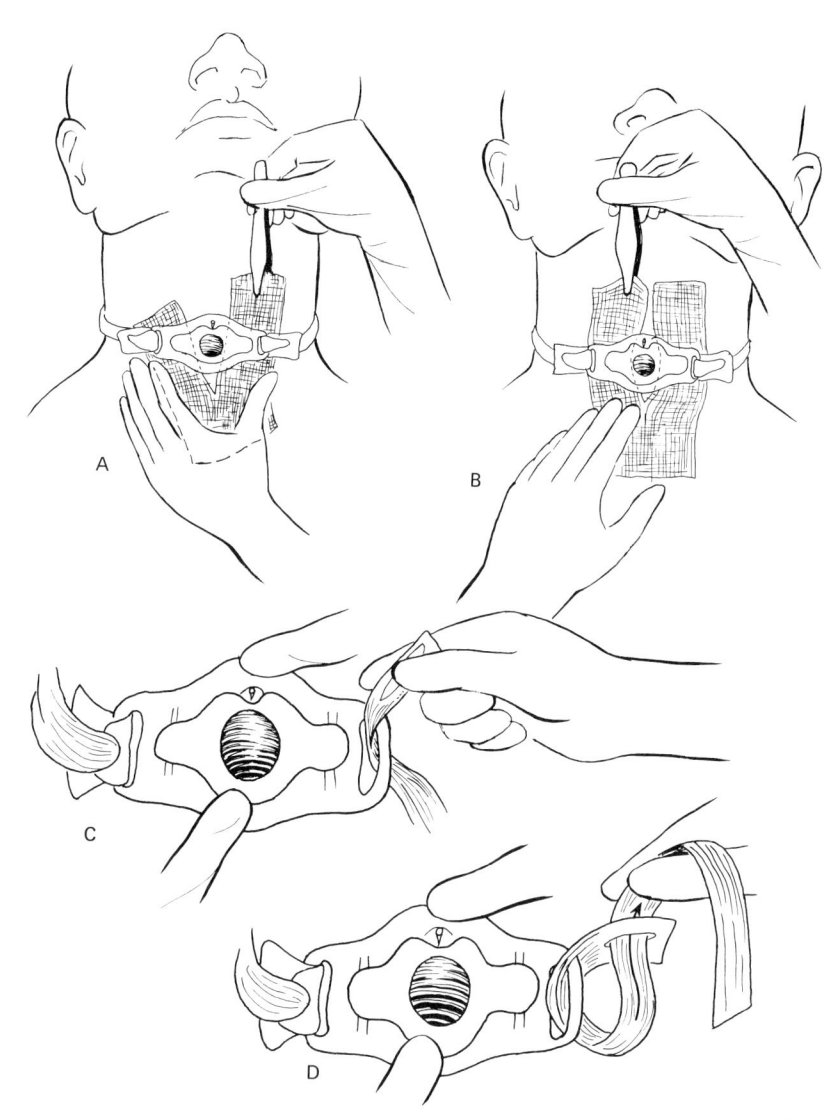

FIGURE 30-12. Tracheostomy dressings and tie tapes. *A.* A prepared bib dressing is placed beneath the tie tapes and under the flange of the tube. *B.* Forceps are useful in positioning the dressing. *C.* An assistant holds the outer cannula to prevent its dislodgment when tie tapes are changed. Prepared tape is slipped through the opening in the flange of the outer cannula. *D.* The method of securing tape through the opening in the flange. Following this, the tapes are securely tied together with a knot at one side of the neck. (Courtesy, Norma Greenler Dison, *An Atlas of Nursing Techniques,* 1st ed. C. V. Mosby Co., St. Louis, 1967.)

322] SUPPLY AND REMOVAL OF GASES

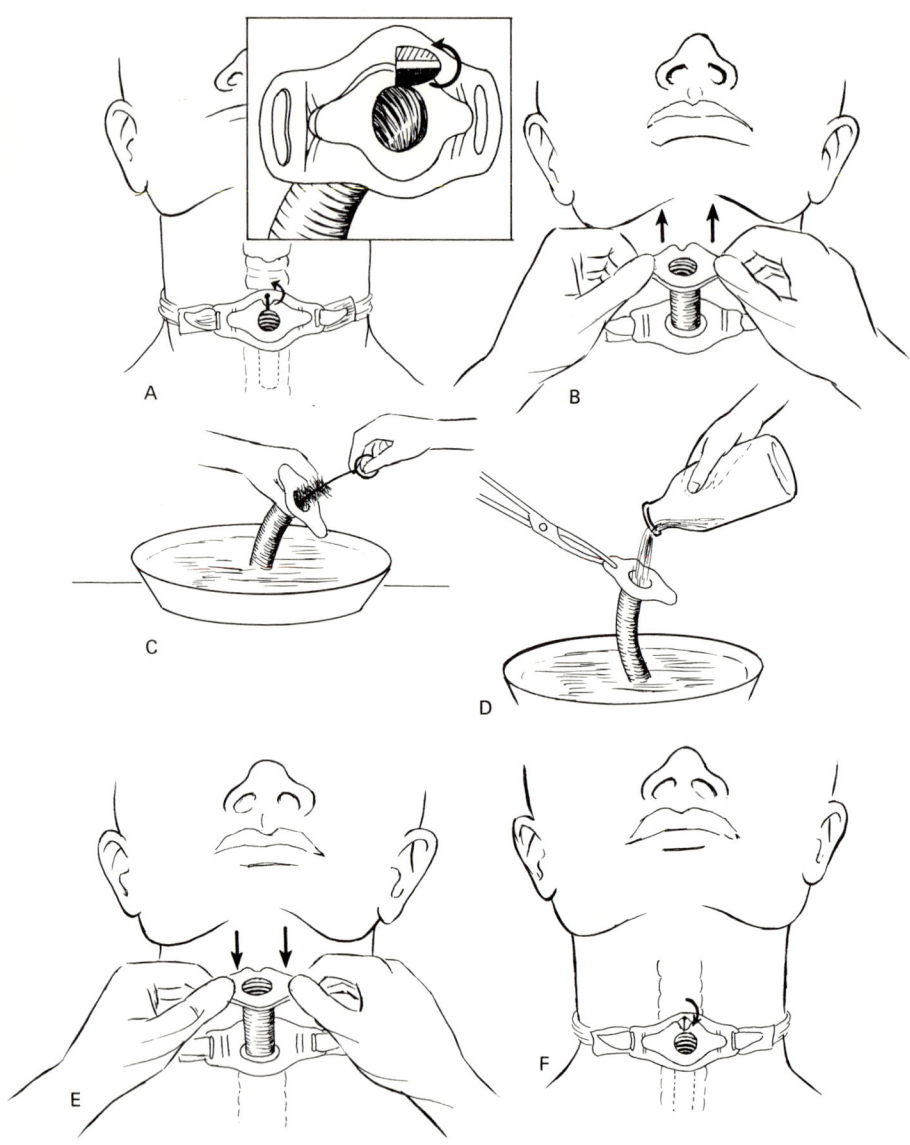

FIGURE 30–13. Care of the inner cannula. *A.* The turn key is unlocked in preparation for removal of the inner cannula. The inset shows turning the key to unlocked position. *B.* The inner cannula is removed. *C.* Cannula is cleansed with brush and cleansing agent. *D.* Cannula is grasped with sterile forceps and rinsed thoroughly with sterile water. *E.* Cannula is replaced. *F.* Turn key is moved to locking position. (Courtesy, Norma Greenler Dison, *An Atlas of Nursing Techniques,* 1st ed. C. V. Mosby Co., St. Louis, 1967.)

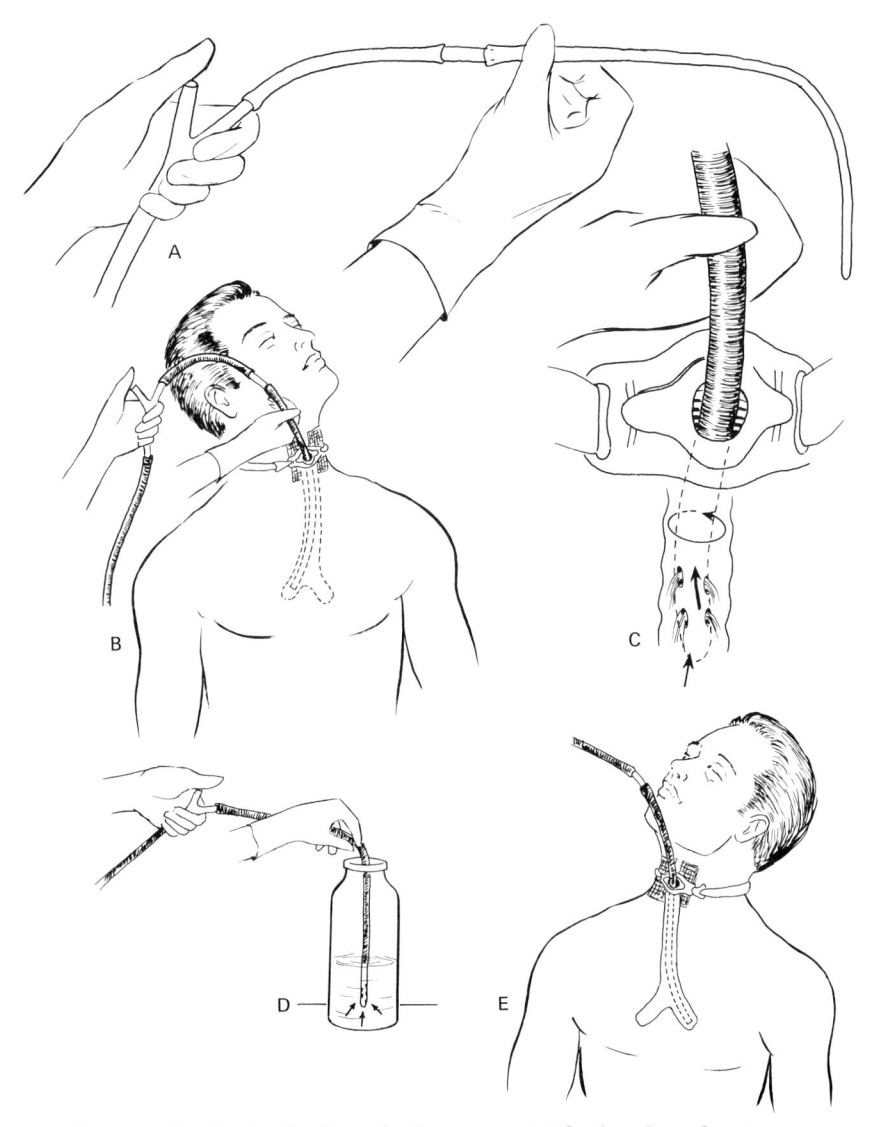

FIGURE 30–14. Tracheobronchial suction. *A.* The hand used to introduce the sterile catheter wears a sterile glove. *B.* If the catheter is to be directed into the main right bronchus, the patient's chest is turned slightly to the right, and his head is turned to the far left. *C.* As the catheter is withdrawn, it is continuously rotated while suction is applied. *D.* Sterile water is aspirated through the catheter, with attention to the amount of secretions removed. *E.* The catheter is directed into the main left bronchus, and aspiration is repeated. (Courtesy, Norma Greenler Dison, *An Atlas of Nursing Techniques,* 1st ed. C. V. Mosby Co., St. Louis, 1967.)

The patient with a fresh tracheotomy is extremely apprehensive. His fear of coughing out the tube and being asphyxiated is compounded by the fact that he cannot talk. He should have almost continuous attendance by the nurse initially and should have access to a pad and pencil. He should be observed for signs of dyspnea or interference with respiration. All efforts are directed toward keeping the tracheotomy tube open. The chief problem is the removal of frequently accumulating mucus, which collects in the tube and must be removed.

Sometimes a laryngectomy must be done. Cancer is a frequent reason. The patient with a laryngectomy has his total larynx removed. He no longer has vocal folds, and he cannot speak in the usual manner. He must learn to swallow air and "belch" it back in a controlled manner so that speech is produced. This is called esophageal speech. It takes time, practice, and patience to learn to control the air so that the sound produced is clear and understandable. The patient with a laryngectomy breathes through the artificial opening in his trachea. Emergency oxygen is administered or mouth-to-mouth breathing is done over this new opening, not over the nose and mouth. The person with a laryngectomy cannot go swimming and must be especially careful when he takes a bath. He is discouraged from smoking. Many states have groups of laryngectomy patients who meet to discuss their mutual problems. Many also teach esophageal speech. Information pertaining to these groups may be obtained from the American Cancer Society, Inc., 521 W. 57th Street, New York, New York 10019.

Other General Measures That Apply to All Patients with Respiratory Involvement

1. Temperature and Humidity. Temperature and humidity influence the comfort of the patient. It is very important to avoid sudden temperature changes and extremes of both heat and cold. The patient should be cautioned to avoid very cold air. Slightly warmed air is usually more comfortable. Dress should provide the maximum in protection out of doors. In the hospital cooling and humidity are provided by oxygen tents, air conditioners, and inhalation of vapor either hot or cold.

2. Position. Positioning, especially at night, with extra pillows and firm support makes breathing easier. Fowler's or semi-Fowler's position increases lung expansion. Let the patient tell you the position in which breathing is easiest.

3. Diet. Diet should be adequate in quality and quantity. Extremes of underweight and overweight are to be avoided. In order to facilitate rest, large evening meals should be avoided. Gas-forming foods may cause distention and interference with movement of the diaphragm during respiration. Examples of gas-forming foods include Lima and navy beans, cabbage, cauliflower, cucumber, onion, radishes, turnips, and melons.

4. *Alcoholic Beverages.* These beverages may affect some patients adversely. Patients with allergies to cereal grains should be very careful.

5. *Fatigue.* Fatigue from overwork or inadequate sleep should be avoided. Emotional stress can also be exhausting. Such things as unpleasant arguments should be avoided or resolved. Exciting "thriller" movies and television programs are best left for others to watch.

6. *Constipation.* Constipation should be avoided. When the patient is constipated, there can be additional respiratory distress. The diaphragm is hindered in its movement when a full bowel presses up against it.

7. *Allergies.* The patient should try to avoid contact with allergens that he is sensitive to. These may include certain foods, animal fur, dust, pollen, and so on. It is important to note a patient's allergies when he is admitted to the hospital.

8. *Colds.* Whenever possible it is advisable for patients with respiratory interference to avoid contact with people who have colds or "flu." Asthma and bronchitis attacks are often precipitated by upper respiratory infections.

9. *Smoking.* The rule is *no smoking*. The importance of this cannot be overemphasized. The lining of the airways is irritated by the fine particles of ash that settle on it. Removal of these particles involves an increase in bronchial secretions. If excessive, these secretions must be coughed out of the lungs. If the cough is inadequate, the secretions plug the small airways and lead to infection and further destruction of tissue.

10. *Environment.* A proposed change in geographic location may be made after careful evaluation. For example, the desert area is not always the perfect home for the patient with chronic bronchitis.

31

INTERFERENCE IN MAINTENANCE OF A PATENT AIRWAY

Allergy

Allergy is a common cause of chronic and acute illness. Allergic responses result when a person comes in contact with some substance to which his tissues are especially sensitive. This contact can lead to discomfort, disability, and fatal reactions. No drug can cure allergy, but they can counteract the allergic symptoms, which include stuffy nose (rhinitis), tearing, and difficult respirations.[10]

Allergy is an antigen-antibody reaction in which the antigen (a substance foreign to the body) stimulates the production of specific antibodies that counteract and neutralize it. In immunity, antibodies that the body has developed react with the antigen to neutralize its toxicity or infectiousness and in this way protect the body from additional harm. A powerful inflammatory response may be involved.

Asthma

Asthma is an example of a disease that is believed to be allergic in origin. The patient is usually sensitive to many offending allergens. The disease is also associated with infection (the patient may be "allergic" to the infecting microorganism) and with emotional stress. Stress causes impulses from the parasympathetic nervous system to constrict bronchioles. There is spasm of the smooth muscle of the bronchioles, and air is trapped in the alveoli. The patient "wheezes" during expiration. He may be in severe ventilatory distress. When the bronchi dilate, the attack subsides and thick mucus is expectorated. Adrenergic drugs such as ephedrine and epinephrine and theophylline and its salts, such as aminophylline, are used as potent bronchodilators. Drugs may be given orally, by injection, or by nebulizer. Aerosol sprays are frequently administered with intermittent positive-pressure breathing treatment. Expectorants such as potassium iodide drops are given in milk or water to thin and loosen bronchial secretions. Bronchodilators such as ethylnorepinephrine hydrochloride (Bronkephrine) relaxe the bronchioles. Tranquilizing drugs may be used to control the anxiety and fear of an attack that are often worse than the actual ventilatory deficit. (See Tables 6–1, p. 48, and 6–2, p. 50.)

Anti-inflammatory steroids may be used in severe cases. A large initial dose may be given. Then the dose is reduced to the point where symptoms are controlled. Examples of anti-inflammatory steroids are cortisone, hydrocortisone, and prednisone. These drugs are potentially toxic and must be used with care. (See p. 350.)

The antihistamine drugs are used to relieve the symptoms of various allergic disorders. These drugs are relatively ineffective for the relief of acute asthma, although they may be used when asthma is associated with hayfever or pollen sensitivity. One explanation for their ineffectiveness is that the histamine released in the lungs during an asthmatic antigen-antibody reaction attaches itself immediately to the smooth-muscle receptors of the bronchioles and thus cannot be blocked successfully by the antihistamine drugs. Examples of antihistamines are chlorpheniramine maleate (Chlor-Trimeton) dimenhydrinate (Dramamine), and diphenhydramine hydrochloride (Benadryl hydrochloride). Most antihistamines are depressants and accidents may occur if the patient drives or handles machinery when taking them.

Decongestant nose drops or aerosol sprays and jellies may be used when rhinitis is present. They should be used only in the prescribed amounts at specified times because they are vasoconstrictors and overdose can cause cardiac stimulation and elevation of blood pressure. Examples of decongestants are cyclopentamine hydrochloride (Clopane) and propyhexedrine (Benzedrex).

Psychotherapy may be advised in conjunction with a medical regimen.

Influenza

Influenza holds special interest for the average man as this is one disease with which he is almost certain to have had personal experience during his life. Usually, the individual has had a mild form of this virus-caused disease that affords him the opportunity to take a brief holiday from work but does not seriously incapacitate him. However, the disease is life-threatening to the elderly and to people who have other chronic illnesses.

The influenza virus can be isolated from a throat culture in its early stages in which fever, general muscular aching, and malaise are experienced. The most important factor to consider is that there are many strains of viruses that produce "influenza-like" symptoms. They are described according to their immunologic or serologic type or their capacity to produce immunity. Infection with one strain of virus does not produce immunity to every other strain. Outbreaks involving various strains of the influenza virus occur regularly. With the present-day ease of travel, the whole world is regarded as a single epidemiologic unit. An outbreak of flu or *la grippe,* as the French call it, travels from one country to another in a matter of months. One has only to remember the Hong Kong flu epidemic of 1968–1969 to realize this. An influenza epidemic occurs when a virus is present, when there is a low level of immunity in a large number of people, and when the climate is suitable. Influenza is a winter disease as a rule. It can be extremely virulent and can result in death. The causes of death are usually reported as influenza and pneumonia.

Control of influenza is possible through the use of vaccine; however, the vaccine is effective only against a particular strain or strains. When the strain mutates (changes), a new vaccine must be developed. Drug companies do not always have sufficient time to prepare enough of the new vaccine before the epidemic spreads. The vaccine induces temporary immunity. Its use is recommended whenever outbreaks of the disease occur. Rest and decreasing the contacts during the three-day incubation period are also thought to help. Medical treatment is directed toward relief of symptomatic complaints such as headache, chills, fever, anorexia, spasm of the abdominal muscles, and prevention of secondary infection.

Bronchiectasis

Bronchiectasis is a chronic condition in which the smooth muscle and elastic tissue of the bronchial tubes are damaged. There is tubular or saccular dilation of the bronchial system. This may be caused by bronchial obstruction, by infections such as bronchopneumonia that cause stagnant exudate to collect, or by degenerative processes.

Atelectasis (airlessness, alveolar collapse) often results.[11] Bronchiectasis can become irreversible. There are a cough and mucopurulent sputum. Large amounts of sputum are expectorated, especially in the morning. There are often hemoptysis and dyspnea. Medical treatment includes use of appropriate antibiotics, postural drainage, aerosol treatment to promote cough and expectoration, moist air to liquefy secretions, tracheostomy to maintain a patent airway, and finally resection of damaged segments of the lung.

Atelectasis

Atelectasis occurs when there is blockage of air to a portion of the lung causing that blocked portion to fail to expand. It collapses. Atelectasis may be caused by obstruction within the bronchi, reduced tone of of respiratory muscles, the presence of mucus or a foreign body in the lung, and so on. It may be mild or severe with death resulting from asphyxiation. Atelectasis can lead to emphysema and spontaneous pneumothorax. Nursing measures include administration of medications to control cough, encouragement of deep breathing, exercises as prescribed by the physician, and ambulation.

Pneumonia

Pneumonia is an infectious disease in which a microorganism, bacterium, virus, or fungus invades the lung tissue. Inflammation follows with decreased ventilatory efficiency. The disease is often caused by immobility in which fluid accumulates in the alveoli (hypostatic pneumonia) and a superb medium for bacterial growth is provided. The increased fluid decreases ventilatory efficiency. Hospital-acquired staphylococcal pneumonia is increasing in incidence.

The patient with pneumonia "feels sick." He is weak. He has a productive cough with rust-colored or bloody sputum and chest pain. He may have a fever as high as 106° F., with chills. Observation may show limitation of movement on the affected side. The patient may use accessory muscles of respiration to help in breathing. One or both lungs may be involved. The microorganism must be identified by culture and an appropriate antibiotic regimen established. Rest and adequate fluid intake are essential. Treatment also includes specific antibiotics, antipyretics for elevated temperature, and analgesics for chest pain. Debilitated patients are especially susceptible to pneumonia.

Bronchitis

Bronchitis is a disease in which there is inflammation of the bronchi. If chronic, the disease may cause permanent structural damage to the bronchioles. The patient has a dry cough initially. Later, there may be mucopurulent sputum. The disease is associated with infection, air pollution, smoking, and allergy. Chronic bronchitis may lead to emphysema (see below). Treatment is much the same as that for asthma. Drugs are used to relieve spasm. Breathing exercises are often encouraged to improve lung ventilation. (See p. 332.) Secondary infection is avoided. A warm, moist atmosphere should be provided.

Emphysema

An early Greek physician coined the term "emphysema": it literally means "blow up" and "full of air." This term is appropriate because when emphysema develops the lungs become blown up and full of gas—stale air.

The underlying problem in emphysema is destruction of the alveolar walls, where oxygen is normally absorbed into the blood and carbon dioxide removed from the blood. Studies have shown that small holes called fenestrations begin to form in the alveolar membrane of the lungs. These enlarge and break into one another, and eventually the membrane of the lungs becomes full of holes. There is loss of functioning surface as the available surface for gas exchange decreases. At this point the transport of oxygen and the removal of carbon dioxide are impaired.

The lung, now riddled with holes, fails to allow for normal filling and emptying of gas. The elasticity of the lung tissue is lost. It becomes flabby, and all the inhaled air does not come out. The residual volume gradually increases. To compensate for the loss of elasticity the lungs tend to overexpand in order to become larger and stretch further to regain some elasticity. This is why patients with emphysema sometimes are "barrel-chested." (See Fig. 31-1.)

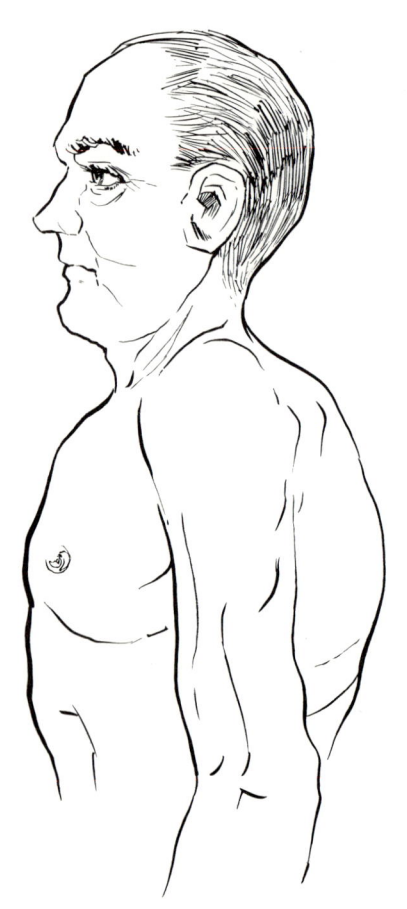

FIGURE 31-1. Diagram of the overexpanded "barrel chest" appearance of the emphysema patient.

Emphysema occurs primarily in older men. It most often develops after age 40, and the death rate increases with each decade thereafter.

Shortness of breath and early morning "smokers cough" are the first symptoms. The patient is in severe distress. He is anxious and pale; he speaks in short, jerky sentences. He exhales slowly and works hard at it. There are an ever-present cough, dyspnea, and orthopnea. In addition there is fatigue, especially in the limbs in the early morning. The patient is easily irritated and may become stuporous as carbon dioxide builds up.[12] This is called carbon dioxide narcosis.

During periods of exacerbation the symptoms are (1) moderate to severe dyspnea during exertion or at rest and (2) cough and abundant expectoration. Physical examination shows a patient with a forward-bending upper trunk and raised shoulders. Distended veins may be seen on both sides of the neck. Pulmonary function tests reveal great respiratory effort and an increased lung volume with a decreased rate of expiratory flow. There is an increased residual volume of air. Treatment is aimed at conserving and increasing pulmonary ventilation. The "stretch" cannot be put back into the inelastic lung; however, exercise can help meet the increased demand placed on the breathing apparatus and can improve the deficient expiratory force by strengthening the internal intercostals, the diaphragm, and the abdominal muscles. (See Table 31–1.)

Bronchodilator drugs are used to increase the patency of the airway. Examples are isoproterenol hydrochloride (Isuprel) by aerosol, or sublingual tablet and protochylol (Caytine) by mouth, injection, or inhalation. Isoproterenol inhalant should not be used if it is brown or contains a precipitate. Steam inhalation, cold-water vapor inhalation, and use of detergent substances such as Alevaire by nebulization help liquefy secretions. Intermittent positive-pressure breathing,[13] e.g., with the Bennett respirator, helps overcome bronchial resistance, helps the patient to cough effectively, and increases ventilatory efficiency. (See p. 316.) A pressure of 12 to 20 cm water applied during inspiration and cycled at a respiratory rate set by the patient helps dilate the bronchi so that trapped carbon dioxide can be expired. This is essential if the patient develops carbon dioxide narcosis from retention of this gas. Oxygen lack actually serves as the stimulus to respiration in this disrupted state. If oxygen is administered it must be given with care because respirations may cease as the oxygen level in the blood rises.

Treatment is long-term and often frustrating for the patient and for his family. It is tedious. Activities must be scheduled to prevent fatigue. Exertion leaves the patient exhausted. He should be taught to use an at-home nebulizer properly. He should be cautioned against contact with known allergens and with people who have upper respiratory infection.

Complications of emphysema include cor pulmonale in which the right

TABLE 31-1. SOME BREATHING EXERCISES FOR EMPHYSEMA

To elevate diaphragm:	Patient sits up at side of bed and inhales deeply while holding a small book against his abdomen. Then he exhales slowly, at the same time bending over and pressing the book as firmly as possible against his abdomen.
To strengthen the abdominal muscles and diaphragm:	Each leg is raised alternately, bringing it as near vertical as possible. Raise slowly and exhale as leg is lifted.
	Lying flat, patient raises head and shoulders from the bed, at the same time exhaling.
	Lying flat, with small book placed on abdomen. 1. Breathe in, puffing out abdomen to raise the book as far as possible. 2. Exhale slowly, pulling in abdomen as far as possible.
To help in contraction of chest:	Lying or sitting—place hands lightly on the lower ribs, fingers almost meeting. Inspire deeply. Then with slow expiration, hands are pressed further together, compressing the lower ribs.
To help maintain bronchial expansion during expiration:	Lips are pursed during expiration, increasing the air pressure in the bronchi to counteract the tendency of the bronchi to collapse on expiration.

heart, affected by the decreased capillary bed in the lung and the resultant increase in pressure in the pulmonary artery, overworks, hypertrophies, and may fail; respiratory acidosis develops because of the retention of carbon dioxide; and carbon dioxide narcosis or "poisoning" develops from retention of carbon dioxide.

The nurse must remember that this patient is in severe respiratory distress. She must wait until he is breathing with less difficulty to carry out related treatments. For instance, go to the patient's bedside with his injection but do not administer it during extreme distress. Make sure the patient can use the intermittent positive-pressure breathing treatment when he needs it. Allow him to assume whatever position is best for him to ease his breathing. Understand the fear invoked by "not being able to get enough air!"

Emphysema, chronic bronchitis, and asthma have the following in common: (1) they are chronic diseases that once established, continue for many years, and (2) the symptoms may come and go but the pathologic and anatomic changes that occur will remain. Viewed on a continuum it appears that first asthma may develop, then chronic bronchitis, followed by emphysema. Chronic bronchitis and pulmonary emphysema are commonly associated. Treatment is toward the bronchitis because it is partly reversible, whereas pathologic changes in destructive pulmonary emphysema are irreversible.[13]

Tuberculosis [15] (Consumption, Phthisis)

Tuberculosis is a serious lung disease caused by the aerobic, rod-shaped tubercle bacillus. The organism is found in the sputum or in other body secretions (urine, feces) of infected persons. It is most frequently transmitted by contact with the secretions from the lungs of an infected individual and through inhalation of droplet nuclei expelled by the infectious person. Bovine tuberculosis is spread to man through nonpasteurized milk. Pasteurization kills the microorganisms.

Tuberculosis can strike people of any age, sex, or race; however, death is more prevalent in white men than white women, especially those living in metropolitan areas where many more men are homeless and have poor dietary habits and where a greater number are employed outside the home. Negroes and Indians have three times greater incidence of the disease than white people. This is attributed to closer living quarters, greater numbers of people housed in one area, poor nutritional status, and general increased susceptibility. There was a decline in the number of new cases reported in 1961; however, the United States Public Health Service reported an increased incidence in 1967.

Pathology of Tuberculosis

Many people are infected with tuberculosis, but, because their resistance is high or the infective dose low, the disease causes few, if any, symptoms. An inflammatory response is invoked, the microorganisms are walled off, and calcified nodules called "primary tubercles" develop. Although the person continues to house the microorganisms in these tubercles, the infection is successfully overcome, and the patient is, for all intents and purposes, healed. He is no longer "communicable." His disease is arrested. He is "sensitized" to the tubercle bacilli, and this sensitization can be determined by skin test with tuberculin. A positive reaction indicates sensitivity—it does not mean an active case of tuberculosis. It simply means the person has developed sensitivity to the tubercle bacilli because he has had a primary case of the disease at some point in his life.

If, on the other hand, the disease is more virulent or if it is a second invading dose, the area of infection becomes larger. A cheeselike "caseated" area develops within the tubercle. It may slough and leave a cavity. At this point, the disease is active. It is infectious and communicable to others especially when contact with the infected individual is prolonged. It takes months and even years to arrest the disease. If the disease spreads to other areas of the body, it is called miliary tuberculosis.

Symptoms include fatigue, anorexia, weight loss, temperature elevation, and a cough. The cough is nonproductive at first but later becomes productive. There is often blood in the sputum. If untreated, the disease causes marked wasting.

How Is TB Diagnosed?

As previously stated, tuberculin testing identifies those people who have been sensitized to the tubercle bacillus. The method of choice, recommended for its accuracy in determining sensitivity, is the Mantoux test, in which a measured amount of tuberculin is injected intracutaneously, usually on the tautly held inner forearm. Weak dilutions of the tuberculin are used first. The test is "read" 48 to 72 hours later. A raised white wheal indicates a negative response, and a stronger concentration of tuberculin may be used. A red area with an indurated center indicates a positive response. People with positive responses then have chest x-rays and sputum examinations for definitive diagnosis. The Mantoux test, using an intermediate strength solution, is effective for mass screening purposes. *A positive Mantoux test does not mean a person has active TB.* Other tests used are the multiple-puncture or Heaf test, the Tine test, and the Vollmer patch test. The patch must be kept dry.

How Is TB Treated?

The development of drugs effective against tuberculosis has brought about many changes in the management of this condition. Patients are no longer confined to sanatoria for very long periods. More are being treated in the general hospital and at home. The surgical procedures used today are not as extensive as they were years ago because treatment with chemotherapeutic agents keeps pulmonary lesions more localized. Mainstays in the treatment are rest and the use of streptomycin, para-aminosalicylic acid (PAS), and isoniazid (INH). (See Table 31–2.)

The tubercle bacilli are grown on culture media to determine which drug they will be most sensitive to. Streptomycin is usually used early in treatment. With it, the patient must be observed for signs of vestibular damage (dizziness, ringing in the ears, deafness, and so on). INH and PAS are then given, usually in combination. Gastrointestinal symptoms may result from use of PAS. In this case, the dosage is decreased or some other drug is selected in its place. The prescribed medications must be taken religiously and for extended periods of time. This must be emphasized because a patient treated at home may stop taking the drug because he "feels well." Frequently microorganisms develop resistance to the drugs. Then newer drugs may be selected. Examples are pyrazinamide (pyrazinoic acid amide) and ethioniamide (Trecator). These drugs are potent

TABLE 31-2. COMMONLY USED DRUGS IN THE TREATMENT OF TUBERCULOSIS

Drug	Abbreviation	Forms Supplied	Usual Dosage	How Used	Toxic Signs
Isoniazid (Isonicotinic acid hydrazide), the least toxic of all chemotherapy	INH	Tablets Ampules	100 mg 3 × day with meals	Oral IM	Visual disturbances Dizziness Twitching Drowsiness Excitability Postural hypotention Convulsions
Streptomycin sulfate and (dihydro streptomycin °)	SM (DSM)	Vials	twice 0.5–1 gm daily or weekly	IM Aerosol	Rash Fever Deafness Staggering gait
Aminosalicylic acid (paraaminosalicylic acid)	PAS	Tablets Granules	4 gm. 3 × daily with meals	PO	Nausea Vomiting Diarrhea
Viocin (Viomycin) sulfate	VM	Vials	1 gm every 3rd day divided into equal doses and given at 12-hour intervals	IM (painful)	Rash Staggering gait Deafness Pallor

° This drug is rarely used because it often produces irreversible deafness.

tuberculostatic agents used for short-term therapy, e.g., before surgery. They, too, invoke microbial resistance. Activity is increased gradually, by physician's order. Nutrition should be adequate. It is suggested that a visiting nurse guide the patient and his family at home. Although rigid isolation precautions are unnecessary once the patient is taking adequate medication, members of the family should be aware of and protected against the major means of spread: the coughing or sneezing of an infected person and his sputum. If possible, the patient should have a bedroom of his own. Burning, boiling for five minutes, and direct exposure to sunlight for several hours kill the microorganisms.

Immunization for TB is possible, although not always successful. BCG (bacille Calmette Guérin) is the vaccine used. This is a solution containing attenuated, live tubercle bacilli. A multiple-puncture disc is used. The vaccine may be given to persons in "high-risk" groups such as elderly people confined to nursing homes and hospital workers who may be exposed to the disease. It is not given to persons who have positive tuberculin skin test reactions.

Complications of Tuberculosis

Hemorrhage and spontaneous pneumothorax are complications of tuberculosis. Hemorrhage may begin with streaking or staining of sputum. It may occur suddenly with no warning. Patients become restless and anxious. When hemorrhage (hemoptysis) occurs, the nurse must stay with the patient and provide a receptacle into which he may expectorate. The patient's position should be adjusted to help prevent aspiration. The nurse should note the patient's color, pulse, and blood pressure because shock may develop. The physician should be notified. Later, mouth care and sips of fluid should be given, as ordered by the physician.[16]

Spontaneous pneumothorax involves sudden uncontrolled escape of air from the diseased lung. The lung collapses. The patient experiences sharp chest pain, dyspnea, faintness, profuse perspiration, fall in blood pressure, and a weak, rapid pulse. He should be placed in a sitting position. Oxygen is administered, if ordered. A thoracentesis is performed in order to remove the air from the pleural space and permit re-expansion of the lung. If air continues to leak into the thoracic cavity, a tube may be placed in the cavity and connected to closed drainage.

Surgical Treatment of Tuberculosis

Surgical treatment of tuberculosis has decreased with the use of chemotherapeutic agents; however, thoracic surgery is important for selected patients and for other respiratory conditions.

32

THE PATIENT HAVING CHEST SURGERY

SURGERY may be instituted for any number of pulmonary conditions. Examples are removal of cysts and tumors, abscess, tuberculosis, and bronchiectasis. Some surgical procedures include:

THORACOTOMY. Surgical incision of the chest wall.
THORACOPLASTY. Removal of portions of the ribs, e.g., to collapse areas of lung.
LOBECTOMY. Removal of a lobe of the lung.
PNEUMONECTOMY. Removal of a whole lung.
DECORTICATION. Removal of pleura or surface lung tissue.

Endotracheal anesthesia makes it possible to work on one lung while keeping the other lung expanded. The physician discusses the surgery with the patient and then institutes preoperative "practice sessions" in which the patient learns to deep-breathe and cough properly (see p. 275) and to do any of the exercises that might be needed later to provide for full shoulder range of motion and lung expansion. He is familiarized with the tubes and bottles that will be in use after surgery and told that oxygen is routinely used for patients having chest surgery.

The patient returns from the operating room with a variety of tubes and bottles. He is fed intravenously and given oxygen usually by nasal catheter. He will have pain caused by severance of the intercostal nerves, and this is controlled with morphine or meperidine hydrochloride (Demerol). He is encouraged to turn from his back to the affected side and to cough and deep-breathe every one or two hours. Medication should be given so that this is not unduly painful, and the wound should be splinted so the patient does not feel like it will "rip apart." If coughing is too shallow, a Bird respirator may be used to assist him. A moderate amount of serosanguineous drainage is expected for the first day. There should not be bright-red, copious bleeding. The patient will have a chest catheter(s) in place for 48 to 72 hours. The catheters are usually placed above and below the resected area in the pleural cavity. The upper anterior catheter allows air to escape; the lower posterior catheter allows fluid to drain. As the patient expires or coughs, the fluid is forced through the catheter into the bottle. The catheters are connected to underwater drainage bottles. They make up a "closed system" so that outside air or fluid cannot get into the lung and collapse it. The tubing must remain under sterile water. About 500 ml of sterile water is placed in the drainage collection bottle, and this is marked on the bottle. Each catheter, properly labeled, is submerged in a separate bottle. There may also be an additional control bottle(s) to regulate the amount of suction transmitted through the drainage bottle to the pleural cavity. The amount of suction is determined by the depth of the submerged tube in water and is ordered by the physician. Submerging the tube 3 to 4 in. draws fluid from the chest.

Points to Remember with Chest Underwater (Closed-Seal) Drainage

1. Keep two Kelly clamps attached to the sheet near the head of the bed for emergency. Clamp tubing close to chest.

2. Never raise the bottle above the level of the bed. Keep them firmly placed in the stand on the floor and be careful not to break them.

3. If the chest catheter is open, as it should be, water will rise and fall in the glass tubing during inspiration and expiration. It will "bubble." If it is blocked, or if the lung has satisfactorily re-expanded, this movement will not occur. The physician should be notified.

4. Put tape around stoppers in bottles to prevent leakage. Milk tubing away from the patient to decrease clotting.

5. If emptying the drainage bottles is a nursing responsibility get adequate instruction! Clamp the tubing with the two Kelly clamps close to the chest, cover the end of the tube with sterile gauze squares, empty and measure drainage (subtract amount of sterile water originally placed in bottle), fill with required amount of sterile water, place stopper in bottle, and reattach.

If a pneumonectomy is performed, drainage tubes are not used. Air and fluid help stabilize the chest pressure imbalance.

Arm and shoulder exercises on the operative side may be ordered to ensure full range of motion of the shoulder and maximum expansion of the lung. Encourage the patient to use the arm on the operative side.

Nursing Observation of the Patient with Pulmonary Surgery

1. Check vital signs frequently. Observe respirations carefully.
2. Check dressings for bleeding.
3. Note any subcutaneous emphysema (leaking from a nonairtight wound).

4. Suction as necessary.

5. Make sure underwater drainage is functioning properly.

6. Be alert for signs of spontaneous pneumothorax: dyspnea, cyanosis, sudden sharp chest pain.

7. Be alert for mediastinal shift: shifting of lung and heart toward affected side.

8. Turn patient from operative side to back every hour unless otherwise ordered. This allows for greater expansion of the remaining lung (s).

9. Encourage deep-breathing and coughing.

10. Place patient in semi-Fowler's position as soon as he has reacted.

11. Begin passive exercise as soon as possible.

12. Record intake and output.

13. Increase activity gradually; observe patient carefully with each increased task.

14. Increase foods, as tolerated.

REFERENCES

1. Kimber, D., Gray, C., Stackpole, E., and Levell, L.: *Textbook of Anatomy and Physiology*, 14th ed. The Macmillan Co., New York, 1961, p. 446.
2. Greisheimer, E. M., *Physiology and Anatomy*. J. B. Lippincott Co., Philadelphia, 1963, p. 549.
3. Kimber, *op. cit.*, p. 447.
4. *Ibid.*, p. 451.
5. *Ibid.*, p 453.
6. Sackheim, G. P., *Practical Physics for Nurses*. W. B. Saunders Co., Philadelphia, 1962, p. 47.
7. Shafer, K., Sawyer, J., McCluskey, A., and Beck, E.: *Medical Surgical Nursing*. The C. V. Mosby Co., St. Louis, 1967, p. 536.
8. *Ibid.*, p. 536.
9. Greisheimer, *op. cit.*, p. 556.
10. Rodman, M., and Smith, D., *Pharmacology and Drug Therapy in Nursing*. J. B. Lippincott Co., Philadelphia, 1968, p. 555.
11. Smith, D., and Gipps, C., *Care of the Adult Patient*. J. B. Lippincott Co., Philadelphia, 1966, p. 469.
12. Secor, J., "The Patient with Emphysema," *Amer. J. Nurs.*, **65**:75, July 1965.
13. Shafer, *op. cit.*, p. 561.
14. Beeson, P., and McDermott, W., *Cecil Loeb Textbook of Medicine*. W. B. Saunders Co., Philadelphia, 1967, p. 532.
15. *Tuberculosis Handbook for Public Health Nurses*. National Tuberculosis Association, New York, 1965.
16. Smith, *op. cit.*, p. 488.

ADDITIONAL READINGS

AHLSTROM, P., "Raising Sputum Specimens," *Amer. J. Nurs.*, **65**:109, Mar. 1965.

BICKFORD, E., and BUDD, E., "Pulmonary Resection, Nursing Care," *Amer. J. Nurs.*, **52**:40, Jan. 1952.

DUTCHER, I., and FIELO, S., *Water and Electrolytes: Implications for Nursing Practice*. The Macmillan Co., New York, 1967.

EASTWOOD, D., and MAHREY, J., "Suction and the Maintenance of an Airway," *Amer. J. Nurs.*, **53**:552, May 1953.

HADLEY, F., and BORDICKS, K., "Respiratory Difficulty: Causes and Care," *Amer. J. Nurs.*, **62**:64, Oct. 1962.

HANAMEY, R., "Teaching Patients Breathing and Coughing Techniques," *Nurs. Outlook*, **13**:58, Aug. 1965.

HARGREAVES, A., "Emotional Problems of Patients with Respiratory Diseases," *Nurs. Clin. N. Amer.*, **3**:479, Sept. 1968.

HELMING, M., "Nursing Care of Patients with Chronic Obstructive Lung Disease," *Nurs. Clin. N. Amer.*, **3**:412, Sept. 1968.

KOONZ, F., "Nursing in Tuberculosis," *Nurs. Clin. N. Amer.*, **3**:403, Sept. 1968.

KURIHARA, M., "Postural Drainage, Clapping, and Vibrating," *Amer. J. Nurs.*, **65**:76, Nov. 1965.

LEVINE, E., "Inhalation Therapy—Aerosols and Intermittent Positive Pressure Breathing," *Med. Clin. N. Amer.*, **51**:307, Mar. 1967.

MURPHY, M., "An Emphysema Clinic," *Amer. J. Nurs.*, **65**:80, July 1965.

MUSSER, R. D., and O'NEILL, J. J., *Pharmacology and Therapeutics*, 4th ed. The Macmillan Co., New York, 1969.

NETT, L., and PETTY, T., "Acute Respiratory Failure, Principles of Care," *Amer. J. Nurs.*, **67**:1847, Sept. 1967.

PETTY, T., et al., *For Those Who Live and Breathe with Emphysema and Chronic Bronchitis*. Charles C Thomas Co., Publisher, Springfield, Ill., 1967.

ROBINSON, F., "Nursing Care of the Patient with Pulmonary Emphysema," *Amer. J. Nurs.*, **63**:92, Sept. 1963.

RODMAN, T., "Management of Tracheobronchial Secretions," *Amer. J. Nurs.*, **66**:2474, Nov. 1966.

———, *Living with Asthma, Chronic Bronchitis and Emphysema*. Riker Laboratories Inc., Northridge, Calif., 1964.

SOVIE, M., and ISRAEL, J., "Use of the Cuffed Tracheostomy Tube," *Amer. J. Nurs.*, **67**:1854, Sept. 1967.

TOTMAN, L., and LEHMAN, R., "Tracheostomy Care," *Amer. J. Nurs.*, **64**:96, Mar. 1964.

UNIT VII

THE PATIENT WITH HORMONAL IMBALANCE

33

BIOCHEMICAL REGULATORS AND ADAPTORS

Many processes within the body take place continuously so that an environment suitable for cell life can be maintained. This dynamic effort is called homeokinesis. Homeokinesis implies an active, "on-the-move" process. Many different adaptive processes help the body to maintain homeokinesis. Some processes involve the body as a whole. Escape from injury is an example. Some take place in individual cells. The intracellular chemical activity of genes, enzymes, vitamins, and hormones is an example. Most physiologic activity is subject to more than one regulatory mechanism, and a disturbance in one mechanism often incurs a disturbance in others.

Hormones

Hormones are chemical regulators that help the body to adapt to internal and external change. Hormones are involved in many physiologic processes. They affect the metabolism of carbohydrate, fats, and protein; water and electrolyte balance; calcium-phosphorus balance between bone and body fluids; growth; sexuality; and so on. Hormones are synthesized by specialized cells of glands found in several body areas. These hormone-producing glands are called endocrine glands.

Endocrine glands secrete hormones directly into the bloodstream. The hormones are then carried to the cells of the body. Some hormones cause a general type of reaction by affecting cells throughout the body. Adrenal steroid hormone and thyroid hormone are examples. Others cause a more specific type of action and stimulate a specific "target" organ. Adrenocorticotrophic hormone of the anterior pituitary gland is an example. It stimulates the cortex of the adrenal glands. The body can react as a whole because hormones can reach all of its cells.

Hormones do not initiate function.[1]* They augment function. They are effective in relatively small amounts.

* References for Unit VII are on pages 392–94.

Classification of Hormones

Hormones are classified as steroids, proteins and polypeptides, and phenolamines. Examples of steroids are those produced by the adrenal cortex (androgens, estrogens, progestins, gluco- and mineralocorticoids). Examples of proteins and polypeptides (like proteins but smaller) are those produced by the pituitary (adrenocorticotrophic hormone, oxytocin) and pancreas (insulin). Examples of phenolamines include those produced by the thyroid gland (thyroxine) and the adrenal medulla epinephrine.) They will be discussed more completely under each specific gland.

Secretion of Hormones

Hormones are not secreted at a precisely uniform rate.[2] Some are secreted daily. The adrenal steroids belong to this group. Some are secreted cyclically. The female sex hormones belong to this group. And some are secreted in response to the level of a constituent in the blood. (See Feedback Mechanism.)

The Feedback Mechanism

Often, the amount of hormone secreted depends on the level of hormone circulating in the bloodstream. When the circulating level is low, the pituitary gland secretes a hormone that stimulates the specific gland to produce more of its own hormone. These pituitary hormones are called "trophic" or "tropic." Trophic means "to nourish." There are many trophic hormones that affect specific gland production. The specific gland is called a target gland. Adrenocorticotrophic hormone (ACTH) is an example. It stimulates the adrenal cortex to produce more of its hormone. If the lengthy word is broken down into its component parts, its action can be deciphered.

Adreno: adrenal
Cortico: cortex
Trophic: to nourish

Thyrotrophic hormone (TSH) is another example. It stimulates the thyroid gland to produce its hormone, thyroxine.

A low level of circulating hormone stimulates the pituitary to secrete its trophic hormone, and this causes increased secretion by the specific target gland involved; conversely, a high level of target gland hormone causes a decrease of the trophic hormone secretion and an ultimate decrease in circulating target gland hormone. This is called the feedback mechanism. Although the specific target glands are able to secrete their hormones in the absence of pituitary stimulation, they cannot maintain a normal rate of hormone secretion. Normally there is a continual secretion of small but varying amounts of trophic hormone which cause a small secretion of tar-

344] HORMONAL IMBALANCE

get gland hormone circulating in the blood. This "feeds back" to regulate the pituitary.[3] The pituitary gland is influenced by the hypothalamus of the central nervous system.

Stimulation of the hypothalamus causes production of a "neurohormone," which, in turn, stimulates the pituitary to produce its trophic hormones. (See Fig. 33–1.)

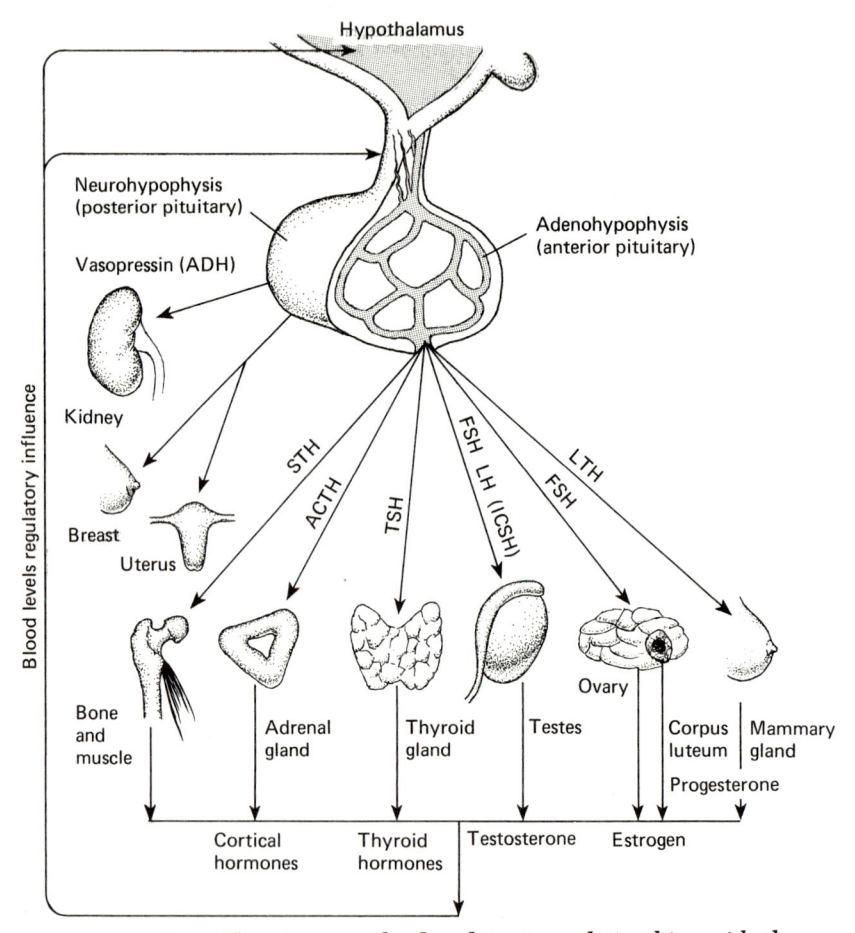

FIGURE 33–1. The pituitary gland and its interrelationships with the brain and peripheral target tissues. (From M. J. Rodman and D. W. Smith, *Pharmacology and Drug Therapy in Nursing*, 1968. Reprinted with permission of J. B. Lippincott Co., Philadelphia.)

The feedback mechanism looks like this:

Hypothalamic stimulation $\xrightarrow{\text{neurohormone}}$ pituitary stimulation $\xrightarrow{\text{trophic hormones}}$ target gland stimulation

In times of physical and emotional stress the hypothalamus-pituitary mechanism is released from inhibition by circulating steroids. The pituitary continues to pump out ACTH, and this, in turn, continues to stimulate the adrenal glands to secrete its hormones, which are essential in meeting the stress situation.[4]

The adrenal medulla is the only gland not under pituitary control. It is more like a part of the autonomic nervous system than the endocrine system. The adrenal cortex is, however, very definitely under pituitary influence.

This normal "feedback loop" is disrupted by disease or by the use of exogenous (from the outside) hormones.

Disruption of Hormone Balance [5]

Symptoms of disease come from an increase or a decrease in hormones and the effect that this change has on the body function that the hormone influences. The glands will enlarge in size (hypertrophy) if the demands made upon it are continuously increased. This hypertrophy is sometimes accompanied by an increase in active secreting cells (hyperplasia) with a concomitant increase in hormone production. Or, the gland can decrease in amount of functioning tissue and hormone production (hypoplasia). Disruption in hormone balance can come from abnormal embryonic development, deprivation of blood supply to the gland, infection, tumor, overgrowth of tissue, or undergrowth of tissue. Stress situations, e.g., fasting, extremes in temperature, undue fatigue, pregnancy, and sudden bouts of unaccustomed exercise, heighten the imbalance.

Some General Suggestions for the Nurse in Caring for a Person with a Hormonal Imbalance

1. *Know the approximate length of time it will take for the effects of hormone to become apparent.* A latent period exists between the administration of a hormone and the time its effect becomes apparent. This period is short for some hormones (regular insulin, 30 minutes) and long for others (thyroxine, 8 to 14 days).

2. *Know the signs of hypo- and hyperfunction of the gland.* Individuals tend to be hypersensitive to hormones they lack, and a small amount of exogenous hormone may cause an excessive reaction.

3. *Encourage the patient to continue medical supervision.* Very often, he must take replacement hormone for the rest of his life, and needs and dosages change.

4. *Encourage the patient to keep a two-month supply of the hormone on hand.* He should use the oldest first.

5. *Encourage the patient to carry an identifying card with him at all times.* (See p. 558.)

6. *Try to avoid stress.*

34

SPECIFIC ENDOCRINE GLANDS AND THEIR MALFUNCTION

The pituitary (hypophysis) is a pea-sized gland located in a cavity of the sphenoid bone below the center of the brain. It is "in back of" the nose. It is composed of an anterior lobe (the adenohypophysis), which is secretory in nature; a posterior lobe (the neurohypophysis), which apparently derives its hormone from the hypothalamus and stores and releases it; and an intermediate lobe, which is involved in skin pigmentation but which has little other importance in medicine at this time. The pituitary gland is often called "the master gland" or "the conductor or the symphony" because of its widespread effect on other endocrine glands. It often "calls the shots!"

Hormones of the Anterior Lobe of the Pituitary [6,7]

1. Adrenocorticotropic Hormone (ACTH). It stimulates the adrenal cortex to produce its adrenal steroids. These steroids are necessary for life.

2. Growth Hormone (GH). Also called somatotropic hormone (STH), growth hormone affects carbohydrate, protein, and fat metabolism and the growth of bone. It influences the rate of growth of the skeleton.

The effect of too much or too little growth hormone depends on the time in life that the under- or oversecretion begins. Insufficient growth hormone before maturity causes dwarfism. The person is perfectly formed for the age at which the decreased amount of hormone occurred, but there is no successive growth. Overabundance of growth hormone before maturity causes an overgrowth of the skeleton (gigantism) with distortion of the normal growth pattern.

When too much growth hormone secretion begins in the adult, most of the epiphyseal bone junctions are already closed. There is enlargement of the flat bones and terminal parts of bones in hands, feet, and head. The forehead and lower jaw enlarge and cause the face to look coarse. There is also enlargement of all the viscera, with the exception of the brain. This condition of overabundant growth hormone in the adult is called acromegaly.

ACRO: terminal   MEGALY: enlargement

These skeletal changes are permanent.

Because growth hormone is "diabetogenic"[8] the patient may develop symptoms of diabetes mellitus. Growth hormone is an insulin antagonist.

No satisfactory drugs have been found to impede an oversupply of growth hormone, but surgical excision or irradiation of the pituitary gland is beneficial.

Human growth hormone is being used to a limited extent to treat some forms of undersecretion. It is extracted, in minute quantities, from the pituitaries of cadavers.[9] It takes the hormone from 150 or more glands to treat one child for one year.

3. *Thyrotropic Hormone (TSH).* This hormone stimulates the thyroid gland to produce thyroid hormone. Thyroid hormone helps maintain normal metabolic rate.

4. *Follicle-Stimulating Hormone (FSH).* In females it stimulates the development of ovarian follicles; in males, together with luteinizing hormone, it causes growth and development of testes and spermatogenesis.

5. *Luteinizing Hormone (LH).* Also called interstitial cell-stimulating hormone (ICSH), it stimulates the production of testosterone from interstitial cells of the testes. With follicle-stimulating hormone it causes follicle ripening and estrogen and corpus luteum formation.

Together, FSH and LH are called gonadotropins. They stimulate the gonads (the ovaries and the testes).

6. *Luteotropic Hormone (LTH).* Also called prolactin, lactogenic hormone, and mammeotropic hormone, it causes development of mammary gland alveoli and stimulates the production of milk in lactating mammaries.

Hormones of the Intermediate Lobe

1. *Melanocyte-Stimulating Hormone (MSH).* This hormone disperses melanocytes of the skin to produce characteristic skin darkening.

Hormones of the Posterior Pituitary

1. *Oxytocin.* Oxytocin stimulates uterine contraction and enhances secretion of milk by the lactating mammary gland.

2. *Antidiuretic Hormone (ADH).* Also called vasopressin, it causes the

reabsorption of water by the renal tubules. Insufficient ADH causes a disease called diabetes insipidus in which the patient voids up to 20 L of dilute urine every day.[10] He is extremely thirsty and becomes hypohydrated. The disease may persist for years with no damage if free ingestion of water is allowed. It can be controlled by administration of extracts of posterior pituitary given subcutaneously, intramuscularly, or by nasal inhalation of dry powder.

If the anterior and posterior lobes of the pituitary fail to function, the patient is said to have panhypopituitarism. This is a disease in which all the organs regulated by the pituitary glands are affected. The complete absence of pituitary function is rare; partial insufficiency affecting one or more of the vital hormones is more frequent. The most common result of partial pituitary insufficiency is the failure of some individuals to reach sexual maturity.[11] The ovaries and uterus in the female and the testes in the male are infantile; there is inadequate development of secondary sexual characteristics, e.g., breast development, pubic and body hair; and the person is infertile. Little can be done to bring about fertility, but some degree of sexual maturity can be achieved with estrogens and androgens.

No medicinal preparation containing all the pituitary hormones has been found practical for use at this time. The patient is treated with the missing target gland hormone instead. Antidiuretic, adrenal cortex, and thyroid hormones are essential to survival and must be replaced for life. Examples of drugs being used are included with the discussion of each target gland.

Because there is no follicle-stimulating hormone available for use, human chorionic gonadotropin (HCG), such as Entromone and Follutein, and pregnant mare's serum gonadotropin (PMSG), such as Anteron and Gonadogen, are used as substitutes.

Hypophysectomy

The excision or obliteration of the pituitary gland is done to achieve remissions in some patients with cancer of the breast or prostate, to stop the rapid progress of nephropathy and retinopathy in some diabetic patients, and to stop the excessive secretion of hormones in some endocrine diseases. One method used to obliterate the pituitary gland is implantation of the radioactive earth metal yttrium 90.[12] It is implanted by means of an yttrium rod surgically passed through the nose and sphenoid sinus to the pituitary fossa. The patient must understand that obliteration of the pituitary will cause cessation of ovarian function in menstruating women (there are usually no menopausal symptoms) and impotence in men. Potency can be restored with doses of testosterone. Both men and women develop sterility as a result of hypophysectomy.

The Adrenal Glands

These are two glands that fit like caps over the tops of each kidney.[13] Each gland is made up of an outer cortex, the hormones of which are essential for life, and an inner medulla, the hormones of which are not essential for life. This inner part is really an extension ganglion of the autonomic nervous system.[14] Its hormones, epinephrine and norepinephrine, regulate functions that enable man to adapt to emergency (stress) situations. They contribute to the ability of the organism to cope with stress. The physiologic effects of norepinephrine and epinephrine are different. Norepinephrine increases peripheral resistance, and this causes an elevation of systolic and diastolic blood pressure. Epinephrine increases blood pressure by increasing the contractility of the heart and its output. Epinephrine has greater overall strength. It has greater influence on metabolism because of its ability to trigger the anterior pituitary gland.

Hypofunction of the Adrenal Medulla

Hypofunction of the adrenal medulla, per se, is not a specific disease syndrome. Even if both glands are removed, the medullary hormones do not have to be replaced. Hyperfunction of the adrenal medulla is, on the other hand, quite serious.

Pheochromocytoma

A pheochromocytoma is a secreting type of tumor that affects the adrenal medulla and results in its hyperfunction. It causes symptoms of excessive sympathetic nervous system stimulation. There are increased heart rate, hyperglycemia, polyuria, tremor, nervousness, headache, nausea and vomiting, and intermittent or, more usually, persistent high blood pressure. The symptoms disappear when the tumor is removed surgically; however, the patient must be observed closely because there may be unusual postoperative blood pressure fluctuations, and drugs must be administered to maintain the blood pressure within a safe range.

Histamine is administered subcutaneously to diagnose pheochromocytoma if the blood pressure is not higher than 170/110. In the normal person, histamine causes a drop in blood pressure. With pheochromocytoma there is a rise in blood pressure. If the blood pressure is over 170/110, the Regitine test is done. An intravenous dose of this drug neutralizes epinephrine and causes a drop in blood pressure. A fall of 35 mm Hg systolic and 25 mm Hg diastolic is considered positive of pheochromocytoma. The drop in blood pressure lasts about ten minutes.

Hormones of the Adrenal Cortices

The hormones of the adrenal cortex fall into the general classification of chemically similar "steroids." They are essential to life because of their widespread effect on protein, fat, and carbohydrate metabolism, on water and salt balance, and on the ability of the body to handle stress.

NAMING OF STEROIDS

Naming of steroids is important. The name indicates the function of the hormone and the placement of elements in its structure. For instance, a *glucocorticoid* affects the metabolism of carbohydrate (glucose); a *mineralocorticoid* affects the metabolism of minerals (salts); oxygen and/or hydrogen are involved in the chemical arrangement of hormones, and the particular name stems from the chemical placement of the oxygen or hydrogen. For instance, *oxy* is the prefix meaning oxygen; *desoxy* or *deoxy* indicates the loss of oxygen from its usual chemical position; *dehydro* indicates the loss of hydrogen from its usual position.

Adrenal cortex hormones are classified as glucocorticoids, mineralocorticoids, and adrenosterones. The first two groups are essential to life. This mixture of hormones influences the whole body. When any tissue is subjected to stress, it needs this mixture of corticosteroids for its restoration. This mixture also has a catabolic-antianabolic overall effect. It speeds up the breakdown of tissue protein to amino acids and prevents them from being readily reutilized in the synthesis of new muscle, skin, and bone.[15] This results in a negative nitrogen balance.

GLUCOCORTICOIDS (CORTISOL, CORTICOSTERONE, CORTISONE, HYDROCORTISONE)

As the name indicates, the glucocorticoids primarily affect the metabolism of glucose. Glucocorticoids antagonize the action of insulin and encourage the formation of new glucose from potein (gluconeogenesis), thereby maintaining and elevating the blood glucose level. Sometimes the blood glucose level is elevated when steroid drugs are administered. This is called "steroid diabetes" and is not the same as diabetes mellitus. It disappears when the steroid drug is withdrawn. Glucocorticoids suppress inflammation, inhibit scar tissue formation, and block some allergic responses. They also influence emotional functioning, and a deficient quantity causes depression. They enhance protein catabolism, inhibit protein synthesis, and regulate melanin (skin-coloring) metabolism.

MINERALOCORTICOIDS (ALDOSTERONE, DESOXYCORTICOSTERONE)

These mineralocorticoids, also called the "electrolyte hormones," regulate the reabsorption of sodium and the excretion of potassium by the kidneys. They cause sodium to be retained and potassium to be lost. This helps to maintain normal blood volume. Without mineralocorticoids, a decreased blood volume would cause circulatory shock. All the steroids have this electrolyte activity. A search is still going on for a steroid that has the antiinflammatory activity of the glucocorticoids without the strong water and electrolyte activity of the mineralocorticoids. Aldosterone is increased following the stress of surgery. This causes a period of postsurgical water retention. Care must be taken to prevent overhydrating the patient at this time.

ADRENOSTERONES (SEX HORMONES: MALE, ANDROGEN AND TESTOSTERONE; FEMALE, PROGESTERONE AND ESTRADIOL)

The rapid increase in androgen production by the adrenals at puberty is called the adrenarche. The adrenal sex steroids are of clinical importance only when secreted in excess in pathologic states, or when their production, even in ordinary amounts, stimulates growth of certain sex-tissue cancers.[16]

Adrenal Cortex Insufficiency

ADDISON'S DISEASE

An insufficient amount of adrenal cortex hormone can stem from a sudden fulminating disease, hemorrhage into the adrenal gland, tuberculosis, and so on. Most often, though, the condition results from the surgical removal of the adrenals or the pituitary gland to treat diabetic microangiopathy (retinopathy, nephropathy) and some types of cancer. If the pituitary gland is removed, the pituitary-adrenal feedback mechanism is no longer intact, and the adrenals eventually atrophy. This same interference with the feedback mechanism can result from long-term use of large doses of steroid drugs. Full adrenal activity does not always return when the steroid is stopped.

Symptoms of Addison's Disease. The symptoms of Addison's disease stem from interference with metabolic processes regulated by adrenal cortex hormones. Because of the interference with sodium and potassium balance there is a drop in blood volume. This causes a drop in blood pressure. The patient feels weak, is easily fatigued, and may faint. His temperature may be low. Because of interference with melanin metabolism, the skin changes to a brown or bronze color. This can occur in exposed or unexposed skin areas. It is seen most frequently in exposed body areas. There may be patchy darkened areas. There is a bluish-black or slate-gray discoloration of the mucous membranes. Growth of hair is suppressed. Because of interference with carbohydrate metabolism there is hypoglycemia, with headache, sweating, visual disturbances, trembling, loss of weight, anorexia, nausea, vomiting, diarrhea, and/or constipation. The patient is irritable, lethargic, and depressed.

Adrenal Crisis. This is a sudden, acute state of adrenal insufficiency. It usually results from increased stress. All the symptoms of adrenal hypofunction are intensified. Vascular shock can cause death unless the patient is treated promptly and vigorously! The level of adrenal hormones in the blood must be elevated, the vascular system must be supported, infection must be controlled, and the nurse must arduously maintain an environment that is quiet and devoid of stress stimuli (changes in room temperature, bright lights, drafts, noise). The patient in adrenal crisis cannot adapt, by himself, to even the most minor of stress. The nurse must do everything for him, with minimal handling. If the patient with Addison's disease is poorly regulated, emergency equipment should be kept at the bedside in case of adrenal crisis. This includes two 50-ml syringes, intravenous hydrocortisone, 5 per cent dextrose in normal saline solution, and so on.

The disease is diagnosed by studying the effect of fasting on the level of glucose in blood (with adrenal insufficiency there is hypoglycemia with fasting); by measuring the quantity of eosinophils in the blood after administration of ACTH (with adrenal insufficiency there is less of a drop in eosinophils than normal); and by measuring the levels of steroids in plasma or urine after the intravenous administration of ACTH over an eight-hour period on two consecutive days (with adrenal insufficiency there is little or no increase in adrenal hormones in response to intravenous ACTH).

Treatment of Addison's Disease. The deficiency is permanent, and the patient must continue hormone replacement therapy for the rest of his life. Hydrocortisone plus sodium chloride may be sufficient; however, most patients require a steroid with mineralocortical activity greater than hydrocortisone. Desoxycorticosterone acetate is an example. It may be given every day by intramuscular injection. Later, this can be switched to a longer-acting steroid with effects that last several weeks after a single injection. These are natural steroids. The dosage is determined by the effects of the daily injections on the blood pressure and on serum electrolyte concentrations. A synthetic steroid with glucocorticoid and mineralocorticoid activity may be given by mouth in small daily doses. Fluorohydrocortisone acetate (Florinef) is an example.

The patient receiving steroid therapy should be weighed daily because of possible water retention. The last dose is usually given by 4 p.m. because the drug may interfere with sleep.[17] Signs of hypercorticalism must be watched for. These include potassium loss (muscle weakness, edema, headache), increase in blood pressure, and cushingnoid features. (See Cushing's disease.)

No patient with Addison's disease should receive insulin by error: he may die of hypoglycemia.

Adrenal Cortex Oversecretion

CUSHING'S DISEASE

In this syndrome there is an overabundance of hormone produced by the adrenal cortex. It is the opposite of Addison's disease. Specific symptoms depend on which of the hormones are in oversupply. Often, there is a mixture. Because corticosteroids tend to speed the breakdown of tissue protein to amino acids and prevent them from being readily reutilized in the synthesis of new muscle, skin, and bone, signs of a "wasting" nature occur. The arms and legs look thin, and there are weakness and pain in the leg muscles. There are characteristic effects on fat distribution, too. Fat is distributed in pads (humps) between the shoulders, above the collarbone, and around the waist. This is called a "buffalo hump" or "girdle obesity." The patient develops typical "cushingnoid features." His face appears full and round; this is called moonface. Excess growth of hair occurs. This is called hirsutism. The skin on the face, neck, and shoulders is flushed: acne-like eruptions occur as well as purplish striae over obese areas. Edema, glycosuria, and hypertension occur. There is an increased susceptibility to infection. The patient has mood swings and often becomes severely depressed. Women frequently develop amenorrhea and signs of masculinization, and men sometimes become impotent.

Treatment of Cushing's Disease. Treatment is aimed at reducing the level of hormones. The pituitary gland may be irradiated; the adrenal glands may be surgically excised. When surgery of the adrenal glands is done, adrenal hormones are given before and after, the amount being decreased if some adrenal tissue is left in the body. The diet should be rich in protein and potassium. Intake and output are recorded. The nurse must observe for signs of hemorrhage, atelectasis, and pneumothorax because the surgery involves the area of the diaphragm and inferior vena cava.

The Thyroid Gland

This gland, also called "the gland of metabolism," is made up of a right and left lobe connected by a narrow isthmus that stretches in front of the trachea, below the larynx. It is popularly called "the Adam's apple." The gland is richly supplied with blood from the superior and inferior thyroid arteries, the latter being associated with the recurrent laryngeal nerve. The gland itself is intimately related to the trachea, larynx, and recurrent laryngeal nerve necessary for speech.

Thyroid Hormones

The two hormones produced by the thyroid gland are thyroxin (tetraiodothyronine, T_4) and triiodothyronine (T_3). The latter is more potent than thyroxin and acts more rapidly, but its action is less sustained. Thyroxin has the more important physiologic activity. It is the principal circulating hormone of the thyroid gland.

The gland synthesizes the hormones from iodine and tyrosine, both of which are usually supplied in sufficient amounts in the daily diet. The normal adult ingests about ⅛ mg of iodine every day. The thyroid gland uses 25 to 35 per cent of this for the synthesis if its hormones.[18] Colloid material within the gland contains enzymes that aid in this hormone synthesis.

Iodine Trapping and Thyroxin Binding

The thyroid gland has a unique ability to pick up iodine from the blood and chemically combine it to form thyroid hormone. This is called "iodine trapping." Once synthesized, the hormones are stored in the gland and are liberated as needed. The thyroxin is secreted into the blood where it is promptly bound to a specific globulin part of the plasma. This is called the thyroxin protein. The binding process is called protein binding.

Production and liberation of thyroxin are regulated by the thyroid-stimulating hormone (TSH) of the pituitary via the feedback mechanism. In the absence of TSH, thyroxin is still produced and liberated but at a much slower rate.

Disorders of the thyroid stem from an increase or decrease in its hormones, or from the effect of an enlarged gland pressing on other structures in the area.

Tests of Thyroid Function

Thyroid function tests are based on the knowledge that the thyroid gland has the unique ability to trap iodine and that its formed hormone is bound to a globulin fraction of the plasma for transport. Products containing large amounts of iodine are withheld for several weeks before the test is done. Examples include the dyes used for gallbladder testing and for intravenous pyelography, cough medicines, nail strengtheners, and iodine antiseptics. The physician should be told if the patient has been taking an antithyroid drug.

PROTEIN-BOUND IODINE (PBI)

Under normal conditions the concentration of protein-bound iodine is about 5 to 8 μg per 100 ml of plasma. Because the thyroid hormones are transported in this bound state their concentration can be determined by precipitating out the protein and measuring the concentration of iodine containing hormone bound to it. Less than 4 μg per 100 plasma is indicative of hypohormone secretion. More than 8 μg per 100 ml serum is indicative of hyperhormone secretion. The patient may be active and may eat prior to the test.

RADIOACTIVE IODINE UPTAKE TEST (I^{131})

A tracer dose of radioactive iodine is given to a fasting patient by mouth. It can be diluted in distilled water or given in capsule form. The tracer dose is small and is harmless to the patient and to those around him. It is odorless and tasteless. The patient eats breakfast 45 minutes after taking the tracer dose. Twenty-four hours after the administration of the radioactive iodine the patient goes to the isotope laboratory. He sits, and a Geiger counter or scintiscanner is positioned in front of the gland. The amount of radioiodine present in the thyroid is determined. A normal thyroid (euthyroid) gland will remove 15 to 50 per cent of the radioiodine in 24 hours. In hyperthyroidism less time is required; in hypothyroidism more time is required. A second Geiger check is often made 36 hours after tracer dose administration. The fate of the radioiodine is also determined by checking the blood and urine. The patient is asked to save all urine voided in the 24-hour period between his first and second appointments with the radiation department.[19] It is checked with the Geiger counter or scintiscanner. Normally, 40 to 80 per cent is excreted.

A "thyroid scan" utilizes a scintiscanner and a recording device. A record of radioactivity concentration is mapped out. This test helps determine if a particular thyroid nodule is benign or malignant. A high uptake in the area of the nodule (a "hot" nodule) is usually benign. A low uptake (a "cold" nodule) can be malignant.[20] A biopsy must be done to verify this.

Usually, no special precautions are required when tracer doses of radioactive iodine are administered. Tracer doses are used for diagnostic purposes, not for therapeutic purposes. Special precautions are always required when large, therapeutic doses are used.

Sometimes a specific laboratory will require special precautions when a tracer dose is used. This should be verified ahead of time. These precautions might include identifying all stool and urine specimens with a "radioactive" label; calling the radioisotope laboratory if clothing or linen has been soiled with urine or feces within 96 hours of the tracer dose administration (they may want to monitor it); saving soiled clothing in a wetproof bag; handling bedpan contents with rubber gloves for 96 hours after the tracer dose administration and washing the gloves afterward (no special precautions are needed if the patient can use the bathroom).[21] Precautions for use of therapeutic doses of iodine are found on page 361.

RADIOACTIVE TRIIODOTHYRONINE (T_3) ERYTHROCYTE UPTAKE TEST

In this test the patient's blood is added to a measured amount of I^{131} tagged hormone triiodothyronine, and radioactivity counts of the whole blood and of red cells are taken. The percentage of the tagged triiodothyronine that adsorbs to the erythrocytes is calculated. If the plasma proteins are already saturated with bound hormone, a greater amount of the tagged hormone will be adsorbed to the red blood cells rather than to the plasma. Thus, the higher the erythrocyte binding, the greater is the amount of naturally occurring hormone bound to plasma. Normal range is 11 to 19 per cent for men and 11 to 17 per cent for women.[22] The test is advantageous because it does not involve any special patient preparation. The patient does not have to be fasting, and he does not receive any exposure to radioactivity.

THYROID SUPPRESSION TEST [23]

If the results of other tests show borderline elevations, the thyroid suppression test is done. After baseline measurement of I^{131} uptake by the thyroid gland, a fast-acting thyroid hormone is given for seven days, and then a repeat measurement of I^{131} uptake is done. In a normal gland, this exogenous thyroid hormone decreases the amount of thyroid-stimulating hormone produced by the pituitary gland and decreases the uptake of I^{131}. Uptake is not suppressed if hyperthyroidism is present because the gland is functioning by itself without the normal thyroid-pituitary feedback controls. It is functioning as an "autonomous gland."

CHOLESTEROL LEVEL

The normal cholesterol level is 150 to 250 mg per cent in a fasting patient. The concentration of cholesterol increases when hypothyroidism is present because the destruction and excretion of cholesterol are so low, and decreases when hyperthyrodism is present.

BASAL METABOLIC RATE (BMR)

This test is gradually being replaced by the more accurate tests already discussed. It measures the rate at which a person consumes oxygen under resting (inert, basal) conditions and compares the results with those of normal individuals. This is reported as the percentage increase or decrease above or below normal. The normal range is -10 to $+10$ per cent. A $+20$ result would mean the patient consumes 20 per cent more oxygen than a normal person of the same size, sex, and age. A patient with hyperthyroidism utilizes a greater amount of oxygen. This indicates a greater metabolic rate. The test involves use of specialized equipment. The patient breathes through a pair of tubes placed in his mouth and attached to bellows that contain the oxygen. His nose is clamped. He must be fasting, quiet, and not anxious. This set of conditions makes the test impractical!

Goiter

This is a condition in which hyperplasia of thyroid tissue produces an unsightly enlargement of the thyroid gland. Hyperplasia results because insufficient amounts of iodine make the gland work harder to produce its necessary hormone. The gland bulges in the neck. This enlarged gland acts like a space-occupying mass. It encroaches on structures in the area (trachea, larynx, esophagus) producing swallowing and breathing difficulties. Goiter may be accompanied by hypo-, hyper-, or normal thyroid hormone production.

CAUSES OF GOITER [24]

Goiter is caused by a deficient intake of iodine. This can come from an absolute lack of iodine, or from a relative lack of iodine when its requirements are increased, as during adolescence, pregnancy, and lactation, but its ingested amount stays the same.

Goiter occurs to some degree in almost every country in the world, where there is a deficient amount of iodine in the water or soil. Areas around the sea contain large, ample amounts of iodine. Soil in sea areas is replenished with air-borne sea iodine. The amount of iodine in inland areas depends on the mineral composition of the rock from which it was formed. Lands exposed to continuous flooding lose iodine. Vast areas of the world were left iodine-poor as a result of the last ice age when the soil was swept away and was replaced by new soil created by grinding of rock. The "goitrous" areas of the United States include the Great Lakes area, the Pacific Northwest, Minnesota, and Ohio. It is interesting to note that thousands of men recruited from these areas to serve in the army in World War I were rejected because the collar of their military tunics could not be buttoned around their enlarged necks.[25]

The disease has largely been eliminated since the introduction of iodinated salt in the early 1920's. Widespread national distribution of food, with foods from nongoitrous areas being utilized in goitrous areas, also decreases the incidence of goiter. Some foods have been found to have a goitrogenic effect. They contain thiocyanates or thiocyanate precursors that block the trapping of iodine by the thyroid. (These are utilized in drugs to decrease hyperthyroidism!) Cabbage, cauliflower, turnips, Brussels sprouts, rutabaga, and thousand-headed kale are examples. Their effects are counteracted by ingestion of more iodine.

Goiter prophylaxis is attained by iodinization of salt (the container is so labeled) in a 1:10,000 proportion. Goiter is prevented by giving 5 mg iodine once a week as potassium iodide in endemic areas.

Hypothyroidism

In this condition the thyroid gland does not produce sufficient amounts of hormone, and all of the body's metabolic processes are slowed. If the deficiency has its onset in infancy, the resulting disease is called cretinism, or congenital hypothyroidism. If the disease is recognized and treated early, the child may develop normally; however, there is a great possibility that mental and physical development will be retarded.

Hypothyroidism that has its onset in adults and in older children is called myxedema. It can result from failure of the gland to develop normally, from failure of the pituitary gland to produce adequate thyroid-stimulating hormone, from infection, from surgical removal or irradiation of the gland with I^{131}, and so on. Sometimes a full-blown myxedema does not occur, but the patient has symptoms of hypothyroidism. This is called borderline hypothyroidism or hypometabolism and responds to administration of thyroid extract.

SYMPTOMS OF HYPOTHYROIDISM

Symptoms stem from decreased metabolism in all body cells. The patient is less able to adapt to any stress situation. He appears dull, sluggish, and lacking in intelligence. He is always sleepy. His speech is thick, halting, slurred, and hoarse. His tongue swells. His skin is thick, puffy, and dry. His hair is brittle and thin on the scalp and eyebrows. He grays prematurely. His nails are also thick and brittle. His muscles are weak. Because of increased capillary fragility he bruises easily. He has an increased susceptibility to infection. He has a reduced tolerance to cold and feels cold regardless of the room temperature. His appetite is decreased, and he tends to gain weight. His heart rate slows, and his blood pressure drops. In the female, there are decreased ovarian function and prolonged menstruation.

TREATMENT OF HYPOTHYROIDISM

A thyroid preparation is administered. Examples include sodium dextrothyroxine (Choloxin), 1 to 2 mg daily, then 4 to 8 mg maintenance; sodium liothyronine (Cytomel, triiodothyronine), 5 μg daily, then 5 to 100μg maintenance; thyroglobulin (Proloid), 60 to 180 mg daily; and thyroid (desiccated thyroid), 15 to 180 mg daily. The aim of treatment is to bring about the greatest possible improvement with the lowest dosage of thyroid.[26] Patients with hypothyroidism are extremely sensitive to thyroid drugs and can easily develop symptoms of hyperthyroidism. A sudden increase in metabolism can cause cardiac strain.

Hyperthyroidism (Graves's Disease, Exophthalmic Goiter, Thyrotoxic Goiter, Toxic Nodular Goiter, Basedow's Disease)

In this condition all metabolic processes are increased because of an increased production of thyroid hormone. The gland can have nodular enlargements, or it can be enlarged diffusely. The latter condition causes more severe symptoms. As the gland enlarges it can press on surrounding structures and act as a space-occupying mass. Cancer of the thyroid gland must be ruled out, especially if the enlargement is irregular, if there is a single nodule, or if there is laryngeal nerve involvement.[27]

SYMPTOMS OF HYPERTHYROIDISM

Symptoms stem from increased metabolic rate in all body cells. The patient has difficulty adapting to any environmental stress. He is intolerant to heat and feels hot regardless of the environmental temperature. His blood pressure, heart rate, and heat production are all increased. There is peripheral vasodilation, and this causes him to appear flushed. The palms of his hands are sweaty and warm. Emotional disturbances frequently accompany hyperthyroidism. The patient tends to be jittery and tense. He is restless and irritable and cries easily. His behavior often mimics the expression of fear or terror generally described as crystallized fright.[28] Reaction time is slower, and there seems to be a latent period between the stimulus and the patient's reaction to it. There is decreased motor ability. The patient with hyperthyroidism often starts a task like a very tired person.[29] Although he may take less time to complete a problem-solving activity, he usually makes more errors than his euthyroid (normal) counterpart. His speech is rapid and excited.

EXOPHTHALMOS

His eyes protrude (exophthalmos, proptosis), and they seem to be continuously "staring." This is because they blink infrequently, and when they do blink, the eyelid moves more slowly than the eyeball. Exophthalmos comes from increased fatty infiltration and edema of the orbit. It develops when there is an increased amount of thyroid-stimulating pituitary hormone. Interestingly enough, it may not develop until after the hyperthyroid condition has been controlled.[30] Control of the hyperthyroidism stops the progression of the exophthalmos, but does not cause its regression. Local injections of adrenocortical steroids under the conjunctiva produce a regression, though the reason is obscure.[31] The patient should wear protective glasses when he is out of doors to prevent corneal irritation, and he should sleep with an eye covering.

Excess thyroid hormone causes excess excretion of calcium, and there is demineralization of bone. Appetite is increased, but the patient continues to lose weight. The female patient has menstrual irregularities.

TREATMENT OF HYPERTHYROIDISM

The goal of treatment is to return the patient to a euthyroid (normal) state; however, this process must not be too rapid because it might be too shocking to a system that has "adapted" to the hyperthyroid condition. Treatment involves use of antithyroid drugs, irradiation of the gland with I^{131}, and thyroidectomy.

DRUGS USED TO CONTROL HYPERTHYROIDISM

Iodine. For years, iodine itself was the only known antithyroid drug. It prevents the glandular excretion of thyroid hormones and in this way decreases metabolic rate and controls the symptoms of hyperthyroidism. Iodine decreases the vascularity of the gland and causes it to shrink (involute). This makes it a very effective drug to use for preoperative preparation of the gland. It has a disagreeable taste, and should be given in milk or juice. It should be given through a straw because it stains the teeth. Effects of iodine last about two weeks. Lugol's solution is an example; 0.1 to 1.0 ml is given.

Thiouracil Derivatives. These drugs inhibit the synthesis of thyroid hormone. They often cause permanent remission of the disease. Their effects may not become evident immediately because the thyroid gland must first "use up" its excess stored hormone.[32] Medication is given about three times each day, and should be given on time. When the symptoms are sufficiently controlled, a maintenance dose is all that is required. Signs of toxicity include sore throat, fever, rash, or jaundice. Agranulocytosis and hepatitis are rare, but serious, possible toxic effects. Periodic blood checks are therefore made. Examples of antithyroid drugs (thiocarbamides) include iothiouracil sodium (Itrumil), 150 to 300 mg each day; methimazole (Tapazole), 5 to 20 mg each day; and propylthiouracil, 50 to 500 mg each day. A preoperative regimen of antithyroid drugs and iodine is used to prepare the patient for thyroidectomy.

IRRADIATION OF THE THYROID GLAND

Sodium iodide (I^{131}), commercially prepared as Iodotope and Radiocaps, in therapeutic doses equivalent to 1 to 100 millicuries,[33] is given orally or intravenously. The dose is based on the estimated weight of the thyroid gland, the patient's age, and the severity of symptoms. I^{131} is "trapped" by the thyroid gland, where it delivers its radiation and destroys thyroid cells. As the cells disintegrate, thyroid hormone that was stored in the gland is released, and the patient may actually experience more hyperthyroid symptoms for four or five days. Remission of symptoms begins about three weeks after the treatment. It is a gradual process that takes several months. If remission is not satisfactory, a second dose may be given. Changes seem to be permanent. I^{131} has a biologic half-life of about eight days; its effects are dissipated rapidly. Radiation sickness following this treatment is rare. The patient is hospitalized for eight days and watched for signs of thyroid storm (exaggeration of the symptoms of hyperthyroidism).

A percentage of thyrotoxic patients who are irradiated with I^{131} develop signs of hypothyroidism and myxedema as long as several years after treatment. Evidence is accruing that 50 per cent of patients so treated will develop hypothyroidism.[34] They must then be treated with thyroid extracts.

I^{131} is not administered to people under 45 years because of the danger of inducing cancerous changes locally.[35] It is not effective in treating cancer of the thyroid gland because cancerous nodes lose their ability to trap iodine. Special safety precautions are used when the patient has a therapeutic dose of radioactive material. These include the following: [36]

1. Perform all nursing care required but be brief and efficient.

2. Visitors are allowed but should stay as far away from the patient as practical for 48 hours following the dose. No pregnant person should come into the room.

3. Call the radioisotope laboratory if the patient vomits within six hours of the dose.

4. Save any bedding or clothing soiled with urine during the 72-hour period following the dose for monitoring. Place it in a wetproof bag and label it "radioactive."

5. If urine is being saved for specimen examination, the container should be labeled with a radioactive sign.

6. The patient may use the bathroom as usual. Suggest that he flush the toilet several times after use. Handle the bedpan with rubber gloves and wash them afterward.

7. Food may be served and returned to the kitchen as usual.

SURGERY OF THE THYROID GLAND

If cancer is found, the total gland and lymph nodes are removed. The patient is given thyroid hormone supplements afterward. Therapeutic x-ray may be used, too.

If surgery is to be done to control hyperthyroidism and to alleviate pressure on and deviation to the trachea because of thyroid enlargement, a subtotal thyroidectomy is performed. Mortality is low in patients who are well prepared for this surgery. This preparation involves administration of antithyroid drugs to control the hyperthyroidism plus administration of an iodine solution for about ten days prior to the surgery to shrink the gland and reduce its vascularity.

A general anesthetic is administered using an endotracheal tube. The patient is positioned so that his head is extended and held firmly in place and the gland is well exposed. A transverse incision is made. Care is taken to avoid injury to the laryngeal nerve, and at least one parathyroid gland must remain in the body. A small Penrose drain is usually inserted on either side of the trachea and brought out through the midline. Sufficient thyroid tissue must be removed to prevent the symptoms; at the same time, sufficient tissue must be left in the body to preserve normal function. About 75 to 85 per cent of each lobe of the gland is removed.[37] The surgeon pays particular attention to controlling bleeding, avoiding injury to surrounding structures, and securing a satisfactory cosmetic result. The patient will have a thin scar across the area.

NURSING MANAGEMENT OF THE PATIENT WITH HYPERTHYROIDISM

Goals are based on the knowledge that there is a great increase in metabolic rate and the patient cannot adapt adequately to changes in his environment. Major objectives include: [38]

1. To modify the physical and emotional environment and foster rest. The patient should, if at all possible, be in a private room. The room should have its own heat-control thermostat. The hyperthyroid patient is intolerant to heat, and the room should be kept comfortable for him. Heavy blankets should be out of sight. Windows should be open. If necessary, an air conditioner can be turned on. The patient should be sponged frequently because he sweats profusely. The room should be quiet. All extraneous noise should be eliminated, and people should be reminded not to talk outside of his room.

2. To provide for increased metabolic needs. The patient with hyperthyroidism on bed rest needs about twice as much food as a normal person not on bed rest.[39] Do not make snide remarks about the quantity of food he eats! Serve him supplementary feedings frequently. His diet should be high in calories, carbohydrate, and vitamins. This helps protect the liver from damage. Liver glycogen tends to be depleted in hyperthyroidism.[40] Help him to eat if fine tremors make this difficult and embarrassing. Keep a glass of juice or eggnog at his bedside and encourage him to sip it. Withhold stimulating drinks (coffee, tea, cola) unless withholding them is very upsetting to him. Weigh him at the same time every day.

3. To understand that the patient will overreact to emotional and physical stimuli and stress. Control the number of visitors allowed at one time and limit the length of their stay. Help the family to understand that the patient's responses are heightened and that offensive remarks are not meant personally. Try to regulate the environment so that stress is at a minimum.

AFTER THYROID SURGERY

Position and Equipment. Immediately after surgery the patient is placed on his abdomen with his head turned to one side, or on his back with sandbags or firm pillows to hold his head still. When he has reacted, the head of the bed is elevated moderately, and he is placed in a low semi-Fowler's position.

An emergency tracheostomy set, a suction machine, and steam inhalation equipment should be near the bedside.

Head Movement; Ambulation. Check with the physician regarding head movement. Usually, the patient is not allowed to extend or flex his neck until the wound has healed somewhat, and side-to-side motions are avoided for two to three days postoperatively. The head should be supported with the patient's or nurse's hands when the patient moves around or sits up. Teach the patient to do this. His head should not be allowed to fall backward with a jerk. He is usually allowed out of bed on the evening of surgery or the following day.

Nutrition. He is allowed a semisolid diet as soon as he can swallow. He will feel some discomfort when he swallows. This is to be expected. Analgesic throat lozenges or medication may be ordered. Intravenous glucose and water is sometimes given on the day of surgery.

COMPLICATIONS OF THYROID SURGERY

Respiratory Obstruction. Respiratory difficulty caused by compression of the trachea from bleeding, from edema, or from increased mucous secretion can occur. An emergency tracheostomy may be required. The patient should be suctioned gently when necessary. Encourage him to cough and deep-breathe once his swallowing reflex has returned. Vital signs should be taken every 15 minutes for the first two postoperative hours, every four hours for the first 24 hours.

Hemorrhage. Pass your hand around the back of the patient's neck to check for bleeding. Blood may run downhill and away from its initial source. If the dressing "feels tight" to the patient, loosen it, but do not remove it. Call the surgeon. Drains may have been inserted during surgery. They drain into the dressing and are removed 24 to 48 hours postoperatively. Be aware of their presence. Watch for signs of bleeding, e.g., fall in blood pressure, increase in pulse rate, and restlessness, and contact the physician if necessary.

Parathyroid Injury. If the parathyroid glands are inadvertently damaged, the patient may develop signs of muscle-nerve hyperirritability (tetany.) These include tremors, muscle spasms, and numbness. Intravenous calcium is administered. (See p. 365.)

Injury to the Recurrent Laryngeal Nerve. During the first 24 to 48 hours after surgery the patient may be hoarse. This is usually caused by swelling in the region of the glottis, and it subsides naturally. Discourage the patient from talking during the first two postoperative days. Sometimes hoarseness results from damage to one or both of the recurrent laryngeal nerves. There may be a crowing sound when the patient speaks. If both nerves are injured, the vocal cords tighten and close off the larynx. This causes severe respiratory obstruction and requires an emergency tracheostomy. If the nerves are injured, healing occurs in a few weeks; if they are severed, permanent paralysis of the vocal cords occurs, and the patient cannot speak. *Report any voice changes to the surgeon.* Hoarseness persisting for more than the first few days suggests damage to the recurrent laryngeal nerve.

Hyperthyroid Crisis (Thyroid Storm). This is a rare complication in which exaggerated symptoms of hyperthyroidism occur. It can happen before surgery or during the first 12 hours after surgery. The heart rate, pulse, and body temperature are so increased that the patient may die. He is placed in an oxygen tent in an effort to supply his cells with oxygen. He is given intravenous and oral solutions and is placed on a hypothermia blanket to control his temperature. (See pp. 273–74.)

Late complications include hypothyroidism (myxedema), recurrent hyperthyroidism, and hypoparathyroidism.

TABLE 34–1. HYPOTHYROIDISM AND HYPERTHYROIDISM COMPARED

System Involved	Hypothyroidism	Hyperthyroidism
CENTRAL NERVOUS SYSTEM 1. Speech	Swelling of tongue and larynx. Halting, slurred, thick, slow speech. Hoarseness	Rapid and excited speech. Hoarseness may exist
2. Affect and thinking	Lethargy, irritability, sleepiness, dullness, "looks stupid." Intelligence remains in adults but thinking is "slow." Myxedema may lead to psychosis	Hyperactive, emotionally labile. Hypersentitive, tense, jittery, restlesss, occasionally depressed. Fine tremor of extended hands or tongue, insomnia
3. Reflexes	Hyporeflexia	Hyperactive reflexes
4. Susceptibility to heat and cold	Very susceptible (intolerant) to cold	Intolerant to heat
CARDIOVASCULAR-RENAL SYSTEM	Bradycardia, hypotension, increased capillary fragility, bruises easily, decreased cardiac output, weak heartbeat, increased circulation time, oliguria	Tachycardia, systolic hypertension, increased cardiac output, palpitation, paroxysmal arrhythmia, dyspnea, wide pulse pressure, decreased circulation time
SKIN, HAIR, NAILS	Skin thick, puffy, dry; hair brittle, dry, sparse. May loose hair on scalp and eyebrows, nails thick and hard	Skin warm, moist, flushed, thin. Hair soft and silky. Nails soft and thin
GASTROINTESTINAL	Constipation. Decreased appetite, low glucose absorption rate, increased weight, increased blood cholesterol	Diarrhea, anorexia. Nausea, vomiting, increased appetite but with tendency toward weight loss, low blood cholesterol
MUSCLE	Weakness; decreased tone	Weakness and twitching; tremors. Muscle wasting

TABLE 34-1. [*Continued*]

System Involved	Hypothyroidism	Hyperthyroidism
EYES		Protruding eyeballs (exophthalmos). Infrequent blinking, lid lag. Failure of convergence; failure to wrinkle brow when looking upward
OVARIAN FUNCTION; MENSTRUATION	Decreased with menstruation prolonged	Altered. Tendency toward oligomenorrhea (decreased menstruation) and amenorrhea (absence of menstruation)

The Parathyroid Glands

There are four, six, or eight glands embedded in and surrounding the thyroid gland. Its hormone, parathormone, regulates the concentration of calcium and phosphorus in the blood and influences the passage of calcium and phosphorus between the blood, bones, and urine. The hormone maintains the concentration of calcium ion activity in the plasma within narrow limits despite wide fluctuations in calcium intake and excretion.[41] The parathyroids affect the rate of calcium metabolism. If they are damaged, as in thyroid surgery, calcium metabolism continues but the serum calcium level is lower.

Hypoparathyroidism (Hypocalcemia, Tetany)

The calcium-phosphorus level in the blood helps to maintain normal neuromuscular excitability. Too little serum calcium with too much serum phosphorus causes increased neuromuscular hyperirritability. There is an abnormal increase in reaction of motor and sensory nerves to stimuli.[42] This is called tetany. The patient experiences painful tonic spasms of muscles. There may be numbness and tingling of the fingers, toes, and lips. There is a positive Chvostek sign. This is a twitching of the facial muscles when the facial nerve is tapped. There is also a positive Trousseau sign. When a manometer is inflated on the arm for one to five minutes, typical flexion-extension spasms of the fingers and hand occur.

WHAT TO DO FOR TETANY

In an emergency, calcium salts (calcium chloride, calcium gluconate) can be administered by slow intravenous drip. Care must be taken to prevent infiltration because sloughing of tissue may occur; care must also be taken to prevent the adverse effects of high calcium concentrations on the heart.[43] Calcium is administered by mouth for milder forms of tetany. It is given in conjunction with large doses of vitamin D, for maximum absorption. The chloride, containing the largest amount of calcium, is also the most irritating to the gastrointestinal tract.[44] Parathyroid hormone extracts are given parenterally.

Hyperparathyroidism (Hypercalcemia)

In this condition there are an increased serum level of calcium and a low serum phosphorus level. There is a loss of calcium from the bones (demineralization), and the patient is prone to pathologic fracture. He experiences muscle weakness (hypotonia), fatigue, nausea, vomiting, anorexia, lethargy, constipation, weight loss, polyuria, thirst, and cardiac arrhythmias. Surgery is done to remove excess parathyroid tissue.

The Thymus Gland

This gland is a major source of lymphocytes before birth and postnatally. Once antigenic stimulation occurs, however, the spleen and lymph nodes become the major lymphocyte producers, and the thymus loses its importance.

35

DIABETES MELLITUS

The Pancreas

This organ, situated behind the stomach and in front of the first and second lumbar vertebrae, has both exocrine and endocrine function. It not only supplies enzymes important in digestion (exocrine function) but also supplies two hormones involved in all cell metabolism. This is its endocrine function. The two pancreatic hormones are insulin (blood-glucose-lowering) and glucagon (blood-glucose-elevating).

Insulin

Insulin is produced by clusters of beta cells within the islands of Langerhans in the pancreas. Insulin enables glucose to pass through cell membranes so that it can provide fuel for energy (cell metabolism). Glucose is obtained from carbohydrate foods, from protein foods, and from fats.[45] Sixty per cent of proteins and 10 per cent of fats provide carbohydrate. It is converted to glucose in the intestines and passes from there into the bloodstream. *Insulin helps the glucose get from the blood into the cells.* It is the blood-glucose-lowering, energy-fostering hormone. It is required for the adequate uptake and storage of glucose by the liver, muscle, and adipose tissue. Glucose is converted to glycogen for storage in the liver and muscle and is reconverted to glucose when it is needed by the body for energy. Glucose is the only form in which carbohydrate can be utilized by the cells for energy, and insulin is necessary to get it into the cells. Although fatty acids and protein can provide energy requirements, the brain depends exclusively on glucose.

In times of stress the body requires additional glucose for energy. This, in turn, requires additional insulin. Stored glycogen in the liver is converted to glucose "in a hurry." Later, additional glucose can be synthesized from nonglucose precursors, e.g., from protein. This new formation of glucose from a nonglucose product is called gluconeogenesis.

If insulin is severely deficient, proteins and fats are burned almost exclusively to provide for energy requirements. Adipose (fatty) tissue releases fatty acids; muscle releases amino acids (catabolism); however, the burning of protein and fats for energy leaves intermediate metabolites circulating in the blood because oxidation simply cannot keep pace with their rapid formation. Circulation of these intermediate metabolites causes severe toxicity. (See Diabetic Ketoacidosis, p. 370.)

Glucagon

Glucagon is the second pancreatic hormone. It is formed in the non-insulin-producing alpha cells. It is the hyperglycemic hormone. It increases the breakdown of glycogen to glucose in the liver. *It is the blood-glucose-elevating hormone.*

In the normal person, a delicate blood sugar level is maintained by insulin, by glucagon, and by other endocrine hormones. Growth hormone (anterior pituitary hormone), glucocorticoids (adrenal cortex hormones), epinephrine (adrenal medullary hormone), and thyroxin (thyroid hormone) are known to be insulin antagonists. Research centers on the study of other body substances that also appear to decrease the effectiveness of insulin, e.g., insulin binding by antibodies.[46]

Diabetes Mellitus

What It Is

Diabetes mellitus is a chronic, incurable disease in which there is a disparity between the amount of insulin needed by the body and the amount of metabolically effective insulin available.[47] Insufficient available insulin prevents the utilization of glucose for energy by all the cells in the body. Without enough insulin, the cells fail to "pick up" enough glucose. The glucose remains in the blood and is ultimately spilled over in the urine. "Sugar in the urine" is the basis for the Greek naming of the disease. Diabetes comes from the words meaning "flowing through," and mellitus comes from "honey."

If glucose is not available to provide for energy needs, fuel must come from another source. Thus, proteins and fats are burned for this purpose. They are not totally oxidized and leave "intermediate products" of metabolism circulating in the blood. These intermediate metabolites, called ketones, cause the severe symptoms of diabetes.

Although primarily a disease of carbohydrate metabolism, diabetes mellitus involves the metabolism of protein and fat as well. It is associated with extensive disease of both the large and small blood vessels, especially the capillaries. This is why gangrene becomes such a potential hazard. It is also why even the controlled diabetic frequently develops changes in the retina (retinopathy) with serious decrease in vision. This can be a rapidly occurring "malignant" type of progression, and excision of the pituitary gland may be done in an attempt to halt it. It is also why the diabetic may develop serious lesions in the kidney (nephropathy) that further decrease his ability to excrete metabolic by-products. Changes in the nervous system (central and peripheral) result from lack of glucose and lack of B vitamins, which are not stored by the body and which are "washed out" with the polyuria of diabetes.

Who Gets Diabetes?

Approximately 3 out of every 1,000 males and 5 out of every 1,000 females in the United States have diabetes.[48] There are about 4 million diabetics in this country today.[49] The incidence [50,51] (rate of appearance of new cases) is highest in women (twice as many females have the disease as males); where the average age is oldest (frequency increases with a maximum of new cases appearing at 45 to 55 years); where obesity is present (obesity increases the need of the body for insulin and may eventually exhaust the islet cells); where occupation is sedentary and income is high; where the Jewish population is highest; and where heredity predisposes the person to getting the disease.

Diabetes mellitus is inherited as a recessive mendelian trait. This means that [52] all the children born to two diabetic parents are genetically liable to diabetes eventually. This is sometimes hard to establish because a child may get the disease before his parents show signs of it.

If a diabetic marries a "carrier" (free of disease but transmits a tendency to it), 50 per cent of their children will be diabetics and 50 per cent will be carriers.

If two carriers marry, 25 per cent of their children will be diabetic; 75 per cent will be carriers.

If a diabetic marries a nondiabetic who is not a carrier, none of their children will develop diabetes, but they will be carriers.

Frank diabetes results from the interaction of this genetic predisposition with environmental factors, e.g., long-term obesity. Long-term modification of environmental factors has a beneficial influence on the course of the disease even if it is certain to develop.

Early diagnosis and treatment mean longer life. The life expectancy of a diabetic is two thirds that of the general population. The highest death rate is in nonwhite females.[53] The severity of the disease is greater when it develops before 30 years of age. Although its incidence is higher in obese people, the severity is greater in lean people. If an obese individual develops the disease, it becomes less severe if he attains normal weight.

Stages of Diabetes Mellitus

Diabetes is described as occurring in three stages.[54]

1. *Prediabetes.* This is the period in the life of an individual who is destined to become a diabetic, before any carbohydrate impairment can be definitely established. The child of two diabetic parents is an example.

2. *Latent Diabetes.* During this period the classic symptoms are not yet present, but there is an increased blood sugar following a glucose tolerance test, or after metabolic stress. This is called "chemical" diabetes. Hyperglycemia and glycosuria may persist for long periods without producing severe symptoms of diabetes (ketoacidosis).[55]

3. *Clinical Diabetes.* This is frank, overt diabetes in which symptoms as well as changes in the blood occur. In its early stages the patient may show elevated blood sugar only after meals.

Diabetes is called juvenile or growth-onset type if it occurs early in life (before 30). It is notoriously difficult to control, and the person with it is very prone to develop ketoacidosis. It is "brittle." Diabetes is called adult or maturity-onset type if beginning symptoms occur after 30 years. It is a relatively stable "ketosis-resistant" type. It is more easily controlled than the juvenile-onset type.

Sometimes, diabetes results from a specific, nonhereditary cause. This is called secondary diabetes. It may follow stress (e.g., pregnancy; surgery; surgical removal of the pancreas; severe infection) or pathology of an endocrine gland other than the pancreas. Hyperthyroidism, hyperpituitarism, and hyperadrenalism are examples.

Symptoms of Diabetes Mellitus

Early symptoms are often vague and can be easily overlooked by the patient. They are caused by the increased glucose circulating in the blood, by its need to be excreted, and by the generalized effects of inadequate cell use of glucose to meet energy requirements. The patient voids very frequently and in large amounts. This is called polyuria and is an attempt by the kidney to excrete excess glucose. The patient is very thirsty (polydipsia) because the glucose utilizes body water for its excretion and the body water must be replaced. He is very hungry (polyphagia) because, regardless of how much he eats, his cells are not getting enough glucose. He loses weight. Note the classic "three P's" of diabetes: polyuria, polydipsia, and polyphagia. The patient feels the effects of the lack of glucose, the energy fuel, throughout his body. He tires easily, is irritable, is weak, and may complain of peripheral nervous symptoms such as numbness and tingling of his hands and feet. He has itching about the genitalia from increased glucose excretion. He may have visual disturbances.

Laboratory study shows an elevation of glucose in the blood (hyperglycemia) followed by an elevation of glucose in the urine (glycosuria) as it is spilled over from the blood. Glucose is found in the urine when it rises to over 180 mg per 100 ml in the blood.[56]

LATER, SEVERE SYMPTOMS OF DIABETES MELLITUS

Ketoacidosis. Uncontrolled diabetes, or diabetes that is thrown out of control because of infections, surgery, thyrotoxicosis, and similar stress situations, can lead to serious symptoms. This syndrome is called diabetic ketoacidosis (acidosis, ketosis, diabetic coma). As the name indicates, this life-threatening condition comes from the severe metabolic acidosis and dehydration that stem from the production, circulation, and excretion of intermediate incompletely oxidized metabolites of fat and protein breakdown. Fats and proteins must be used to provide fuel for energy because glucose is unavailable to the cells. The kidney, however, cannot "keep up with" the excretion of the metabolic by-products, and they circulate in the blood. Following is the sequence of events that lead to diabetic ketoacidosis: [57]

1. Decreased available insulin causes increased glucose in the blood. This, in turn, causes increased glucose concentration in the glomerular (kidney) filtrate.

2. Increased glomerular filtrate requires water for its excretion. Water is drawn from the plasma first; then it is drawn from the cells. It removes potassium, magnesium, and phosphate with it. There is a loss of water and electrolytes. The patient is dehydrated.

3. There is a drastic increase in circulating by-products of incompletely oxidized proteins and fats (beta-hydroxybutyric acid, acetoacetic acid, and acetone). Fats and proteins must be burned because glucose is not available to the cells for energy.

4. Increased circulating ketones require fixed base in order to be excreted. They "latch onto" base leaving a relatively acid body pH. The patient is now in metabolic acidosis.

5. Blood volume decreases as more water is drawn from it to excrete substances. Circulatory shock may develop. The dehydration coupled with the metabolic acidosis may cause coma and death.

Another Look at This Acute Diabetic Syndrome [58]

Inadequate usable insulin
　↓
hyperglycemia
　↓　　↗polyuria
glycosuria→polydipsia
　↓　　↘polyphagia
mobilization and breakdown (catabolism) of proteins and fats for energy
　↓　　　　↗ketones in urine
weight loss, ketosis→urinary loss of cations (fixed base)
　↓
ketoacidosis, coma, death

The patient with developing ketoacidosis has all the symptoms previously discussed. In addition, he is extremely dehydrated. His skin is flushed, dry, and hot. His lips are parched. He has a decrease in blood pressure and temperature. His respirations increase in depth (Kussmaul respirations) in an attempt to "blow off" excess carbon dioxide (acidosis), and his breath has an acetone smell. He complains of chest pain (potassium imbalance), abdominal pain (distention), and bowel atony. He is anorexic and nauseated and may vomit coffee-ground vomitus. This color comes from the presence of changed blood. Laboratory study of the urine reveals moderate amounts of sugar, diacetic acid, and acetone. The patient becomes progressively drowsy, and if not treated quickly and vigorously, he loses consciousness. Diabetic ketoacidosis may progress rapidly in a matter of hours, or, more often, over a period of days. (See p. 387 for management.)

How Is Diabetes Mellitus Diagnosed?

Changes in carbohydrate metabolism can be observed in the blood and in the urine.

BLOOD SUGAR

The normal range in a fasting patient is 60 to 90 mg per 100 ml blood by the Somogyi-Nelson method, and 80 to 120 mg per 100 ml by the Folin-Wu method. A venepuncture is done. Diabetic patients should not receive insulin until after the blood is drawn.

The newer Somogyi-Nelson method (see above) and the autoanalyzer measure glucose exclusively. Older methods measure other carbohydrates as well. A paper-strip enzymatic method for direct blood glucose determination (the strip is dipped into the blood) is in the testing stage.[59]

POSTPRANDIAL BLOOD SUGAR TEST

This is one in which the specimen is drawn one to two and one-half hours after a meal. This seems best for diagnostic purposes because many early diabetics have blood sugar elevation only after meals. Developing diabetes is characterized by fluctuating, intermittent elevations.

STANDARD GLUCOSE TOLERANCE TEST

This test is used only if the diagnosis is indefinite after blood sugar determinations are made. It is used to diagnose less overt clinical diabetes. It determines the physiologic response to a standard amount of glucose. The patient is allowed an unrestricted diet containing at least 150 gm of carbohydrate each day for three days before the test. Any agents likely to affect blood glucose are withheld for a period equal to their duration of action, e.g., hormones, oral hypoglycemic agents, thiazide diuretics, and large amounts of aspirin. The patient fasts the night before the test, and a venous blood specimen is drawn the morning of the test. Then, he is given 100 gm of glucose dissolved in 200 ml of water and flavored with lemon juice to make it more palatable. He should drink all the solution within five minutes.[60] Venous blood and urine specimens are obtained one-half hour after ingestion of the glucose, and each hour thereafter for four to five hours. *Carefully check the hospital's procedure manual for glucose tolerance testing* because it varies, slightly, with the laboratory method used. The patient is allowed water but no other food or beverage throughout the test. He should not smoke because smoking is stimulating and may alter test results. He should remain in his room so that he is available at the prescribed times.[61] All specimens should be marked with the time drawn.

Insulin is secreted in response to the elevated blood glucose level and causes the blood glucose level to fall below the fasting level. This phenomenon occurs about the second or third test hour and may cause transitory symptoms such as weaknesses and sweating. It should be recorded, and the patient should rest in bed to prevent accidents.

A commercially prepared bottle of a carbonated measured-carbohydrate load drink is now available. It contains 7 oz of a flavored corn syrup beverage containing 75 gm of glucose (Glucola, Ames Company). It can be used in mass diabetes screening programs. The person drinks the beverage, and two hours later a drop of finger blood is drawn and tested. It is a more sensitive indicator of early diabetes than mass urine testing.

RAPID INTRAVENOUS GLUCOSE TOLERANCE TEST [62]

This test is especially valuable for ambulatory outpatients. The patient fasts for 14 hours before the test and eats a high-carbohydrate diet (two extra slices of bread at each meal) for three days before coming to the laboratory. A single glucose injection is given intravenously over four to six minutes. Blood samples are obtained from an indwelling needle in the opposite arm prior to the glucose infusion, and then every five minutes between 15 and 50 minutes after the infusion. The test is quick, and the patient does not experience the nausea associated with drinking the glucose.

CO_2-COMBINING POWER

The normal range is 52 to 58 volumes per 100 ml of venous blood. This is a test that demonstrates the presence of acidosis. If protein and fat are metabolized because of inadequate utilization of glucose, the by-products of its incomplete breakdown latch on to bases for their excretion. This produces a decreased CO_2-combining power indicative of acidosis. No special preparation of the patient is required.

URINE TESTS

Urine is tested for sugar, and if sugar is present, it is tested for acetone. These are tests that the patient must learn to do himself, at home. They are usually performed before breakfast and before supper in the controlled diabetic.

Glucose. No glucose is normally present in urine. Positive results, reported as trace and 1+ to 4+, indicate amounts of glucose found. This is a color test with the degree of positivity indicated by changes in color. Tablets, tapes, or paper sticks are used. If Clinistix, Urostix, or Testape is used, it is dipped into the urine, and the color change is read according to a scale shown on the bottle or dispenser. The Testape dispenser looks like a tape measure dispenser.

If Clinitest tablets are used, 5 drops of urine is added to 10 drops of water in a test tube, and the tablet is dropped into the solution. The solution "boils," and the color change is read 15 seconds after the boiling stops. Clinitest color changes are:

0 %	black	negative
¼%	dark green	trace
½%	green	1+
¾%	brown	2+
1 %	rust brown	3+
2 %	orange	4+

The Clinitest tablet should have a spotted bluish-white color. It should not be used if it has turned dark blue or has changed color in some other way.

Acetone in Urine. Acetone is one of the ketones produced when fatty acids are burned for energy in place of glucose. A strip of paper impregnated with reagent is "dipped" into the urine. A purple color indicates a positive test. Acetest tablets may be used, too. The tablet is placed on a piece of white paper. A drop of urine is put on the tablet, and its color is compared with the color chart 30 seconds later. If the response is negative, the tablet remains unchanged or appears cream-colored. The color is lavender (purplish) if the response is positive.

TEACHING THE PATIENT

The patient should learn to do these tests while he is still in the hospital. He should be shown how to keep a record of the results. A stenographer's notebook with a column for the date and time the test was done is satisfactory.

Remember, glycosuria does not always mean diabetes mellitus! Other conditions produce these symptoms, too. Examples include hyperthyroidism, stroke, severe liver disease, obesity especially just after a high carbohydrate meal, and chronic illness.

Management of the Patient Who Has Diabetes Mellitus

Diabetes is a lifetime, "forever" disease. The treatment program becomes a necessary, integral part of the patient's everyday existence. Some people are psychologically equipped to accept this changed health status and incorporate it in their self-image. They adjust readily to the therapeutic program. Others have a great deal of difficulty doing this. Many still feel that "having sugar" should be hidden from relatives and friends. The words are whispered.

The patient is usually hospitalized during diagnosis and establishment of an individualized control regimen. The nurse plays a vital role as teacher and as psychotherapeutic agent during this critical transition period.

GOALS IN MANAGEMENT

1. To Maintain an Internal Physiologic Environment Capable of Supporting Cell Life. The error in metabolism of carbohydrate, fats, and protein must be corrected exogenously (from the outside). The three standard tools in the therapeutic armamentarium include diet modification, use of insulin, and/or use of oral hypoglycemic drugs. The patient with diabetes mellitus will always require diet modification; he may not require insulin or a hypoglycemic drug.

The physician chooses the degree of control suitable. For chemical control emphasis is on establishing and maintaining a normal blood sugar concentration. This requires a rigid, strictly enforced therapeutic regimen. On the other hand, clinical control places emphasis on attaining and maintaining absence of symptoms. As long as the patient remains symptom-free, a moderate blood sugar elevation is acceptable. Clinical control involves a less rigid program and an easier one for the patient to follow. It is believed that this less rigid program will be more astutely adhered to on a long-term basis than a strict regimen that might predispose to frequent "binges" by the patient.

2. To Educate the Patient So That He Can Manage to Live with the Disease Safely. The more the patient understands about the disease, the better he can care for himself. The nurse plays an important role here. The diabetic association's monthly magazine *The Forecast* helps keep patients informed. The following checklist for patient instruction was developed by the American Diabetes Association:

1. Diet
2. Urine testing
3. Action of insulin and other hypoglycemic agents
4. Technique of insulin injection and sites to use
5. Care of syringe and needle
6. Symptoms of hypoglycemia
7. Symptoms of uncontrolled diabetes
8. Care of the feet
9. What to do in case of acute complications

3. *To Avoid the Immediate Consequences of Uncontrolled Diabetes.* Prevention of diabetic ketoacidosis is the rule, here. This involves continuous medical supervision, a strong teaching program, awareness of beginning signs of acidosis, the effect of stress (infection, surgery) on the course of diabetes, and so on.

4. *To Avoid Harm Induced by Therapy.* Emphasis is on signs of too much insulin causing hypoglycemia. This often occurs when the patient suddenly exercises much more than usual. Exercise decreases the need for insulin. The condition also occurs when the patient skips meals and so on.

5. *To Prevent or Postpone Long-Term Complications of Diabetes.* Emphasis is on the changes caused by "microangiopathy," changes of the small blood vessels. This predisposes the patient to gangrene, retinal changes, kidney changes, and so on. Continuous medical supervision along with maintenance of an adequate control program is the rule here.

Diet Modification in Control of Diabetes Mellitus

The dietary prescription is determined by the physician. It is then converted by the dietitian or nutritionist into daily food allowances and a pattern of meals and refreshments based on the need to have the food eaten at appropriate times throughout the day and on the patient's customary eating habits. The patient's economic level and the availability of foods must also be considered. It is important to know what foods the patient dislikes as well as what foods he finds it difficult to live without. For instance, he may require the equivalent of a pint of skim milk a day. He may be nauseated by skim milk, but may adore buttermilk. Skim milk certainly would not be selected! Meal plans are designed to meet nutritional needs, compensate for the metabolic defect, and overcome weight problems. The physician's prescription lists the amount of protein, fat, and carbohydrate required in grams. Then, the nutritionist or dietitian uses a variety of food value tables to convert this into a daily meal and snack plan. Occasionally the nurse is called on to do this if a dietitian is not available. Use of the exchange list plan has made this a relatively simple task. (See p. 377.)

The average United States adult diet [63] contains about 60 to 70 gm of protein; 100 to 125 gm of fat; 250 to 350 gm of carbohydrate; and about 2,900 calories. It supplies 1 to 1½ gm of protein per kilogram of body weight; 1 to 2 gm of fat per kilogram body weight; and 4 to 6 gm of carbohydrate per kilogram body weight.

The average United States adult *diabetic* diet should contain 60 to 90 gm of protein (essential as a tissue builder), 85 gm of fat (a proportion supplied as a polyunsaturated fat), and 150 to 300 gm of carbohydrate. This supplies a high-normal amount of protein (at least 1 gm per kilogram of body weight); a low-normal amount of fat; and about 50 to 70 per cent of the usual amount of carbohydrate. Carbohydrate ingestion should never fall below 125 gm each day or ketogenesis occurs.[64] The carbohydrate should be derived from breads, cereals, potatoes, rice, flour, and so on. *It should not be derived from highly concentrated sugars such as syrups, table sugar, candies, and frosted cakes.* These highly concentrated forms of carbohydrate are digested very rapidly and tax the already overburdened glucose disposal mechanisms of the body. Concentrated carbohydrates also fail to supply nutritional value and serve as "empty calories." Alcohol must be counted calorically if it is ingested.

A diet relatively high in protein and fat and relatively low in carbohydrates will be associated with the greatest tendency to stability of blood sugar.[65]

As a general rule, the protein, fat, and carbohydrate should be evenly distributed throughout the day. Proper combinations of protein and fat with carbohydrate greatly lessen the hyperglycemic effect of a given amount of carbohydrate. When diet alone is required (no insulin), the total daily food allowance is divided into approximately three equal parts spaced five to six hours apart; when the patient is taking insulin, he has three regular meals plus intermediate "supplementary" feedings determined by the physician.

THE EXCHANGE LIST PLAN

The vast majority of meal plans are now based on six standardized food-exchange lists that have been developed by the American Dietetic Association in conjunction with the American Diabetes Association and the United States Public Health Service. For copies write to the American Dietetic Association, 620 North Michigan Avenue, Chicago 11, Illinois.

The patient is told how many exchanges he can have from each list every day and how many he should select from each list for each meal. This spaces the food appropriately. He can exchange foods within each list, but not between lists. Portions of food are measured with standard household measuring devices rather than weighed. The only kind of food listed in ounces is meat. Bread is listed in slices; fruits by the piece or size of piece. Patients readily learn to recognize sizes of portions.

There are six exchange lists and a variety of meal plans to fit the physician's prescription. The individual plans range from 1,200 to 3,000 calories and contain varying amounts of carbohydrate, fat, and protein in each plan using the exchange list method of food selection.

The six lists include the following:

List 1. Milk (*not* cheese). One exchange of milk contains 8 gm protein, 10 gm fat, 12 gm carbohydrate, and 170 calories. Whole milk and skim milk are listed, e.g., powdered skim milk, buttermilk, evaporated milk. If the patient selects his number of milk exchanges from skim milk rather than whole-milk products, he is allowed two additional fat exchanges.

List 2A. Vegetables containing little carbohydrate and protein and few calories. Examples include asparagus, cucumber, green beans, and cauliflower. The patient is allowed these vegetables *ad libitum* and need not count them; however, he should not eat more than 1 cup at any one time.

List 2B. Vegetables containing 2 gm protein, 7 gm carbohydrate, and 35 calories in each ½-cup portion. Examples include beets, carrots, onions, peas, collards, and turnips.

List 3. Fruit exchanges. One serving contains 10 gm carbohydrate, 40 calories. Examples include a small apple, ½ small banana, 1 cup of strawberries, and ¼ large cantaloupe.

List 4. Bread exchanges. Each exchange contains 2 gm of protein, 15 gm carbohydrate, and 70 calories. Examples include 1 slice bread, ½ to ¾ cup cereals, ½ cup rice, ½ cup grits, ½ cup macaroni, 5 saltine crackers, 2 tablespoons flour, ¼ cup baked beans, ½ cup dried peas and beans, and 1 small potato. The patient may use Italian or French bread, Jewish rye bread, pumpernickel, bagels, biscuits, cornbread, and so on, as long as each slice or piece is equal in weight to 1 oz of American packaged bread.

List 5. Meat exchanges. One meat exchange contains 7 gm protein, 5 gm fat, 75 calories. Examples include 3-oz servings of fish, beef, pork, lamb, chicken; 1 slice of cold cuts; 1 frankfurter; 1 egg; 1 slice of cheese; and 2 tablespoons peanut butter.

List 6. Fat exchanges. Each fat exchange contains 5 gm fat, 45 calories. Examples include 1 teaspoon butter or margarine, 1 teaspoon mayonnaise, 1 tablespoon cream cheese, 1 crisp slice bacon, 1 tablespoon French dressing, and 5 small olives.

Each of the exchange lists contains pictures of the servings of foods frequently selected.

SOME ADDITIONAL POINTS REGARDING FOODS

1. Avoid overeating or undereating. Eat meals and snacks at about the same time every day. Never skip a meal.

2. Add water to reconstitute condensed soups. If milk is used, it must be included as a milk exchange.

3. Select at least one citrus fruit from the fruit-exchange list each day.

4. Many exchanges may be combined to make up special dishes, e.g., macaroni and cheese, beef stew. The ingredients must conform to the total number of exchanges allowed. They must be counted. Beef stew is an example. It might contain:

2 meat exchanges
1 bread (potato) exchange
2 fat exchanges
1 vegetable, list 2B (½ cup peas)
1 cup vegetable, list 2A (green pepper)

TABLE 35–1. A DIABETIC MEAL PLAN USING THE EXCHANGE LIST METHOD *

Meal Plan for _____

Carbohydrate_____ Protein_____ Fat_____ Calories_____

Your Food for the Day

Amount	Kind of Food	Choose From
_____	Milk	List 1
Any Amount	Vegetable exchanges A	List 2A
_____	Vegetable exchanges B	List 2B
_____	Fruit exchanges	List 3
_____	Bread exchanges	List 4
_____	Meat exchanges	List 5
_____	Fat exchanges	List 6

Divide this food as follows:
Your Meal Plan

Breakfast:

Lunch or supper:

Dinner or main meal:

Bedtime meal:

---

* American Dietetic Association and American Diabetes Association, *Meal Planning with Exchange Lists*. American Diabetes Association, New York, 1950.

Coleslaw is another example. It might contain:

1 cup group-A vegetable (cabbage)
1 fat exchange (1 teaspoon mayonnaise)

5. Desserts can be calculated so that the patient feels less restriction in his diet. Fruit shortcake is an example. It must be included as part of the daily allotment; avoid use of concentrated sugars.

6. Many foods are unrestricted. Seasonings such as oregano, pepper, parsley, allspice, and lemon rind are examples. Dill or sour pickles, unsweetened gelatin, and sugar substitutes are included. Sugar substitutes, e.g., saccharin, come in tablets, **powder, and liquid form and can be used**

in cooking. Cyclamates, e.g., Sucaryl, should only be used with physician's prescription.

7. Use alcoholic beverages only with the physician's permission. A drink often "delays" a meal, and it is important that the patient eat about the same time each day, especially if he is taking insulin. If alcohol is used, it must be calculated as part of the daily food allotment.

8. A source reference for calculation of foods not commonly found in the American diet is A. Bowes and C. F. Church, *Food Values of Portions Commonly Used* (J. B. Lippincott Co., Philadelphia, 1963). For gourmet recipes see E. and J. Gibbons, *Feast on a Diabetic Diet* (David McKay Co., Inc., New York).

DIETETIC FOODS

These are specially prepared foods that contain no sugar. They may, however, contain other carbohydrate, protein, and fat. Most contain some calories. Therefore, they must be calculated as part of the daily food allotment if they are used. Some dietetic foods include water-packed fruits, puddings made with artificial sweeteners, sodas, and special breads and cakes. They may aid in varying the diet but they do tend to be expensive. *They cannot be used ad libitum!* Their labels should be scrutinized carefully to determine content.

Insulin

Insulin is the hormone produced by the beta cells of the islets of Langerhans in the pancreas. It is commercially derived from beef or pork pancreas. Discovered in 1921 by Sir Fredrick Grant Banting and Dr. Charles Herbert Best, it has prolonged and saved the lives of diabetics who were otherwise doomed to a sick, nonproductive life and an early death. It has recently been synthesized chemically. This is beneficial to the small percentage of people who develop an antigenic response to the injection of the natural animal protein.[66]

The production and packaging of insulin are universally standardized. Each bottle has a specific amount (10 ml), shape (round for regular, PZI, and globin; square for NPH; and round with six-sided shoulders for the lente), and label color. Concentrations containing 80 units per 1 ml have green and white labels and a green stopper. Concentrations containing 40 units per milliliter have red and white labels and a red stopper. Insulin comes in greater concentrations; however, the U40 and U80 are the most frequently used. If more than 40 units are to be injected, the U80 concentration is selected so that the total volume for the single injection is not too great.

Insulin should not be submitted to extremes in temperature. It should be stored in the refrigerator. The bottle being used can be kept at room temperature. It should be protected from extremes in light.

RAPID-ACTING INSULINS

Regular; Unmodified; Regular Iletin. The oldest form of insulin has nothing added to it to prolong its action in the body. It is a clear solution and works rapidly. It has its onset in one to one and one-half hours and lasts six to eight hours. It is frequently used when the patient is being initially regulated for insulin dosage. It does not have to be mixed because it is not a suspension.

Prompt Insulin Zinc Suspension; Semilente Insulin; Semilente Iletin. This insulin has an "S" superimposed on the colored printing. Its action is similar to that of regular insulin with onset in one and one-half to two hours and a duration of 12 to 18 hours. It does not come from pork pancreas and is, therefore, suitable for people who are allergic to pork products. It should be mixed by rotating it in the hands.

INTERMEDIATE-ACTING INSULINS

These and long-acting insulins have substances (protamine, globin, histone) added to them to extend their duration of action.

Isophane Insulin Suspension; Neutral Protamine Hagedorn Insulin (NPH). This is a cloudy suspension of crystals of insulin, protamine (a protein), and zinc. It must be mixed (rotated in the hands, not shaken) before use. It best suits the needs of the greatest number of diabetics. Its onset of action is one to two hours and its duration is 20 to 32 hours.

Insulin Zinc Suspension; Lente Insulin, Lente Iletin. This is a cloudy solution that has an "L" superimposed on its label. It must be mixed. Its action is similar to that of NPH, but it contains only insulin and zinc, no protein. Therefore, it tends to be less allergenic. It does not come from pork pancreas. It has its onset of action in one to two hours and lasts 26 to 30 hours.

LONG-ACTING INSULINS; EXTENDED INSULIN ZINC SUSPENSION; ULTRALENTE INSULIN, ULTRALENTE ILETIN

This is a cloudy, milky suspension that must be mixed. It has a "U" superimposed on its label. Its action is slower and longer than lente insulin. It has no protein added to it and is less allergenic than other insulins. It does not come from pork pancreas. Its onset is five to eight hours and its duration 34 to 36 hours.

Protamine Zinc Insulin Suspension, Protamine Zinc Iletin, PZI. This is a cloudy, milky suspension that must be mixed. It has its onset in seven hours and a duration of 24 to 36 hours.

REGULATING THE PATIENT ON INSULIN

This is a tricky task. The patient is usually hospitalized for initial therapy and instruction. To begin, about 10 units of regular, unmodified insulin is given before breakfast. Tests of blood and urine are done. If indicated, then, additional small amounts of regular insulin are given before other meals and at bedtime. If tests indicate that the patient cannot be maintained on diet alone, or on diet and an oral hypoglycemic agent, the total amount of regular insulin administered is calculated, and the physician tries a single before-breakfast dose of one of the intermediate-acting forms. The goal is to decrease the number of injections needed on a daily basis while maintaining adequate control.

If the patient continues to spill sugar after meals, he may require supplemental injections of regular insulin, or if he spills the sugar after breakfast, a mixture of regular and intermediate insulin. If the blood sugar rises during the night, a long-acting form may be used. The program is custom-designed for the individual patient. It is not a static, once-and-for-all program. Insulin needs change, and the patient must always continue to have medical supervision.

Quick-acting insulins are given about 20 to 30 minutes before meals; longer-acting insulins may be given at the time of the meal or immediately after it.[68]

COMBINING INSULINS

Insulins may be mixed in a single syringe. Strengths used should be the same. Unmodified, regular insulin is drawn into the syringe first so that it is not contaminated by a modified form. If regular insulin is mixed with PZI insulin, the proportion must be at least 2 parts regular to 1 part PZI or the regular insulin does not act. This proportion is not required if regular and NPH insulins are mixed, or if lentes are mixed.[69]

ROTATING THE BOTTLE OF INSULIN

All insulins except regular and globin are cloudy suspensions and should be rotated in the hands before use. The bottle should not be shaken.

INSULIN AND EXERCISE

Insulin dosage is regulated according to the patient's normal exercise pattern. If exercise should increase, the amount of insulin required decreases. The physician usually advises the patient to eat an additional amount of food if he knows he is going to exercise more than usual.

INSULIN AND STRESS

Any stress situation increases the amount of insulin required, and the patient should always have medical supervision during stressful periods. Examples of stress include illness and infection, pregnancy, and surgery.

INSULIN AND MEALS

When regular insulin is used, the patient is allowed three meals a day, five to six hours apart. When intermediate and long-acting forms of insulin are used, an additional midmorning, midafternoon, and bedtime snack may be used. Fruit and a glass of milk are examples. The bedtime snack, especially if the patient is taking a long-acting form of insulin, should contain a combination of carbohydrate, protein, and fat. A bowl of cereal and milk or crackers and cheese serve well. These snacks must be included in the total amount of food allowed. No meals should be skipped.

INSULIN REACTION (HYPOGLYCEMIA, TOO MUCH INSULIN)

An insulin reaction occurs when the patient has too much insulin in his body, or too little food. This is a hypoglycemic reaction. Hypoglycemia develops when there is less than 60 mg of glucose per 100 ml of blood. Symptoms may occur quickly if the reaction stems from a quick-acting insulin. They occur more insidiously when caused by a longer-acting preparation. *Never ignore a patient's subjective statement,* "I don't know what's the matter; I just don't feel right!"

An insulin reaction may develop as a result of a missed meal or delay in eating the meal, from undue amounts of exercise especially in hot weather, from an error in measuring insulin dosage, or from gastrointestinal upset with vomiting and/or diarrhea, and so on. The patient may be brought to the hospital looking drunk. Symptoms include nervousness, fatigue, weakness, sweating, tremors, hunger, blurred or double vision, tingling in hands, pallor, a decrease in blood pressure with an increase or decrease in pulse, headache, and nausea.

As an immediate measure, if the patient is conscious, the nurse should give some form of concentrated carbohydrate. It takes about 20 to 25 gm of carbohydrate to overcome an insulin reaction.[70] This amount is contained in 4 teaspoons of granulated sugar, or in the juice of two oranges. Orange juice or grape juice with an added teaspoon of sugar is satisfactory, as is Coca-Cola.

If the patient is not conscious, a blood specimen is taken immediately. The physician administers 1 ml of intramuscular or intravenous glucagon (the hyperglycemic pancreatic hormone), epinephrine (it promotes glycogenolysis and hyperglycemia), and intravenous glucose solutions. Five per cent glucose in 1,000 ml Ringer's solution is an example.

Sometimes the diagnosis of hypo- or hyperglycemia is difficult to make; however, insulin is not administered until two successive urines show sugar, or there is a blood sugar elevation.

ADMINISTERING INSULIN

Official insulin syringes are available in long and short types (long are easier to read); 1- and 2-ml sizes; exclusively for U40 or U80 concentrations, or containing a U40 and a U80 side; disposable or permanent. Needles should be ⅜, ½, or ⅝ in. long, 25 to 26 gauge. (See Fig. 35–1.)

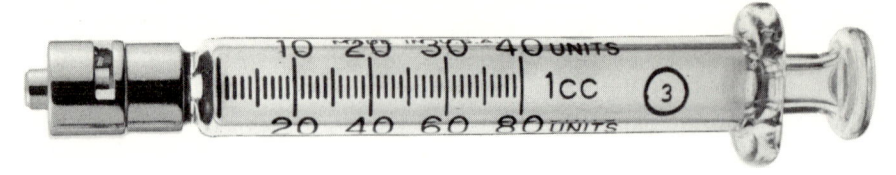

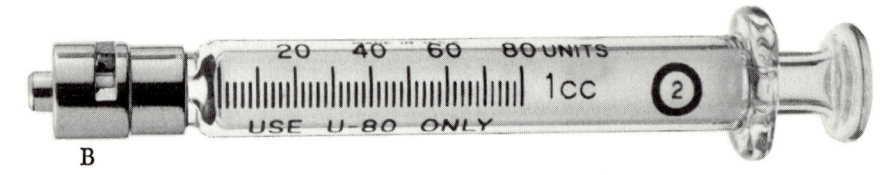

FIGURE 35-1. Insulin syringes. A. Syringe has a U40 and a U80 side. B. Syringe has only a U80 side. (Courtesy of Becton-Dickinson, Rutherford, N.J.)

If U40 concentration is used, only the U40 side of the syringe can be used to draw up the insulin. If U80 concentration is used, only the U80 side of the syringe can be used to draw up the dosage.

Insulin is injected subcutaneously, but at a right 90-degree angle with the needle perpendicular to the skin. This angle decreases the chance of developing lipodystrophy, a common sequel to long-term injections. There is swelling in the subcutaneous fat followed by tissue atrophy.

No two injections should be closer than 1 in. to each other within a two-week period.[71] The same injection site should not be used again for two weeks. Redness, stinging, and itching after injection may indicate an allergic response. Seen most often when the patient first begins injections, it is self-limiting and not serious.

Injection Sites. The upper arms, thighs, abdomen, and buttocks are good sites. If the thigh is used, count about five fingers above the knee and use the anterior or lateral aspect. If the upper arm is used, start about three fingers below the shoulder to about five fingers above the elbow; any area of the abdomen can be used below the umbilicus; and any area of the buttocks can be used. The same site should not be used again for two weeks. Sites are rotated. (See Fig. 35-2.)

Teaching the Patient to Administer Insulin. Most patients, given proper instruction and a patient instructor, can learn to inject themselves. This is advantageous because it avoids the need to be dependent on someone else. The patient must show some evidence that he is ready to learn. Then, the nurse works with him to develop mutual goals. Goals cannot be met all at once, and a schedule of appointments with the patient over several days with the same nurse best accomplishes them. Several appointments

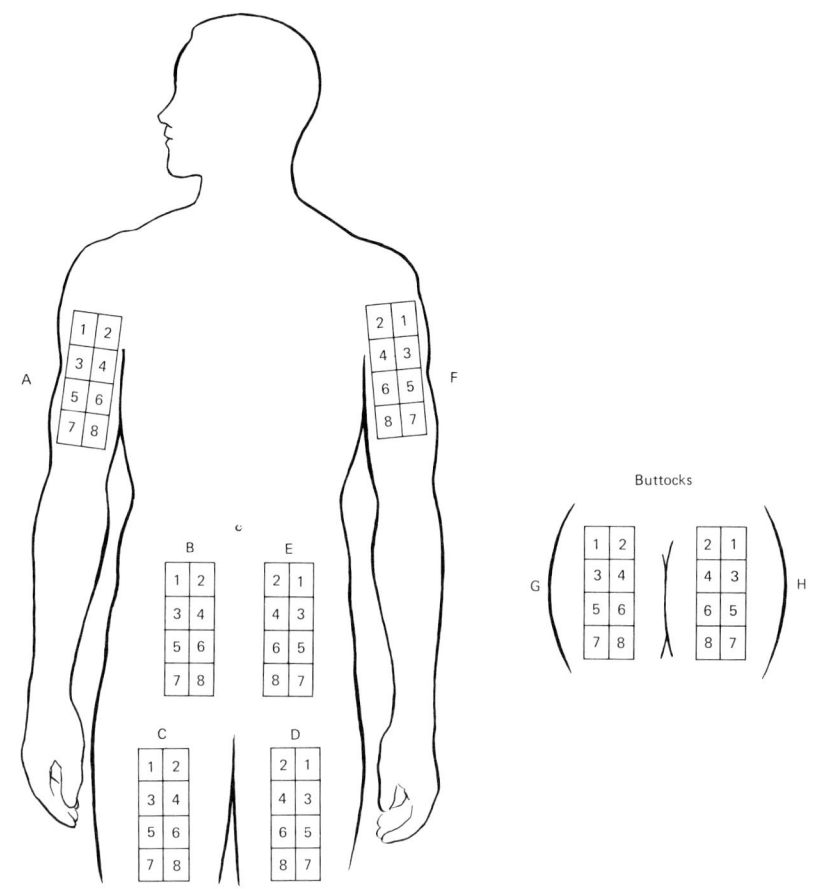

FIGURE 35-2. Insulin injection sites should be rotated using a planned pattern.

are needed to talk about how the patient feels about diabetes, what the disease means physiologically, what the diet is all about, how to test the urine, and so on.

When the patient is ready to begin learning how to give himself the insulin, bring him a bottle of real insulin, show him the label, and explain what U40 (or U80) means. Show him the syringe so that he can see what 1 ml really means (this is a strange measurement to him) and let him see the U40 and U80 side. Let him begin handling the syringe and show him how to draw up solution. Label a bottle of physiologic saline "contaminated" and leave it and the syringe at the bedside so he can practice with them. Remember how long it took you to feel comfortable with the skill! This author has found it valuable to inject herself with ½ ml of sterile normal saline as a method of showing the patient the technique and showing him that "someone can really do it to himself." If he seems ready, let him draw up and inject his own insulin into his thigh the next morning. Be positive. A statement like, "You try it today, Mr. Brown." is better than, "Do you want to try it?" If he refuses, do not punish him by your disapproving attitude. Try again the next day. Let him feel that you really believe he can do it. When he does inject himself, praise him.

Once the patient is home, the visiting nurse should provide follow-up guidance. Equipment is an individual matter. Discuss this with the physician first. He may have some preferences. Disposable syringes and needles are available. The patient may purchase a package containing one disposable syringe and 30 needles, or 30 needles and syringes. A nondisposable syringe should be boiled for five minutes at least once a week (a strainer and saucepan are all that is needed) and stored in a syringe holder containing 70 per cent ethyl or isopropyl alcohol. Kits are available containing everything the patient needs to inject the insulin and store the syringe.

An automatic insulin injector called the Busher syringe is available. (See Fig. 35-3.) The physician may want the patient to use this if he is extremely reluctant to inject himself with the regular insulin syringe. The patient needs practice in setting the Busher syringe if he is going to use it.

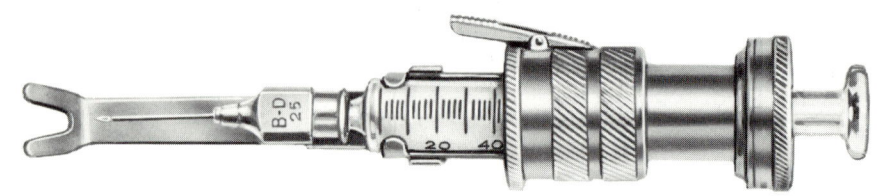

FIGURE 35-3. Busher automatic insulin injector. (Courtesy, Becton-Dickinson, Rutherford, N.J.)

Oral Hypoglycemic Drugs

These drugs, used in conjunction with proper dietary control, are effective in lowering blood sugar in some diabetic patients. Older, maturity-onset diabetics seem to be the best candidates. Oral hypoglycemics are not effective if the diabetes is "brittle" or "juvenile-onset" type. Oral hypoglycemics may be used in conjuction with insulin. Remember:

They are not oral insulins.
They do not replace insulin if insulin is needed.
They do not eliminate the need for dietary control.

The sulfonylureas (acetohexamide, Dymelor; chlorpropamide, Diabinese; tolazamide, Tolinase) and tolbutamide (Orinase) were the first to be utilized. These drugs stimulate release of endogenous (within the person's body) insulin by the pancreatic beta cells. The patient must have some functioning pancreatic tissue.

The more recent biguanides (phenformin; DBI) do not seem to require remaining pancreatic function. They may act on other tissues to step up utilization of glucose, but their action remains uncertain. DBI is given after meals because it may cause nausea. Others are given before meals.

Hypoglycemic reactions are not seen often; however, they may occur when hypoglycemic drugs are combined.

The patient should understand that a stress situation might require the temporary use of insulin to re-establish control.

Special Needs of the Diabetic

CARE OF THE FEET

The feet are affected by the condition of the circulation more than any other part of the body. Any unusual condition of the feet should be reported to the physician. This includes swelling, pain, soreness, changes in color of the skin, burning, and cramping. Gangrene is always a threat.

Feet should have a daily soak in warm soapy water for five minutes. They should be dried thoroughly with a soft Turkish towel and powdered well between the toes. Toenails should be cut straight across. Clean socks or stockings should be used every day. They should be ½ in. longer than the length of the foot. They should not be bulky. Shoes should fit properly. They should allow the feet to rest in the natural position for freedom of movement and support of body weight. New shoes should be "broken in" by wearing them only for short periods of time initially. No rolled stocking or circular garters should ever be used. No corn remedies should be used unless specifically advised by the physician. If the feet tend to be dry, lanolin can be massaged in gently; however, it should not be used between the toes where remaining moisture predisposes to bacterial growth. The physician may order daily Buerger-Allen exercises to improve circulation. (See p. 287.)

The Diabetic Emergency

KETOACIDOSIS (HYPERGLYCEMIA; DIABETIC ACIDOSIS; DIABETIC COMA)

In this condition (already described on p. 370) the diabetes is completely out of control. The condition may have been caused by gross indiscretions in diet, omission of insulin, diarrhea or vomiting, or severe stress. Or, the patient may have been unaware he was a diabetic. In any event, he is brought to the hospital extremely sick and possibly unconscious. He is dehydrated and is in severe electrolyte imbalance.

The physician must ascertain, through blood analysis and clinical symptoms, whether the patient is in acidosis or whether he is experiencing a reaction to too much insulin. (See Table 35–2.)

TABLE 35–2. SYMPTOMS OF HYPO- AND HYPERGLYCEMIA

	Hypoglycemia *Too Much Insulin* *Insulin Reaction* *Insulin Shock*	*Hyperglycemia* *Too Little Insulin* *Ketoacidosis* *Diabetic Acidosis*
Onset	Sudden or slow	Slow
Skin	Pale, moist, cool	Flushed, hot, dry
Behavior	Excited, nervous	Drowsy
Breath	Normal	Smells of acetone
Respirations	Normal to rapid; shallow	Air hunger; Kussmaul respirations
Pulse	Increased or decreased	Rapid, weak
Blood pressure	Elevated or normal	Low
Vomiting	Absent	Present
Hunger	Present	Absent
Thirst	Absent	Present
Urinary sugar	Absent in second specimen	Large amounts

Immediate goals of treatment include controlling overproduction of ketone bodies, restoring the ability of the cells to use glucose, and overcoming the water and electrolyte imbalance. Intravenous solutions are started. Five per cent glucose in Ringer's solutions is an example. Potassium may be added. Once the diagnosis is definitely ketoacidosis, quick-acting insulin is given intravenously or intramuscularly. B vitamins are given because they are not stored by the body and are lost with the polyuria. Blood pressures are taken every 30 minutes to determine the state of the circulation; and electrocardiograms may be done to determine the effect of hypopotassemia on the heart. The patient may be catheterized so that hourly urine samples can be checked for glucose. Sometimes, gastric aspiration with warm physiologic saline is done to decrease the chance of aspiration of vomitus and to facilitate earlier oral intake.[72] If the patient has not had a bowel movement in the last 24 hours, a low physiologic saline enema might be administered.

Unless treatment for acidosis is instituted promptly, the water and electrolyte losses and the drop in blood volume from dehydration may lead to irreversible coma and death.

36

SEX STEROIDS

A Word About the Sex Steroids

Under the influence of anterior pituitary gonadotropins the ovaries produce the female sex hormones estrogen and progesterone, and the testes produce the male sex hormone (androgens) testosterone. Because of their effect on functioning of all body tissue, as well as their specific genital effect, they will be briefly discussed in this text.

Female Hormones

Estrogen and progesterone set the stage for childbearing. Estrogen is secreted by the maturing ovarian follicle. Increasing estrogen levels cause the proliferative "priming" stage of uterine endometrium development. The endometrium is made thicker and more vascular. The peak estrogen level occurs at about day 14 of the menstrual cycle at which time the ovarian follicle ruptures and an ovum is discharged. After the ovum is discharged, the ruptured follicle is transformed into a small body filled with yellow fluid called corpus luteum.[73] Corpus luteum produces another hormone, progesterone. Also called "the pregnancy hormone," it further prepares an estrogen-primed endometrium for possible implantation with a fertilized ovum. If fertilization occurs, progesterone continues to be secreted throughout the pregnancy, now by the placenta. Whether or not fertilization occurs, the progesterone causes a "secretory stage" in which the endometrium of the uterus is especially suited for implantation and nourishment of a fertilized ovum. Then, rising levels of estrogen and progesterone signal the pituitary to cease gonadotropic hormone secretion (the feedback mechanism), and the corpus luteum shrivels and dies. This is called the "sloughing state." Menstruation occurs.

Female sex hormones also stimulate tissue-building (anabolic) processes, aid in maintaining the mineral content of bones, tend to keep plasma cholesterol levels low and skin elastic, maintain the thickness of the vaginal tract mucosa, and stimulate growth of the mammary gland ducts and alveoli. Estrogens tend to cause sodium and water retention; progesterones tend to cause sodium and water excretion.[74]

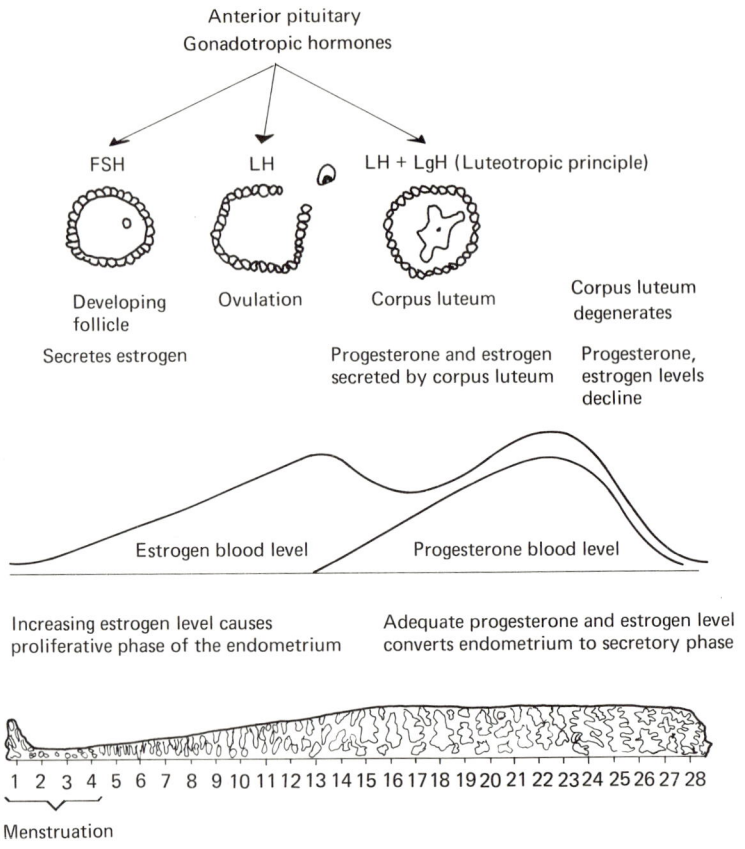

FIGURE 36–1. Simplified version of the normal menstrual cycle. (Courtesy, Upjohn Co., Kalamazoo, Mich.)

Male Hormones

Testosterone is produced by the testes. Responsible for much of the sexual development and growth seen in boys at puberty, testosterone has both sexual and metabolic function. With pituitary gonadotropins, it helps maintain sperm production and male characteristics (deep voice, body hair, etc.), and it stimulates tissue-building processes (anabolic activity) while decreasing tissue breakdown (catabolic activity).

Knowledge of these sexual and general metabolic hormonal functions has led to the use of hormones for treatment of menstrual disorders, infertility, menopause (natural and artificial), abortion, and contraception. Hormones are used to cause remissions and relief of the pain in carcinoma, to treat undersecretion of male sex hormone (hypogonadism), and to promote an anabolic, protein-building effect. It is used to counteract the catabolic effect of corticosteroids that cause osteoporosis. Some hormones currently in use include estrogens (estradiol, estriol, mestranol), synthetic estrogens (benzestrol, diethylstilbestrol), progestational steroids (progesterone), and androgenic agents (testosterone, Ethylestrenol). Testosterone is especially indicated for women in instances where estrogen therapy would be dangerous. The patient who has carcinoma with bony metastasis is a prime candidate. Large amounts of testosterone may cause masculinization signs.

A Word About Menopause

The average woman outlives her ovaries by 25 years.[75] There is ovarian hormone deficiency. Menopause occurs when these hormones are insufficient to ripen the endometrial tissue. It can occur as a natural process of aging or can be caused artificially by removal of the ovaries (bilateral oophorectomy, panhysterectomy) or radiation therapy. Menopause can be a rapid or a gradual process. In either case, symptoms stem from suppression of circulating estrogen and include patchy redness of the skin, disturbed sleep, fatigue, emotional lability (the person tends to "fly off the handle") and hypersensitivity, "hot flashes," and so on. Some women cope with these changes more easily than others. Long-term effects of estrogen deficiency include the degeneration and atrophy of the urogenital tract, breasts, blood vessels, and bones. The patient becomes "atherosclerosis-prone." Ovaries used to be removed with much the same freedom as tonsils and appendices;[76] however, removal of the ovaries at hysterectomy was found to cause a fourfold increase in degree of coronary artery degeneration.[77]

Many physicians view menopause as a needless syndrome and prescribe long-term estrogen therapy, often continuing for the patient's entire life. Others believe menopause to be a normal physiologic period that requires no exogenous replacement of hormones.

If estrogen is used, enough must be given to achieve well-being and prevent body changes. If endometrial shedding (menstruation) is desired (if the patient has a uterus), a progesterone compound is added to the estrogen for about five days in the month. Menstruation is an excellent monitor of ovarian and uterine function and is usually accepted by older women being treated with the combined hormone. Menstruation occurs two or three days after the progesterone-containing tablet is taken. The patient knows when she will menstruate.

Steroid Combinations to Prevent Conception

These agents mimic the normal estrogen-progesterone cycle. They suppress ovulation by reducing the secretion of gonadotropic hormones produced by the anterior pituitary gland. They contain a progestin in combination with an estrogen. They are prepared as single tablets taken orally for 20 days beginning on the fifth day after the onset of menstruation and ending on the twenty-fourth day, or as two tablets with one containing only estrogen and one an estrogen-progestin combination. They are taken in a "sequential" regimen. The estrogen is taken for 15 days and is followed by the combined tablet for five days. When the tablet is withdrawn, the endometrium, prepared by the progestin, sheds, and the patient menstruates. Examples of these oral contraceptives include chlormadinone and mestranol (C-Quens); ethynodiol and mestranol (Ovulen); and norethynodrel and mestranol (Enovid E). They are contraindicated in patients with thrombophlebitis or who have a history of cancer.

REFERENCES

1. Beland, I., *Clinical Nursing: Pathophysiological and Psychosocial Approaches*. The Macmillan Co., New York, 1965, p. 1021.
2. *Ibid.*, p. 1021.
3. Brown, J., and Barker, S., *Basic Endocrinology*. F. A. Davis Co., Philadelphia, 1966, p. 2.
4. Rodman, M., and Smith, D., *Pharmacology and Drug Therapy in Nursing*. J. B. Lippincott Co., Philadelphia, 1968, p. 4.
5. Schaeffer, K., Sawyer, J., McCluskey, A., and Beck, E., *Medical-Surgical Nursing*. C. V. Mosby Co., St. Louis, 1967, p. 729.
6. Beland, *op. cit.*, p. 1026.
7. Brown, *op. cit.*, p. 23.
8. Frohman, L., Mac Gilliuray, M., and Aceto, T., "Acute Effects of Human Growth Hormone on Insulin Secretion and Glucose Utilization in Normal and Growth Hormone Deficient Subjects," *J. Clin. Endocr.*, **27**:561, Apr. 1967.
9. *Time Magazine*, Time, Inc., New York, Aug. 2, 1968, p. 53.
10. Brown, *op. cit.*, p. 52.
11. Di Palma, J., "The Pituitary Hormones: Potential Wonder Workers," *RN*, **29**:72, Jan. 1966.
12. Hawken, P.: "Hypophysectomy with Yttrium 90," *Amer. J. Nurs.*, **65**:122, Oct. 1965.
13. Rodman, *op. cit.*, p. 13.
14. Brown, *op. cit.*, p. 14.
15. Rodman, *op. cit.*, p. 15.
16. *Ibid.*, p. 16.
17. Smith, D., and Gipps, C., *Care of the Adult Patient*. J. B. Lippincott Co., Philadelphia, 1966, p. 787.
18. Hazard, J., and Smith, D. (eds.), International Academy of Pathology Monograph, *The Thyroid*, Williams and Wilkins Co., Baltimore, 1964, p. 49.
19. French, R., *Nurse's Guide to Diagnostic Procedures*. McGraw-Hill Book Co., New York, 1962, p. 19.
20. Sister Mariana Garde, "Cancer of the Thyroid," *Amer. J. Nurs.*, **65**:100, Nov. 1965.
21. *Ibid.*, p. 100.
22. French, *op. cit.*, p. 22.
23. Smith, D., *op. cit.*, p. 777.
24. Hazard, *op. cit.*, p. 100–107.
25. *Ibid.*, p. 102.
26. Rodman, *op. cit.*, p. 425.
27. Derby, A., "Surgical Approach to Disease of the Thyroid Gland," *Canad. Nurse*, **61**:878, Nov. 1965.
28. Artunkal, S., and Togrol, B., "Psychological Studies in Hyperthyroidism," in *Brain-Thyroid Relationships*. Little, Brown and Co., Boston, 1964, p. 92.
29. *Ibid.*, p. 95.
30. Brown, *op. cit.*, p. 36.

31. Smith, S., "Drugs and the Thyroid Gland," *Nurs. Times*, **63**:186, Feb. 10, 1967.
32. Smith, D., *op. cit.*, p. 777.
33. Rodman, *op. cit.*, p. 428.
34. Derby, *op. cit.*, p. 878.
35. Smith, S., *op. cit.*, p. 35.
36. Sister Mariana Garde, *op. cit.*, p. 98.
37. Derby, *op. cit.*, p. 37.
38. Beland, *op. cit.*, p. 1048.
39. Smith, D., *op. cit.*, p. 39.
40. Beland, *op. cit.*, p. 1050.
41. Rasmussen, H., "Parathyroid Hormone—Nature and Mechanism of Action," *Amer. J. Med.*, **30**:41, 1961.
42. Dutcher, I., and Fielo, S., *Water and Electrolytes: Implications for Nursing Practice*. The Macmillan Co., New York, 1967, p. 120.
43. Rodman, *op. cit.*, p. 637.
44. Dutcher, *op. cit.*, p. 121.
45. Rosenthal, H., and Rosenthal, J., *Diabetic Care in Pictures*. J. B. Lippincott Co., Philadelphia, 1960, p. 1.
46. Martin, M., "Diabetes Mellitus: Current Concepts," *Amer. J. Nurs.*, **66**: 510, Mar. 1966.
47. *Ibid.*, p. 511.
48. Brown, *op. cit.*, p. 175.
49. Ralli, E., *The Management of the Diabetic Patient*. G. P. Putnam's Sons, New York, 1965, p. 1.
50. Brown, *op. cit.*, p. 175.
51. Joslin, E., Root, H., White, P. and Marble, A., *The Treatment of Diabetes Mellitus*. Lea and Febiger, Philadelphia, 1959, p. 19.
52. Rosenthal, *op. cit.*, p. 4.
53. Ralli, *op. cit.*, p. 2.
54. Martin, *op cit.*, p. 512.
55. Root, H., "Diabetic Ketoacidosis and Coma," *Hosp. Med.*, **2**:69, Sept. 1966.
56. Smith, D., *op. cit.*, p. 794.
57. Dutcher, *op. cit.*, p. 50.
58. Joslin, *op. cit.*, p. 101.
59. Hamwi, G., and Danowshki, T. (eds.), *Diabetes Mellitus: Diagnosis and Treatment*. American Diabetes Association, New York, 1967, p. 45.
60. *Ibid.*, p. 48.
61. French, *op. cit.*, p. 66.
62. Hamwi, *op. cit.*, p. 52.
63. Ralli, *op. cit.*, p. 6.
64. Hamwi, *op. cit.*, p. 52.
65. *Ibid.*, p. 97.
66. Martin, *op. cit.*, p. 510.
67. Rodman, *op. cit.*, p. 437.
68. Ralli, *op. cit.*, p. 48.
69. Hamwi, *op. cit.*, p. 102.
70. Rosenthal, *op. cit.*, p. 138.
71. Smith, D., *op. cit.*, p. 801.
72. Dutcher, *op. cit.*, p. 49.
73. Smith, D., *op. cit.*, p. 819.
74. Rodman, *op. cit.*, p. 405.
75. McEwen, D., "Estrogen Replacement Therapy at Menopause," *Canad. Nurse*, **63**:34, Feb. 1967.
76. Fortier, L., "The Role of Hormones in Gynecology," *Canad. Nurse*, **61**:815, Oct. 1965.
77. McEwen, *op. cit.*, p. 35.

ADDITIONAL READINGS

BECK, R., "Synthetic Progestational Compounds," *Canad. Nurse*, **61**:953, Dec. 1965.

BIRNSTINGL, M., "Subtotal Thyroidectomy," *Nurs. Times*, **63**:1332, Oct. 6, 1967.

BLANCHET, J., "Estrogen and the Menopause," *Canad. Nurse*, **63**:38, Feb. 1967.

CAMERON, M., and O'CONNOR, M. (eds.), *Brain Thyroid Relationships with Special Reference to Thyroid Disorders*. Little, Brown and Co., Boston, 1964.

DUNCAN, G., "Management of Diabetes During Surgical Complication," *Hosp. Med.*, **1**:14, Sept. 1965.

HAGANS, H., "Some Offbeat Techniques of Postthyroidectomy Care," *RN*, **27**:51, Oct. 1964.

KAUFMAN, M., "The Many Dimensions of Diet Counseling for Diabetics," *Amer. J. Clin. Nutr.*, **15**:45, July 1964.

KAUFMAN, M., "A Food Preference Questionnaire for Counseling Patients with Diabetes," *J. Amer. Dietet. Ass.*, **49**:31, July 1966.

KUMAHARA, Y., IWATSUBO, H., MIYAI, K., MASUI, H., FUKUCKI, M., and ABE, H., "Abnormal Thyrotropic Substance in the Pituitaries of Patients with Graves Disease," *J. Clin. Endoc.* **27**:333, Mar. 1967.

LAPOINTE, R., "Premenstrual Tension," *Canad. Nurse*, **61**:805, Oct. 1965.

NEVINS, C., "Acute Tracheal Collapse Following Thyroidectomy," *J. Amer. Ass. Nurs. Anesth.*, **35**:287, Aug. 1967.

SCHLETTER, F., CLEFT, G., MEYER, R., and STREETEN, D., "Cushing's Syndrome in Childhood: Report of Two Cases with Bilateral Adrenocortical Hyperplasia Showing Distinctive Clinical Features." *J. Clin. Endocr.*, **27**:22, Jan. 1967.

WHITELOCK, D. (ed.), "The Effects of the Sulfonylureas and Related Compounds in Experimental and Clinical Diabetes," *Ann. N.Y. Acad. Sci.*, **71**:71, July 10, 1957.

WOLSTENHOLME, G., and PORTER, R. (eds.), *The Human Adrenal Cortex: Its Function Throughout Life*. Little, Brown and Co., Boston, 1967.

UNIT VIII

THE PATIENT WITH A PROBLEM IN NEUROLOGIC-ORTHOPEDIC CONTINUITY

37

REHABILITATION

What Is Rehabilitation?

Neurologic-orthopedic problems stem from interference with the smooth-functioning "sending-receiving-interpreting-fulfilling" message system of the body. There is interruption somewhere in this administrative network. The patient cannot command his body to function easily and with little thought as to "how." The fulfillment of familiar, routine tasks becomes a major endeavor. Mobility is jeopardized, exposing the patient to the life-threatening hazards of immobility. Many disease entities, though of diverse cause, produce comparable neurologic-orthopedic deficits.

The patient is a candidate for rehabilitation if, after thorough evaluation, it is estimated that his disability can be modified to the extent that he can learn to function in a satisfactory, although very different, manner. He is helped to make maximum use of his residual abilities. This process may involve strengthening commonly used muscles or learning to harness the power of infrequently used muscles for routine tasks. It may mean protecting or assisting weak muscles with braces, crutches, or other similar devices. In any case, the goals set are flexible and are realistic for the patient. *Goals are based on the understanding that some injuries leave permanent, irreversible disability.*

Rehabilitation involves the coordinated effort of many people and requires active involvement and participation by the patient. Because people vary in their response to disability, it is difficult to determine the point at which they become actively involved and truly accept the purpose of rehabilitation. The team is headed by the physiatrist, a physician who specializes in the use of physical agents (water, heat, electricity) in working with enduring, pervasive disabilities. Also participating on the team are other physicians and surgeons, rehabilitation nurses, physical therapists, psychologists and psychiatrists, nutritionists, vocational, recreational and speech therapists, and social workers. The joint effort of these members is directed toward increasing the patient's assets and substituting new methods for achieving old activities. The work is hard and tedious. The most minor achievements require tremendous effort and unbelievable patience.

The field of rehabilitation medicine is a growing one. More people reach and must contend with the disability diseases of old age; more people are involved in fast-moving vehicular accidents; and more men receive disabling war injuries. The process of rehabilitation begins as soon as the patient is admitted to the general hospital, for it is here that many of the disabling residual effects of immobility can be prevented, and an optimistic attitude can be nurtured. Rehabilitation then progresses to involve treatment in an extended-care hospital, a specialized hospital, and/or an outpatient department. The major goal is the return of the patient to his home and community. Long-term dependence on the rehabilitation agency is discouraged.

Rusk [1] has summarized basic principles of rehabilitation treatment, regardless of the cause of the disability, as follows:

1. Evaluate each person and plan an individualized program for him, by prescription.
2. Prevent deformities by immobilizing affected parts in optimal position, supervising bed posture, avoiding unnecessary fixation of joints, maintaining function of uninjured parts, and stimulating muscles that cannot move.
3. Mobilize as early as possible without jeopardizing healing because mobility preserves joint range, prevents permanent scar formation, retards atrophy, and disperses edema.
4. Relieve pain before doing therapeutic exercise with heat, massage, and medication.
5. Protect muscle weakness by avoiding activities of which there is no chance of accomplishment, by splinting and bracing, and so on.
6. Treat weak muscles specifically with selective re-education and avoidance of muscle fatigue.
7. Treat joints gently by avoiding forced motion, by not placing resistance against swollen joints, and by combining rest with short periods of motion.
8. Begin weight bearing as early as possible.

Evaluating the Patient

The evaluation is a lengthy procedure that includes a careful history and physical examination. The musculoskeletal system is inspected carefully for deformity, atrophy, hypertrophy, and muscle spasm. Specific groups of muscles are tested for strength and for their ability to perform motor tasks. Prehension, the ability of the thumb to oppose other fingers for grasp, is an example. Joint range of motion is evaluated with a goniometer, a simple instrument that measures the angle through which the joint may be moved. It resembles the instrument used to measure angles in geometry.

Electrodiagnosis is used to determine the electrical activity of specific nerves and muscles. The muscles are stimulated and their electrical response is shown on a scope. A physiatrist must perform this test and evaluate it as it is in progress.

The evaluation also includes a thorough neurologic examination with testing of reflexes, observation of gait (how the patient walks), and determination of mental orientation. The physician might ask the patient what his name is, where he is, what the date is. He observes the patient's ability to understand and use language.

Therapies Used in Rehabilitation

Therapies are prescribed by the physician. They include the use of superficial heat (whirlpool baths, hot packs, paraffin); deep heat (shortwave diathermy, ultrasound); exercise; muscle re-education; and massage. Massage relaxes the muscles and causes vasodilation. It is not a substitute for active exercise nor is it used to develop muscle strength. Short periods of exercise repeated during the day are preferable to prolonged periods once a day.[2] Motions utilized include those that are done for the patient by the therapist or by a mechanical device (passive); those that are done by the patient with the assistance of the therapist or mechanical device (active, assistive); those accomplished wholly by the patient (active); and those that are accomplished by the patient with the application of additional resistance (resistive). If the patient experiences pain after exercising, and if the pain lasts longer than three hours, or if there is a decrease in range of motion or strength, exercising has been too long or too strenuous.[3] Exercise is accomplished on mats, with parallel bars, with crutches, and so on. The patient may be placed in an upright position gradually by use of a tilt table. He usually remains on the tilt table for 30 to 60 minutes each day.

Activities of Daily Living

Abbreviated A.D.L., these are major endeavors in rehabilitation, for they teach the patient to become as independent as possible within his own limitations. Activities are listed and "checked off" as they are accomplished. At that point, the patient is expected to do them himself. Facilities are structured so that they look like facilities found in real life. The patient practices in a room designed like a bedroom-bathroom complex or in a kitchen adapted for use by the handicapped. The patient learns ways of caring for his personal needs. He learns to eat, bathe, and go to the toilet himself. He learns to move about his house, move outside of his house, and use public transportation. Basic to all of these activities are transfer procedures. These are specified, repeated patterns of movements that the patient must learn so that he can get from one surface to another safely. The movements include transfer from bed to wheel chair, and from wheel chair to toilet, bathtub, or car and then back again. (See Fig. 37–1.)

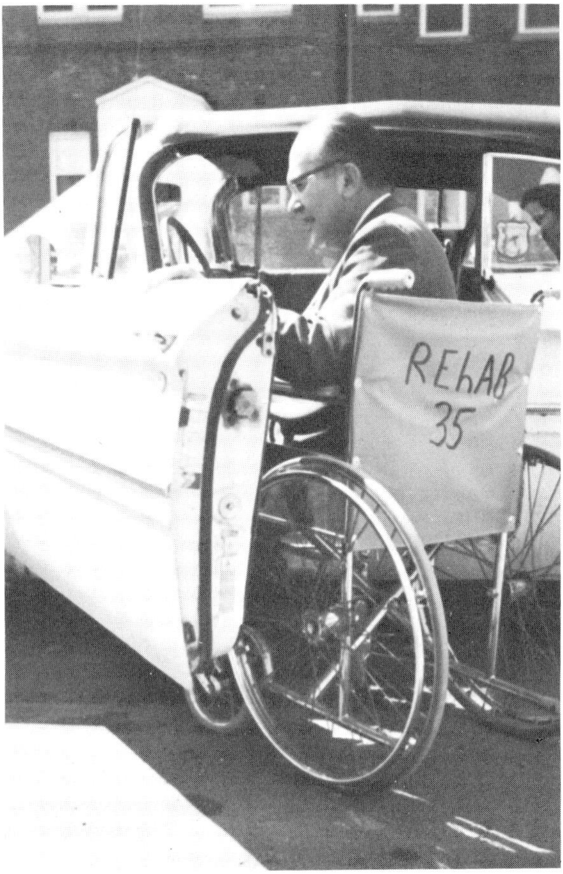

FIGURE 37–1. Wheel-chair-to-car transfer. This car has hand controls.

There must be a stable take-off point and a stable landing platform. The process of transfer training begins as soon as the patient is able to balance in the sitting position. Most transfers are made toward the more normal side. When the lower limbs are paralyzed, the patient may use a sliding board to assist in the transfer. Two corners of the boards are placed on the bed and two corners are placed on the wheel chair. Using the board, the patient moves his legs over the side of the bed with his arms and slides to the edge of the bed in position for sliding transfer to the chair.[4]

Leaning on his right forearm, the patient places one end of the sliding board under himself and moves across the board to the wheel chair. Hydraulic lifts can be used for patients who cannot accomplish the transfer without extensive assistance.

Many self-help devices have been designed using simple, easy-to-obtain ten-cent-store supplies. Examples include a long-handled bath brush that can be strapped to the patient's hand and an electric razor with a strap. Patients also learn how to conserve their energy and simplify their work. Many rehabilitation centers have specially designed kitchens for men and women to work in. Some of the modifications include doors left off the cupboards so that supplies are easy to get, space for a wheel chair (see Fig. 37–3) to be pushed underneath the sink, gas knobs away from the front of the stove, suction cup devices to hold mixing bowls steady on a surface, and nails on a cutting board to hold vegetables to be peeled. The patient is taught to use fixed work stations with special places to do a

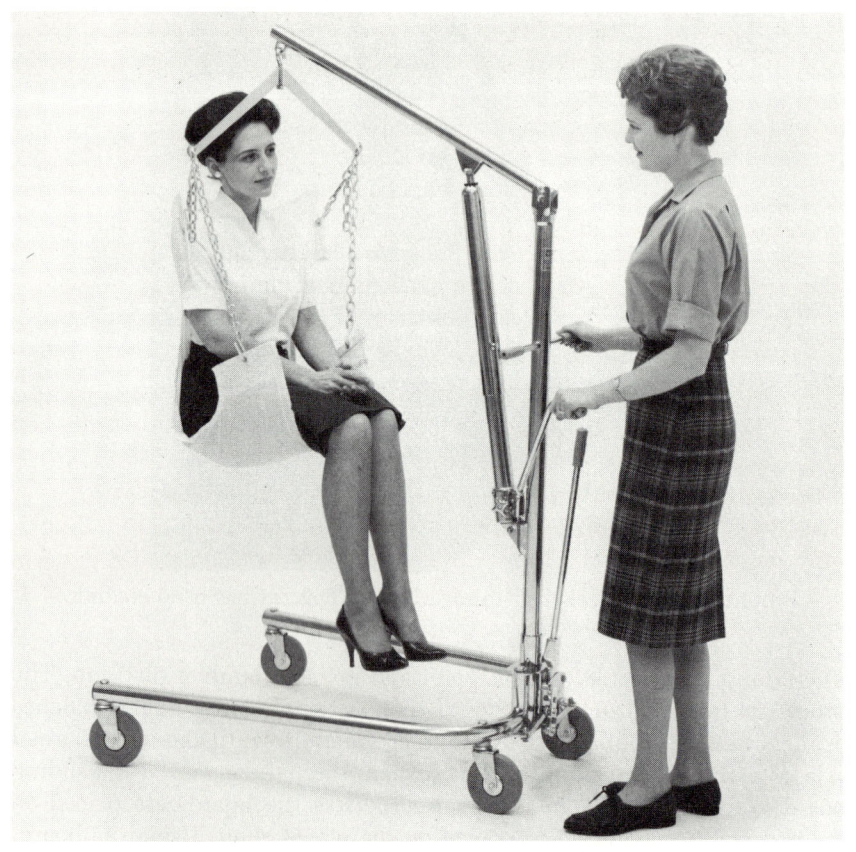

FIGURE 37–2. A patient lifter. (Courtesy, Ted Hoyer and Co., Inc., Oshkosh, Wis.)

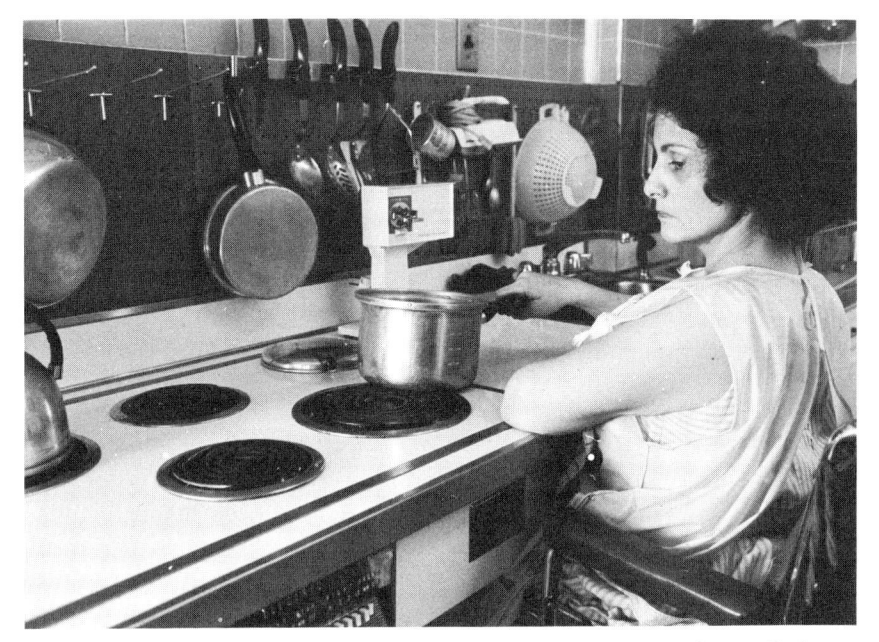

FIGURE 37-3. Electric cooking top provides a burner almost flush with surrounding work surface, enabling homemaker with weak arms to slide, rather than lift, pans onto burner. Open undercounter permits closer access to working surface. Peg board on wall stores utensils within easy reach. (From Rehabilitation Monograph XXVII, *Planning Kitchens for Handicapped Homemakers*, by Virginia Hart Wheeler, IRM, New York University Medical Center, 1966, reproduced with permission.)

particular job. Equipment used should be adaptable for a variety of different jobs and should be stored so that it is placed for immediate use. The patient sits whenever possible.

In dressing, some minor adaptations may mean the patient can be independent, e.g., large flat buttons in the front rather than at the side or back, zippers, and use of Velcro instead of buttons or snaps. Special extension hooks and reachers are available. *Enough time must be allowed for dressing.*

Some Major Problems of the Patient with a Neurologic-Orthopedic Disability

Grief

The patient who experiences a disabling disease progresses through the phases of grief, though the length of time through each phase varies with the individual and with the meaning of the loss to him. He "mourns" the loss of the part or function. If nothing important to him has been lost, or if the disability is time-limited, the response will probably be one of comfortable acceptance.[5] A boy in a body cast may be in this category. However, grief and denial follow change in body image, and in a society that values physical strength, beauty, and dexterity, it is difficult to make the necessary switch from a comparative to an individual-asset value system. Psychologic shock is followed by denial that the disability has occurred, and this is followed by a period of "mourning the loss." Grief should not and cannot be hurried or interrupted; progressing through its various phases has advantageous prognostic value. On the other hand, long-term, continued denial of the loss indicates poor rehabilitation potential. (See p. 9.)

Role Modification

The patient is the same person he has always been, and will react with the same characteristic personality traits that have been his for his lifetime. The degree of response, though, may be exaggerated. He must assume new roles that are "different from" those he is accustomed to and frequently are in conflict with those prescribed by society. The principal developmental task of the disabled person is attaining a compromise between his own shifting self-image [6] and the expectation of society that he is crippled and should therefore be nonproductive and should assume passive activity. The patient may also have to accept role reversal with his mate in which he maintains the home and she becomes the wage earner. This is a difficult adjustment. She may have worked prior to his disability but he could rationalize it as being "her wish." With his disability it becomes a necessity.

There is change in his (or her) biologic sex role. Barriers include lack of sensation, lack of the capacity to ejaculate, inability to assume positions, and lack of the availability of sex partners. Very often, psychologic satisfaction is gleaned if the disabled partner can satisfy his mate even if he feels no sensation himself. Women seem to have less of a problem in this area because of their accustomed passive role. They can usually conceive and bear children with the disability.

Roles can be modified so that they become acceptable to the patient and to his family. The person who is intelligent and educated fares better than his less endowed brother.

Difficulty in Communicating [7,8]

The ability to utilize language effectively involves a vastly intricate and interrelated neurologic-orthopedic mechanism that requires hearing, learning, mental ability, muscular ability, personality, and so on. Speech is one single facet of language, as are articulation (the ability to pronounce words so that they are understood) and rhythm (flow of speech; rate, pause, and pattern). Patients who cannot properly understand the spoken words of others and cannot select the right words and arrange them appropriately have language disorders. These occur in many neurologic conditions such as stroke, increased intracranial pressure, and cranial nerve disease. Language disorders are called *aphasias* and are classified as receptive aphasia and expressive aphasia. In receptive aphasia there is a problem in comprehending written or spoken symbols, and the defect is in "input" (auditory comprehension, reading comprehension, visual recognition). Receptive aphasias have been called sensory aphasia, agnosia (inability to comprehend sensation), and Wernicke's aphasia.

In expressive aphasia there is inability to convey ideas through speech, writing, and gesture. The defect is in language output. Expressive aphasias have been called motor aphasia, dysphasia, and apraxia (inability to control voluntary movements of speech). The patient has difficulty in finding words and naming objects. He confuses letters, has disturbance in word order, makes grammatical mistakes, and uses gibberish.

Many patients have *mixed aphasias* involving expressive and receptive disability. *Global aphasia* indicates extreme disability in all areas of language. The patient has difficulty communicating on any level.

The speech therapist works with the patient to develop a profile of language performance. Then she employs a variety of techniques to help the patient. She uses mirrors so that he can observe his lip and tongue activity; flash cards so he can practice recognizing letters, numbers, and words; and so on. The better-educated patient seems to make the best linguistic recovery. The nurse must remember that "words have not been lost; but they are less available."[9] The earlier treatment is begun, the better are the chances of recovery.

Problem with Skin Breakdown

When a patient is immobilized for any length of time, he tends to lie with pressure in areas of weight bearing. Some susceptible body areas include the backs of the heels and the sacral area in the supine position; the bony prominences on the outside of the ankles and the area over the trochanter of the femur in the side-lying position; and over the two bony prominences (the ischial tuberosities) in the sitting position. This pressure decreases the lumen of blood vessels, decreases the supply of blood to that area of the body, and produces ischemia in the area of the pressure. Decubitus ulcers form. It is a well-known fact that these ulcers are much more easily prevented than cured! *Patients should have their positions changed more frequently than every two hours* because they cannot feel pressure or pain when there is neurologic involvement. Round doughnut-type devices are not suggested because they only divert the pressure from the center to the periphery. There should be complete elimination of pressure by proper bed positioning, keeping sheets wrinkle-free, using splints and other special devices, using lamb's wool or synthetic substitutes under pressure areas, and using alternating air-pressure mattresses. The Stryker frame and the Circ-O-Lectric bed are used when the patient cannot be turned easily. The Stryker frame permits turning from front to back-lying positions. The Circ-O-Lectric bed allows horizontal, vertical, and sitting positions. (See Figs. 37–4, 37–5, and 37–6.)

Ultraviolet treatment is sometimes used. Scrupulous cleanliness is essential. The patient should be instructed in the use of a long-handled mirror so that he can inspect every portion of his body. He should be reminded to wash all areas. Too often, he divorces the paralyzed areas from his mind because he cannot feel them and fails to include them in his daily cleansing routine. Periodic whirlpool baths are effective in decreasing the chance of decubitus formation. The Hubbard tank is an example of such a device. There are a variety of preferred treatments for decubitus ulcers once they are evidenced. Tincture of benzoin and Dermoplast sprays are often chosen to help toughen areas around the ulcer; hydrogen peroxide is often used to irrigate and clean the ulcer itself. Telfa and abdominal pads may be used to cover the ulcer areas after treatment.

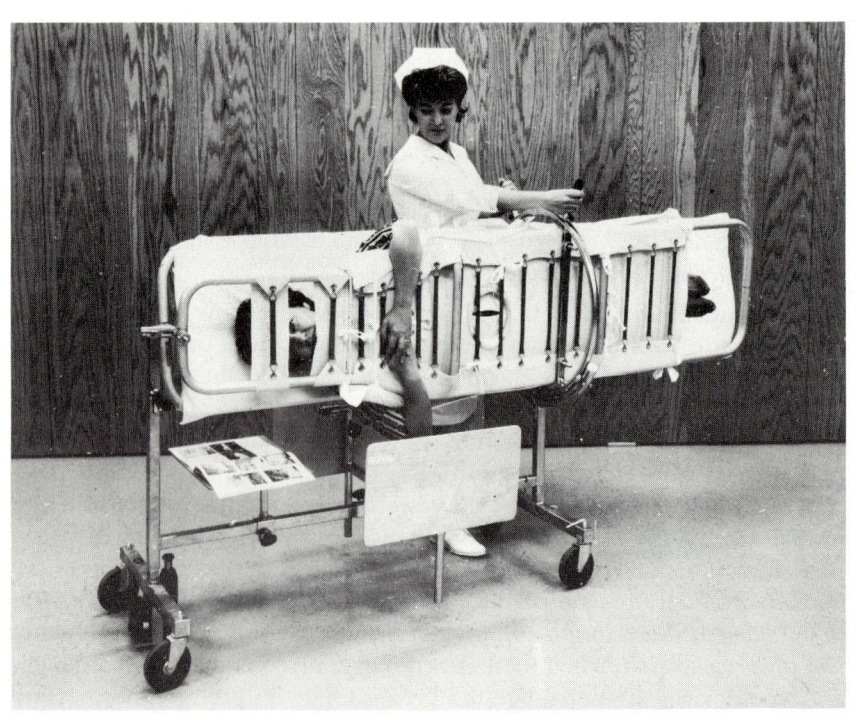

FIGURE 37–4. The Stryker turning frame. Patient being turned on frame. (Courtesy, Stryker, Kalamazoo, Mich.)

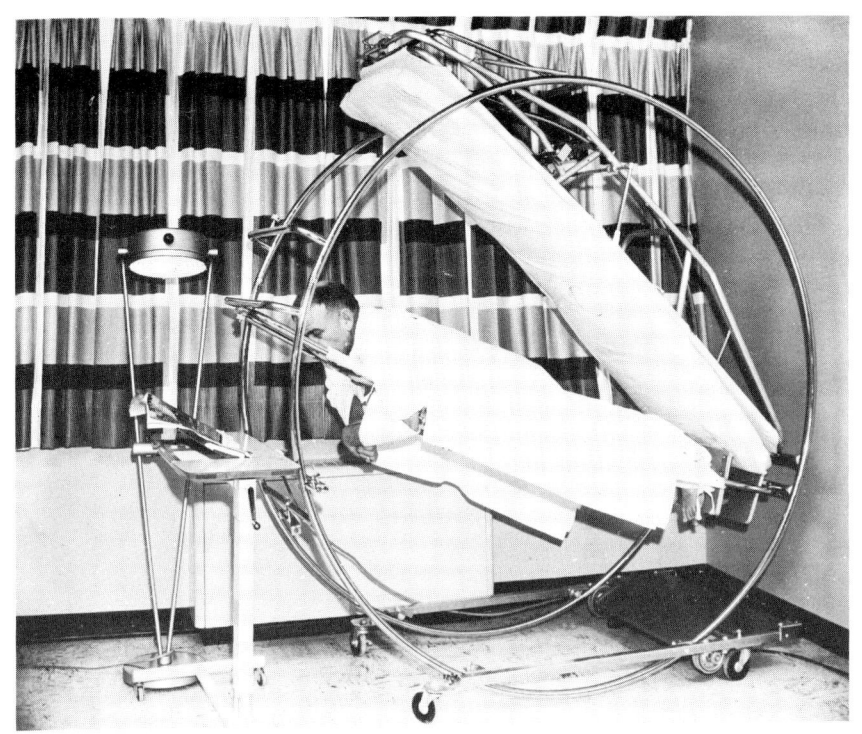

FIGURE 37-5. Circ-O-Lectric bed turned for patient to read and rest. (Courtesy, Stryker, Kalamazoo, Mich.)

They are held in place by special plastic tape. Sometimes the ulcer must be débrided. This involves the surgical removal of all dead tissue to encourage growth of healthy tissue. Plastic repair of decubiti is sometimes done. In this surgical technique decubiti are covered with full-thickness skin flaps. Grafting is considered only after maximum response has been attained through adequate diet high in protein, frequent change in position, and so on.

Profuse perspiration above the level of a spinal cord injury, combined with absence of perspiration below the level of the injury, is another reason why frequent and adequate bathing of all parts of the body is necessary for patients with neurologic injury.

Prevention of Contractures and Ankylosis

Contractures and ankylosis involve shortening of the muscles and stiffness in the joints. This causes decreased range of motion and leads to deformity. Proper body alignment combined with frequent changes in position constitutes the major method of preventing these deformities in patients who are confined to bed for long periods of time. Patients tend

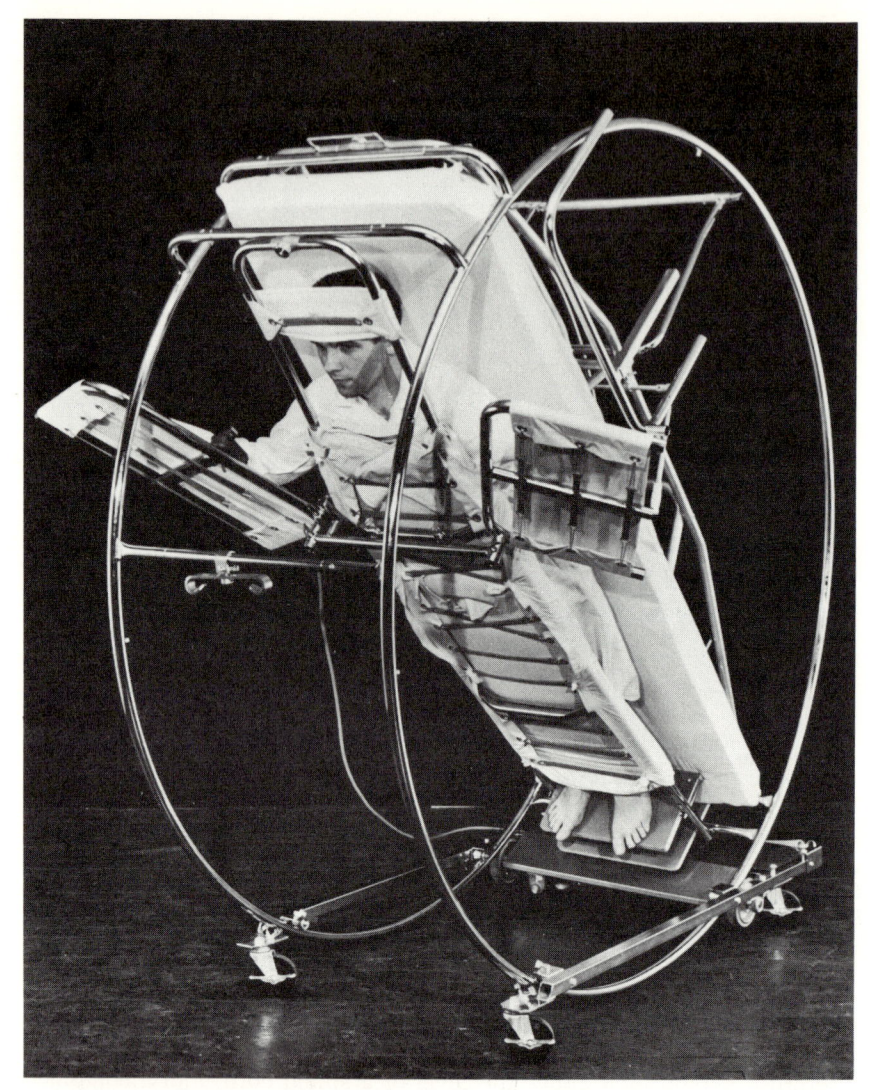

FIGURE 37–6. Circ-O-Lectric bed with patient positioned to rest arms and body. (Courtesy, Stryker, Kalamazoo, Mich.)

to assume the position that affords them most comfort and the least amount of pain. The muscle positions that allow for this comfort involve the stronger of the muscle groups. For instance, the flexors and adductors dominate the upper extremities. If the patient is not aligned properly, he will assume a position in which the arms will be very close to the chest and bent at the elbow; the fingers will be almost entirely clenched. In the lower limbs there will be external rotation of the legs with flexion and adduction at the hip joint. His foot will assume the familiar "foot-drop" position. This is called talipes equinus. It is a condition in which the foot can be plantar-flexed (sole toward the floor) but not dorsiflexed (sole toward the ceiling). It can easily be prevented by use of a footboard.

Three Optimum Bed Positions [10,11]

Use a firm, nonsagging mattress for each.

SUPINE (BACK LYING)

Head. In a position that allows the neck to maintain its normal curve in relation to the rest of the spine. A small pillow may be used, if approved by the physician, to support natural curve.

Shoulders. In a neutral or slightly depressed level, flat against the bed in a relaxed position.

Arms. Abducted and internally or externally rotated with forearms supported on pillows. Elbows only slightly flexed, wrists slightly dorsiflexed. Fingers in "functional" position: slightly flexed with thumb in position to oppose fingers (prehension). A rolled washcloth or a splint may be used to maintain this position.

Back and Hips. Flat in bed. A small pillow may minimize lordotic curve. If the backrest is elevated, hips should be well back in the angle of the bed with the weight of the body firmly on buttocks and posterior thighs, not on lumbosacral curve. Change backrest level frequently with flat position for equal period of time. Prevent external and internal rotation of hips with trochanter roll, sandbags, pillows between the legs.

Legs. In neutral position with knee slightly flexed in position for walking. A small pillow under the calves lessens pressure on the heels and relaxes knee joint (no pressure on popliteal space). A rectangle of foam rubber, 4 by 8 in., may be used just back of the heels. Feet flat against footboard to prevent foot drop.

IN THE PRONE POSITION (FACE LYING)

After building up tolerance, a neurologic patient may use this position for eight hours of sleeping without signs of excess pressure.

Head. Small pillow or foam-rubber rectangle under head may make patient more comfortable. Do not hyperextend head with "bunched-up" pillows.

Shoulders and Hips. Both should be flat on bed with pillows under abdomen to prevent hyperextension of the lumbar and cervical spine.

Arms. Abducted and externally rotated with elbows flexed; this allows full expansion of the chest.

Legs. Feet extended over the foot of the bed or supported with rolled blanket or pillow under the ankles.

IN THE LATERAL POSITION (SIDE LYING)

Head. Not hyperextended or flexed on sternum. Use small pillow or foam-rubber rectangle.

Back. The back should be straight with weight evenly distributed. Patient should feel secure. Use pillows rolled along length of back.

Arms. Upper arm supported on a pillow.

Legs. Use pillow or pillows lengthwise to remove tension from the hip and back. Do not allow one leg to lie on top of the other causing pressure on underneath leg. Feet should be in neutral position with help of pillows.

Be creative. Use a variety of devices (pillows, blanket rolls, washcloths) to establish and maintain adequate body alignment. Positioning a patient properly takes time. It should not be done haphazardly. Do not allow patients with dorsal spine involvement to lie with their arms above their heads unless specific permission is given by the physician.[12]

Renal Involvement

One of the most life-threatening complications of immobility, especially in patients with spinal cord lesions resulting in paralysis of the limbs (quadriplegia and paraplegia), is the formation of renal calculi and the development of urinary tract infection. *Urinary tract infection is the killer of patients with paraplegia and quadriplegia.* These patients tread a well-known path to renal destruction [13] in which immobility fosters stasis of urine in the kidney; static fluid provides an optimum medium for bacterial growth; bacteria gain entrance to the urinary system through catheters that are required for long periods of time; and calculi form, obstructing the kidneys and causing gradual loss of kidney function. The cycle is a vicious one. The physician studies kidney function through intravenous pyelograms done every three to six months for at least two years after the incidence of neurologic involvement. Measures utilized to decrease renal involvement include mobilizing the patient as early as possible, using the tilt table, and keeping the urine acid (bacteria thrive in an alkaline urine). This is accomplished by encouraging the ingestion of foods high in acid ash, such as breads and cereals, cranberries, plums, prunes, cheese, fish, meats and poultry, corn and lentils, and eggs, and discouraging foods that are potentially alkaline ash, such as all other fruits, jams and jellies, honey, milk, vegetables except corn and lentils, and carbonated beverages.[14, 15] Juices with high citric acid content (orange, grapefruit, tomato, pineapple, lemonade) are avoided. Mandelic acid may be prescribed, and the patient is encouraged to drink between 3,000 and 4,000 ml of water every day. Because of the tendency to formation of renal calculi, eggs are restricted to one a day; milk to 1 pt a day; and no spinach, turnip greens, collard greens, kale, rhubarb, or cabbage is permitted. The nutritionist must balance the diet so that the patient receives all the essential nutrients, especially protein for tissue repair and vitamin C for healing.

CATHETER CARE

A retention catheter is necessary during the early period following injury to the spinal cord. This period is called the period of spinal shock. The bladder is flaccid and has no reflex ability to empty. Special precautions must be taken when a patient has an indwelling retention catheter. Cleanliness is of prime importance. Bladder irrigation is done twice a day to decrease the introduction of microorganisms through the catheter. A variety of solutions are used, e.g., Zephiran 1:5,000 and Furacin 1:10; a 1 per cent acetic acid solution may be instilled and allowed to remain in the bladder for 30 minutes. The catheter should be carefully cleaned at its junction with the genitalia. Zephiran 1:700 is often selected for this purpose. In the male patient the foreskin should be pushed back and the penis cleaned carefully and regularly. The catheter should be taped to the abdomen to decrease the constant downward pull by straightening the penoscrotal angle. This decreases the possibility of fistula or abscess formation at the penoscrotal junction.[16] Women should be instructed about special attention to cleanliness at the time of the menses.

If the urine remains clear, with a minimum of white blood cells, the catheter is changed every two weeks. In the presence of persistent cystitis, it may have to be changed every five to seven days.[17]

BLADDER TRAINING

Immediately following injury to the spinal cord the bladder is atonic; however, there is gradual return of bladder reflex ability. The major goals in bladder training are: [18]

1. Freedom from use of a catheter
2. A bladder capacity of 200 to 400 ml of urine
3. A bladder that empties completely at each voiding

Bladder training is instituted as soon as there is reasonable chance for catheter-free voiding. Injuries result in two types of residual bladder function. If the bladder reflex center at the end of the lumbar cord is not functioning, the bladder is called autonomous. It is not under any reflex control. Nearly all patients with autonomous bladders become catheter-free.[19] An automatic bladder, on the other hand, is one in which reflex activity remains. Sixty per cent of the patients with automatic "reflex" bladders become catheter-free.

Theoretically the patient cannot feel a desire to void when the cord has been severed; however, many patients say that they have vague sensations of bladder fullness. This sensation is probably the result of autonomic nervous control. The patient will say he feels "vague abdominal discomfort" or "burning pain around the pubis" when he has to empty his bladder.

In bladder training for reflex control, the catheter is intermittently clamped and then unclamped. Tone is recovered this way because the detrusor fibers of the bladder, which cause reflex emptying, gradually lengthen as the bladder fills and shorten when the catheter is released. The patient begins training by clamping the catheter every hour during the day and remaining on straight drainage at night. Records are carefully kept of the amount of urine released at each unclamping. The length of time between "unclampings" is increased until a bladder capacity of about 300 ml is reached. Then, the catheter is taken out in the morning. The patient drinks water every hour and then attempts to trigger reflex-detrusor emptying by such methods as tapping above the pubic area, stroking the genitalia, and scratching the inner thigh. Once voiding begins the patient puts manual pressure over the pubic area and strains abdominally until he is certain the bladder is empty. Following catheter removal, the patient rigidly controls his fluid intake so that voiding will occur at times that are convenient to him.

Autonomous bladder training begins as soon as the patient's physical condition permits him to assume a comfortable physiologic position for expression of urine. The catheter is removed in the morning; the patient drinks a glass of water every hour, and then when 300 to 400 ml of urine has accumulated, he sits or stands at the toilet, and by manually compressing the lower abdomen and by straining, he empties his bladder. Residual urine is measured in the afternoon, and if it is less than one third the capacity of the bladder on three successive days, the catheter is left out.

Tidal drainage, once widely used in many centers to help maintain bladder ability to continuously fill and empty itself, has been largely abandoned in favor of this simple clamping and unclamping procedure.

The length of time to acquire bladder control varies with individual patients. Some patients are never successful and must wear a condom or leg-bag urinal. A woman has a more difficult problem and must resort to use of sanitary napkins and rubber protective pants.

BOWEL CONTROL

Bowel training begins with the routine establishment of a daily time for evacuation. Usually, this is one-half hour after a meal, so that use is made of the gastrocolic reflex. Coffee often stimulates defecation, as does nicotine. The goal is to encourage adequate peristalsis. Adequate fluid intake, foods that contain roughage, and a mobile patient foster peristalsis. Enemas and the manual removal of stool sometimes must be used; however, these methods tend to discourage normal peristalsis. A program may be tried in which the patient drinks 1 oz of mineral oil and 6 oz of prune juice before bedtime, and then inserts a Dulcolax or glycerin suppository about one-half hour before the bowel evacuation. The program is customized for the patient, and a variety of methods are often tried before a successful regimen is discovered. Since the regimen must be followed for several years, the least irritating substances should be selected. Normal sitting position on a toilet or commode helps in bowel control. If the toilet has been elevated to make it easier to transfer from the wheel chair, a footstool should be provided to allow for the physiologic "squatting" position. A toilet with a water spray attachment for cleansing helps.

The most profound frustrations of patients with spinal cord injuries stem from loss of control of bladder and bowel function. Many become reluctant to leave the protective environment of the hospital because of these excretory problems.

Spasms

Spasms are involuntary contractions of large groups of muscles. They serve no functional purpose, and because they are so uncontrollable and cause such muscle rigidity they frequently interfere with the rehabilitation process. They may seriously mask voluntary motor power. Spasms are a problem in a variety of neurologic-orthopedic conditions, some of which include cord damage, multiple sclerosis, vascular lesions and neoplasms of the brainstem, stroke, and cerebral palsy. The question frequently arises, "if the patient is paralyzed, how can he have spasms?" Doesn't this mean a return of muscle activity? The answer is a firm "no," although this is difficult for the patient to accept because a spasm indicates movement and this movement serves as remaining proof to him that the limb is very much alive. This is basically what happens: Limb movement is under dual control. First, it is under voluntary control through the pyramidal motor tract. The nerve cells of this tract are called upper motor neurons, and they convey impulses from the motor area of the brain down through the brainstem and spinal cord to a lower motor neuron. The lower motor neuron serves as the final common pathway, and it is essential for motor activity. *A lesion in the upper motor neuron results in spasms.* It separates efferent neurons from central control. *A lesion in the lower motor neuron results in muscle flaccidity.*

Second, limb movement is under the very basic, involuntary control of reflex arcs that cause a stimulus-response action. The stimulus (e.g., pain) occurs at the receptor organ (e.g., the skin). It travels by means of an afferent pathway (sensory) that goes toward the central nervous system to the posterior (dorsal) part of the spinal cord. Here it synapses (meets, joins with) another nerve cell and then travels an efferent (motor, away from the central nervous system) pathway out the anterior (ventral) root of the cord to the effector organ, which results in some muscle activity.

It all sounds very involved, but it is a commonly occurring, not-thought-about activity. Think of what happens when a hand is accidentally placed on a hot stove. Pain is felt and the hand is instantly pulled away from the source of heat. This is reflex activity. The sequence looks like this:

Pain in skin (receptor) → sensory impulse via afferent pathway to the posterior (dorsal) root of the cord → synapse with efferent neuron → stimulus via efferent pathway through anterior (ventral) root of cord to effector organ → muscle activity

Even though the cord may be isolated from the rest of the central nervous system because of injury, spasms will occur below the injury if the reflex arcs have not been damaged. *Any lesion that separates the efferent neurons from central control causes spasticity.*

Management of spasms is difficult and must be individualized. Sometimes, decreasing sensory cord bombardment is effective. For instance, a bladder infection would increase sensory cord stimulation, as would decubitus ulcers, severe cold, anger, extreme excitement, and pain. Daily stretching is done to maintain full range of motion and prevent contractures. Bracing frequently helps. In severe cases the physician may inject dilute procaine solution or may elect to have the reflex arc surgically destroyed. This surgical procedure stops the spasms and produces permanent flaccidity.

38

EVALUATION AND INITIAL MANAGEMENT OF DISORDERS OF THE NERVOUS SYSTEM

A Review of Anatomy

The nervous system is composed of two major portions: the central nervous system, which is made up of the brain and the spinal cord, and the peripheral nervous system, which is made up of the 12 pair of cranial nerves, 31 pair of spinal nerves, and the autonomic nervous system. The autonomic nervous system is also called "visceral." The voluntary nervous system is called "somatic."

Nerve Regeneration

Cells of the nervous system include the nerve cell itself, called a neuron; cells that provide nourishment and support for the nerve cells, called neuroglia; and cells that carry impulses from one part of the nervous system to another, called internuncial or associational neurons. Each neuron contains short fibers (processes) called dendrites that are afferent in nature and bring sensory impulses to the nerve cell, and long fibers (processes) called axons that are efferent in nature and take impulses away from the cell to join muscle, gland, or dendrite of another neuron.

The axon can be covered with a fatty sheath of myelin when fast, discrete function is required of the nerve. The axon can also be covered with a very delicate sheath called neurillema. Neurillema is very special because its presence allows the fibers of nerves to regenerate if they have been severed and are cut off from their neurons. Regeneration takes place if conditions are favorable, for instance, if the distance between the two ends of axon is not too great, or there are no bone chips or scar tissue to interfere. The process of regeneration is diagrammed in Figure 38-1. *Neurillema is found in only part of the peripheral nervous system (none in cranial nerves). Nerve fibers in the central nervous system do not contain neurillema and therefore cannot regenerate.*

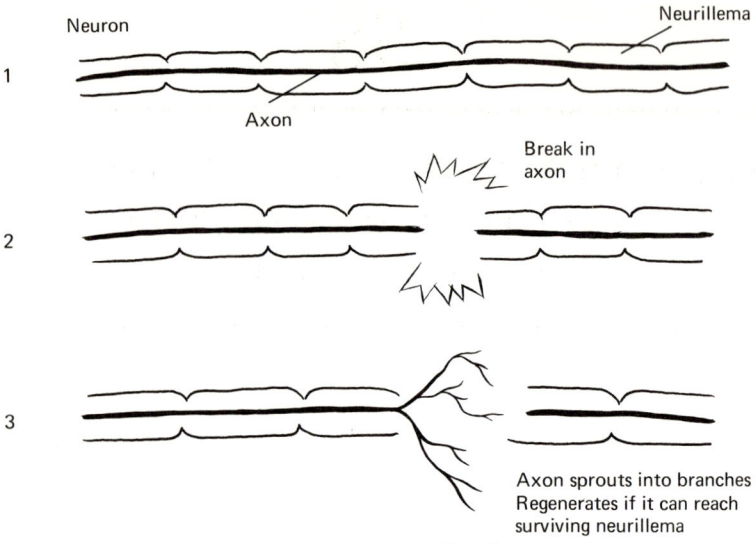

FIGURE 38-1. Regeneration of peripheral nerve processes.

The Spinal Cord

The spinal cord is housed in the canal formed by consecutive central canals of the vertebrae. The vertebral column is made up of seven cervical, 12 thoracic, and five lumbar vertebrae, plus the sacrum and the coccyx. The cord is continuous with the medulla oblongata in the brainstem. It becomes "spinal cord" at the large opening in the base of the skull called the foramen magnum and runs from the superior border of the first cervical vertebra to the upper border of the second lumbar vertebra.

Meninges

The brain and spinal cord are covered by layers of tissue called meninges. The tough, outermost layer is the dura mater. The middle layer is the arachnoid, and the innermost layer is the pia mater. Compartments are formed between the layers. The subdural compartment is between the dura mater and arachnoid; the subarachnoid space is between the arachnoid and pia mater. The subarachnoid space is extremely important. The cerebrospinal fluid circulates over the surface of the brain and cord through it. This same compartment serves as a roadbed for the vascular system of the brain. Veins lie here; cerebrospinal fluid is absorbed through wartlike nodules here; and arteries supplying the brain are carried with the pia into the cortex here.

Meninges serve as protection for the nervous system structures and, by folding in and out, separate and support structures. For instance, a double fold of the dura mater separates the occipital bones and the cerebellum and is called tentorium. All structures above this dural layer are referred to as being supratentorial; those below it are infratentorial.

Circulation to Brain and Cord

The brain requires 20 per cent more oxygen than any other organ.[20] It can only survive anoxia for four minutes without permanent organic damage. In the absence of oxygen symptoms will occur in ten seconds. The brain receives about 750 ml of blood from arteries rich in newly oxygenated blood from the heart. It is supplied by two internal carotid arteries anteriorly and two vertebral arteries posteriorly. These arteries "communicate" at the base of the brain through the basilar artery and the circle of Willis. The anterior, posterior, and middle cerebral arteries stem from the internal carotids that supply the cortex. The cerebellum and cord are supplied by the vertebral arteries, and the meninges are supplied by meningeal arteries.

Veins drain into sinuses that run in the dura mater and ultimately into the internal jugular veins and back to the heart.

Circulation of Cerebrospinal Fluid

The circulation of cerebrospinal fluid is often referred to as "the third circulation." There are four cavities in the brain involved in the formation of this fluid. They are called ventricles. Cerebrospinal fluid is formed from blood by choroid plexuses (clusters of blood vessels) that project into two lateral and a third and fourth ventricle. Cerebrospinal fluid protects nervous system tissue by acting as a shock absorber. It circulates in the subarachnoid space of the brain and the spinal cord.

Schematic Representation of Cerebrospinal Fluid Circulation

Fluid formed by choroid plexus in lateral ventricles → through foramen of Monro → to third ventricle → through aqueduct of Silvius → to the fourth ventricle → through foramen of Luschka and Magendie → to cisterna magna → to the subarachnoid spaces of the brain and cord

The Brain

The outer area of cortex contains nerve cells that appear gray in color, hence the term "gray matter." The inner areas contain nerve processes that, because of being myelinated, appear white in color, hence "white matter." There are two identical cerebral hemispheres. The right hemisphere controls the left side of the body, and the left hemisphere controls the right side of the body. One hemisphere becomes functionally more important to the individual than the other and is thus called "the dominant hemisphere." This is especially important for speech. In right-handed people the left hemisphere is usually dominant. Motor speech is handled in the premotor cortex of the left hemisphere. Injury to this area of the brain in a right-handed person would result in speech disability.

The brain is divided into four areas called lobes. Each hemisphere contains all four lobes. The frontal lobe controls elaboration of thought, handling abstract information, problem solving, judgment, personality, behavior, thinking, planning, and "acting rationally." It is called "the disciplinary center." It also contains a "motor strip" in front of the fissure of Rolando. Upper motor neurons are found in this area. They control voluntary motor activity. The top of this "motor strip" controls the bottom of the body. Functions progress upward so that the bottom of the strip controls the face and the tongue. The frontal lobe also contains the higher centers for autonomic functions, e.g., gastrointestinal, respiratory, and cardiovascular activity.

The parietal lobe controls sensation with the exception of smell, taste, sight, and hearing. It contains a "sensory strip" at the back of the fissure of Rolando.

The temporal lobe controls three special senses: hearing, taste, and smell. It is also important for understanding the spoken word.

The occipital lobe controls vision.

Other Areas of the Brain

The hypothalamus is found in the inferior part of the cerebrum. The pituitary body is attached to it. This influences carbohydrate, water, and fat metabolism; growth; body temperature; sexual maturity; vital signs; and sleep. The thalamus modifies and controls primitive emotional responses, e.g., pain, rage, fear, love, and hate. It is also a "relay station" for sensation-carrying impulses between the spinal cord and brain cortex. All sensory impulses end in the thalamus.

Basal Ganglia

The basal ganglia are large cell masses slightly caudal to the thalamus at the base of the brain. These cell masses control automatic-associated body movements such as swinging the arms when walking. They also exert a steadying influence on muscular activity. Injury to them might cause tremors, rigidity, and loss of automatic movement. Parkinson's disease is an example of a syndrome involving the basal ganglia.

Internal Capsule

This is a broad band of white substance "squeezed" between the thalamus and some of the basal ganglia. It consists of ascending and descending tracts. Tracts are groups of fibers that have the same related function. They convey impulses between the cord and brain. There are ascending and descending pathways on both sides of the cord. Tracts are named according to where they start and where they end. For instance, the pyramidal tract, a voluntary motor tract, is called corticospinal. It begins in the cortex of the brain and goes to the spinal cord. The extrapyramidal tract, involved with automatic-associated movement, is extracorticospinal. It begins in the basal ganglia and goes to the cord. The reticulospinal tract begins in the reticular formation (diffuse nerve cell fiber system between the top of the cord and the thalamus) and goes to the cord. The spinothalamic tract starts in the cord and goes to the thalamus. All tracts enter the cord and cross over (decussate) to the other side. Some cross high in the cord; some cross in the midbrain. Knowledge of where the pathways decussate helps determine which side of the body will have symptoms.

Brainstem

The brainstem is composed of the medulla, the pons, and the cerebellum. It begins at the cerebral hemispheres and ends at the foramen magnum where it merges with the spinal cord. The brainstem contains the nuclei of ten of the cranial nerves and the ascending and descending tracts. The medulla is extremely important because it contains several vital centers that control heart, circulation, respiration, and vomiting. If the medulla is accidentally "pulled down" and squeezed in the foramen magnum, the patient would probably die because of vital center interference. The cerebellum is involved in coordination. It controls muscle tone and movement and helps in maintaining balance and equilibrium. This is called "posture in space." The patient who has interference in cerebellar function would be ataxic.

Cranial Nerves

There are 12 pair of cranial nerves, which are both motor and/or sensory in function. They do not contain neurillema and therefore cannot regenerate. Their nuclei are paired along either side of the top of the cord (bulb) and the pons. They are tested carefully in the neurologic examination. (See p. 420.)

Autonomic Nervous System

This is an involuntary part of the peripheral nervous system, also called "vegetative" or "visceral." It contains a series of ganglia and nerve fibers that form a chain on each side of the vertebral bodies, and that are influenced by higher cells in the cortex. There are two divisions to the autonomic nervous system: the sympathetic or adrenergic system with ganglia originating in the thoracolumbar cord areas; and the parasympathetic or cholinergic system with ganglia originating in the craniosacral regions of the cord. Sympathetic stimulation causes a mass emergency response. Parasympathetic stimulation causes a discrete response.

TABLE 38–1. ACTION OF THE SYMPATHETIC AND PARASYMPATHETIC NERVOUS SYSTEMS *

	Sympathetic	Parasympathetic
Heart	Accelerates	Retards
Iris	Dilates pupils	Constricts pupils
Bronchi	Dilates	Constricts
GI peristalsis	Inhibits	Stimulates
GI secretion	Inhibits	Stimulates
Bladder emptying	Inhibits	Stimulates
Internal urinary sphincter	Constricts	Relaxes
GI sphincters	Constricts	Relaxes
Salivary secretion	Causes viscid flow	Causes watery flow
Adrenal secretion	Stimulates	Inhibits
Coronary arteries	Dilates	Little effect
Other arteries	Constricts	Little effect
Sweat glands	Stimulates	No supply
Pilomotor muscles	Stimulates	No supply

* From C. de Gutiérrez-Mahoney and E. Carini, *Neurological and Neurosurgical Nursing*, 4th ed., 1965, reprinted with permission of The C.V. Mosby Company, St. Louis.

The Neurologic Evaluation

The fundamental clinical picture of neurologic dysfunction depends on the location of the lesion. The symptoms are the same regardless of the particular cause. A complete physical examination and detailed history precede the more specialized components of the neurologic procedure. The nurse assists the physician with the examination. She uses the same tools of observation in his absence. *Observation is particularly important when there is neurologic involvement because a patient's condition may change very, very rapidly.*

Equipment for the Examination

The examination tray should contain all equipment required for a general physical examination plus the addition of a tuning fork, substances labeled for testing taste (sweet, sour, bitter, salty), substances with distinctive odors for testing smell, a pin for testing sensation to pain, cotton, and a dynamometer for testing hand grip.

Special Neurologic Aspects of the Examination

LEVELS OF CONSCIOUSNESS

The consciousness center is thought to be in the pons. Interference with its function may cause a change in the level of consciousness. Unconsciousness is a state of depressed cerebral function in which the appreciation of stimuli is lost; response, if present, is on a reflex level.

Somnolence (Drowsiness). The patient sleeps when he is left alone. He may be restless or still. He can answer questions but may be confused. When awakened he is usually cooperative. The nurse must record the stimulus that awakened the patient.

Stupor. The stuporous patient responds by becoming restless and irritable when stimulated. He may be combative. There may be twitching or picking motions. He responds to tactile or loud auditory stimuli and to bright lights. He may answer simple questions if roused sufficiently with repeated stimuli. Record such things as, "responded when shouted at."

Semicoma. In the semicomatose patient spontaneous motion is uncommon unless the patient is aroused. He may groan or mutter. He withdraws from painful stimuli. He is incontinent.

Coma. The comatose patient responds to only the most painful stimuli. There is no spontaneous movement. Muscles are still and flaccid. Supraorbital pressure is used to demonstrate coma. The thumb is pressed firmly upward in the groove between the eyeball and eyebrow. The patient in coma is the farthest from alertness.

MENTAL STATUS

This includes knowledge of whether the patient is unduly anxious, whether he has rapidly changing extremes in mood (mood lability), what his memory for recent and past events is, his speech, his stream of thought (is he hallucinating? does he have delusions?), and his orientation to time, place, and person (does he know his name? the date? where he is?).

MENINGEAL IRRITATION

Stiff neck (nuchal rigidity) results when there is meningeal irritation. Meningeal irritation is indicated when there is a positive Brudzinski and/or Kernig sign. In the former test the patient has pain when he tries to flex his head on his chest, and this is accompanied by involuntary flexion at the hip and knee joints. In the latter test, there are restricted leg extension and pain when the thigh is flexed.

MOTOR FUNCTION, COORDINATION, AND EQUILIBRIUM

The motor function, tone, and strength of muscles are tested. Muscles are observed for wasting, and the joints are observed for degree of range of motion. The physician observes for coordination. He may ask the patient to repeatedly touch his index finger to the tip of his nose and then to the examiner's finger. He watches the patient walk and observes his gait. He tests equilibrium; e.g., in the Romberg test the patient stands with his heels and toes together and his eyes closed. Increased swaying in this position might indicate neurologic dysfunction.

SENSATION

To test for pain the physician uses a pin; for temperature sensation he uses warm and cold water; for touch he uses the stroking of a wisp of cotton; for vibration he uses the ability to feel the "buzz" of a tuning fork placed on a bony prominence. Sensation is tested with the patient's eyes closed.

REFLEXES

Many abnormalities of the sensory and motor pathways can be discovered because of the absence or presence of reflexes. The knee jerk and biceps jerk are tested by striking the tendon of the muscle firmly with the percussion hammer. These are normal reflexes. The plantar reflex is tested by stroking the outside of the sole of the foot from the heel toward the toes with a wooden applicator. Normally there is a downward movement of the big toe. This is called plantar flexion. If the big toe is flexed upward and outward this is called dorsal flexion. This is an abnormal reflex and is called a positive Babinski sign.

Examination of the Cranial Nerves

I OLFACTORY, SENSORY NERVE

Each nostril is tested, one at a time, with a familiar strong-smelling substance such as coffee, tobacco, vanilla, or oil of cloves. One nostril is pinched closed while the substance is held under the other nostril.

II OPTIC, SENSORY NERVE

Gross visual acuity is tested by having the patient count the number of fingers held up or read. The Snellen chart may be used for testing finer visual acuity, and a screen and object followed with the eyes may be used to check visual fields. The physician wants to see what the patient can see straight ahead; he also wants to check vision at the periphery of the eyes by having the patient hold his head still, look straight ahead, and tell when he can see an object coming in from the side.

The fundus of the eye is carefully examined with the ophthalmoscope. Retinal vessels can be seen, as can the optic nerve head. If this nerve is swollen, this is called papilledema or choked disc. Papilledema is frequently found with increased intracranial pressure.

III OCULOMOTOR, IV TROCHLEAR, AND VI ABDUCENS, MOTOR NERVES TO THE MUSCLES OF THE EYE

These three nerves are examined together. The patient may be asked to follow a moving finger. The ability of the pupils to constrict is examined by shining a light into the eyes from the side. Accommodation is checked by noting convergence and pupillary change when the patient follows objects brought from a distance up close. The following conditions are noted:

PTOSIS. Lid drop
STRABISMUS (SQUINT). Crossing of eyes
DIPLOPIA. Double vision
NYSTAGMUS. Involuntary back-and-forth, up-and-down, or rotating movement of the eye

V TRIGEMINAL, MOTOR AND SENSORY NERVE

This nerve has three large branches. The ophthalmic division supplies the forehead, eyes, nose, temples, meninges, and paranasal sinuses; the maxillary division supplies the upper jaw, teeth, lip, cheeks, hard palate, maxillary sinuses, and nasal mucosa; and the mandibular division supplies the lower jaw, teeth, lip, buccal mucosa, tongue, part of the external ear, auditory meatus, and meninges. Sensation to the face is examined by pinprick for pain and cotton for light touch. Corneal sensation is checked. A wisp of cotton brushing the cornea will normally cause the eye to promptly close. Muscles of mastication are checked by seeing if the patient can chew.

The disease syndrome that affects this fifth nerve is called trigeminal neurolgia or tic douloureux. With it, there is excruciating pain and a burning sensation anywhere in the areas supplied by this nerve but most frequently in the lower part of the face. The spasm that causes the pain is often "triggered" by brushing the teeth, by feeling a blast of cold air, by chewing, and so on. The patient realizes what triggers the spasm and does everything he can to avoid this. The pain lasts anywhere from a few seconds to a minute. Flushing of the face, watering of the eyes, and running nose are also present. Injecting the peripheral branches of the nerve with 95 per cent alcohol gives relief for several months. Drugs such as methantheline (Banthine) and diethazine (Diparcol) are now being used. Sometimes, fifth-nerve resection is done; however, the resulting numbness is often unbearable.

VII FACIAL, MIXED NERVE, MAINLY MOTOR

Symmetry of the face is noted. Any asymmetry at rest or when the patient is asked to perform a facial movement is noted. The patient is asked to raise his eyebrows, close his eyes, show his teeth, whistle, and smile. Taste to the anterior part of the tongue is checked by holding the tip of the tongue with a piece of gauze and then rubbing a cotton-moistened applicator along the tongue. The patient indicates whether it tastes sweet (sugar used), sour (citric acid used), bitter (quinine used), or salty (table salt used).

Bell's palsy (peripheral facial paralysis) is a disease of the facial nerve in which there is flaccid paralysis. There may be drooping of the mouth with the mouth drawing to the opposite side, food collecting between the cheeks and gums, and dribbling. The eye cannot be closed and it waters. It must be protected to prevent corneal ulceration. Sensation may be lost. Bell's palsy may be caused by chilling of the face, middle-ear infection, tumors, fractures, or meningitis. The patient should wear an eye shield to protect the cornea from dust. Outside, he should wear glasses to protect the cornea from flying particles.

VIII ACOUSTIC, SENSORY NERVE

This nerve controls hearing and balance. Hearing is tested at the bedside by seeing if the patient can hear the ticking of a watch or the whisper of a voice, and by using the tuning fork. The audiometer is used for more accurate testing. Attention is paid to:

TINNITUS. Ringing, buzzing, hissing, singing, or roaring in the ear
HEARING SCOTOMAS. Deafness to certain pitches and noises
RECEPTIVE APHASIA. Ability to hear but not comprehend

Equilibrium is tested by the caloric test in which hot or cold water is injected into the external auditory canal. Normally, stimulation of the canal with cold water produces rotary nystagmus (involuntary circular movement of the eye) away from the side of the ear being irrigated; hot water normally causes rotary nystagmus toward the irrigated side.

IX GLOSSOPHARYNGEAL AND X VAGUS, MIXED SENSORY AND MOTOR NERVES

These two nerves are tested together. They are usually both involved when there is disorder of either. The tongue is depressed and the posterior pharynx is touched with an applicator to determine if sensation is present and if the gag reflex is active. Swallowing is tested by having the patient drink water, and taste to the posterior third of the tongue is tested with sweet, bitter, sour, and salt substances. The larynx, controlled by the vagus nerve, is tested by having the patient speak and cough. If he is hoarse or if his cough is ineffectual, there is vagus nerve involvement.

XI SPINAL ACCESSORY, MOTOR NERVE TO THE STERNOCLEIDOMASTOID AND TRAPEZIUS MUSCLES IN THE NECK AND SHOULDERS

These muscles are inspected for atrophy. They are tested for strength by having the patient rotate his head and shrug his shoulders against resistance.

XII HYPOGLOSSAL, MOTOR NERVE TO THE TONGUE

The tongue is observed for atrophy. The patient is asked to stick his tongue out and move it from side to side. Lateral deviation indicates paralysis on one side. Its strength is tested by having the patient put it in his cheek and resist pressure applied by the examiner on the outside.

Special Neurologic Tests

Signed permission must be obtained for all the following special tests.

LUMBAR PUNCTURE

Cerebrospinal fluid may be obtained through a lumbar puncture. The patient lies at the edge of his bed on his left side with his legs flexed and his back rounded. His neck is bent so that his chin is resting on his chest. In this position the vertebrae are widely separated. The area is anesthetized with 2 to 5 per cent procaine hydrochloride. A needle with stylet is inserted between the fourth and fifth lumbar vertebrae into the spinal subarachnoid space. The stylet is removed and spinal fluid drips out. *No cord damage is done because the cord ends at the upper aspect of the second lumbar vertebra.*

Samples of spinal fluid are collected for laboratory analysis and culture to isolate specific microorganisms. Normal spinal fluid is clear, colorless, and odorless and contains a minimal number of cells, 20 to 40 per cent protein, 720 to 750 mg per cent chloride, and 60 to 80 mg per cent sugar. Red blood cells in the sample would indicate bleeding although there may be blood in the first sample obtained as a result of the puncture wound. For this reason, several samples are collected and labeled. Increased numbers of leukocytes might indicate infection; elevated protein might suggest degenerative diseases or tumor.

A manometer is attached, and pressure of the cerebrospinal fluid is measured. Normal pressure is 80 to 180 mm H_2O. If a blockage of cerebrospinal fluid is suspected, the physician may do the Queckenstedt test in which the nurse places pressure over the jugular veins with her fingers flat against the patient's neck for ten seconds. Readings are then taken at five-second intervals from the time the jugular veins are compressed until the pressure drops and becomes stabile. There is normally a rise of 100 ml H_2O with a fall to the previous level within 30 seconds.[21] A sluggish, poor rise with a delayed fall suggests a partial obstruction; no rise indicates complete block.

The patient must lie still when lumbar puncture is performed. Even with injection of an anesthetic he will experience some pain and pressure as the dura is entered. He may feel a shooting pain down one leg when the needle comes close to a nerve; however, the nerve is floating in fluid and is safe from injury.[22] Headache is fairly common following lumbar puncture. It is thought to be caused by leakage of cerebrospinal fluid through the dura. For this reason, the patient is usually kept flat in bed with one pillow for several hours after the test. The physician will specify the length of time the patient is to lie flat.

When increased intracranial pressure is suspected (from tumor or a space-occupying lesion), lumbar puncture is not done. The rapid release in pressure when cerebrospinal fluid is removed combined with the elevated pressure in the cranium might cause "coning." This is a herniation or pulling down of brainstem and cerebellum through the foramen magnum. The vital centers are "squeezed" and respirations may cease.

PNEUMOENCEPHALOGRAPHY (LUMBAR AIR ENCEPHALOGRAPHY)

A lumbar puncture is performed and air or oxygen is injected to replace spinal fluid that is withdrawn. About 20 to 30 ml of air is injected. The gas rises to the ventricles in the brain, and x-rays are taken. The ventricles are not outlined by x-ray unless air or oxygen is used. The patient is not permitted anything by mouth for four to six hours before the test. He is given a sedative about one hour before. The test is done in the x-ray department. Afterward, the patient must remain flat with one pillow for 12 to 48 hours, until all the air is absorbed. There are often severe headache and vomiting. The patient must be turned every two hours and encouraged to drink fluids after the nausea and vomiting subside to hasten the absorption of air and stimulate production of cerebrospinal fluid. Intramuscular injection of caffeine sodium benzoate relieves headache. Ice bags help, too. The patient is observed carefully for signs of increased intracranial pressure (see p. 430) as well as chills, fever, shock, and convulsions.

VENTRICULOGRAPHY

In this test air is injected directly into the ventricles through a bur hole drilled in the skull. This procedure is used if increased intracranial pressure is suspected, to prevent coning. This procedure is done in the operating room. An intravenous or general anesthetic is used.

CISTERNAL PUNCTURE

In this test a short beveled hollow needle with a stylet is inserted below the occipital bone into the cisterna magna. This test is selected when it is impossible to obtain cerebrospinal fluid by lumbar puncture. The back of the patient's neck may be shaved, and he is placed on his side at the edge of the bed with his head bent forward and held firmly by the nurse.

MYELOGRAPHY

In this test gas or a radiopaque liquid is injected into the subarachnoid space of the spinal canal through a lumbar puncture, and x-rays are taken in an attempt to visualize a lesion of the spinal cord. This test is done when slipped disk is suspected although it does not always indicate the lesion even when it is certainly present. The test is done in the x-ray department on a tilt table that is tilted to various degrees. After fluoroscopic and x-ray examination the physician removes the dye by doing another lumbar puncture. The dye must be removed or it will cause irritation to the meninges. If it is all removed, the patient lies flat for a few hours. If some of it remains, care is taken to keep the patient's head elevated to decrease gravitation of the dye to the brain. Repeated attempts are made to remove the dye under fluoroscopy. The patient is not permitted anything by mouth for four to six hours before the test. Sometimes a cleansing enema is administered to decrease the chance of gas shadows interfering with the x-ray pictures.

ANGIOGRAPHY

In this test contrast medium is injected into the carotid arteries in the neck and x-rays are taken. Blood vessels within the cranium are outlined. Intracranial aneurysms, anomalies, or ruptured vessels are discovered. The patient is given a sedative the night before the procedure and atropine sulfate and meperidine or morphine sulfate one-half hour before the procedure.

ELECTROENCEPHALOGRAPHY

In this test, the electrical activity of the brain is recorded. It is a painless procedure in which about 16 tiny electrodes are attached to the scalp with collodion. The hair does not have to be cut. The patient sits in a comfortable chair or lies on a bed. He must be very still and very quiet and is told to keep his eyes closed. Every five minutes the record is interrupted to allow him to move. The room must be devoid of external distraction. The patient need not be fasting.

ECHOENCEPHALOGRAPHY

In this test reflected ultrasound from the bones of the skull and some structures in the head is recorded and projected on a screen. The time taken is indicative of structural shifts in the brain. If general anesthesia is to be used, the test is done in the operating room. Otherwise, it is done in the x-ray department.

RADIOISOTOPE UPTAKE (BRAIN SCAN)

A radioactive substance such as mercury or iodinated serum albumin is injected intravenously. Three to four hours later radioactivity emanating from the head is recorded and projected onto x-ray films of the skull. Abnormal concentration of the radioactive material indicates a lesion. The test is done in the x-ray department.

The Neurologic Emergency

Initial Management of Spinal Cord Injury

All unconscious patients and all patients with back injury should be treated as if there were spinal cord injury. Injuries to the cord are usually found in the cervical or lumbar areas. The thoracic area is protected by the rib cage.

Scrupulous care must be taken to protect the cord from any further damage and the patient from paralysis. The patient is paraplegic if both lower limbs are involved; he is quadriplegic if both arms and legs are involved; he is hemiplegic if the arm and leg of one side of the body are involved.

Here are the rules for the initial management of spinal cord injury:

1. Never place the patient in a sitting or a semireclining position as this might flex the cord and cause further damage. Transport him with his head and his hips parallel.
2. Maintain normal vertebral alignment by using boards, sticks, rolls of newspaper, or clothing.
3. Move the patient as one rigid piece with several people assisting. Do not change the vertebral alignment.
4. Question him regarding paralysis and loss of sensation. If he can move his hands but not his legs, place him on the stretcher fully extended with his face down. If he cannot move his arms, the injury is to the cervical cord. Keep him in face-up position.

The degree of injury is estimated when the patient arrives at the hospital. Skeletal traction to the vertebral column is the treatment of choice for fracture dislocations of the cervical spine. Crutchfield tongs are used. They look like ice tongs. Local anesthetic is injected into the scalp in the lateral parietal areas.[23] Stab wounds are made down to the skull and then bur holes are drilled in the outer part of the skull. Tong points are inserted, the tongs are then tightened to secure them in place, and weights are attached. Piano wire (Hoen) is sometimes placed in grooves made in the skull, with the ends securely intertwined and traction secured to the wire union.

Bracing is necessary if the lesion is partial, if it is in the healing stage, or if it is at the fifth cervical level even in incomplete lesions because accidental damage could be fatal.[24]

Head Injuries

Automobile accidents account for most head injuries. All patients with acute head injuries should be put to bed immediately. If unconscious, they should be placed on their side with the mouth slightly dependent and the head slightly raised to decrease the chance of aspirating mucus. The most serious aspect of head injuries is the possible damage to the brain. Loss of consciousness comes from actual physical damage to its cells and fibers. In general, the depth and duration of unconsciousness are indicative of the degree of trauma. The more serious the injury, the longer and deeper is the depressed level of consciousness. (See p. 427.)

SKULL FRACTURE

Skull fracture can be a simple, linear break in the continuity of the skull (a crack); a comminuted break (fragmented); or a depressed break in which slivers of bone are driven into the brain substance. Fractures are "open" if there is a break in the scalp, skull, and meninges. This may cause serious infection. A fracture may cause injury to the cranial nerves as they pass through the foramen magnum in the skull. Cerebrospinal fluid or blood may leak through a nasal sinus or ear if there is a break there. The patient may be in shock.

TYPES OF HEAD INJURIES

Concussion. This is a "shaking" injury to the brain that may cause damage to nerve fibers. The patient loses consciousness momentarily. There are usually no demonstrable neurologic signs.

Contusion. More serious than concussion, a contusion implies bruising of the brain. Neurologic damage may be present. There is a longer period of unconsciousness. Recovery is usual.

Compression. This is the most serious in the group. Vessels are torn. Hemorrhage follows. There can be congestion in the brain with pressure on vital areas.

COMPLICATIONS OF HEAD INJURY

Extradural hematoma is a buildup of blood between the skull and the dura mater. It develops as a result of tearing of the meningeal vessels and may cause increased intracranial pressure with eventual compression of brain substance. The clot must be removed through bur holes drilled in the skull.

Subdural hematoma is a buildup of blood between the dura mater and the arachnoid from small vessels being torn. There is ultimate increase in intracranial pressure. The process is slow. Symptoms show up weeks or months after the injury. Fluid-filled cysts form. There are headache and drowsiness. Bur holes must be drilled and fluid from the cysts drained.

Subarachnoid hemorrhage involves bleeding in the space formed by the arachnoid and the pia mater. Although it can result from injury, it more frequently results from spontaneous rupture of an aneurysm.[25] The patient experiences headache, stiff neck, and photophobia. There is no surgical treatment.

OBSERVATION

Initial observations of the patient are extremely important because they establish a "baseline" against which further deterioration or improvement can be measured. Observation includes:

1. *Level of Consciousness.* If the patient is drowsy it may be necessary to awaken him during the first 24 to 36 hours following injury to evaluate

his alertness and his general response to stimulation. The specific stimulus that awakens him should be charted, e.g., "responded to loud talking" or "responded to tapping his cheek."

2. *Mental State.* Ascertain whether the patient is oriented to time, place, and person. What is his behavior like? Is he hallucinating?

3. *Vital Signs.* Vital signs are sensitive indicators of neurologic status, especially increasing intracranial pressure and brainstem damage. An elevated temperature (hyperthermia) is a frequent complication of injury to the hypothalamus. Vital signs are taken every 30 to 60 minutes during the first 12 to 24 hours.

4. *Convulsions.* (See p. 437.) If convulsions are present, they must be observed and recorded accurately because they give vital clues about where the brain damage is. The patient must be protected from injuring himself. If convulsions occur shortly after injury, they may cause cerebral anoxia and further brain damage. They are controlled with drugs such as phenobarbital.

5. *Speech.* Is it clear? Mumbled? Confused? Is expressive or receptive aphasia present?

6. *Pupils.* Note whether they are equal in size, whether they constrict when light is shone into them, and what their shape is.

7. *Presence of Blood.* Report the presence of blood or cerebrospinal drainage from any orifice. Emergency surgery may be necessary.

8. *Stiff Neck.* Nuchal rigidity is present when there is irritation to the meninges. This should be reported.

Care of the Unconscious Patient

Unconsciousness is a state of depressed cerebral function in which appreciation of stimuli is lost. If response is present, it is on a reflex level.[26] Loss of consciousness may result from a variety of causes, some of which include injury and falls, drug or alcohol overdosage, stroke, subarachnoid hemorrhage, epilepsy, and diabetes mellitus.

The unconscious patient cannot do anything for himself. All his needs must be met by other people to prevent the complications of immobility.

Maintain Patent Airway

Position the patient on his side with his mouth dependent so that mucus and other secretions will drain out and not be aspirated. A suction machine should be at the bedside. Careful suctioning should be done with the catheter passed through the nose or mouth with the suction turned off. The suction is turned on once the catheter is in place. The catheter should be twisted with the thumb and forefinger to prevent prolonged contact of the open end with any one part of the mucosa. Irritation might cause bleeding and increased amounts of secretion. An emergency tracheotomy set should be ready. If the patient's tongue is paralyzed, an oral airway should be inserted with the tongue pulled forward.

Maintain Water and Electrolyte Balance and Meet Nutritional Requirements

The patient is usually fed by vein during the first 48 hours. He is given a daily intake of 2,000 to 2,500 ml of fluid with 5 to 10 gm NaCl and about 40 to 80 mEq potassium, determined according to serum electrolyte levels, if intravenous feedings must be continued for several days.[27] If the patient cannot eat by the second or third day, gastric tube feedings are instituted. It is not possible to maintain adequate caloric intake by vein. Formulas containing fluids, proteins, and calories are mixed in a blender and are made thin enough to pass through the tube. Eggs, cooked cereal, juices, crust-free bread, salad oil, strained or puréed meats, and vegetables are all passed through the gastric tube. Feedings of 400 to 500 ml are given several times each day. The patient's head should be elevated and the feeding should be given slowly. The tube should be rinsed with 20 ml water after each feeding. The gastric tube should not remain in the same nostril for more than five days and should be kept well lubricated with a water-soluble lubricant at the nostril to lessen the chance of crust formation. Feedings by mouth are begun when the swallowing reflex returns.

Control Urinary Retention and Incontinence

Incontinence may be the result of impaired consciousness rather than bladder dysfunction. Intermittent catheterization or an indwelling catheter is used initially, but is discontinued by the third or fourth day unless the patient remains greatly distended. In this way an attempt is made to prevent permanent impairment of the bladder muscles. Output is measured and the patient is kept clean and dry to prevent decubitus ulcer formation.

Prevent Muscle Atrophy and Contractures

Passive range-of-motion exercise is done several times a day while the patient is unconscious. He is turned at least every two hours, by planned schedule.

Eye Care

Special care must be given to the eyes if corneal reflexes are absent. Corneal irritation is likely to occur from scratching on a pillow, dust particles and dryness, because of decreased secretion and incomplete eye closure. The eyes should be examined frequently for inflammation and irrigated with suitable solutions ordered by the physician, e.g., sterile saline. They should be covered with eye shields or closed with butterfly dressings made of gauze and collodion. Neglect of the eyes of the unconscious patient can cause corneal irritation, keratitis, and blindness.

39

INCREASED CRANIAL PRESSURE

An increase in pressure in the cranium is very serious because it causes compression or "pressing" on vital centers in the brain, and may result in death. Pressure can stem from tumors, bleeding, inflammatory disease, thrombi, or any space-occupying lesion. Because the brain is housed in a rigid skull, it cannot expand as the space-occupying lesion grows. The bigger the lesion, the greater the pressure on the vital brain centers. The more crowded the nonexpansible space becomes within the cranium, the more limited is the blood-oxygen supply to the individual neurons. This oxygen deficit causes the cerebral symptoms. Tumors will be discussed as an example of space-occupying lesions.

Tumors

One third of the total number of brain tumors are slow-growing, benign, and compatible with life for ten years or more. The remainder are rapidly growing, malignant, and kill within a month or two after first symptoms.[28] Some benign tumors, because of their rapid increase in pressure on brain tissue, may have a malignant effect. Tumors arise in any part of the nervous system and are named according to the area of involvement. For instance, a meningioma is a benign tumor that grows in the coverings of the brain and spinal cord; a glioma derives from the supporting tissue (neuroglia) of the brain and grows within its very substance. It can be benign and very slow-growing, or malignant and very rapid. It is a difficult type of tumor to remove surgically because of its infiltrating nature. More than half of brain tumors are gliomas and meningiomas. Tumors can also spread from other primary sources, especially from the lungs. Initial symptoms are often so subtle that they are overlooked.

Tumors are called supratentorial if they are located in the cerebrum or anterior two thirds of the brain. They are above the tentorium. The tentorium is a double fold of dura mater between the occipital lobes and the cerebellum. Tumors are designated as being infratentorial if they are located below the tentorium. These include tumors of the cerebellum, brainstem, and posterior third of the brain.

The treatment of choice, of course, would be the complete surgical removal of the tumor; however, this is not always possible. If the tumor is in the ventricular system the Torkildsen procedure, in which a catheter is placed between the lateral ventricles and the subarachnoid space in the region of the foramen magnum, may be attempted. This allows the ventricular fluid to bypass the obstruction through the catheter.[29] X-ray therapy is often used to control the spread and symptoms by shrinking the tumor. See page 432 for further discussion of surgery.

Symptoms

Regardless of the type of tumor, symptoms are caused by increased compression to the area on which the tumor is pressing. For instance, a tumor of the auditory cranial nerve would cause decreased hearing acuity; one of the optic nerve would cause decreased visual acuity, diplopia, and so on. The major symptoms of the increased pressure within the cranium include the following:

HEADACHE AND VOMITING

The patient awakens in the morning with a severe throbbing headache. It decreases in intensity as the day progresses and is frequently relieved by vomiting, which also occurs in the morning, is not accompanied by nausea, is unrelated to eating, and does not have to be "projectile." Elevating the head of the bed to a 30- to 35-degree angle increases venous return and helps decrease the headache.

PAPILLEDEMA

The rise in intracranial pressure is transmitted along the optic nerve and causes it to swell. This "swelling" is called optic nerve edema, choked disk, or papilledema. It can be seen with an ophthalmoscope. It causes vision to fail.

CHANGES IN VITAL SIGNS AND LEVEL OF CONSCIOUSNESS

Pressure on the brainstem, especially on the medulla, which controls many vital body functions, causes changes in vital signs. Although there may be an initial rise in pulse rate, there follows a drop in pulse rate to less than 50 beats per minute. The physician should be notified if the pulse rate falls to 60 or below. The more rapid the increase in intracranial pressure, the greater the decrease in pulse rate. There is an elevation in blood pressure and a change in the rhythm of respirations with a decrease in the rate of respirations. Cheyne-Stokes respirations may develop. *A consistent slowing of pulse rate and respiratory rate with a concomitant rise in blood pressure is grave. The physician should be notified immediately!*

Hiccuping and cardiac irregularities may develop. With the decreased supply of oxygen to brain cells there is often a change in level of consciousness. The patient may be comatose.

CHANGES IN MENTAL STATUS

Concentration and memory are poor. The patient may seem "absent-minded," slow, and lethargic. There may be personality change and slowing of speech processes.

FOCAL SIGNS

These vary according to the area of brain being compressed. There may be hemiparesis with weakness and loss of sensation to the leg and arm of one side of the body. There may be receptive and/or expressive aphasia. The patient may be unable to read, write, calculate, or recognize the size, shape, weight, or texture of objects. His movements may lack coordination, and there may be unusual eye movements and visual defects.

Observation of the patient at admission is of critical importance for establishing a baseline against which further comparative observation may be made. Every contact the nurse makes with the patient should include observation and recording of same.

Conservative treatment for increased intracranial pressure [30] involves a dehydrating routine. Fluid intake is limited to 800 to 1,200 ml for 24 hours. Hypertonic solutions that draw fluid toward themselves and increase their excretion through the kidneys may be used; 250 ml of 25 per cent glucose, 50 ml of 50 per cent glucose, concentrated proteins, and mannitol (Osmitrol) in 5, 10, 15, or 20 per cent concentrations are examples. An administration set with a filter is recommended for infusing the 20 per cent concentration of mannitol. Dehydrating drugs such as 30 ml of saturated solution of magnesium sulfate may be given by mouth before breakfast or by retention enema. An intramuscular injection of caffeine sodium benzoate may be used. In any case, the head of the bed is kept at a 30- to 45-degree angle to increase venous drainage from the brain.

Surgery of the Brain

In many instances surgical removal of the space-occupying lesion is the treatment of choice. Brain surgery requires the greatest gentleness and patience. Rough handling might injure surrounding neurons and leave the patient with other permanent damage. Unless surgery is of an emergency nature, preoperative assessment takes several days. Many tests are done to locate the exact area containing the lesion. Cerebral angiography, pneumoencephalography, and ventriculography help determine the presence or absence of a space-occupying lesion. Certain brain tumors selectively accumulate radioactive isotopes such as radioactive iodine combined with serum albumin. A Geiger counter over the area or a brain scan indicates this increased density and in this way outlines the tumor area. Electroencephalography is useful, too. Bursts of slow-wave activity frequently indicate tumor sites. A normal EEG, however, does not rule out the presence of a tumor.

Preoperative Preparation for Brain Surgery

A dehydrating regimen may be instituted before surgery in an attempt to decrease intracranial pressure. This is usually done if operative bleeding is suspected. The patient's hair is washed and his head is shaved. The hair should be put in an envelope, properly labeled, and kept safely. An enema may be ordered so that the patient will not have to strain at stool postoperatively. Any straining would cause an increase in intracranial pressure. Morphine sulfate is usually *not* given to any patient with brain involvement as it tends to mask pupillary reaction and depress respirations. If there is preoperative pain, meperidine (Demerol) and/or aspirin is usually ordered.

The Craniotomy

The scalp is incised and reflected back and a flap is made. Bur holes are made in the skull, a wire saw is inserted, and the bone between the holes is cut. The bone remains attached to the muscle, which acts as a hinge when the flap is turned.[31] The dura mater is exposed and it, too, is reflected back to expose the space-occupying lesion. If the tumor is supratentorial (in the anterior two thirds of the brain), the incision is usually made in the area overlying the tumor site in the frontal, parietal, temporal, or occipital region. When the tumor is infratentorial (in the brainstem and cerebellum), the incision is made above the nape of the neck. Sometimes, the physician inserts a vacuum drain during surgery to help eliminate serous fluid and blood, and to decrease the facial edema. The drain remains in place for 24 to 48 hours postoperatively.

After Craniotomy

The bed is made up so that its foot becomes its head. It is easier to handle and to observe the head from this position. Side rails are kept up. A mouth gag, suction apparatus, tracheotomy set, airway, and lumbar puncture tray should be close at hand. The patient is usually placed on his side with a small pillow under his head and his mouth downward so that fluid drains out and there is less chance of aspiration. Maintenance of a patent airway is a major goal. When the patient awakens and can swallow, the head of the bed is elevated 25 to 35 degrees to help decrease cerebral venous pressure and edema. However, the position of the patient varies according to the location and extent of the surgery. This must be clarified with the physician. If a particularly large space-occupying lesion was removed from the cerebrum, a large open cavity will remain. Until the body's natural processes have a chance to fill in this space with new tissue, the patient is kept on the nonoperated side so that the brain does not "shift" to the vacant space. A sign on the bed helps prevent confusion, e.g., "do not turn patient on right side." After surgery to the brainstem or cerebellum the patient is kept off his back. He is placed flat, on either side, with one small pillow under his head. In any case, the head should remain in alignment with the rest of the body. The nurse must make sure she has adequate help when she turns the patient. She must be sure that no tension is placed on the suture line.

Dressings are observed carefully. A moderate amount of serous drainage is expected the first 24 to 48 hours postoperatively; however, the presence of yellowish-clear drainage indicates leakage of cerebrospinal fluid, and this should be reported to the physician immediately. Dressings can be reinforced with sterile towels or sponges. If a drain has not been inserted the dressings may become saturated and may be changed on a daily basis. Usually, though, dressings are reinforced but not changed until the sutures are removed about the fourth postoperative day. The dressing is an encircling one and may get too tight and cause constriction and edema. In this case, the physician would slit the dressing to relieve the pressure. If a bone flap has not been replaced, extra care must be taken to prevent compression to that area. The patient must be told that there will always be a slight indentation in that area and that he must protect it from injury. When the final dressings are removed, special scalp care is given to cleanse the head and remove dried blood and crusts. This may be done with mineral oil, petroleum jelly, or hydrogen peroxide followed by a shampoo. Care must be taken not to rub the operated area or put tension on the suture line. The head is covered with some type of cap.

Medications that depress respirations or mask pupillary signs (e.g., morphine) are used sparingly, if at all. Most patients are given anticonvulsants, paraldehyde, diphenylhydantoin (Dilantin) postoperatively.

Intake and output are measured. Sometimes fluid intake is limited postoperatively to decrease the chance of cerebral edema. The patient is fed intravenously in the early postoperative period with the drops administered no faster than 40 per minute. Nasogastric feedings begin as soon as it is feasible. They are administered every two hours. Oral foods and fluids are initiated as soon as the patient is able to swallow.

Vital signs are taken frequently. The physician indicates an acceptable range for a given patient, and the nurse notifies him if there is deviation.

An increase in blood pressure and a decrease in pulse might herald an increase in intracranial pressure from cerebral edema and bleeding. Vital signs also indicate shock, hemorrhage, and recovery from anesthesia.

Frequent rectal temperatures are taken to make sure the heat-control center in the hypothalamus has not been disturbed. Continuous, long-term elevations of temperature (hyperthermia) are destructive to the brain. The physician should be notified if the temperature is 102° F. or over. He may order tepid water or alcohol sponge baths, aspirin suppositories, or a hypothermia blanket to decrease the patient's temperature and maintain it at a designated level. (See p. 274.)

The patient often complains of severe headache one to two days after surgery. This is common. Headache is controlled by codeine sulfate given hypodermically every four hours and by aspirin either orally or rectally. An ice cap to the head helps. Movements must not be jarring. When the patient is turned, the nurse might use a turning sheet and certainly should get sufficient help. Noise should be kept at a minimum.

Enemas are usually not ordered postoperatively because they may increase straining, which in turn might increase intracranial pressure.

The patient is often allowed out of bed on the second to fifth postoperative day. Ambulation must be gradual. The patient begins by having the head of the bed elevated to a high Fowler's position, progresses to sitting on the edge of the bed with his feet resting on a stool, and is then assisted to a chair later in the day if he was able to tolerate the sitting position. He must be observed carefully for signs of increasing intracranial pressure when he is up. His pulse and blood pressure should be taken before the activity and upon return to bed.

To prevent complications of immobility, range-of-motion (ROM) exercises are done at least twice a day. The patient is encouraged to deep-breathe and he is turned frequently. He usually goes home by the end of the second week.

Complications of intracranial surgery include shock, cerebral edema with elevated intracranial pressure, clot formation due to postoperative bleeding (further surgery must be done to locate and remove clots), convulsions, and infections.

Nursing Observation

Observations made by the nurse are of utmost importance. Changes occur very rapidly and can be fatal. An alert, cooperative patient may become confused, drowsy, and unconscious in a matter of minutes.

Report any deterioration in level of consciousness or changes indicating elevating intracranial pressure immediately. The patient may have to be returned to surgery.

Specific Observations	Reason
Rectal temperature	Elevation may indicate interference with hypothalamus. Drop may mean shock
Respiratory rate and rhythm, pulse, blood pressure and vomiting	Change in vital signs and vomiting may mean pressure on the medulla. Report pulse less than 60 beats per minute with rise or fall in blood pressure. Vomiting may mean increasing intracranial pressure
Elevation of bone flap	May indicate edema; increasing intracranial pressure
Level of consciousness	Report any changes; physician may order that the patient be continuously stimulated, e.g., by talking to him even if he does not appear to hear or by having him grasp the nurse's hand
Mental status	There are usually some confusion and memory lapses in early postoperative period. Check patient's orientation to person, time, place. Speak clearly and slowly to him
Convulsions	Caused by electrical imbalance in the brain, they can lead to permanent brain damage. Observe and report when convulsion started, precipitating factors, pattern and progression of activity, etc. Protect patient from injury
Paresthesias, muscle strength, motor dysfunction and coordination	May indicate interference with pyramidal tracts, further brain involvement
Eyes	Is corneal reflex present? Does eye close completely? Are the pupils equal? A large, nonreactive pupil may be present on the operative side. Report whether patient complains of visual disturbances. May indicate cranial nerve involvement, interference at the optic chiasm

Following intracranial surgery, and depending on the individual need of the patient, the physician solicits the help of the physical, occupational, and speech therapists, the visiting nurse, the nutritionist, and the psychologist.

40

CONVULSIVE DISORDERS

THE functioning ability of the brain depends on the electrical activity of its cells. Normally, there is balance between electrical excitation and electrical inhibition. In a convulsion or "seizure" this balance is disturbed and the bursts of electrical energy are irregular. A convulsion, then, is a disturbance in electrical balance within the brain. Any normal brain has a threshold for convulsions. It can be made to convulse with chemicals or electricity. The threshold seems to be lower in the patient with a convulsive disorder. The convulsion originates in an area of abnormal cerebral tissue. It may be localized (focal) or may spread to involve normal brain cells as well. The signs that are seen during the convulsion depend on the area of the brain involved in the irregular electrical activity.

Types of Convulsions

A *grand-mal convulsion* is one in which there is complete loss of consciousness and a classic sequence pattern, which includes:

1. Aura (not always present)
2. Tonic phase: contraction and spasm of muscles
3. Clonic phase: alternate contraction and relaxation of muscles; "jerking activity"
4. Deep sleep (not always present)

There may be a "prodromal" period lasting several hours in which the patient experiences some sensation that warns him of the coming convulsion. He may be unusually tense, depressed, or excited. Immediately before the convulsion there may be an "aura." This lasts only a few seconds but warns of the coming convulsion by some unusual body sensation such as tingling in a limb, feelings of unreality, an odd smell, or a flash of light. If there is an aura, the patient has time to protect himself by removing his dentures and eyeglasses and lying down on the floor. During the tonic phase muscles contract and go into spasm. The patient may utter a sudden cry caused by the forcing of air through the larynx, which is itself in spasm. Limbs become rigid. Breathing may cease for about one half of a minute and the patient becomes cyanotic. He falls and there is loss of consciousness. During the clonic phase the limbs seem to "jerk." There appear to be alternate contraction and relaxation of the muscles. The tongue is often bitten, and blood-stained foam appears at the mouth. The patient becomes incontinent of urine and stool. This lasts only about one minute. The patient remains unconscious. He becomes "limp" and breathes deeply. The whole convulsion lasts only about three minutes. The patient may go into a deep sleep afterward, or be confused. This lasts about a half hour. He has no recollection of the convulsion.

If one grand-mal convulsion follows right after another in a continuous sequence, the patient is said to be in status epilepticus. This is very serious because it may cause permanent brain damage. The patient becomes exhausted. Intramuscular anticonvulsants and intravenous sodium pentathol are administered to stop the convulsions.

Petit-mal convulsions are sometimes unnoticed. They cause a very brief interruption of consciousness. The patient momentarily stops what he is doing. He is usually unaware that he has stopped eating, talking, and so on. His eyelids may flutter, and he seems to be temporarily staring vacantly into space. Sometimes there is slight jerking of the limbs.

Jacksonian Convulsions

Described by a British neurologist, Hughlings Jackson, these are convulsions that begin in a specific area of the motor or sensory cortex, usually where there is scar tissue, and spread to normal brain cells. The convulsion typically starts with a jerking in a thumb, tongue, or leg, and then progresses to a whole side of the body, corresponding to the spread of electrical discharge from one part of the cortex through other parts, in succession. The patient usually remains conscious throughout.

Psychomotor Convulsions

These convulsions are called psychomotor or psychomotor-equivalents because some unusual mental and/or motor activity takes the place of the usual tonic-clonic pattern of a convulsion. There is a transient disturbance in mental, emotional, and motor activity.[32] The behavior is inappropriate for the situation. It is automatic. The patient may stop what he is doing and stare. He may begin repetitive movements such as stroking his hair or clutching at linen. He may mumble and begin chewing motions with his jaw. He may walk out of his house and "wake up" without any idea of how he got where he finds himself. The convulsion lasts from 15 seconds to several minutes and is extremely varied in its symptoms. Amnesia occurs. The attack may end with a period of confusion.

All types of convulsions may be precipitated by stimuli such as bright flickering lights, noise, pain, hyperventilation, ingestion of alcohol, irregularity in taking prescribed medications, increase in age and body weight, severe emotional strain, fever-producing illness, changes in blood sugar level and blood-gas concentration, and upset in body fluid equilibrium and pH.

Epilepsy

Epilepsy is a group of disorders characterized by recurring convulsions. About 2 million Americans are affected by it. Although it has been considered an inherited disorder, no specific genetic mode of transmission has been established. It is therefore called "familial" and the patient is said to have a "hereditary predisposition" to the disease. Epilepsy is called *idiopathic* if the cause is not known. Most epileptics fall within this category. Epilepsy is called *symptomatic* if the cause can be traced to some brain injury. Examples include difficult births, postnatal head trauma, nutritional or toxic disorders, cerebral anoxia, tumors, alcohol intoxication, and febrile states. The patient with idiopathic epilepsy will more than likely have grand-mal and/or petit-mal convulsions. The patient with symptomatic epilepsy will probably have jacksonian or psychomotor convulsions.

Precautions and Management of the Patient with Convulsions

The patient must be protected from injury. If he is already in bed, side rails should be used to prevent falls. If he is out of bed, he should be placed in bed if there is time or laid on the floor if there is not. The bed should be positioned so that his head can be seen easily. The door should be left open unless a nurse remains with him. The nurse must close the door and stay with the patient if he does convulse. He should have a small, firm pillow rather than a thick, fluffy one. He should use paper rather than glass straws, and his temperature should be taken rectally rather than orally. If he smokes, the nurse should stay with him. A padded tongue blade (or wooden spoon at home) should be taped to the head of the bed and inserted between his upper and lower molars if a convulsion begins. This prevents him from biting his tongue and provides a means of getting to the tongue if it slips back and obstructs the airway. Once the teeth have clamped shut, attempts should not be made to force the tongue blade between them. This may cause additional damage. If the patient begins to convulse, the nurse should pull the bedcovers from his body so that she may observe his position, the first movement she sees, the chronologic order of motor activity, and the last movement. These observations give the physician clues as to the area of brain involvement.

Scott [33] outlines the observation and recording of a convulsion this way:

A. Events preceding it
   1. Activity
   2. Change in mental state or behavior seconds, minutes, or hours before
   3. Precipitating event
B. The convulsion
   1. Aura
   2. First event, e.g., "loud cry"
   3. Posture during attack, e.g., "almost fell off chair"
   4. Movements and their spread, e.g., "jerking of arms and then legs"
   5. Level of consciousness, e.g., "did not respond to loud auditory stimulus"
   6. Changes in appearance, e.g., color of skin, salivation, sweating, pupils constricted or dilated
   7. Incontinence, e.g., "incontinent of urine"
   8. Injury, e.g., none
C. Events following the convulsion
   1. Speech, e.g., "slurred"
   2. Confusion, e.g., "drowsy," "no recollection of attack"
   3. Weakness of limbs
   4. Abnormal behavior
   5. Other, e.g., "stated he had headache"

The duration of the convulsion should also be noted, e.g., "lasted three minutes."

The goals of treatment include:

1. Find and treat the underlying cause
2. Control or prevent convulsions by use of anticonvulsants and/or surgery
3. Understand the total problem facing the patient regarding living with the disease

To localize the area of cerebral electrical imbalance, electroencephalography is done. The area of brain involvement and the type of convulsion can be established by observation of type of brain waves. For instance, petit-mal epilepsy shows a typical spike and wave discharge. See Figures 40–1, 40–2, and 40–3 for the various brain waves: normal, grand mal, and petit mal.

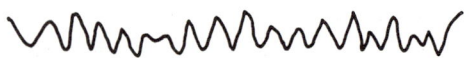

FIGURE 40–1. Schematic drawing of normal alpha brain waves.

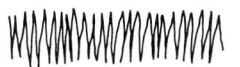

High Voltage Fast Waves

FIGURE 40–2. Grand-mal epilepsy as shown on the electroencephalographic recorder.

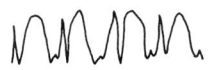

Spike and Dome 3 Per Sec

FIGURE 40–3. Petit-mal epilepsy as shown on the electroencephalographic recorder.

Use of Anticonvulsants

With properly regulated amounts of anticonvulsant drugs 75 to 80 per cent [34] of patients become convulsion-free; however, some patients still have convulsions though their frequency is decreased. Ideally, anticonvulsants should develop stability in the cerebral tissue so that it can withstand "provoking" factors and at the same time they should not sedate the patient or cause severe untoward effects. The physician begins by trying a small amount of one drug and gradually increases the amount until convulsions are controlled or toxic symptoms develop. The majority of patients are treated with one or a combination of phenobarbital, methylphenylethyl hydantoin (Mesantoin), diphenylhydantoin sodium (Dilantin), and trimethadione (Tridione, Trimetin). The latter is especially effective for petit-mal convulsions. Because many of the drugs must be administered three times a day, they are given at mealtime so that the patient does not forget to take them. If phenobarbital is used, it is usually given at night because of its sedative effect. Phenobarbital remains one of the oldest and most successful anticonvulsants; however, if a patient has been taking it for a long period of time, he must be warned not to stop taking it abruptly or he will precipitate an attack of status epilepticus. Anticonvulsants are continued for one to three years following the last attack, or for the lifetime of the patient if convulsions continue. Because these drugs affect the blood-forming mechanism in the body, laboratory studies should be done when the drug is initially instituted, every two weeks until maintenance dosage is established, and then once a month for the first year.[35] Other side effects include hypertrophy of the gums, hirsutism, lymphadenopathy that resembles Hodgkin's disease, kidney problems, dizziness, photophobia, and rashes.

Surgery for Epilepsy

In symptomatic epilepsy surgery is sometimes elected to remove the causative tissue. Patients are candidates for this kind of surgery [36] if they have focal seizures that always begin in the same restricted area of cortex; if the involved area can be removed without producing paralysis or other serious neurologic disability; and if the seizures have not been satisfactorily controlled by an adequate trial of drugs. A thorough neurologic examination is done with special attention placed on observation and recording of the pattern of the convulsion. Sodium amytal may be injected into the patient's common carotid artery to make sure which side of the brain is dominant for speech and thus to ensure that it will not be tampered with during the surgery. Although right-handed patients almost always have their speech centers in the left hemispheres, the opposite is not always true in left-handed people. They may have their speech centers in the left side, too. If sodium amytal injected into the left common carotid artery produces temporary right hemiplegia plus inability to talk, left-sided speech dominance is ascertained.[37]

The surgery is done under local anesthesia injected into the scalp and into sensitive areas of the dura mater. General anesthesia distorts the brain waves and does not allow the patient to answer questions and follow commands during the surgery. Use of a local anesthetic also provides opportunity for accurate brain mapping by electrical stimulation so that vital areas are not touched.

Postoperative measures are the same as those for craniotomy. (See p. 432.) Corticosteroids are used during the first ten postoperative days to decrease cerebral edema. The patient is out of bed by the third postoperative day and home the third postoperative week. He is advised to allow two months for recuperation without any strenuous physical or mental activity. He must avoid excess fatigue. Anticonvulsants are continued for at least one year after surgery, and periodic electroencephalograms are done.

Living with Epilepsy

The great majority of people with epilepsy are completely normal except for the problem of their convulsions. Yet, they find adjustment difficult because of social pressures that still dictate a feeling of prejudice, fear, and misconception concerning the disease. Many people still believe that people with epilepsy are, in some magical way, being punished for a sin.

The person with epilepsy does not have an inferior intellect. The intellect of epileptics varies in exactly the same way that it varies in people who do not have this handicap: some are very bright and others are less so. Epilepsy and mental illness are not synonymous. The epileptic does not automatically have mental illness because of the epilepsy. If he develops mental illness it is a result of the stress of living with the disease in the same way that other people without epilepsy develop the symptoms of mental illness.

The controlled epileptic should be able to compete successfully in the labor market; yet, many employers have regulations that preclude the possibility of hiring the handicapped even though there is conclusive proof through Workmen's Compensation Insurance statistics that epileptic employees working alongside nonepileptic employees have no greater claims experience than would be expected from that particular occupational class.[38] The person with epilepsy is often faced with the heinous job of determining whether he should conceal his condition so that he can get the job, or reveal it honestly and probably be refused the job.

For those epileptics whose disease cannot be controlled, most states run sheltered workshops.

The consensus of opinion among authorities is that marriage has an advantageous stabilizing and integrating effect for epileptics. Yet, some states still have archaic laws concerning the rights of epileptics to marry. One prohibits epileptics from marrying under any circumstance; two require that epileptics be sterilized before a marriage license is issued.[39]

Issuance of driver's licenses seems a more logical area of concern. States have various laws concerning the driving rights of people with convulsive disorders. Most feel that a person should be seizure-free for two years before driving alone.

41

VASCULAR DISEASES OF THE BRAIN

DEGENERATIVE changes in the vessels that supply the brain impede blood flow and cause anoxia to the neurons. Complete absence of blood supply to an area in the brain causes necrosis to those neurons.

Cerebral vascular disease (stroke) is classified as being "impending, transient, or incipient" if there is intermittent cerebrovascular insufficiency usually resulting from deteriorative changes and spasm of the walls of the arteries. This is often called a "little stroke." There are episodes of neurologic disturbance related to the area of the brain that is deficient in oxygen. The "episode" lasts 5 to 30 minutes and the patient is neurologically normal between attacks; however, transient cerebrovascular deficiency indicates the ongoing nature of the disease process, and a serious stroke is often the end result.

The patient may experience dizziness, confusion, numbness on one side of the face, weakness of an extremity, and garbled or thick speech. He should be placed in a supine position. The head should not be rotated, extended, or flexed. It should be kept in a neutral position until symptoms disappear. This allows for optimum blood flow through vessels. Symptoms are often unnoticed.

Cerebrovascular disease is classified as being "stroke in evolution, advancing, evolving, or progressing" if there is evidence of gradually accumulating neurologic deficit within a few hours to 48 hours. This is the stroke as it is happening. If symptoms last more than an hour, the physician suspects developing brain infarction (death to cells) rather than transient ischemia (lack of oxygenated blood). Usually, by the time the physician sees the patient the stroke has passed from the evolving stage to the "completed" stage.

Cerebrovascular disease is classified as "completed, established" when the disease is no longer extending its anatomic confines. Maximal involvement has been reached. The damage is done and neurologic symptoms remain. Symptoms are primarily hemiparesis (paralysis of one whole side of the body from the top of the head to the toes), speaking and swallowing difficulties, and intellectual or memory defects.[40]

Causes of Stroke (CVA, Apoplexy)

Thrombosis of the artery with blockage by a clot or fatty plaque is the most frequent cause of stroke. It is often seen after unusual fatigue or when the blood pressure drops during sleep. Not enough blood is pushed through the sclerosed arteries, the blood tends to "stagnate," and clots form. This condition is seen in people between 50 and 70 years of age. Onset of symptoms is usually slow and there is often pre-existing vascular disease, e.g., hypertension.

Embolus is a condition in which a particle or piece of clot breaks off and lodges in a cerebral vessel causing infarction to the surrounding cells. The embolus may come from a piece of a clot, tumor, fat, a clump of bacteria, or air. The condition is particularly common in patients who have a history of rheumatic heart disease, bacterial endocarditis, and coronary artery thrombosis. The majority of emboli arise from the mitral valve and atria of hearts of patients who have had rheumatic heart disease.[41] It is also frequently seen in patients who have had cardiac fibrillation. When the fibrillation stops there is a sudden strong beat that mobilizes stagnant blood and clots. The condition is frequently seen in patients under 40 years of age. The onset of symptoms is rapid.

Cerebral thrombosis and embolus are the most frequent causes of stroke.

Cerebral hemorrhage is caused by injury to the brain with concomitant bleeding, or by rupture of a vessel, especially rupture of an aneurysm (vessel "outpouching"). The vessel wall becomes weakened and ruptures, and blood is pushed into the surrounding brain tissue causing damage to the cells in that area. Sometimes the pool of resulting blood acts like a tumor causing symptoms of increased intracranial pressure. Hemorrhage can be into the cortex, in the subarachnoid space, into the meninges, and so on. Catastrophic effects of cerebral hemorrhage are seen in people from 30 to 60 years of age. Cerebral hemorrhage can be fatal. It is the most serious type of stroke.

Cerebral edema is always present to some degree with infarction. If serious, it may compress the brainstem and cause death from respiratory failure. Initial mortality from stroke due to atherosclerotic vascular disease is 25 per cent.[42] For those who survive the initial phase, the most common causes of death during the first three months are pulmonary infarction, cardiac failure, and recurrent stroke. The prognosis is least good for older patients with severe stroke and evidence of vascular disease in other areas of the body. It is best for young patients with mild stroke and no evidence of vascular disease in other sites.

Symptoms of Stroke

Sometimes, the patient has "premonitory" warning signs of coming stroke that include dizziness, headache, unusual fatigue, and disturbances in speech or vision; but often stroke occurs suddenly without any warning. It often occurs during normal activity or when the patient is at rest. Shock may follow. The patient may be unconscious. His face may appear brick red. His breathing may be stertorous or difficult. Cheyne-Stokes respirations may be present. His cheek "blows out" on the involved side with every expiration. If brainstem centers have been disturbed, the pulse may be slow, full and bounding, or feeble and irregular. The blood pressure is usually elevated. If an aneurysm has ruptured, there will probably be severe headache in the area near the rupture. If there is meningeal irritation, there will be generalized headache and stiff neck. During the early shock stage it is not possible to determine what parts of the brain have suffered anoxia and may recover and what parts of the brain have suffered infarction and will not recover. There is always cerebral edema, too. As the edema fluid is absorbed, the pressure on brain cells is decreased, and symptoms decrease. This process of edema absorption takes up to six months. Residual symptoms are those seen with any patient who has hemiplegia. If the stroke occurred on the left side of the brain, there is weakness of the whole right side of the body. If the stroke occurred on the right side of the brain, then weakness is to the left side of the body. Although the arm and leg of one side are both involved, one is often relatively "more affected" than the other. This is the reason some patients are walking before they have use of their involved hand and arm. Speech is affected in a right-handed person if the stroke was on the left side of the brain. The opposite is not always true, however, in left-handed people. Often, the left side of their brain is dominant for speech, too.

Medical Management of Stroke

Medical management is palliative, symptomatic, and supportive. It is based on the severity of the stroke and the extent of damage. Drugs such as reserpine (Serpasil) are used to maintain the blood pressure at a prescribed range. The pressure must be monitored carefully because if it gets too low there is an increase in ischemia to the brain, and if it gets too high there is increased intracranial pressure. Anticoagulants are used cautiously in the presence of thrombosis or embolus; they are never used when hemorrhage is the cause of the stroke. If anticoagulant therapy is instituted, daily prothrombin times are done the first five to seven days to determine proper dosage, then every week for four weeks, and then, if it is stable, every two to four weeks.[43] The patient should be advised to carry a supply of vitamin K tablets in the event of bleeding.

Surgery

Surgery should be considered if the presence of a localized intra- or extracranial lesion can be isolated. A clear picture of the vessels is obtained with cerebral angiography. Radiopaque media are injected through the carotid, vertebral, or brachial arteries, under local or general anesthesia. If a local anesthetic is injected, the patient will feel a brief burning sensation of the head and face as the substance is injected. Aneurysms are outlined this way. They can be surgically sealed off so that they cannot rupture and cause cerebral hemorrhage. The neck of the aneurysm is clipped or tied. If this is not feasible, the main artery feeding the aneurysm can be clipped. If no direct surgery is possible because of the size, shape, or location of the aneurysm, it can be "reinforced" by surrounding it with muscle or with a plastic material. This type of surgery is done on an anesthetized patient using surface hypothermia. The patient's temperature is lowered to 30° C. (86° F.). At this temperature the brain is relaxed and the exposure of the aneurysm is made easier. The brain can tolerate manipulations in this state that might cause secondary residual damage at the normal temperature.[44] Endarterectomy may be done to remove an atheroma from an artery.

Sometimes, extracranial surgery is done. This involves gradual occlusion of one of the arteries supplying the circle of Willis with the eventual aim of total occlusion. A special clamp is inserted surgically[45] around the carotid or vertebral artery on one side of the neck. The clamp has a detachable screwdriver that is used by the surgeon to adjust the clamp tightness. The clamp is gradually tightened around the vessel.

Nursing Management of the Patient with Stroke

Martin[46] divides the management of the patient with stroke into five major phases: initial acute phase, diagnostic phase, planned special therapies, later special therapies (convalescent), and transition to an environment beyond the hospital. Rehabilitation is an integral part of each phase. The active program begins as soon as the clinical state has stabilized. The quality of care during the acute phase influences recovery and the ability of the patient to progress toward maximum health.

The time immediately following a stroke is very trying. The patient is afraid of being left alone; he often cannot communicate his needs; sometimes he seems unreasonable. The nurse must develop unlimited patience when caring for a patient during this early period. Positioning is extremely important in helping to prevent aspiration of mucus. A side-lying position with the head of the bed elevated to about 20 degrees is appropriate. Flexion or rotation of the neck compresses the veins and should be avoided because it interferes with return of blood from the head. Suction apparatus should be at the bedside. If oxygen is needed it should be administered by nasal catheter or cannula so the face is always easily visible. The nurse must watch for signs of further developing pathology, especially evidence of increasing intracranial pressure. Assessment of the patient should include degree of responsiveness (describe how and what he responds to), speech ability, vital signs (decreased pulse and increased blood pressure may signal rising intracranial pressure), visual ability, cranial nerve functioning, sensory and motor ability, continence, and the subjective statements made by the patient.

During the first 48 hours after stroke the nurse carries out passive joint range-of-motion activity several times during the day. (See p. 465.) After the initial 48 hours the patient wtih stroke from thrombosis or embolus can assume more active involvement in range-of-motion activity, with permission by the physician; and the patient with stroke from hemorrhage assumes more active involvement in five to six days. Physical activity must be prescribed, in detail, for the physical therapist. Range-of-motion exercise is usually begun in the upper limbs and progresses to include the lower limbs. The patient is turned or asked to turn at least every two hours. Unless properly positioned at regular intervals throughout the day and night the patient will assume the "typical hemiplegic posture" with adduction and internal rotation of the arms; flexion of the elbow, wrist, and fingers of the affected limb; external rotation of the leg; and later flexion and adduction of the hip joint and knee, and plantar flexion of the foot.[47] Because the patient may have lost his sense of balance, sitting up must be a gradual process, first with the bed just slightly elevated. He should be taught to balance himself while sitting with the unaffected arm extended, his hand flat on the bed, and his feet on the floor. When the physician allows him to begin standing, he is taught to do this using two chairs, back to back at the bedside. He stands between them. The affected hand can be "attached" to the top of one chair with Ace bandage if it is totally paralyzed. The patient grasps the back of the other chair with the unaffected hand. The nurse presses against the affected knee to keep it from buckling. Parallel bars or any firm support may be used for this purpose.

When the patient begins to ambulate, the nurse tells him to step forward with the right foot and swing the left arm forward at the same time. This is called "reciprocal arm movement" and is difficult for the patient to relearn. Pointing to the right foot and looking at the point of the right shoe helps. The patient tends to drag the affected foot along and must be taught to lift it up and put it down.

The nurse begins to work with the patient in using his unaffected arm and hand to care for himself. He begins to regain some lost independence in this way.

When the clinical state has stabilized, an active program of rehabilitation is started. Approximately 90 per cent [48] of all hemiplegics who enter active programs of rehabilitation can be taught ambulation and self-care; 30 per cent can be taught to do gainful work.

Working with the Family

Many people do not go to a rehabilitation hospital after discharge from a general hospital. They go directly home. It is important to help the family plan for this period of time.

A daily schedule should be developed and followed. This includes a specified time for bathing, eating, resting, exercise, and other activities. The patient should be up, dressed, and in regular shoes every day. He should do as much as he can for himself. Eating sometimes is a problem because the paralyzed side has lost feeling and there is a tendency for the food to drip from the corner of the mouth. A large "lobster" bib helps protect the clothing. The patient may be able to feed himself with an adapted device that straps to his hand. A metal plate-guard attached to his plate helps him to get peas, beans, and other food onto his fork or spoon. Emphasize the point that improvement will be noted but the patient must practice chewing, swallowing, and manipulating his food. This is often a very frustrating experience.

Vision may be temporarily affected because of involvement of the muscles of the eye. The patient may have diplopia (double vision). The eyes gradually correct themselves, though there is sometimes permanent loss of vision in part of the visual field in the affected eye. For instance, the patient may be able to see directly in front of him but may be unable to see to one side.

Personality problems seem to be the most difficult to cope with. Normal mood swings become exaggerated. The patient indulges in very impulsive behavior, especially when he finds that he cannot communicate his needs easily. He may know what he wants to say but it may come out "all wrong," and he may impulsively throw the dishes from the table in anger. He has "one-track thinking." To get his point across he may continuously return, again and again, to a single topic. His innate intelligence is usually unaffected; however, his ability to concentrate and to remember are often impaired. He has difficulty grasping abstract ideas, and it is best to use concrete examples when talking to him, e.g., show him a tool to be used rather than describe it verbally to him. Make sentences short, direct, and specific. Encourage him to talk regardless of how the sentences come out. Mental coordination must be achieved gradually, one step at a time.

Patients often ask whether they will be able to drive again. This is a decision that the physician must make based on each individual's status. Some do drive again.

Many ask about the ability to have sexual relations. Although reactions are slower and it takes a longer time to reach orgasm, the patient can have a completely satisfactory sexual relationship. This, too, should be discussed with the physician.

Return to work is also a very individual matter and depends on the patient's functional progress and the type of work he did. Career changes are sometimes necessary.

There are many agencies who help the families of handicapped people. The visiting nurse and physical therapist go into the home on a regular basis to guide, support, and evaluate progress. Many states have rehabilitation commissions that provide money and facilities for a variety of related activities including training for employment.

42

PROGRESSIVE NEUROLOGIC DISEASES

THE patient who has a progressive neurologic disease is a candidate for rehabilitation just as is the patient whose disease process has stabilized. The major difference is that the ongoing nature of the disease requires frequent modification in rehabilitation methods and goals. Hope is given the patient because many disease processes develop slowly over 10 to 20 years. During this time the patient can remain functionally able. Rehabilitation goals focus on maintenance of maximum functional ability according to the individual's current status with development of minimal secondary complications derived from immobility. Two frequently encountered progressive neurologic diseases are Parkinson's disease and multiple sclerosis.

Parkinson's Disease (Paralysis Agitans, Shaking Palsy)

This is a disease in which there is loss of cells and fibers in the basal ganglia of the brain. These cells and fibers normally exert a steadying influence on muscular activity and control automatic movement. Extrapyramidal, involuntary motor tracts are involved. Major symptoms, which are very slow to develop, are tremor and muscle rigidity.

The patient who has Parkinson's disease has rhythmic, alternating, rapid, fine tremors, which may start in the fingers, move to the arms, and then spread to the whole body. They occur in resting muscle, often increase during purposeful activity,[49] and disappear in sleep. There is a characteristic "pill-rolling" movement as the thumb beats against the fingers. Tremors are exaggerated under stress.

There is also widespread muscular rigidity with some flexion of the limbs. Reflexes and the power of contraction are not affected, but balance, speed of movement, and coordination are. Coordinated acts must be thought out deliberately. Walking becomes a problem. The patient is fearful of falling; he cannot regain his balance to protect himself if he stumbles. He walks with a typical "shuffling gait," on his toes. There is bending forward of the trunk and stooping, and the stride consists of very rapid short steps. The patient cannot control the involuntary acceleration of stride. There is loss of reciprocal arm-leg movement (swing of the arm and opposite leg) as he walks.

The patient has difficulty communicating his feelings through facial expression, and he develops the typical "masklike rigidity" common to people with Parkinson's disease because he cannot raise his eyebrows or twist the corner of his mouth in a quick smile or frown. As the disease advances the muscles of the jaw, tongue, and larynx become involved, and the patient has difficulty eating and speaking. His speech becomes slurred. He swallows with difficulty and drools at the mouth. He has difficulty blinking his eyes and may occasionally develop oculogyric crisis in which the eyes roll up or down and remain that way for hours or days. This is extremely frightening.

There is no disorder of sensation or clouding of the mind. Symptoms are very slow to develop. The actual cause of the disease is unknown but its symptoms have been known to follow in the path of epidemics of Spanish influenza and encephalitis. The disease is also associated with arteriosclerotic changes affecting the basal ganglia of the brain. Carbon monoxide poisoning is implicated.

The peak onset is in people over 50 years of age. The person continues to work as long as he is able.

Treatment with drugs that control the tremors and relax the muscles is only palliative. Drugs belonging to the belladonna group, such as atropine, were once used exclusively; however, in order to get the desired effect, large doses had to be used and unpleasant side effects resulted. The patient experiences dry mouth, blurred vision, and skin reactions. Newer synthetic antispasmodic agents are currently in favor. They include trihexyphenidyl HCl (Artane, Tremin), benztropine methanesulfonate (Cogentin), biperiden HCl (Akineton), diphenhydramine HCl (Benadryl), and many others.

Treatment with L-dopa,[50] a new drug still being used experimentally, has had some success. The cells involved in Parkinson's disease secrete the amino acid dopamine. The patient with Parkinson's disease has diminished amounts of dopamine and is given dihydroxyphenylalanine (L-dopa), a synthetic substance produced from fish flour or extracted from broad beans and velvet beans that are used to feed horses, and this is converted by the brain into dopamine. The drug is given in gradually increasing doses over several days until 5.0 to 8.0 gm is attained. Forty per cent of the patients treated so far have had dramatic results with few or no residual symptoms of Parkinson's disease; forty per cent have had good results with some residual symptoms; and twenty per cent have had no detectable results.

Surgical intervention for parkinsonism aims at destroying tissue in the basal ganglia to control rigidity and tremor. This can be accomplished with electrocoagulation, radiofrequency current, alcohol injection, excision, or, more recently, freezing techniques (cryogenic surgery) using liquid nitrogen. Not all patients are candidates for this type of surgery. Results seem best in young people who have unilateral involvement following other diseases and who have marked tremor and rigidity.[51] For pre- and postoperative care see page 433.

Multiple Sclerosis

Known as "the crippler of young adults," this disease strikes men and women in their most productive years, between 20 and 40. It destroys the myelin (fatty sheath) around the axon fibers of tracts in the brain and spinal cord leaving patches of sclerotic tissue and causing degeneration of the nerve fibers. Symptoms are as varied as the variety of nerve tracts involved. Usually there are acute exacerbations of the disease with periods of remission, probably resulting from partial healing in the areas of degeneration. Exacerbations are triggered by fatigue, emotional stress, acute respiratory infection, chilling, and so on. There is no cure for the disease; however, people are known to live with it for 20 years or more. Its cause is unknown though metabolic and enzymatic disorders, allergy, and viral infection have been considered.

Symptoms [52, 53] may be transient or long-lasting. They include:

1. Paresthesias: sensory impairment, tingling and numbness.
2. Muscular weakness: usually one side of the body is more affected than the other. This may progress to full paralysis of extremities. There may be spasms.
3. Poor coordination, impaired position sense, loss of balance, ataxia, difficulty in walking.
4. Visual disturbances, especially nystagmus (involuntary movement of the eyeball in any direction), blurring, diplopia (double vision), scotomas (spots before the eyes), and loss of vision.
5. Defects in articulation; slurred, hesitant speech.
6. Intention tremor: the hand trembles when the patient uses it.
7. Urinary and fecal incontinence or retention.
8. Emotional lability: inappropriate emotional affect; mood swings.

The course of the disease is unpredictable. There may be long periods of remission during which the patient is almost free of symptoms; however, he becomes increasingly disabled and physically incapacitated. At home, a routine with planned rest periods is suggested. The patient exercises, but must not exercise beyond the point of fatigue. Because he is usually tired, he learns to recognize some sign that he is fatigued, e.g., a tightening in the chest. He is told to avoid precipitating factors such as a rundown physical condition and excess stress. His environment should be relaxed, his diet well balanced. Vitamins B and E are sometimes supplemented for their systemic effect. Drugs that relieve spasticity are prescribed. Mephensin (Tolserol) is an example. Some patients benefit from warm, relaxing baths, physical therapy, and psychotherapy.

43

SOME SPECIFIC ORTHOPEDIC PROBLEMS

Orthopedic Injury

Orthopedic injuries include injuries to the bones and joints, fractures, dislocations, injuries to the tendons and ligaments (soft-tissue injuries), and others. If not treated properly, injuries to these soft tissues cause a longer period of disability than those to the bone. Fractures will be discussed as an example of management of any orthopedic injury.

Fractures

Fractures are breaks in bone. They are classified in the following ways:

1. CLOSED, SIMPLE. One in which the skin is not broken.
2. OPEN, COMPOUND. One in which the skin is broken. There is communication between the fracture and the outside air.
3. INCOMPLETE, GREENSTICK. One in which the continuity of the bone is not entirely interrupted.
4. COMPLETE. One in which the continuity of the bone is entirely interrupted.
5. COMMINUTED. One in which fragments of bone are broken into many small pieces.
6. IMPACTED. One in which fragments are driven one into the other so that the fracture is stabilized. A Colles wrist fracture is an example. The lower fragment at the end of the radius is displaced backward and tilted to the radial side.
7. MULTIPLE. One in which there is more than one separate fracture.
8. ARTICULAR. Fracture of the joint surface of a bone.
9. PATHOLOGIC. One resulting from minor injury to a bone already weakened by disease, e.g., osteoporosis.

Fractures are also described according to the direction of the line of break (see Fig. 43–1).

1. Transverse, across the bone
2. Oblique
3. Spiral

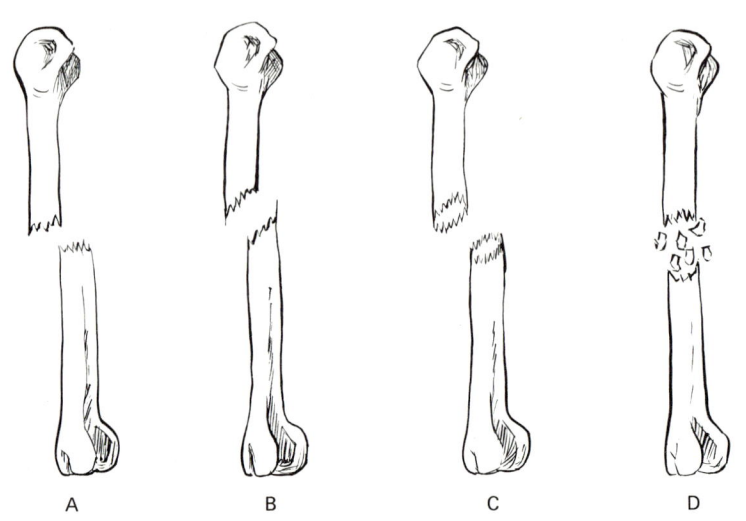

FIGURE 43-1. Types of fractures: *A.* Transverse. *B.* Oblique. *C.* Spiral. *D.* Comminuted.

EMERGENCY TREATMENT

Splint them where they lie; do not attempt to push the ends of bones back in place. The wound should be covered and the part immobilized by splinting with any available firm item. A first-aid wooden splint, a telephone book, and a board are examples.

REDUCING THE FRACTURE

X-rays are always taken; then, the fracture is "reduced." It is put back in place, to correct the deformity and restore normal anatomic alignment. Usually the physician does this under general anesthesia, with his hands. This is called manual manipulation or closed reduction. However, if this type of manipulation fails or is likely to fail, the part is reduced in the operating room by exposing the bone. This is called open reduction. If open reduction is to be done, the limb must be specially prepared. Each hospital has its own procedure for an "orthopedic prep." It is more involved than a regular preparation because of the potential danger of bone infection. The part is usually scrubbed for one and one-half minutes with pHisoHex or green soap, rinsed, shaved, and scrubbed again for ten minutes. Then, donning sterile gloves, the nurse wraps the limb in two thicknesses of sterile towels and secures them in place with bandage or stockinette. If the fracture is compound, the adjacent area may be prepared away from the operating room, but the area itself is prepared in the operating room. The ends of the bones are also scrubbed.

Once the fracture has been reduced, it must be immobilized to maintain the reduction. This can be done in the operating room by internal fixation of the part with nails, screws, wires, and plates; by application of traction; by casts; or by a combination of methods.

IMMOBILIZATION WITH CASTS

Casts are made of plaster of Paris. Rolls of bandages and splints, in a variety of widths and lengths, are impregnated with the plaster of Paris and are stored in dry form. When the bandage is submerged in tap water it swells and sets rapidly to form a hard cement. Hot water hastens the setting and usually fails to give the physician enough time to apply it properly. The part to be immobilized is covered with stockinette. Felt is placed over bony prominences if a body cast is used. The bandage is saturated in a pail lined with newspaper so that the plaster that settles to the bottom can be easily lifted out and discarded. The bandage is dropped into the pail and left undisturbed until bubbles cease to rise. Then it is gently grasped at each end and squeezed toward the middle. Most physicians prefer doing this themselves.

The injured part is held with the fracture reduced as the plaster bandage is applied. The edges are trimmed with a sharp knife. The cast then becomes a fixed type of traction. A long piece of gauze may be placed under the stockinette as a "scratcher." It extends out beyond the cast.[54] Excess plaster can be removed from the skin with warm water, but no soap. As the plaster "sets," the patient will feel a marked warmth. An ice bag held to his head makes him more comfortable. A fan can be used, but not directly on the cast. Extremity casts "set" in ten minutes but do not completely dry for two days. Body casts take about three days to dry.

Care of the New Cast. If the damp cast must be touched, the palms of the hands should be used so that finger indentations do not harden and cause pressure. The cast is supported in physiologic position on pillows while damp. Pillows prevent indentation of the damp cast, which would also cause pressure. Pillows are not used under the head of a patient in a body cast because they thrust the patient forward against the cast and the cast then digs into the body.

Drying is hastened if the cast is left exposed to the air. The patient is covered, but the cast is left uncovered. The physician may specifically order the use of a commercial dryer with controlled heat or a heat cradle with 25-watt bulbs; however, heat to a newly operated-on area may cause hemorrhage and the patient must be observed carefully. Stronger bulbs are not used because they would rapidly dry the outside of the cast while the inside remained moist and prone to mildew formation. The cast is dry when the plaster is white, shining, odorless, hard, firm, and resonant when tapped.[55] Weight bearing is not allowed until the cast is dry. The cast can be kept clean with stockinette coverings that can be removed and washed. A waterproofing substance such as shellac can be applied after the cast is dry. Strips of plastic can be inserted around the buttock opening in a body cast to protect it from being soiled. The cast may be scoured with an almost dry cloth or sponge and a cleanser such as Bon Ami. *Do not wet the cast.* If the stockinette at the inner edges of the cast becomes soiled, it can be pulled down and cut off with a razor.

Itch is a common problem. Do not allow the patient to insert an object like a hanger to scratch a hard-to-reach spot. The scratcher might break the skin and predispose to infection or it might "bunch up" the stockinette and cause it to act like a tourniquet and cause gangrene!

Observation of the encasted part is essential in preventing gangrene and permanent nerve paralysis. A cast that becomes too tight causes pressure on blood vessels and may ultimately cause gangrene. It may also press on nerves and cause nerve paralysis.

Observe frequently for the following:

1. Cyanosis	This may indicate interference with venous return.
2. Pallor or blanching	This may indicate arterial vasospasm and impairment of circulation.
3. Temperature and color	The part should be warm to touch and exposed areas rosy; if it feels hot this may mean the presence of inflammatory response and infection; compare encasted limb with nonencasted limb.
4. Odor	These should be no odor once the case is dry. A musty smell indicates gas bacillus infection or mildew.
5. Mobility	Make sure the patient can move his fingers and toes.
6. Sensation	Never ignore a complaint! Always report a limb that feels hot, cold, or numb. Some throbbing is normal after cast application and can be relieved, by physician's order, by elevation and by application of ice bags placed along the side of the cast, not on top of it.
7. Excess swelling	The physician may order elevation of the limb above the level of the heart to decrease swelling.

8. Plaster sores — These are sores that come from pressure, friction, trapped items like crumbs. A window may have to be cut in the cast to treat it. The opening is then packed with felt and the piece of plaster is reapplied and secured in place with tape.

If the cast is causing undue pressure, the physician will split the plaster and padding along the full length of each side of the cast. This is called bivalving and can be done by the nurse as an emergency procedure. While the patient is in bed the injured limb is elevated on pillows to help prevent edema.

TYPES OF CASTS AND SPLINTS

A *cylinder cast* encompasses an extremity. It becomes a "walking cast" by the addition of a walking heel or caliper, added at the time of application. This heel allows the patient to bear weight on the cast.

A *body cast* is one that encompasses the entire trunk.

A *hip spica* cast is one that encompasses all of one leg and either all of the other leg or to the knee of the other leg.

A *splint or mold or plaster jacket or collar* is used if the goal is protection rather than correction. If used on a limb it does not encompass the entire extremity but supports a particular part, e.g., the knee following surgery. It provides some immobilization and provides a fixed point from which traction may be applied. The Thomas splint is an example.

TURNING THE PATIENT IN A BODY CAST

Turning the patient in a hip spica or body cast requires at least three people as long as the cast is not thoroughly dry. When it is dry, the patient can be taught to help turn and lift himself. A trapeze on a frame over the bed helps him, especially when he must lift himself onto a fracture bedpan.

The cast must be turned as one rigid unit to prevent twisting of the patient's body.

The patient is moved to the side of the bed toward the leg in plaster or, if both legs are encased, toward the operated side. If he is in a body cast, move him to either side of the bed. Pillows are arranged to conform to the contour of the cast to be received.

For Hip Spica. One nurse supports the leg in plaster, one supports the patient's back, and one stands at the other side of the bed with her hands on the patient's shoulder and hip and pulls him toward her.

For Body Cast. One nurse stands near the head of the bed next to the patient and places one hand under the patient's neck to gently grasp the opposite shoulder and one hand under the rib cage. One nurse stands near the foot of the bed next to the patient with one hand under the buttocks and one under the knees. One nurse stands on the opposite side of the bed with her hands on the patient's shoulder and hip. Together they lift and roll the patient as the third nurse pulls him toward her.

Align the patient so that there is no pressure on his toes. Make sure there is no foot drop. If the patient is lying prone, make sure the cast extends far enough over the edge of the bed to avoid pressure on the dorsum of the foot.

The patient in a cast may be moved as frequently as is necessary for care and comfort. He may lie on his back, abdomen, or side without endangering the immobilization of the injured part.[56]

BONE HEALING

Healing progresses through several stages. Granulation tissue forms. The hematoma between the bone ends is invaded by calcium salts and transformed into immature bone called callus. This callus eventually matures and becomes new bone. Healing is more rapid with fewer complications in healthy young adults. Elderly or debilitated patients recover slowly. Oblique and spiral fractures unite more rapidly than transverse, and impacted fractures unite more rapidly than those in which there is a wide gap between the bone ends. If the fracture unites in a deformed position it is called malunion. This happens if soft tissue (muscle, nerve) gets caught between the bone fragments. Further surgery is done if the malunion interferes with functional activity. Recently, patients have been encouraged to place weight on the fractured extremity before it is completely healed. They are "walked" early in the healing process. This method follows Wolff's law that states: "Bone will respond to stress by becoming thicker and stronger." This law can be applied to non-weight-bearing bones by use of a compression plate technique. The compression plate is fixed on one side of the fracture with screws, and a clamp is placed between an outside screw and the inner adjacent end of the plate. When the clamp is closed, the gap at the fracture site is closed with added compression to the bone ends.[57]

Fractures involving joint surfaces such as the upper end of the tibia and those involving the knee, ankle, elbow, or shoulder cause stiffness if immobilized for long periods of time because blood in the joint leads to scar formation, which in turn leads to intra-articular adhesions and contraction of the joint capsule. Early active exercise is advised in these types of fractures.

CAST REMOVAL

Casts are removed by being "bivalved" first. Cuts are made along the two lateral lengths of the cast. This is done with a cast saw. An electric cast saw with vacuum attached is now used. It sucks in the plaster for ease of disposal. After the cast is removed, the skin may be washed with pHisoHex. Some physicians prefer several gentle soaking and washings. Lubricating creams are applied. Joints will be stiff and painful for a while. They should be mobilized gradually and not forced. The limb should be kept elevated on a chair except when the patient is walking. This helps diminish the swelling.

Traction [58,59]

Traction is a pull exerted on a limb to gain or maintain body alignment, to ensure immobilization of a part, or to correct a deformity. The continuous pull maintains the length and position of an extremity until healing takes place. Weights varying from 1 to 20 lb are used. Manual traction is applied with the hands. A discussion of mechanical traction follows.

MECHANICAL TRACTION

1. *Skin (Nonoperative).* Traction is applied to the skin and exerts its pull indirectly on the muscles and bone. Strapping is applied parallel to the long bones. Spiral twists "trap" skin and may cause necrosis. The material used for the traction straps should be hypoallergenic and should allow for evaporation of perspiration. Fastrac is an example of a cotton-backed sponge rubber strip impregnated with a special adhesive solution that does not require use of an adherent under it. It can be removed and replaced up to five times. Some strips are made of sponge rubber with perforated plastic backing or moleskin with adhesive backing. If the traction is to be maintained for extended periods of time, an adherent and tincture of benzoin may be applied. The traction strips are held in place by a wrapping material such as bias-cut stockinette or woven bandage and are attached around the footplate. Head halters are used for cervical traction. They should be padded if they cut into the patient along the jaw. Pelvic belts are used for pelvic fractures or for low back pain. (See Fig. 43–2.)

2. *Skeletal Traction.* This is the most effective type of traction. It is applied directly to the bone. Metal pins, nails, wires, or tongs are driven into the bone. Weights are attached to these devices. The ends of pins or wires can be incorporated in casts. The wire ends do not protrude from the plaster but the pins do and should be covered with cork. Use of Krutchfield tongs in the skull is an example of skeletal traction.

Internal fixation of bone with wire, pins, or nails may be utilized without cast application or additional weight applied. This is frequently done for elderly patients who have had fractures from seemingly trivial accidents because of degenerative (osteoporotic) processes in the bone. When a fractured femur is internally fixed (pinned), the patient can be mobilized much earlier and is not prone to the secondary hazards of immobility. With hip pinning, the patient is turned from side to side, although this is

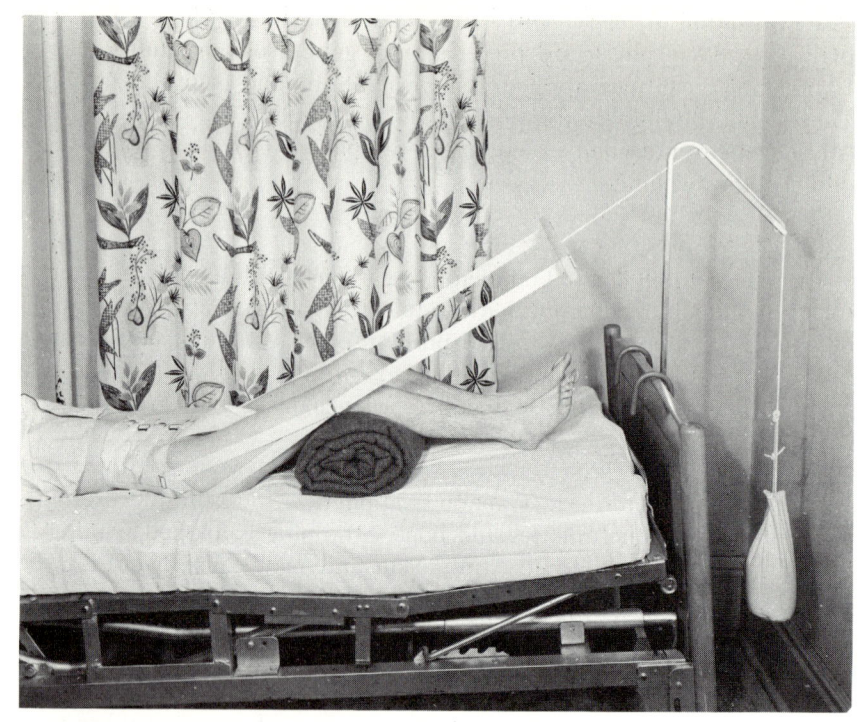

FIGURE 43–2. Pelvic traction. (Courtesy, S. H. Camp & Co., Jackson, Mich.)

painful, on the day of surgery. He is usually allowed out of bed in a chair the morning after surgery. The leg is elevated. Weight bearing is not allowed for six months, however, and the patient must be carefully assisted or lifted into the chair. Early weight bearing may be allowed with some devices, and this order must be explicitly clarified by the physician.

Devices used for internal fixation are made of inert metals that should not cause tissue reaction. They can remain in the body indefinitely or can be removed when the fracture heals. They do have a "fatigue life" and will break from unusually severe or prolonged strain.[60] The implants come in a variety of sizes. They may be stored in multipocket wrappers especially designed for them, are used only if sterile and unmarred, and are never reused because their "fatigue life" has been expended.

3. *Pulp Traction.* A suture is placed through the pulp of a finger or toe and fastened to an extension piece incorporated in a plaster cast.

TYPES OF PULL IN EXTREMITY TRACTION

1. *Straight or Running Pull.* This provides a pull on the affected part by a weight attached to pulleys. The pull is against the weight of the body and its friction on the bed. Straight traction is not "balanced" by a ham-

mock support. The lower end of the bed may be elevated on blocks to supply "countertraction" and keep the patient in proper alignment. Buck's extension is an example. (See Fig. 43–3.)

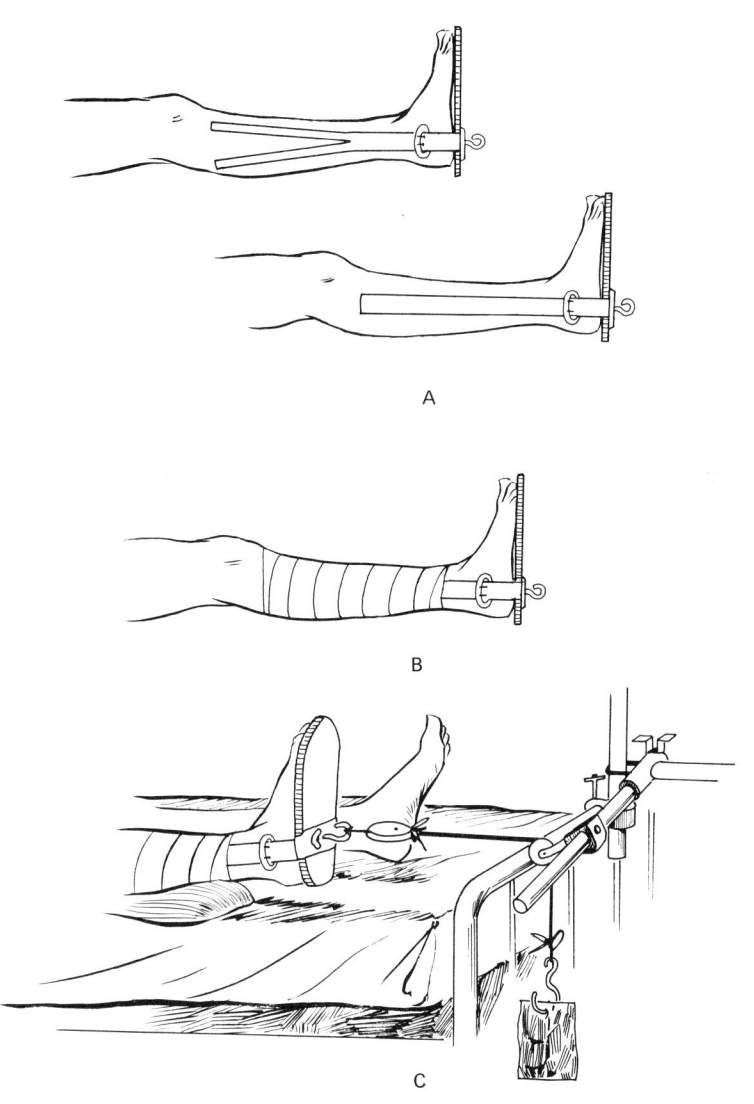

FIGURE 43–3. Buck's extension. A. Two equally good methods of applying traction strips. B. Wrapping is started high enough to avoid pressure on the tendon of Achilles and extends to below the knee so that there will be no wrinkling or pressure in popliteal area. C. Weight is attached. (Redrawn from A. Kerr, *Orthopedic Nursing Procedures*, 1960, and used with permission of Springer Publishing Co., New York.)

2. *Balanced Traction.* This is straight traction with the addition of a balance for countertraction, usually in the form of a hammock under the knee. Pull is from the hammock attached to a pulley overhead, to a pulley at the foot of the bed, to a pulley on the footplate, or to a pulley from which the weight hangs. Russell's traction is an example. (See Fig. 43–4.)

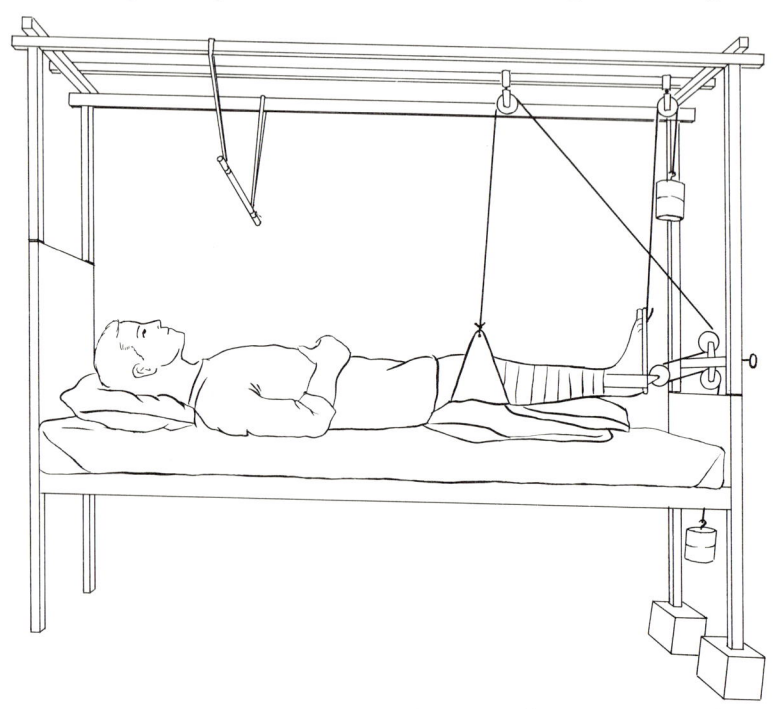

FIGURE 43–4. Russell traction. Note that the Balkan frame is attached to the bed, the leg is supported on pillows, and the heel extends beyond the pillow. (Reproduced from K. Schafer, J. Sawyer, A. McCluskey, and E. Beck, *Medical-Surgical Nursing*, 4th ed. C. V. Mosby Co., St. Louis, 1967.)

3. *Fixed Traction.* This is traction between two fixed points. The Thomas splint is an example. It is frequently used in conjunction with balanced traction because it is slightly suspended over the bed and allows the patient more freedom in moving about in bed without altering the line of traction. The pull of the extension tapes tied to the end of a Thomas splint is countered by pressure of the ring against the ischial tuberosity. The Thomas splint makes it possible to have two separate lines of pull on the same extremity. This is advantageous when there are fractures on the upper and lower leg. The ring of the Thomas splint should not be padded because it tends to become wet. It should be polished with saddle soap to prevent cracking.

Each traction setup is "custom-designed" for the individual patient. It is the responsibility of the physician to apply the traction. The nurse collects the necessary equipment. This includes pulleys, rope, traction arms, footplates, and spreader bars. The physician orders continuous or intermittent traction. Sometimes, he allows traction to be on and off at the patient's discretion. If continuous, the traction should not be removed for any purpose! When the patient is moved up in bed, the weight should not be lifted. The amount of pull remains the same as he moves up in bed.

Alignment is maintained only as long as the traction is functioning properly. The patient cannot be turned. He usually is allowed only the recumbent position. Balanced traction, with use of an overhead trapeze, allows him more movement than straight traction.

Here are some pointers:

1. Keep the patient pulled up in bed so that the "line of pull" is not changed.
2. Keep the weights off the floor.
3. Make sure the ropes are running freely.
4. Prevent foot drop. Make sure the footplate is supporting the foot properly and not resting against the foot of the bed.
5. Observe for signs of circulatory impairment: coldness or burning sensation; numbness, pain, edema, color of nails; compare the limbs.
6. Keep noninvolved parts of the body moving.
7. If the physician wants pillows to be used, have him show you where and how he wants them placed; otherwise, pillows are not used.
8. Leg traction is usually not disturbed as long as the hips remain on the bed in proper alignment. Have the patient lift himself with the trapeze when bathing him, and when making his bed. It is easier to make the bed from top to bottom. Use a small orthopedic (fracture) bedpan.
9. The headrest can usually be raised and lowered though the effectiveness of running traction is decreased when this is done. Make sure the bed is rolled flat at least half the day.
10. The traction strips can be removed only if specifically ordered by the physician. Inspect the area carefully for signs of skin irritation or breakdown.
11. Make sure there is no pressure at the popliteal space under the knee and at the Achilles tendon at the ankle.

Joint Range of Motion for the Bedridden [61]

Joints are articulations at which point bones are connected to one another. These are beautifully constructed mechanisms, clothed and lubricated by a synovial membrane and fluid, surrounded by capsules, and bound together by ligaments.

Normal joint motions include flexion or bending; extension or straightening; abduction or being brought away from the midline of the body; adduction or being brought toward the midline of the body; internal rotation or rolling toward the midline; external rotation or rolling away from the midline; and circumduction, which is a combination of all these movements.

The joints are interdependent in that deformity or limitation of movement of one joint often imposes unnatural mechanical strain on others.

SOME SPECIFIC JOINTS AND THEIR MOVEMENTS

Vertebral Column. This is a flexible rod capable of flexion, extension, side bending, and rotation.

Shoulder Joint. This is a ball-and-socket joint capable of flexion, extension, abduction, adduction, and circumduction.

Elbow Joint. Capable of supination (turning forearm with palm up) and pronation (turning forearm with palm down), flexion, extension, internal and external rotation.

Wrist Joint. Capable of palmar flexion (in the direction of the palm), dorsiflexion (in the direction of the ceiling), abduction and adduction.

Hip Joint. A ball-and-socket joint capable of flexion, extension, adduction, abduction, rotation, and circumduction.

Knee Joint. A hinge joint capable of flexion and extension and some rotation.

Ankle Joint. Capable of flexion (dorsiflexion, toward the body) and extension (plantar flexion, toward the ground), abduction and adduction.

Foot Joints. Capable of inversion (turning up inner border of the foot) and eversion (turning up outer border of foot).

The joints can be exercised either passively, with the nurse taking them through their ranges of motion, or actively, with the patient taking them through their ranges of motion with the nurse guiding the exercise. *Range of motion should be gentle and gradual. It should not cause pain.*

SOME THERAPEUTIC EXERCISES FOR THE BEDRIDDEN [62]

Quadriceps Setting. This exercises muscles on the top, anterior aspect of the thigh whose main function is to extend the leg. Activate them by having the patient press the back of the knee against the bed and try to lift the heel from the bed.

Gluteal Setting. This exercises muscles of the hip which abduct, adduct, extend, flex, and rotate the leg. They enable a person to stand erect by holding the pelvis over the femur. Activate them by having the patient pinch the buttock together and attempt to lift the hip while recumbent; try to bring the leg out to the side of the bed while recumbent.

For Foot Motion. This exercises foot extensors. Have the patient circle the foot in both directions, bend the foot toward and away from the knee.

Crutch Walking

Many people must leave the hospital with crutches to assist walking. The physical therapist teaches crutch walking; however, in the absence of a physical therapist the nurse must assume this responsibility. She must also guide crutch walking when the patient practices and the physical therapist is not present. It is advisable to have the nurse learn to walk with crutches herself so that she can effectively guide the patient. Handing the patient a pair of crutches and saying, "Here they are, now walk with them," is like expecting an infant to get up and walk without any preliminary activity. It is wrong. It can foster ineffective technique, poor functional mobility, and inaccurate body alignment.

Crutches are made of a variety of materials (wood, aluminum) and designs, and the type to be used is selected on an individual basis. The standard crutch can be used in all instances. Crutches must be measured for the patient.[63,64]

MEASURING CRUTCHES

1. In the erect or supine position crutches should reach from about 2 in. below the axilla to a point 6 to 8 in. out from the foot with the patient wearing shoes, or the distance from the patient's axilla to the sole of his foot plus 2 in.

2. The patient's elbow should be approximately 30 degrees in flexion when he grasps the handbar and should be at a level for practically complete extension of the elbow with the wrists hyperextended and the weight on the palms. Handles should be adjustable.

3. Crutches should not be so long that there is pressure in the axilla. This can cause nerve paralysis of the arm.

4. Crutches require tips that are securely attached.

The patient is prepared for the use of crutches by preliminary muscle strengthening and balancing exercises. He may use his overhead trapeze for exercise or do push-ups from the prone position. He must learn to balance with the crutches before ever trying to walk with them. He starts by standing in a corner of the room. This gives him the feeling of protection if he should fall backward. The therapist stands in front of him. He begins by shifting his weight (if weight bearing is allowed) from one foot to the other. Then he shifts his weight from his legs to his arms. Then he moves his hips in a rocking motion. He is taught to hold his shoulders at a normal or slightly depressed level, not hunched. He is taught to walk with his foot flat on the floor, to take short, equal steps, and not to hurry. The crutches are placed 4 in. to the side and 4 in. ahead.

The weight is taken on the hands, not in the axillae. If only one cane or crutch is ordered, it is used on the side opposite the involved extremity to better balance the weight. The most frequently used crutch gait is the three-point gait. This is used if one leg is in a cast. A description of the various gaits follows.

FOUR-POINT CRUTCH GAIT

This is used when the patient may bear some weight on each leg. The patient with arthritis is an example. The weight is first balanced on both feet and both crutches. Then, in a four-point sequence, the patient puts one crutch forward, then the opposite foot; he puts the other crutch forward, and follows with the opposite foot. For speed, the four-point gait may, with practice, become a fast two-point gait. The crutch and opposite leg are brought forward at the same time.

THREE-POINT CRUTCH GAIT

This is used when little or no weight is allowed on one leg. With the weight on the nonaffected leg, the affected leg and both crutches are brought forward. The weight is transferred to the two crutches and the affected leg, and then the nonaffected leg is brought forward.

SWING-THROUGH CRUTCH GAIT

This gait is used when the patient must stand on both feet at once in order to support his weight. The patient with quadriplegia is an example. It is the least like a normal walking gait and can lead to atrophy of the legs if it is used for extended periods of time. It is the crutch gait most frequently seen in the street. The patient stands with his feet together and with the weight on both feet and both crutches. He swings both crutches forward together; then he pushes hard on the hand grips, and with his weight balanced on the crutches, he swings both feet through no farther than 12 to 15 in. beyond the crutches. He regains his stance by arching his back and pulling his hips forward and repeats the sequence rhythmically.

MANEUVERING STEPS [65]

To get up steps using a three-point gait the body weight is taken on the hands and the crutches, and the normal limb is advanced to the upper step. The body weight is then taken on the normal extremity and the crutch and involved limb follow.

To get down steps the crutches are placed on the lower step, the weight is taken on the hands, and the normal extremity is brought down to the lower step with the crutches. Then, with the body weight on the normal extremity, the crutches are placed on the next step.

With a hand rail, the patient may elect to place both crutches under one side and use the banister for the hand on the other. (See Fig. 43–5.)

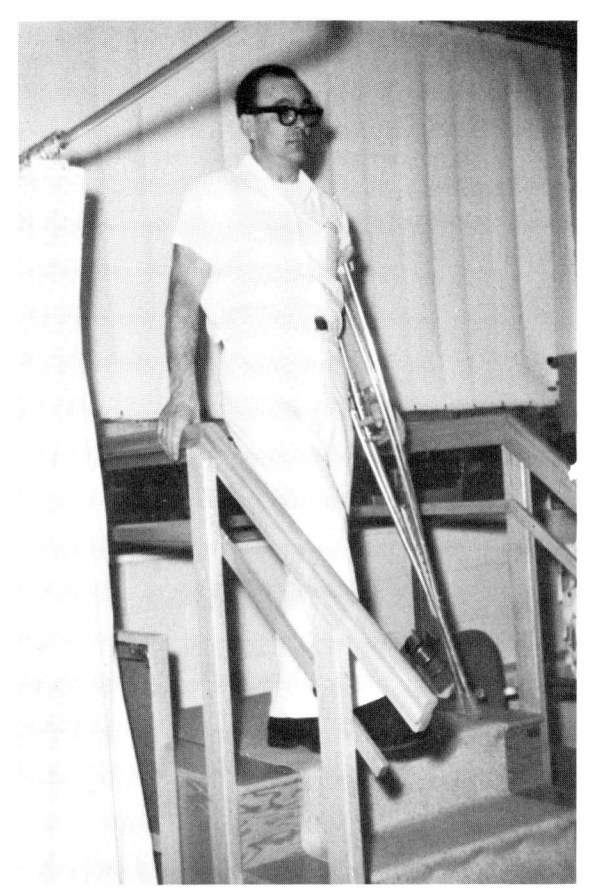

FIGURE 43–5. The physical therapist demonstrates a method of going down stairs with crutches.

Amputation

Surgical removal of a limb is often required when the limb has been deprived of an adequate blood supply and becomes gangrenous, when a malignant tumor is discovered, and in other cases. The most commonly occurring type of amputation is one-sided, above-the-knee leg amputation, although prosthetic devices are found to work better when the amputation is below the knee.[66] There are three recognized stages in amputation. The first involves the actual surgery to eliminate the pathology and leave a healed stump of adequate length, shape, comfort, and function. A below-knee amputation, best for later use of a prosthetic device, is only feasible if adequate circulation in the skin flaps and major vessels is found at the time of surgery.

The second stage involves the stump and preprosthetic stage during which the stump and remaining limb are conditioned through exercise and range of motion. The third stage is learning how to be an amputee.

The first two stages usually take place in the general hospital. When the patient returns from the operating room, there will be a drain at the lower end of the stump to eliminate accumulated fluids. This is left in for two days following the surgery. The patient experiences some discomfort for the first three days after surgery. He may have "phantom sensation" in which he experiences pain or some feeling in the distal area of the missing limb. This would be in the foot causing "phantom foot" or in the hand of an arm amputation causing "phantom hand." It may be caused by nerve-ending excitation in remaining scar tissue, or in the "body image theory," it is the result of the patient's having been made aware of the limb through multiple sensory impressions during his growth and these sensory impressions continue to give him an image of himself with the limb.[67]

The second stage begins after the stitches are removed, about the fourth postoperative day. The stump is washed daily with warm water and mild soap or with a liquid antiseptic like pHisoHex. It should be rinsed and dried thoroughly. Elastic compression bandages or socks are used to shape and shrink the stump. They are changed and washed and dried once or twice a day. If bandages are used rather than elastic socks, care must be taken to prevent the bandage from acting like a tourniquet. It is applied with six or seven diagonal turns. The greatest pressure should be at the tip of the stump and should decrease as it approaches the proximal end. A 6-in. bandage is used for an above-the-knee stump. It should be carried high into the groin. A 4-in. bandage is used for below-the-knee stumps. It should reach the patella. The physician may want the stump elevated on pillows to hasten absorption of edema fluid. The stump and remaining limb must be conditioned so that it is ready to receive a prosthesis. *The main goal for any amputee is to prevent flexion contractures:* more specifically, to prevent abduction, flexion, and external rotation at the hip and flexion at the knee. Steps to prevent contractures should be instituted by the third to fifth postoperative day. The patient should be taught to avoid prolonged sitting, especially in the wheel chair. The head of the bed should not be raised continuously. The patient is taught to lie flat with no pillow under the stump and to lie face down part of every day with the pelvis level with the rest of the body. A graded program of exercise is begun, first gently active, later resistive. (See p. 466.) The patient is taught crutch walking as soon as he is able. If he can "swing through" in crutch walking and can negotiate steps, he will probably use an artificial limb satisfactorily.[68]

The patient is usually measured for a prosthesis eight to ten weeks after surgery when most of the stump shrinkage has taken place. In some instances a temporary plaster of Paris prosthesis is fitted immediately after the surgery and early ambulation is ordered. This prosthesis acts like a pressure dressing and tends to decrease postoperative edema and pain.

Not all patients find use of a prosthesis necessary. People over 55 seem less adaptable for using an artificial limb.

In stage 3 the patient learns how to use his prosthesis advantageously. The prosthesis, or "artificial limb," is not an over-the-counter item. It is prescribed for a specific individual with a specific objective for its use. It is made up of a socket that should be washed daily, a knee joint and shin, an ankle joint, and an articulated foot. It is suspended from the body with a strap or halter. The stump should fit snugly into the socket with a virgin-wool sock on. If the prosthesis must be left off for a period of time, the original elastic-compression sock is used. It takes about 12 training sessions for the person with a below-the-knee amputation to learn to use his prosthesis properly, 18 if the amputation is above the knee.[69]

Arthritis

Arthritis is a disease of the connective tissue. It is called a "collagen disease" because connective tissue contains collagen. The word itself means inflammation of a joint. Joints are normally clothed by a synovial membrane, lubricated with synovial fluid, and surrounded by a joint capsule. The pathologic process in the joint that leads to arthritic deformity progresses this way:

1. Inflammation of the synovial membrane
2. Synovial fluid effusion
3. Pain, heat, distention within the joint capsule
4. "Functional splinting" of the joint to prevent pain
5. Tendon and capsule tightening
6. Decrease in the range of motion of the joint

The pain is greatest when the joint is moved in extremes of ranges of motion, so that the patient guards against those motions. This enforced immobility, or "functional splinting," causes shortening of the supporting tissues around the joint. Eventually actual fibrosis of muscle and tendon and ankylosis of bone may develop. There is muscle weakness around the joint from disuse and distortion in joint alignment. This disease is seen more frequently in women than in men.

Types of Arthritis

Rheumatoid arthritis, also called atrophic arthritis or arthritis deformans, is a disease of unknown cause that has its highest incidence in people in the third and fourth decades of life. It causes the greatest toll in crippling because it ultimately leads to ankylosis and deformity. The peripheral joints are most frequently affected, though it can strike any joint. Joints become red, painful, swollen, and shiny. Nodules often develop over the bony prominences. If the disease involves the spine, it is called rheumatoid spondylitis or Marie-Strumpell disease. It leads to kyphosis (hunchback), an increase in the posterior curve of the thoracic vertebrae.

Degenerative arthritis, also called hypertrophic arthritis, osteoarthritis, senescent arthritis, or the "arthritis of attrition," [70] is a disease process that begins later in life, probably as a result of wear and tear of the joints. It is present to some extent in all people over 50. The joints are enlarged but are not swollen or red. Most frequently involved are the weight-bearing joints and the joints that are subjected to the greatest continuous trauma. The interphalangeal joints of the fingers develop typical knobby enlargements called Heberden's nodes.

The knees, hips, lumbosacral spine, and cervical spine are the weight-bearing joints involved. When the spine is involved, there is partial destruction of the intervertebral disks, and "spur formations" that project and encroach on the intervertebral foramina press on the spinal cord. There is some limitation of motion with degenerative arthritis but little ankylosis or deformity.

Arthritis may also result from direct trauma to the joint such as from a fracture that extends into the joint and causes permanent disruption to its architecture. More often, the trauma results from repeated "microtraumas" associated with a particular occupational stress.

Arthritis can also result from metabolic disturbance in which there is a deposit of uric acid crystals in the joint causing "gouty arthritis," or from infection, although this is infrequent since the use of antibiotics.

Patients have periods of exacerbation and remission of arthritis that appear to be related to emotional stress, lowered resistance, increased trauma, and other factors.

Treatment of Arthritis

The major goals in treatment are:

1. To maintain mobility of the involved joints,
2. To protect the power in those muscle groups upon which the joints depend for stability and mechanization,
3. To protect the joints against progression of the arthritis,
4. To suppress the inflammation,
5. To relieve the pain,
6. To increase the patient's overall resistance.

The basic ingredients of a treatment regimen include use of heat, range-of-motion and muscle exercises, rest, a well-balanced diet, analgesics to relieve pain, and anti-inflammatory drugs to decrease inflammation. A program of exercise is established for the individual. Stretching exercises are done only by specific written order. Some form of heat is used to relax the muscles before exercise begins. Paraffin is often selected. It is an excellent insulator of heat. The paraffin is melted in a double boiler if used in the home. It is ready to use when it is removed from the stove, cooled, and a thin film appears on its surface. The arthritic part is immersed in the liquid paraffin several times. When it hardens, it forms a "glove of wax." The paraffin can be brushed on inaccessible parts. Waxed paper is placed over the "glove," and this is wrapped in a bath towel and left on for about a half hour. It is peeled off easily when the treatment is finished, remelted, and reused. Paraffin is inflammable and must be handled with care if gas or other open flame is used for heating. It can be purchased in the drugstore.

Salicylates, especially aspirin, are used almost universally for the pain of arthritis. Large doses of 5 to 10 gm every day may be ordered. Sodium bicarbonate may be given with the aspirin to balance its acid effect.

To decrease inflammation phenylbutazone (Butazolidin) may be used, and gold salts seem to control inflammatory symptoms. Solganal-B and Myochrysine are examples. The nurse must be alerted to skin reaction and liver or kidney toxicity when gold salts are used. Jaundice should be reported immediately. The steroids are very effective anti-inflammatory agents but are potentially dangerous drugs that can lead to chronic steroid toxicity. They may be administered orally or injected directly into the joint, but are usually given only for short periods of time to relieve acute exacerbations. They are discontinued as soon as possible. Adrenocorticotropic hormone and hydrocortisone are examples. They cause a marked feeling of well-being. Because they tend to cause retention of fluids, dietary sodium is often restricted when they are used. They also have potent endocrine side effects, and the patient must be watched for moonface, hirsutism (hair on the face), voice changes, and so on.

To control gouty arthritis colchicine (Benemid) may be used for its anti-inflammatory properties, and uricosuric agents such as probenecid are used to increase renal excretion of uric acid.

The joints should be protected against progression of the deterioration by relieving them of as much work as possible. This is accomplished by weight reduction if the patient is overweight, by restriction of weight-bearing activities, by the use of self-help devices such as wheel chairs and canes, and by use of properly fitted shoes with adequate support. Postural faults are corrected, and occupational and other avoidable sources of trauma are eliminated.

The patient must be cautioned against the use of advertised "quick cures" or miracle drugs. They are costly, the advertising is "half true," and it takes advantage of people who are prey to these tactics because of their desire to be rid of chronic illness.

Surgery for Arthritis

Surgery is done to correct deformity and improve functional ability. *Arthrotomy* is the operative exploration of a joint. *Arthrodesis* in the fixation (stabilizing) of a joint by fusion. It may be used to stabilize an affected part such as a knee that has become distorted because of joint disease and muscle spasm. Bones in the foot may be fused to correct deformity and allow the patient to wear shoes again without severe pain. *Arthroplasty* is the operative creation of a new joint to replace an ankylosed joint; for instance, a "cuplike prosthesis" may be inserted into the acetabulum after the head of the femur has been removed from the socket and spongy ankylosing bone has been scooped out.[71] For cervical and lumbosacral spine arthritis, diseased intervertebral disks may be removed and bone grafts inserted in their place.

Postoperatively, the fixation-immobilization must be safeguarded. The physician specifies the details of activity allowed and immobilization required. Sandbags may be used on either side of the entire leg so that it is in neutral rotation and slightly abducted. The nurse must carefully execute such activities as change of body position and exercise of uninvolved parts. Traction may be ordered in some instances. Exercise of the affected part is often begun during the second or third postoperative day, with ambulation from five days to six weeks postoperatively. The patient usually uses a walker during the early stages of ambulation.

The arthritic disease process is not halted by the surgery, and the patient must continue his regimen of exercise, heat, and so on when he returns home. This is often very discouraging because he expects "great things" from the surgery.

It is very frustrating to have arthritis. The discomfort, though minimal some of the time, is chronic. The patient cannot "shake it"; it is always there. The nurse must be very patient in working with a person who has arthritis.

Ruptured Intervertebral Disk

There is a space between the bodies of the vertebrae that contains a disk made up of a cartilaginous core called the nucleus pulposus and surrounded by an elastic fibrous capsule. When the fibrous capsule of the disk loses its elasticity, its content, the nucleus pulposus, can protrude out into the spinal canal and press on spinal cord and spinal nerves. This is called herniation, rupture, or slipped disk. The lumbar and cervical regions of the spine are the two most mobile areas. They are subjected to maximum flexion and extension and are the areas most prone to disk herniation. Herniations occur most frequently between the fourth and fifth lumbar vertebrae, between the fifth lumbar and first sacral vertebrae, and between the fifth and sixth or sixth and seventh cervical vertebrae. Slipped disk is the major cause of low-back pain. (See Fig. 43–6.)

Slipped Disk

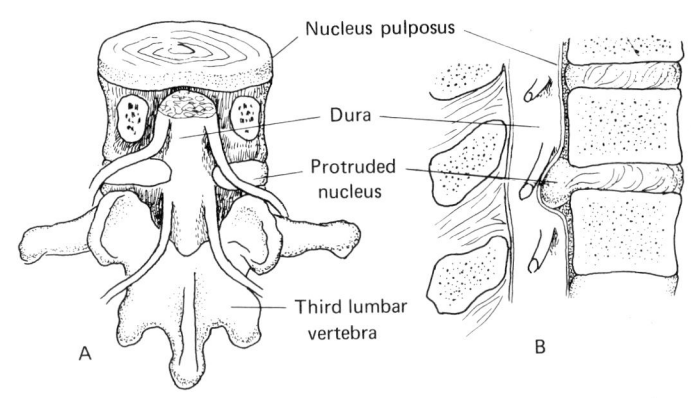

FIGURE 43–6. Slipped disk. Lumbar spine showing compression of nerve root. A. Posterior view. B. Lateral view. (From E. Sachs, *Diagnosis and Treatment of Brain Tumors and Care of the Neurosurgical Patient*, 2nd ed., 1949. Reprinted with permission of the C. V. Mosby Co., St. Louis.)

Causes of Disk Problems

Injury to an intervertebral disk usually is caused by stress on the back while it is in acute flexion. Poor body mechanics is definitely implicated. For instance, a person who lifts a heavy weight by bending from the waist rather than stooping with the knees flexed and the back straight is lifting the weight while the spine is in acute flexion. Cervical disk injury can come from a sudden stop with brutal flexion, then extension of the neck (whiplash). This causes strain on the ligament and may precipitate ruptured disk. Often, herniation cannot be traced to any specific trauma.

Symptoms depend on the area of involvement and the particular nerves that are being compressed. There are motor and sensory losses along the course of the impinged nerves. If the lumbar area is involved, there is usually pain radiating down the leg toward the foot and even including the heel and toes. There is numbness or tingling in the area, decrease in reflexes, and often decreased tone in the muscle of the leg. If the herniated disk presses on the sciatic nerve, there is pain along its length. The pain is increased when the leg on the affected side is raised straight up without bending the knee. This is called Lasègue's sign. Pain is increased when the patient coughs, sneezes, strains at stool, and so on. The patient limps. There is often acute low-back pain. If the herniation is in the cervical region, there is pain in the neck and adjoining portion of the scapula. This gradually irradiates along the upper limb. There is muscle spasm with difficulty in turning the neck (torticollis). Movement of the head increases the pain.

To specifically diagnose a ruptured disk, the physician will perform a myelogram. This involves the injection of a radiopaque dye through a lumbar puncture, followed by fluoroscopic and x-ray visualization. Occasionally a slipped disk will not be seen with myelography. The patient is allowed to eat because a general anesthetic is not used. He is kept in a horizontal position with one small pillow for 24 hours following the test to decrease the seepage of spinal fluid and thereby lessen headache. (See p. 424.)

Conservative Management of Slipped Disk

Conservative management of slipped disk focuses on rest, immobilization, heat, and muscle relaxation. The goal is to increase the intervertebral space with traction so that the herniated disk can fall back in place. The bed should be prepared before the patient arrives at the hospital. It should have a firm mattress and often a full-length bed board. The patient is placed on bed rest and usually kept flat. Sometimes, a semisitting position is effective. The lumbar spine should be supported with a firm flat pillow, folded sheet, or similar device. Mechanical traction to the cervical or pelvic region is used. It is ordered for intermittent or continuous use. The amount of weight varies. For continuous pelvic traction 4 to 10 lb is used.[72] Sometimes, this is increased and up to 20 lb of weight is used,[73] if intermittent traction is prescribed. A brace or corset is used between traction periods. For cervical traction 10 to 15 lb may be used for half-hour treatments, according to individual tolerance. Less weight is used for continuous traction. It can be applied in the sitting position. A collar is worn between treatments.

Drugs are used to decrease pain, e.g., codeine and aspirin, and to decrease muscle spasm, e.g., methocarbamol (Robaxin). The drugs are administered before onset of traction so as to obtain maximum muscle relaxation. Physical therapy, using warm water and exercise, may be ordered to decrease spasm. The patient is taught the need to keep the spine in proper alignment and not flexed. He "log-rolls" when he turns in bed by crossing his arms over his chest, bending the uppermost knee to the side to which he wants to roll, and rolling over. He is also "rolled" onto an orthopedic (flat-backed, fracture-type) bedpan. If he has sensory loss, heating pads and hot-water bottles should not be used.

When the patient leaves the hospital, he is advised to refrain from any movements or positions that cause poor body alignment. Lifting and bending are forbidden for six weeks. It is suggested that the patient sit in a straight-backed hard chair rather than a soft one; that he not elevate his feet on a footstool or cross his knees; that he not drive a car because this stretches the legs; that he not climb stairs frequently; that he shower rather than bathe in a tub; and that he refrain from bowling, handball, and golf because they are instigators of low-back pain.[74]

Manual Manipulation

There is controversy as to whether manual manipulation of the spine is advantageous. If done correctly, it seems to reduce muscle spasm; if done incorrectly, it may rupture the disk completely.[75] Manual manipulation has recently regained some favor for diskogenic disease. The patient lies on his right side at the edge of a table with his left leg dropped over the edge of the table and his left arm behind him. The manipulator places one hand on the left shoulder and the other on the iliac crest and twists the torso by pushing the shoulder backward and pulling the iliac crest forward. This maneuver is repeated on the other side. Then, the patient lies on his back, and the hips and knees are hyperflexed sufficiently to flex the lumbar spine forcibly. A "crunching" sound is heard.

Laminectomy

Laminectomy is the removal of a piece of the bony part of the vertebra (the lamina) so that the physician can get to the intervertebral area. This "approach to the intervertebral area" is used to remove ruptured disks and tumors and is used as a preliminary step in operations for the relief of intractable pain, e.g., a chordotomy, in which pain-conducting tracts are divided, or a rhizotomy, in which spinal nerve roots are divided. The skin incision is made directly over the involved spinous processes.

To remove a ruptured disk, a unilateral or bilateral laminectomy is performed, the nerve roots are retracted away from the ruptured material, and the ruptured material is removed. If the vertebral bodies have maintained their rectangular shape and are found in mechanically sound alignment, this is the extent of the surgery. If, however, there is unusual instability of the spine or if more than three intervertebral disks are ruptured, a fusion may be necessary. If this is the case, a graft of spongy tissue from the patient's iliac crest is used and the spinal vertebrae are ankylosed. This permanently prevents movement to this area of the spine. The postoperative regimen [76] depends on the extent of the surgery. For instance, the patient is often allowed out of bed the day of the surgery if a unilateral laminectomy was done at only one level for disk removal. However, if a spinal fusion was done, complete immobilization must be maintained during the initial 48 hours after surgery. Spine alignment must be as straight as possible so that healing of the bone graft can take place in proper position. A Hemovac is often used to remove excessive wound drainage. Vital signs, sensation, motor power of the extremities, and signs of hemorrhage from the surgical site and from the donor site are checked. The nurse must record the location and degree of pain carefully. Turning by log-rolling technique is usually ordered for at least the first 12 hours, longer if fusion was done. The patient is thus turned in one plane without twisting the hips. Pillows are kept between the legs when the patient is turned to maintain straight alignment. A turning sheet and at least two nurses are needed. If the patient is to be in bed for more than 24 hours, muscle-setting exercises are done. (See p. 466.)

When the patient begins to sit up and ambulate, he wears a back support that is custom-made for him and that is applied in the supine position. He is taught the procedure for sitting up and ambulating to prevent twisting and strain on the operative area. One method involves the following sequence: [77]

1. The patient lies prone.
2. The nurse supports his legs as he eases around to lying across the side of the bed with his hips at the edge of the mattress.
3. The limbs are lowered to rest firmly on the floor while the body is still on the bed.
4. Using each hand alternately the patient pushes his body to the erect position.

Although the patient may leave the hospital eight to ten days after surgery, less when a fusion is not done, the convalescence is lengthy and lasts six to ten weeks. This is the reason many patients do not elect to have the surgery. For some, though, it is better than having frequent disabling and recurring attacks during the year.

44

THE EYE

Major Factors in Eye Anatomy

THE eyeball is housed in the orbital cavity of the skull. Six extrinsic muscles are attached to it and to the wall of the orbit, for movement of the eye in all directions. The eye is protected by the eyelids, which act like movable curtains. The points where the eyelids meet are called the inner canthus, closest to the nose, and the outer canthus, farthest from the nose. There is a plate of fibrous tissue in each eyelid called a tarsal plate. It gives consistency and shape to the lids. The inner surfaces of the lids are covered by conjunctiva. It is reflected onto the eyeball. A lacrimal gland found in the frontal bone of the skull close to the side of the upper lid secretes tears. It empties through canals and ducts into a conjunctival sac between the lids and the anterior surface of the eyeball. It eventually drains through the nose.

There are three "layers" of the eyeball. The tough, outer layer is called the sclera. It is protective in function. It is modified in front of the eyeball to form the transparent cornea. The middle layer is called the choroid. It is vascular and nutritive in function. It includes the ciliary body and the iris. The ciliary body is formed by a thickening of the choroid layer. It is primarily muscular in function. The iris, or colored part, of the eye is made up of muscle, too. Together, these muscles are called the intrinsic muscles. They regulate pupillary size (the opening in the iris) in response to light. The pupil constricts to keep out bright light and dilates to bring more light in. The lens is suspended from the ciliary body of ligaments, also called zonules of Zinn. The space anterior to the lens contains aqueous humor. This space is further divided into an anterior chamber, bounded by the cornea in front and the iris and lens behind, and a posterior chamber, bounded by the iris in front, the ciliary processes and suspensory ligaments on the side, and the lens behind. The space behind the lens contains vitreous body.

The inner coat of the eye is called the retina. It has two layers: an outer, colored layer attached to the choroid and an inner, "nerve" layer, which contains cells sensitive to light. These cells are called rods and cones. The cones are functional in color vision, the rods in dim light vision. The rods and cones are the nerve receptors. The optic nerve, which leaves the retina at a circular disk (the blind spot; no rods or cones are present), is the afferent nerve pathway. It takes the visual impulses to the brain. The macula lutea is an area at the center of the retina. The fovea centralis is at its depressed center. This is the area of the retina that is adapted for the most acute vision because only cones are found here. The retina adjusts to changes from light to darkness. The power of adjusting its sensitivity to variation in light intensity is called adaptation. Adaptation requires a short period of time. That is why it "takes a while to get used to" a bright sunny day after being in a darkened room such as a movie theater.

Accommodation

This is the mechanism by which objects at varying distances from the eye can be seen. To see near objects the lens bulges and becomes more convex (fat, bulbous). This is accomplished because the ciliary muscle contracts and pulls the choroid coat forward. This loosens the tension of the suspensory ligaments, which, in turn, loosens the tension in the capsule of the lens.

To see far objects, the lens becomes less convex. It "flattens out." This is brought about by relaxation of the ciliary muscles with tension on the suspensory ligaments and lens capsule. As a person gets older the power of accommodation decreases because the lens and capsule lose their elasticity.

Examination of the Eyes

The eyes should be examined by an ophthalmologist at regular intervals throughout life. In adults before 40 years of age the eyes should be examined about every five years; after 40, when the lens begins to lose its ability to accommodate to changes in distant vision, the eyes should be checked every two years. Many nurses confuse the titles of the various people involved in the care of the eyes. The ophthalmologist or oculist is the physician who has had specialized training in care and treatment of the eye; the optician, like the pharmacist, fills prescriptions, grinds lenses, and fits glasses according to the physician's order; the optometrist can examine eyes for refractive errors and their ability to accommodate and can prescribe, grind, and adjust lenses. He is not a physician and cannot use or prescribe medications or treat eye diseases.

Inspection of the Eyes

The ophthalmologist inspects eyes carefully. He looks for any inflammation. For instance, he checks for conjunctivitis (inflammation of the conjunctiva) and blepharitis (inflammation of the lids). He checks the lids for drooping (ptosis) and the pupils for their ability to contract and dilate. If he suspects a corneal abrasion he instills a drop of 2 per cent solution of fluorescein. This is a dye that stains any abraded areas green. Individually packaged dye-impregnated filter papers are also available. They are moistened and gently placed on the lower lid. The ophthalmoscope is used to examine the fundus (interior) of the eye. It contains a light and is battery- or house-current-powered. It is not sterilized by boiling or autoclaving because of its many delicate lenses. Its parts can be cleaned with a disinfectant solution if necessary. The lights are turned off, and the physician will ask the patient to look toward a point at the opposite side of the room, directly forward and over his shoulder. This usually brings the optic nerve into view. The physician may wear a combination of lenses and prisms on a headband or on a pair of eyeglass frames to illuminate and magnify the eye. They look like a bizarre pair of glasses. For greater accuracy he may use a machine called a slit lamp. This provides a beam of light that gives intense illumination and magnification of the eye and also serves as a biomicroscope, which permits the study of microscopic changes in limited portions of the eye.

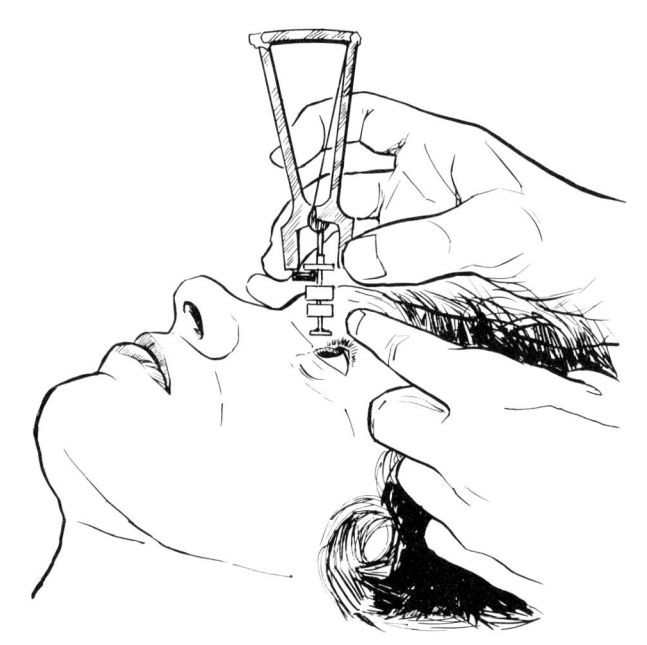

FIGURE 44–1. Measurement of intraocular pressure with a tonometer. (From W. Havener, W. Saunders, and B. Bergersen, *Nursing Care in Eye, Ear, Nose and Throat Disorders,* 1964. Reprinted with permission of C. V. Mosby Co., St. Louis.)

Measurement of intraocular pressure has become a common part of the eye examination, especially in people over 40. The cornea is anesthetized with a drug such as tetracaine (Pontocaine), 0.5 per cent. With the lids held apart a delicate instrument called a tonometer is placed on the cornea. The needle on the tonometer indicates pressure in the eye. The normal pressure is 15 to 30 mm Hg. A four-minute pictorial graph of intraocular pressure can be obtained. This is called tonography. The tonometer is attached to an electric recording device, and a record of intraocular pressure is obtained.

Refraction

Refraction is one of the most common eye examinations. Refraction means "bending light." The eye has several areas that serve to refract light so that it can be focused properly on the retina. Proper focusing of light makes accurate near and far vision possible. The refractive surfaces of the eye are the cornea, aqueous, lens, and vitreous. Refractive errors account for the largest number of impairments to good vision. More than half the people in the United States suffer from some degree of visual impairment.

Terminology

Emmetropia refers to a normal eye; ametropia means a refractive error is present. Myopia (nearsightedness) indicates an unusually long anteroposterior dimension of the eyeball with light rays focusing in front of the retina. Hyperopia (farsightedness) indicates a short anteroposterior dimension with light rays focusing behind the retina. (See Fig. 44–2.) Astigmatism indicates irregular curve of the cornea so that rays in the horizontal and perpendicular planes do not focus at the same point. Presbyopia indicates a decreased ability to accommodate because of a less elastic lens so that the person has good far vision, but poor near vision.

Before refraction is performed, drops may be instilled to temporarily paralyze the muscles of accommodation (cycloplegia) and dilate the pupil (mydriasis). Cyclopentolate (Cyclogyl) may be used. This drug is effective in a half hour and its effect is worn off in six hours. It has largely replaced homatropine, which requires one hour to take effect and lasts up to 24 hours. *Drugs that dilate the pupils are not used in persons over 40 because of the possibility of the increase in intraocular pressure that may be caused by the dilatation of the pupil.* Actually, cycloplegia is not required in people over 40 because their power of accommodation is sufficiently weak to permit satisfactory examination.

The Snellen chart contains square-shaped letters in diminishing sizes. The largest letter is at the top of the chart. It is so large that a person with a normal eye can see it when he is 200 ft from it. The next row is

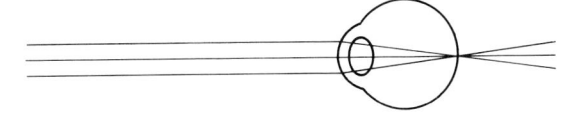

A. Normal (emmetropia)

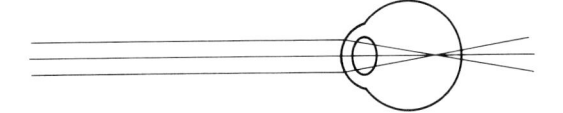

B. Myopia (nearsightedness)

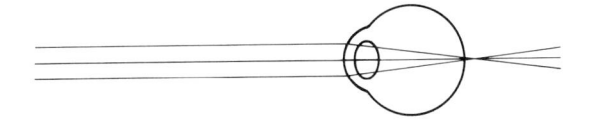

C. Hyperopia (farsightedness)

FIGURE 44–2. The focus of light rays.

seen by the normal eye at 100 ft, then 70 ft, and so on down each line. The patient sits 20 ft from the chart because rays of light from this distance are practically parallel.[78] Each eye is tested separately. The result is expressed as a fraction. The numerator is always 20, indicating the distance of the patient from the chart. The denominator corresponds to the number indicating the distance at which the smallest letters seen by the patient are seen by the normal eye. For instance, 20/100 means that the patient can see at 20 ft what the normal eye can see at 100 feet. *The bigger the denominator, the poorer the vision.* 20/20 is normal. 20/200 is considered legal blindness if it cannot be corrected with lenses.

Lenses are prescribed to correct the errors of refraction. The patient then wears glasses containing the prescribed lenses. Bifocal lenses are frequently prescribed for people over 40 who have presbyopia. Bifocal lenses are really two pair of glasses in one. The lower part of the glass is used for near vision, the upper part for distance vision. Sometimes, bifocals contain a plain-glass upper portion if the person needs no correction for distance vision. Trifocals are three lens strengths in one. They sometimes are helpful in viewing objects from various distances. If a person desires sunglasses and wears corrective glasses, he should also wear corrective sunglasses ground to his own prescription. If he does not wish to go to this expense, he can clip sunglasses onto his own corrective glasses. Any sunglass should be carefully ground and should be large enough to exclude bright light around their edges and dark enough to exclude about 30 per cent of the light.

Contact Lenses

Contact lenses are tiny plastic lenses inserted over the iris. They are suitable for some people. They are difficult to "get used to" because they act like foreign bodies in the eye, initially. They must be fitted properly and then checked by the ophthalmologist regularly. The patient is taught how to insert and remove them and then is supervised in doing this. No artificial lubrication is needed because the normal conjunctival secretions accumulate in sufficient amounts. The contact lenses are, however, cleaned with a special contact lens solution before they are inserted and then when they are removed. They are stored in a special receptacle that protects them from scratching. The person gradually increases the amount of time they are worn. They may sometimes be worn all day, but are never worn during sleep! Occasionally they are worn with protective glasses over them. For instance, on a very windy day dust and particles of soot may "get stuck" underneath the lenses, rub the cornea, and cause corneal abrasions. The person may have pain in the eye. This should be examined by the ophthalmologist, who usually will have the patient leave them out for several days and may prescribe an antibiotic or anti-inflammatory drug for instillation. Bifocal contact lenses are available.

Testing Field of Vision

The field of vision is tested. Peripheral (side) vision occurs when the image falls on some part of the retina outside of its central portion. Peripheral vision is essential to complete vision. Poor peripheral vision is the cause of many automobile accidents because the person is not able to see someone or something coming toward him from the side unless he turns his head toward it. One eye is tested at a time. The physician may move his hand from the side inward and ask the patient to tell him when he starts seeing the hand. A more accurate method is through use of the perimeter or tangent screen. The head is supported on a chin rest in both instances. One eye is covered and the other is fixed on a white spot at the center of a revolving metallic semicircular arc, which is marked in degrees. The test object, a white or colored disk, is moved along the inner surface of the arc on the end of a black rod. The point at which the test object is seen is noted. The tangent screen is a large black curtain on a frame. The patient fixes his eye on a white spot in the center of the screen. A test object is moved from the periphery toward the center, and the patient indicates when he sees it.

Other Tests of the Eye

The physician may test for color recognition. Field for color is smaller than that for white; it is largest for blue and smallest for green.[79] He may wish to know if the person is color-blind. This indicates inability to identify one or more of the primary colors (red, blue, or green).

Rules for Daily Eye Care

1. Normal, healthy eyes require no proprietary drops to "refreshen and cleanse" them. They cleanse themselves. Although drugstore preparations are generally harmless, they serve little useful purpose and do cause an allergic reaction in an occasional person.
2. Hands should be kept away from the eyes. Many bacterial infections of the eyes stem from hand-to-eye transfer.
3. "Eyestrain" is a much overused term. In actuality, using the eyes does not strain them. Sometimes, when there is difficulty in accommodation, the ciliary muscles are strained. This does not cause any permanent eye damage. The eyes cannot be "overused"!
4. A good light directed over the shoulder and placed so that a shadow is not cast by the hands [80] should be used for reading, writing, sewing, or any close work.
5. When fine work is being done, the muscles should be rested periodically by looking at something far away. This relaxes the muscles of accommodation.
6. Make sure the diet is well balanced. Changes in the conjunctiva and corneal epithelium, which can lead to blindness, are often traced to a deficiency of vitamin A, as is difficulty in adapting to night vision. Pathologic changes occur in the retina from deficiency of vitamin B.
7. Avoid excess exposure to direct sunlight and sunlamps. They can burn the lids and the cornea.

The Eye Emergency

Accidental injury to the eyes is commonplace. When an acid or any type of irritating substance gets into the eye, flush it copiously with water from the tap. Have the person bend over the sink, hold his eyelids open, and let the water run over the eye. If sterile saline is available, it should be used; however, time should not be wasted searching for it. The longer the substance is in contact with the eye, the greater is the damage. The same method is used if the wrong medication is accidentally instilled into an eye. Following the irrigation the patient is told to close his eye and an eye pad is placed over the lid and secured with cellophane tape. The patient is taken to the hospital or to the ophthalmologist immediately.

Foreign Bodies in the Eye

The nurse may remove a foreign body from the eye if it is not on the cornea and if it does not appear to have penetrated the eyeball. She asks the patient not to further irritate the eye by rubbing it. She washes her hands and then carefully inspects the eye, including the inside surfaces of the upper and lower lids, to see where the foreign body is. She must evert the upper lid to inspect it. This is tricky. An applicator or a toothpick with cotton wrapped on its edge is placed at the border of the upper lid close to the lashes. The lashes are grasped with the other hand. Gentle pressure is placed on the applicator, and the lid is then rolled back over it. The particle is removed by gently touching it with an applicator moistened with sterile saline or tap water if the saline is not available. If the particle is not removed easily, the attempt is discontinued and the patient is taken to the ophthalmologist. Damage can be done if it is "picked at." Keeping the eye closed and covering it gently with an eye pad secured in place with cellophane tape decreases the irritation and the pain. The patient will experience some discomfort from irritation for a while after the particle has been removed. Entrance and lodgment of a foreign body within the globe usually cause severe inflammation and destruction of the eyeball unless the foreign body is removed promptly. The gravity of the accident depends on the nature and the size of the foreign body. For instance, a fragment of copper almost invariably leads to destruction of the eye, whereas lead, gold, silver, and glass become encapsulated and may not cause trouble for a long time. Metal particles are removed with magnets.

Sympathetic Ophthalmia

Two weeks to one year after injury to an eye a dread condition called sympathetic ophthalmia sometimes occurs. Although not seen frequently today, this is a situation in which the noninjured eye reacts with such a severe inflammatory uveitis that its function may be lost completely. Once sympathetic ophthalmia has begun its progress, removal of the injured eye will not halt it, although steroids may help save it. To prevent this from happening the physician may have to remove the originally injured eye to save the noninjured eye. This is called an enucleation. If the contents of the eyeball are removed leaving the sclera in place, it is called an evisceration. If possible, the eyeball alone is removed leaving the surrounding membrane and muscle attachments. A metal or plastic ball or a piece of fat is inserted in the capsule. It serves as a permanent stump that provides support and motion for the artificial shell. The shell is made of glass or plastic and resembles the patient's other eye. The "ball" remains in the socket; the shell eye is removed at night. It is fitted, like any other prosthetic device, about six weeks after surgery, and the patient is instructed in its use.

To remove the artificial eye, one hand is cupped underneath it; the lower lid is pulled down; the lower edge of the eye is slipped out and with gentle pressure on the upper eyelid it is pushed out. To insert the eye the upper lid is raised and drawn slightly outward. The eye is slid under the upper lid and held with one finger while the lower lid is pulled down and the lower edge of the eye is slipped behind it. The more pointed side of the artificial eye is placed nearest the nose. It looks like and moves like a regular eye, but its pupil, of course, does not dilate and constrict. It is stored in a clean, dry place after cleansing. It can also be stored in a container of normal saline.

Nursing Management of the Patient Having Eye Surgery

The adult patient having eye surgery is usually in good health when he enters the hospital. His surgery is usually scheduled ahead of time so that he has an opportunity to arrange for his home responsibilities. The surgery is usually aimed at preserving or restoring vision. The patient is rational, alert, and awake. He often brings his medications from home, and the physician leaves specific orders concerning their use. Sometimes the patient will be on a previously prescribed medication in one eye, and a preoperative medication will be ordered for the other eye. The nurse must be very careful to use the correct drops in each eye. The abbreviation for right eye, is o.d.; for left eye o.l. or o.s.; for each eye (both eyes) o.u.; of each āā.

Drugs used preoperatively include sedatives, tranquilizers, analgesics, antibiotics, and anti-inflammatory agents. Frequently drugs are prescribed to reduce intraocular pressure. These include miotics such as pilocarpine, 0.5 to 4 per cent, and carbachol, 0.75 to 3.0 per cent; or more powerful miotic agents such as isofluorophosphate (Floropryl, DFP), 0.1 per cent, and echothiophate iodide (Phospholine), 0.06 to 0.25 per cent. Hypertonic solutions that draw water toward themselves for excretion include oral glycerin, 1 ml per kilogram body weight, and intravenous mannitol (Osmitrol), 5 to 20 per cent. If mannitol is used, it should not contain crystals and should be administered with filter tubing if the 20 per cent concentration is used. Acetazolamide (Diamox), 200 to 500 mg, may be used. It tends to produce a mild acidosis and potassium depletion. This electrolyte must be replaced if the drug is used for any length of time. Mydriatic-cycloplegic drops may be instilled to dilate the pupil and paralyze the muscles of accommodation. Examples are homatropine, 1 to 2 per cent, and cyclopentolate (Cyclogyl), 0.5 to 1.0 per cent. Once the patient is medicated, or if his vision is severely restricted, the side rails should be kept up. The patient may be instructed to wash his face with a hexachlorophene soap for ten minutes three times on the evening before surgery.[80] He is allowed nothing by mouth from midnight if general anesthesia is to be used; he may have a light breakfast the morning of surgery if a local anesthetic agent is to be used.

The nurse must find out which eye(s) is to be operated on. She should be able to tell the patient whether one or both eyes will be covered postoperatively. Many physicians ask that dentures be left in if a local anesthetic agent is used so that facial contour is maintained. This must be clarified beforehand.

Much eye surgery is done under local anesthesia to decrease the chance of postoperative vomiting, which so greatly increases intraocular pressure. The patient is sufficiently sedated so that he sleeps intermittently throughout the procedure. His head is immobilized and his arms restrained. A few drops of a sterile ophthalmologic anesthetic solution such as lidocaine (Xylocaine), 4 per cent, or proparacaine (Ophthaine), 0.5 per cent, are placed in each eye. Sometimes, retrobulbar filtration anesthesia is also used. If the lashes are to be cut, a small amount of petroleum jelly on the blades of the scissors catches them. The patient is asked to close his eyes gently and his face is cleaned. If a lens is to be removed, the operating team is alerted so that the blood pressure cuff is not inflated at that time. This would cause an increase in pressure.

When the patient returns to his room, he is very sensitive to sounds and to odors. If both his eyes are covered, he may fear blindness and be very anxious. There is some discomfort after intraocular surgery; however, if the patient complains of severe pain, it may mean hemorrhage and/or wound rupture, and the physician should be called immediately. The patient is not allowed solid foods immediately after surgery to lessen the chance of vomiting. Sometimes drugs are used to control vomiting. The patient remains quiet, in a position ordered by the physician. He need not be absolutely still and immobilized with sandbags along the sides of his head, as was the custom a few years ago. Pillows are sometimes used for slight immobilization. The patient must not lift, bend, or participate in any vigorous activity. He should be kept quiet in a darkened room. He must not smoke in bed. He is usually allowed bathroom privileges the day after surgery, but shaving and teeth brushing require specific orders. Women should not comb or set their hair immediately after surgery.

Glaucoma

The normal pressure within the eye is 15 to 30 mm Hg. This range is maintained because of a delicate balance in the amount of aqueous humor formed and the amount ultimately reabsorbed through the general circulation. Aqueous humor nourishes the lens and cornea. It is drained through a meshwork filter system at the outer margin of the anterior chamber, into the canal of Schlemm. If the amount of aqueous produced is greater than the amount drained, intraocular pressure increases.

Glaucoma is a disease in which there is an increased intraocular pressure. Glaucoma is called "closed-angle" if the faulty removal of aqueous comes from a narrowing of the angle leading to the drainage channels. This is a mechanical problem and is almost always binocular. Glaucoma is called "open-angle" if the angle is adequate but there is obstruction in the drainage system. In any case, the disease is most prevalent in people over 40, and it can lead to blindness if it is uncontrolled because it destroys the optic nerve. Glaucoma is a major cause of blindness in the United States. There seems to be a family predisposition to it.

Acute Glaucoma

In the "prodromal" stage of acute glaucoma the patient has transitory attacks during which his visual acuity decreases and his sight seems obscured by fog. He may see a halo (circle) of rainbow tints around artificial lights and have a feeling of dullness or slight pain in his eye and head. The symptoms last for a number of hours and then disappear with the eye returning to normal except for a decrease in the power of accommodation. The attacks are often precipitated by insomnia, worry, emotional excitement, overeating, or the use of a mydriatic drug that dilates the pupil and decreases the area available for fluid drainage. The attacks gradually become more frequent and the patient is then said to be in the stage of acute glaucoma. There is a great increase in intraocular pressure. The onset of the attack is sudden, and the patient experiences severe pain and headache. There may be nausea and vomiting. The eyelids become swollen, the pupils dilated and immobile, and the cornea cloudy. With each attack there is greater decrease in sight as the optic nerve is impinged upon. Immediate treatment is necessary! Drug therapy includes the use of miotics, such as pilocarpine, sometimes instilled as often as every 15 minutes to increase the drainage of aqueous by constricting the pupil and pulling the iris away from the drainage channels; the use of carbonic-anhydrase inhibitors such as acetazolamide (Diamox) to decrease the production of aqueous; and the use of hypertonic solutions such as mannitol (Osmitrol) and urea to decrease edema. Analgesics are used to decrease the pain. Emergency surgery may be indicated for closed-angle glaucoma to halt the rising intraocular pressure and prevent irreversible optic nerve damage. Surgery is done when the glaucoma cannot be controlled medically.

Chronic Glaucoma

This occurs more frequently than acute glaucoma. Symptoms may begin so slowly that they remain unnoticed by the patient. There is often a decrease in peripheral vision. The patient cannot see objects to the side, and this often results in automobile accidents. He may have blurred vision and an aching sensation in his eyes, especially after seeing a movie or watching television for a long period of time. He may have headache and confuse this with sinusitis. He may see halos (rings) around artificial lights. If he starts having to have his glasses changed frequently, having difficulty adjusting to darkness, or having any of the above symptoms, he should be directed to an ophthalmologist. Treatment includes the use of miotics, analgesics, hypertonic agents to reduce fluid pressure, and rest. The patient may be advised to limit the amount of fluid ingested at any one time and to avoid heavy lifting, straining at stool, or any activity that would cause a rise in intraocular pressure. Surgery is indicated if the intraocular pressure cannot be reduced and controlled medically.

Surgery for Glaucoma

The goal of surgery, regardless of the procedures selected, is to produce an increased filtering channel so that there is more efficient outflow of aqueous.

IRIDECTOMY

This is the removal of a piece of iris thereby preventing it from bulging out and encroaching upon the drainage channels. An iridectomy creates a permanent entrance to the drainage channel ensuring passage of aqueous from the posterior chamber to the anterior chamber. It is called a peripheral iridectomy when a small piece of iris is removed at the periphery, and a total or keyhole iridectomy if a larger piece of iris is removed. It looks like a keyhole after removal.

TREPHINATION, IRIDENCLEISIS

Trephination is the removal of a button of cornea and sclera to allow aqueous to seep under the conjunctiva, and iridencleisis is the cutting and inverting of iris to provide a wick that filters fluid out under the conjunctiva.

All patients who have glaucoma, with or without surgery, must have periodic eye examinations by an ophthalmologist.

Cataract

A cataract is a clouding or opacity of the normally transparent lens. As the "clouding" progresses, vision decreases. Cataract is the leading cause of blindness in older people. Cataracts may be congenital, they may be associated with other diseases of the eye such as iritis or uveitis, or they may be the result of the degenerative processes of aging. Usually, both eyes are affected, with one in advance of the other. Surgery is the only effective treatment. It can be done successfully in very old people. Surgery involves removal of the lens. An incision is made at the junction of the cornea and sclera and extends through the entire 180-degree circumference. If the intracapsular technique is used, the lens is extracted within its capsule. This is facilitated by the use of cryosurgery (freezing) techniques in which a cryoprobe is inserted, cooled to temperatures of $-25°$ to $-40°$ at which point an iceball forms and the lens is slid out. If the extracapsular technique is used, the lens is lifted out of the capsule and the capsular membrane is left in place. This is not done very often. A partial or complete iridectomy may be included in the procedure to form an additional opening through which aqueous can flow. This is done because vitreous tends to come forward and block the flow of aqueous through the pupil. The surgery is often done under local anesthesia. Both cataracts are not removed at the same time. This is a precautionary measure to protect the other eye in case of some unexpected emergency or complication. Both cataracts may, however, be extracted during a single hospital admission, one week apart.

The cataract passes through many stages, which cannot be hurried or slowed down. It is said to be "mature" or "ripe" when the lens loses its excess fluid, shrinks, and is perfectly opaque. A patient need not wait until his cataract is "ripe" to have it extracted. Often, the physician will instill the enzyme alpha-chymotrypsin to dissolve the lens ligaments (zonular fibers) and facilitate removal. Surgery is done when vision cannot be corrected adequately with eyeglasses, and when the cataract interferes with the patient's work. The eye operated upon is covered with a dressing and a protective shield. The patient is usually allowed out of bed the day after surgery.

The eye without a lens is called aphakic. When the lens is removed, the patient can see only light and dark without corrective glasses. This may frighten him! Everything seems out of focus, fuzzy, and unrecognizable. Cataract glasses have thick lenses with edges that tend to curve straight lines. Any sudden movement of the eyes sets the curves in motion, and lines seem to "writhe like snakes." The patient feels as if he were looking into a carnival trick mirror.[82] He must relearn depth perception. For instance, he has difficulty walking through an open door because the opening looks too small. The nurse can help him by letting him feel the opening and by guiding him through it and encouraging him to look forward moving his head rather than his eyes.

The corrective lens causes the patient to see objects about one third larger than a normal eye sees them. The patient must understand that he will have to have frequent eyeglass adjustments made because cataract glasses are easily put out of focus if the frames slip.

If the lens has been removed from one eye and not from the other, the patient will use one of his eyes at a time, but not both together, because of a great difference in what each eye sees. Contact lenses are helping to solve this problem by lessening the difference in the size of the image seen by both eyes and making binocular vision possible.

Other Commonly Occurring Eye Conditions

Stye

Stye (hordeolum) is a circumscribed infection at the edge of the eyelid that originates in a lash follicle. It starts as a red, painful swelling, increases in size, and then usually ruptures and releases pus after which the pain diminishes and the lesion heals spontaneously. Sometimes the stye must be incised so that it will drain. Hot compresses and antibiotics may be ordered.

Chalazion

Chalazia are pea-sized nodes that stem from infection of sebaceous (meibomian) glands in the eyelids. The ducts become blocked and the nodes develop. Chalazia sometimes disappear after applications of antibacterial ointments, massage, and hot compresses. When they are large or multiple, they are removed surgically. This can be done in the hospital or in the physician's office.

Conjunctivitis

Often called "pink eye," this is an inflammation of the conjunctiva from bacterial or viral infection, an allergic reaction, irritation from smoke or dust particles, and so on. Antibiotics are used if a causative organism is found.

Uveitis

Uveitis is an inflammation of the middle, vascular coat of the eye, which contains the iris, ciliary body, and choroid. These structures are so intimately associated that disease frequently involves all parts. Symptoms include redness, tearing, pain, photophobia, and blurred vision. The cause of uveitis is frequently unknown, and the inflammation is difficult to control and often recurs. It can lead to cataract, glaucoma, or permanent destruction of the eye.

Keratitis

Keratitis is an inflammation of the cornea, frequently resulting from infection with a virus. The symptoms include redness, tearing, photophobia, and pain.

Keratoplasty is a corneal transplant. When injury to the cornea is so severe that vision is no longer possible, a transplant is considered. The opaque portion of the cornea is removed and the donor cornea is sutured in its place. People may will that their corneas be used after their death. They should be removed within six hours after death. The Eye Bank for Sight Restoration, Inc., collects and distributes donated corneas throughout the country. A certain amount of immobilization is required after surgery, depending on the type of graft done. This may mean that the patient is kept flat in bed with both eyes covered for 48 hours.

Retinal Detachment

The retina is the innermost layer of the eye. It is composed of a pigmented outer layer, which is closely aligned to the vascular, nourishing choroid, and a sensory inner layer, which receives visual impulses and transmits them to the brain. In detached retina, the two layers become separated. As the inner layer fails to receive adequate vascular nourishment it fails to receive a clear image, and vision decreases. Fluid (vitreous humor) seeps between the separated layers through tears and holds the layers apart.

Retinal detachment occurs most frequently in people over 40 years. Its incidence is higher in those who are myopic. It is associated with a hole or tear in the retina resulting from degenerative changes or trauma. The patient has flashes of light in part of the visual field; then, days or weeks later, he will complain of a dark cloud before the eye, or loss of central vision. He has "gaps" in vision where the retina is detached. There is usually no pain.

If the detachment occurs in the central part of the retina, visual loss will be greater than if it occurs at the periphery. Diagnosis is more accurate than it once was. Although use of the conventional ophthalmoscope shows only a small portion of the retina, the stereoscopic indirect ophthalmoscope produces an image of a much larger retinal area with less distortion. The examination takes more than an hour, and a map of the retina, with its breaks, is drawn.

Surgical repair is now successful in 85 per cent of patients with retinal detachment.[83] Goals of surgery include draining fluid from the retinal space so that it can return to its normal position and sealing the retinal break firmly to the choroid to prevent future leakage. This is done by scleral buckling. A section of sclera and choroid that overlies the retinal detachment is treated with diathermy. This produces an inflammatory response that helps to seal holes in the retina by causing the formation of adhesions. The subretinal fluid is released. Then, the treated sclera and choroid are indented or "buckled" inward toward the vitreous cavity by making a fold of the treated area and actually suturing this fold in place. This "seals" the retinal break to the choroid to prevent further leakage. Silicone-rubber implants are placed under the scleral sutures to assist in the creation of a buckle. Cryosurgery is also used. Replacement of the diseased vitreous with donor vitreous that has been dried and then remoistened and the use of synthetic vitreous are in developmental stages.

During recovery from anesthesia the patient should lie with the unoperated eye down so that no undue pressure will occur on the operated eye. A light pressure dressing of cotton balls over an eyepad is used to decrease edema. The patient may be allowed out of bed the day after surgery or may have to remain in bed flat on his back up to ten days. This must be clarified with the physician. Movement of the head and eyes does not jeopardize the sealing of the retinal break though any sudden jerking motion or increase in pressure as from coughing or vomiting could be serious.

The operated eye is opened three to four days after surgery when the lid edema begins to subside. Mydriatic drops are instilled several times each day and are continued from four to six weeks postoperatively to dilate the pupil and prevent the formation of adhesions between the iris and lens. Steroids are used to decrease intraocular inflammation. The patient can usually return to sedentary work three to four weeks after surgery and to heavy work about two months after surgery.

Blindness

A person is considered legally blind when the vision in the better eye is 20/200 even with corrective lenses. With the increasing number of older people in the United States blindness associated with degenerative diseases (e.g., arteriosclerosis) is a major problem. Many blind people can learn to be self-supporting and independent. Many learn to read Braille, a system of raised dots arranged to signify letters of the alphabet. Many learn to move about in city traffic with a specially trained dog or with a cane. Many do productive work. Blind people learn to live in and be a part of a sighted world. Each state has an agency that helps the blind person in all phases of his rehabilitation. The individual state addresses can be obtained from the American Foundation for the Blind, Inc., 15 West 16th Street, New York, New York 10011.

Here are some hints for caring for the blind patient at home or in the hospital:

1. Do not pity him or treat him as though he were a child.
2. Let him tell you how he is accustomed to managing. Respect his methods and honor them.
3. Tell him where his food is on his plate; e.g., the meat is at 9 o'clock, the vegetable at 6 o'clock, and the potato at 3 o'clock. Try to arrange the food in this order regularly.
4. Keep the furniture in exactly the same place all the time. Make sure the cleaning personnel maintain this rule.
5. If your patient is newly blind, allow him to go through the phases of grief at his own pace. Do not rush him.
6. Encourage and guide him to care for his own body needs, e.g., shaving, combing his hair, bathing. Modify equipment if necessary, e.g., an electric shaver instead of a razor with blade.

7. Suggest the availability of talking books and newspapers. The *New York Times* Review of the Week section is recorded every week and mailed to blind subscribers. Information concerning loan or purchase of talking books can be obtained from the Library of Congress, Washington, D.C., and from individual state agencies for the blind.

8. Speak to the patient before touching him so that he knows you are there. Do not speak loudly because he cannot see. Tell him what you are going to do.

9. If you give a blind person directions, do not use visual landmarks such as "the large gas station on the corner." Counting the number of streets that he will cross is effective. If you are leading a blind person, let him hold your arm. Walk slightly ahead of him so that he has time to feel when you stop at a curb.

45

THE EAR

The ear is the organ of hearing and balance. The external ear is made up of an auricle and a canal. It contains wax and sweat glands. It provides a channel for the passage of sound waves on their way to the tympanic membrane (ear drum). The middle ear is directly behind the tympanic membrane. It is an air-filled space. The air pressure in this space is regulated by opening and closing of the eustachian tube, which opens into the nasopharynx from the middle ear. The eustachian tube opens when we yawn or swallow in order to maintain the equalization of air pressure between the middle and outer ear. Changes in balance of pressure, such as occur when we ascend or descend in an airplane, cause some discomfort. The eustachian tube is also involved in the spread of infection from the nasopharynx to the middle ear. This is called otitis media. It is seen more often in young children because the eustachian tube is short and widely open. Forceful nose blowing, especially with one nare closed by the thumb, forces nasopharyngeal secretions into the middle ear.

The middle ear contains the three smallest bones in the body: the malleus (hammer), the incus (anvil), and the stapes (stirrup). These bones vibrate and conduct sound to the membrane of an oval window that brings the sound to the inner ear.

The inner ear is the organ of hearing and equilibrium. The vestibular labyrinths with three semicircular canals are involved in maintenance of equilibrium. The organ of Corti, found within the cochlea, is the end organ for hearing. It contains tiny hair cells, which are bent by sound waves and convert them from a mechanical force to an electrochemical impulse that travels to the brain via the acoustic nerve. Sound can then be interpreted and we say we can hear.

Symptoms of disease of the ear include pain, tenderness, tinnitus (ringing), vertigo (dizziness), headache, discharge, and change in hearing acuity. The pain of an earache is exquisitely severe. A thorough examination by an otologist is essential.

Cerumen (Wax)

Very often people ask the nurse how to remove wax from the ears. Usually, wax does not have to be "cleaned out." A normal amount of wax helps decrease itch, and it is beneficial. It is sterile when produced in the external canal. Occasionally, wax becomes hardened and impacted. This "old" wax serves as a breeding ground for microorganisms, causes discomfort, and can cause temporary deafness. It should be removed by a skilled person, not by the patient. The wax is often softened with warmed oil or warmed hydrogen peroxide first and is then irrigated out with a pomeroy syringe. The irrigating solution is directed toward the upper wall of the canal so that the wax is not forced further back toward the eardrum. The external canal of an adult is straightened by grasping the auricle within the index and third fingers and gently pulling it upward and backward. Sometimes the physician lifts the wax out with a hooked instrument.

Foreign Bodies in the Ear

Vegetable products such as beans or corn should never be irrigated. The solution causes them to swell, and they become more tightly lodged in the ear. They are removed by the physician with a hooked instrument. Insects are killed by filling the canal with mineral oil to smother them and then removing them with irrigation or forceps.

Ototoxic Drugs

Streptomycin, kanamycin, neomycin, and Gentamicin are known to have ototoxic effects in some people. If a patient is to have the drug for more than two weeks, auditory testing is suggested before and after treatment. The nurse should watch for vertigo, nystagmus (uncontrolled movement of the eye in any direction), and blurred vision.

Noise

Some persons are subject to hearing loss when different amounts of frequency, duration, and intensity of sound are present. The noise causes the basilar membrane to vibrate, and this can injure the organ of Corti. Acoustic damage is influenced by the length of exposure, by the age of the person (older people are more prone to trauma than young), by the type of frequency (low-frequency sounds are less damaging than high), and by the presence of previous ear disease. Special ear protectors, e.g., padded helmets and earplugs, should be worn if the person is exposed to noise for long periods of time.

Surgery of the Ear

Because of the tiny size of the parts of the ear, surgery is done with an operative microscope. The incision is endaural if it is made through the ear canal; it is postaural if it is behind the ear.

Myringotomy

This is a procedure in which the tympanic membrane is incised so that pus can drain out of the middle ear. Myringotomy relieves the throbbing pain and pressure caused by the bulging eardrum and prevents its spontaneous rupture, which would leave jagged edges and cause slower healing with scar tissue formation. The procedure was done frequently before the advent of antibiotics to control middle-ear infection.

Mastoid Cell Infection

There is also a possibility of the spread of infection to the mastoid cells in the mastoid process of the temporal bone. The middle ear connects with the mastoid process through involved passages. Mastoiditis is serious because it can spread to the brain and it can cause permanent loss of hearing. Occasionally cells of the mastoid process must be removed. This is called mastoidectomy. A radical mastoidectomy to eradicate stubborn infection involves removal of mastoid cells along with removal of the incus, malleus, and eardrum. The stapes is left in place to protect the entrance to the inner ear. The middle ear is reconstructed in a procedure called tympanoplasty. The extent of the surgery for removal of mastoid cells and repair depends on the extent of the infection.

Tympanoplasty

This is a group of reconstructive procedures involving the eardrum and/or middle ear. It is designed to improve hearing in people with conductive (external or middle ear) hearing loss. For instance, a vein graft may be used to replace a tympanic membrane (myringoplasty) or a polyethylene joint may take the place of one of the tiny bones (ossiculoplasty).

Stapedectomy or stapes mobilization is done for otosclerosis. Otosclerosis is a condition in which there is loss of hearing from gradual immobilization of the footplate of the stapes bone (the stirrup) in the oval window. New growth of bone around the stapes blocks its movement so that it is no longer free to vibrate. Both ears are usually affected though not necessarily in equal degrees. The disease is seen more frequently in women, tends to be familial, and becomes apparent in the second and third decades of life. The patient experiences a buzzing tinnitus and a diminished hearing acuteness. The surgeon may break the bone loose so that it is free to move again (stapes mobilization), or he may remove the bone completely and replace it with a prosthetic device (stapedectomy). After the surgery, hearing usually improves, though it is not necessarily "normal" hearing. The patient hears with one ear at a time. He may be dizzy after the surgery. A most frustrating complication arises when the patient is able to hear after the surgery and weeks later becomes suddenly deaf because of infection or scar tissue formation.

INSTRUCTIONS FOR THE PATIENT AFTER A STAPEDECTOMY *

First 24 hours following surgery, it is important for you to

    Stay *flat* in bed, even for meals.

    † Keep your head movements to a minimum. When you do move, do so very slowly.

    † Keep fast moving objects, even those on television, out of your field of vision.

    10 Avoid blowing your nose or sneezing.

        Tell the nurse about sensations of pain, nausea, taste changes, other sensations, such as the "sloshing" in the ear, and so on.

Second 24 hours it is important for you to

    Call the nurse to your bedside before attempting to rise.

    † Rise slowly to a sitting/standing position.

    † Keep your head level.

    † Look at the floor for orientation in space.

    † Walk slowly, move your head and upper trunk together.

    Be sure a member of your family gets instructions from the nurse on how to change your ear dressing before you leave the hospital.

During convalescence remember that you should

    † Close your eyes while riding in traffic.

    10 Not take showers, go swimming or get water on the ear dressing after surgery to prevent water from contaminating the ear.

    30 Stay away from people with upper respiratory infections.

    30 Avoid elevators and other sudden movements.

    30 Avoid flying in airplanes or going to high altitudes.

    30 Stay in quiet surroundings and especially avoid jet noises at airport.

Key:

    † After third day, gradually redevelop normal patterns.

    10 Approximately ten days observe the instruction.

    30 Approximately thirty days observe the instruction.

* Reprinted with permission from De Laney, R. E., "Stapedectomy," *Amer. J. Nurs.,* **69:**2409, 1969.

Care of the Patient Regardless of the Type of Surgery

1. The external ear and surrounding skin must be kept meticulously clean.

2. Observe and report signs of injury to the facial nerve; e.g., can the patient wrinkle his forehead, close his eyes, pucker his lips? Paralysis may indicate damage to the nerve or edema causing pressure on the nerve.

3. The surgeon changes the dressing. The nurse observes it for drainage and reinforces the dressing.

4. Aseptic technique is essential because of the closeness of the ear to the brain. Instruct the patient to keep his hands away from the dressing.

5. Because vertigo is a common occurrence, the patient must be protected from falls. Use side rails, help him from bed to chair, and so forth.

6. To prevent nasopharyngeal secretions from traveling from the eustachian tube to the middle ear, and to protect the delicate surgery, nose blowing is not permitted during the early postoperative period. The nose can be wiped with a tissue.

7. Hearing may not return immediately. The patient should understand this and should be encouraged to discuss his fears with his physician.

Hearing Impairment

There are four types of hearing impairment.

1. Conductive Loss. This is a mechanical difficulty in the conduction of sound waves in the outer ear, middle ear, or both. The inner ear can still analyze clearly the sound that it receives, but for some reason the sound "is not getting through." People with conductive losses benefit most from surgery and from use of hearing aids. These are battery-operated devices that increase the volume of the sound and therefore make speech comfortably loud for the patient. Hearing aids consist of a microphone to receive sound waves and convert them into electrical signals, an amplifier to increase the strength of the signals, and a receiver to convert the amplified signals into acoustical signals. Hearing aids can be built into the temples of eyeglasses, worn in the ear or behind the ear, or worn on the torso.

2. Sensorineural Loss. Also called "nerve deafness" or "perceptual deafness," this type of loss involves the inner ear and/or its central connections. Sounds get to the inner ear adequately but are not analyzed correctly. For instance, speech may sound distorted regardless of the articulation or volume; there may be an abnormal sensitivity to loud sounds or intolerance to noice. If the loss is to both ears, the patient's voice is usually louder and more strained than normal. He has more difficulty understanding speech in a noisy than in a quiet environment. The most common cause of sensorineural deafness is presbycusis, the gradual reduction in hearing with advancing age. Sensorineural losses are irreversible and are not benefited by surgery. These patients are poor candidates for hearing aids although some may benefit to some degree.

Many patients have combined conductive and sensorineural losses.

3. Functional Loss. This implies an underlying psychologic problem. There is no organic damage to the auditory system.

4. Central Loss. This implies damage in the central nervous system at some point between the auditory nuclei in the brain.

The patient who has a hearing impairment should be thoroughly examined by an otologist (a physician who has had specialized training in diseases of the ear). This includes accurate measurement of hearing with use of an audiometer, a machine that produces pure tones of controlled loudness and pitch. It also includes a variety of tests with a vibrating tuning fork. Measurements of bone conduction loss are determined in this manner.

Often a nurse will be the first person to detect a partial hearing loss when she observes that the patient asks her to repeat statements frequently, or when she receives inappropriate answers, or when she finds that the patient hears much better if he watches her face when she is speaking. Deviations in articulation sometimes point to a hearing loss.

The major goal for the patient with hearing loss is efficiency in oral communication. If the patient has been deaf since birth and has never heard speech, this is very difficult to attain. Methods used include prevention of loss of speech following hearing impairment, auditory training to improve the person's listening skills and residual hearing, and speech therapy with focus on "speech reading" (lip reading). In speech reading the patient watches the speaker and utilizes visual clues for effective communication. He not only "reads lips" but responds to facial expression, position, and so on. If the patient will benefit from the use of a hearing aid, he is advised to go to a hearing center where he will be guided in the selection of an aid best suited to his needs. He is taught how to use the aid and encouraged to be patient, for it takes time to "get used to it."

Suggestions for Nursing the Patient with Hearing Impairment

1. Speak clearly and naturally. Do not shout.
2. Face the patient so that he can speech-read; have sufficient light.
3. Use uninvolved sentences and keep a pad and pencil available for writing key words.
4. Protect the patient's hearing aid from damage.
5. The ear mold is the only part of the hearing aid that is washed. Mild soap and water and a pipe cleaner can be used. It should be thoroughly dry before being reconnected to the receiver.

REFERENCES

1. Rusk, H., *Rehabilitation Medicine*. The C. V. Mosby Co., St. Louis, 1964, p. 376.
2. *Ibid.*, p. 104.
3. *Ibid.*, p. 104.
4. Krusen, F., Kohke, F., and Ellwood, P., *Handbook of Physical Medicine and Rehabilitation*. W. B. Saunders Co., Philadelphia, 1965, p. 421.
5. *Ibid.*, p. 150.
6. Christopherson, V., "Role Modifications of the Disabled Male," *Amer. J. Nurs.*, 68:290, Feb. 1968.
7. Krusen, *op. cit.*, p. 112.
8. Rusk, *op. cit.*, p. 267.
9. Krusen, *op. cit.*, p. 134.
10. Kerr, A., *Orthopedic Nursing Procedures*. Springer Publishing Co., New York, 1960, pp. 17–28.
11. Culp, P., "Nursing Care of the Patient with Spinal Cord Injury," *Nurs. Clin. N. Amer.*, 2:452, Sept. 1967.

12. Kerr, *op. cit.*, p. 28.
13. Rusk, *op. cit.*, p. 515.
14. Cooper, L., Barber, E., Mitchell, H., Rynbergen, H., and Green, J., *Nutrition in Health and Disease.* J. B. Lippincott Co., Philadelphia, 1958, p. 67.
15. Krusen, *op. cit.*, p. 623.
16. Culp, *op. cit.*, p. 453.
17. Rusk, *op. cit.*, p. 519.
18. Culp, *op. cit.*, p. 454.
19. Krusen, *op. cit.*, p. 624.
20. de Gutiérrez-Mahoney, C. P. and Carini, E., *Neurological and Neurosurgical Nursing.* The C. V. Mosby Co., St. Louis, 1965, p. 15.
21. *Ibid.*, p. 58.
22. Schaeffer, K., Sawyer, J., McCluskey, A., and Beck, E., *Medical Surgical Nursing.* The C. V. Mosby Co., St. Louis, 1967, p. 750.
23. de Gutiérrez-Mahoney, *op. cit.*, p. 382.
24. Culp, *op. cit.*, p. 447.
25. Scott, D., Dodd, B., and Lamb, G., *Neurological and Neurosurgical Nursing.* Pergamon Press, New York, 1966, p. 74.
26. de Gutiérrez-Mahoney, *op. cit.*, p. 163.
27. McDowell, F., "Initial Treatment of Cerebrovascular Diseases," *Mod. Treatm.*, **2**:27, Jan. 1965.
28. Fairburn, B., "Brain Tumours," *Nurs. Times*, **63**:108, Jan. 27, 1967.
29. Leavens, M., "Brain Tumors," *Amer. J. Nurs.*, **64**:80, Mar. 1964.
30. de Gutiérrez-Mahoney, *op. cit.*, p. 105.
31. *Ibid.*, p. 367.
32. Scott, *op. cit.*, p. 97.
33. *Ibid.*, p. 94.
34. Robb, P., "Epilepsy and Its Medical Treatment," *Canad Nurs.*, **61**:172, Mar. 1965.
35. *Ibid.*, p. 172.
36. Branch, C., "Surgical Treatment of Epilepsy," *Canad. Nurs.*, **61**:174, Mar. 1965.
37. Robertson, C., and Murray, P., "Nursing an Adolescent with Seizures," *Canad. Nurs.*, **61**:178, Mar. 1965.
38. de Gutiérrez-Mahoney, *op. cit.*, p. 180.
39. *Ibid.*, p. 179.
40. *Ibid.*, p. 259.
41. McDevitt, E., "Treatment of Cerebral Embolism," *Mod. Treatm.*, **2**:52, Jan. 1965.
42. McDowell, F., "Initial Treatment of Cerebrovascular Diseases," *Mod. Treatm.*, **2**:22, Jan. 1965.
43. Whisnaut, J., "Anticoagulant Treatment of Transient Ischemic Attacks and Progressing Strokes," *Mod. Treatm.*, **2**:28, Jan. 1965.
44. Fairburn, B., "Neurosurgery Today: Subarachnoid Hemorrhage," *Nurs. Times*, **63**:177, Feb. 10, 1967.
45. Martin, M., "Nursing Management of a Patient with Cerebral Aneurysm," *J. Nurs. Educ.*, **6**:36, Aug. 1967.
46. *Ibid.*, p. 46.
47. Covalt, D., "Rehabilitation of the Patient with Hemiplegia," *Mod. Treatm.*, **2**:84, Jan. 1965.
48. *Ibid.*, p. 84.
49. de Gutiérrez-Mahoney, *op. cit.*, p. 218.
50. Fangman, A., and O'Malley, W. E., "L-Dopa and the Patient with Parkinson's Disease," *Amer. J. Nurs.*, **69**:1455, July 1969.
51. Schaeffer, *op. cit.*, p. 758.
52. Smith, D., and Gipps, C., *Care of the Adult Patient.* J. B. Lippincott Co., Philadelphia, 1966, p. 400.
53. de Gutiérrez-Mahoney, *op. cit.*, p. 216.
54. Kerr, *op. cit.*, p. 116.
55. *Ibid.*, p. 121.
56. Eaton, P., and Heller, F., "Therapeutic Nursing Care of Orthopedic Patients," *Nurs. Clin. N. Amer.*, **2**:429, Sept. 1967.
57. Roberts, J., "New Developments in Orthopedic Surgery," *Nurs. Clin. N. Amer.*, **2**:383, Sept. 1967.
58. Kerr, *op. cit.*, p. 149.
59. Powell, M., *Orthopedic Nursing.* Williams and Wilkins Co., Baltimore, 1965, p. 10.
60. Peers, J., "The Care and Handling of Orthopedic Implaints," *RN*, **28**:67, Oct. 1965.

61. Powell, M., *op. cit.*, p. 5.
62. Eaton, *op. cit.*, p. 429.
63. Kerr, *op. cit.*, p. 288.
64. The Middlesex Rehabilitation Hospital mimeographed material, North Brunswick, N.J.
65. Larson, C., and Gould, M., *Calderwood's Orthopedic Nursing.* C. V. Mosby Co., St. Louis, 1965, p. 124.
66. Sarmiento, A., "Recent Trends in Lower Extremity Amputation," *Nurs. Clin. N. A.*, 2:399, Sept. 1967.
67. Krusen, *op. cit.*, p. 108.
68. *Ibid.*, p. 106.
69. *Ibid.*, p. 107.
70. Krusen, *op. cit.*, p. 558.
71. Schaeffer, *op. cit.*, p. 825.
72. Krusen, *op. cit.*, p. 608.
73. Bertrand, C., and Martinez, S., "Herniated Discs," *Canad. Nurs.*, 61:200. Mar. 1965.
74. Krusen, *op. cit.*, p. 611.
75. Bertrand, *op. cit.*, p. 200.
76. Musick, D., and MacKenzie, M., "Nursing Care of the Patient with a Laminectomy," *Nurs. Clin. N. A.*, 2:437, Sept. 1967.
77. *Ibid.*, p. 437.
78. Allen, J., *May's Manual of the Diseases of the Eye.* Williams and Wilkins Co., Baltimore, 1963, p. 25.
79. *Ibid.*, p. 30.
80. Smith, *op. cit.*, p. 1011.
81. Brockhurst, R., and Odonnell, C., "Detachment of the Retina," *Amer. J. Nurs.*, 64:90, Apr. 1964.
82. Nordstrom, W., "Adjusting to Cataract Glasses," *Amer. J. Nurs.*, 66: 1579, July 1966.
83. Brockhurst, *op. cit.*, p. 96.
84. Smith, *op. cit.*, p. 1011.

ADDITIONAL READINGS

BALLEN, P., "Care of Ophthalmological Patients, What the Surgeon Expects of the Nurse," *Hosp. Topics*, 45:101, June 1967.

BASTROM, J., "Treatment of Muscular Dystrophy," *Mod. Treatm.*, 3:298, Mar. 1966.

BROOKS, L., "Post-Op Care of the Brain Surgery Patient," *RN*, 27:65, Aug. 1964.

CATFORD, G., "An Introduction to Eye Disease," *Nurs. Times*, 62:1280, Sept. 30, 1966.

COLLINS, E., *A Guide to Diseases of the Nose, Throat, and Ear.* Williams and Wilkins Co., Baltimore, 1964.

CRAWFORD, E., and DEBAKEY, M., "Surgical Treatment of Occlusive Cerebrovascular Disease," *Mod. Treatm.*, 2:36, Jan. 1965.

DYCH, P., and STILLWELL, G., "Hereditary Neurogenic Muscular Atrophies and Allied Disorders," *Mod. Treatm.*, 3:254, Mar. 1966.

GRIFFIN, C., "Social Factors in Epilepsy," *Canad. Nurs.*, 61:185, Mar. 1965.

HADDAD, H., "Drugs for Ophthalmologic Use," *Amer. J. Nurs.*, 68:324. Feb. 1968.

HALL, E., "The Care of Eye Patients," *Hosp. Manage.*, 103:88, May 1967.

HAVENER, W., SAUNDERS, W., and BERGERSEN, B., *Nursing Care in Eye, Ear, Nose and Throat Disorders.* C. V. Mosby Co., St. Louis, 1964.

HOLLIDAY, J., "Bowel Programs of Patients with Spinal Cord Injury: A Clinical Study," *Nurs. Res.*, 16:4, Winter 1967.

HOWARD, F., "Treatment of Myasthenia Gravis and Other Disease with a Defect in Neuromuscular Transmission," *Mod. Treatm.*, 3:278, Mar. 1966.

Langan, E., "Nursing Care of Neurosurgical Patients: Post-operative Care," *Nurs. Times*, p. 111, Jan. 27, 1967.

Moody, L., "Nursing Care: Patient with Herniated Discs," *Canad. Nurs.*, 61:204, Mar. 1965.

Mulder, D., "The Treatment of Anterior Horn Cell Disease," *Mod. Treatm.*, 3:243, Mar. 1966.

Rodman, M., and Smith, D., *Pharmacology and Drug Therapy in Nursing*. J. B. Lippincott Co., Philadelphia, 1968.

Rogers, C., "Care of Ophthalmological Patient: Nurse Describes Routines in Surgery," *Hosp. Topics*, 45:102, June 1967.

Sataloff, J., *Hearing Loss*. J. B. Lippincott Co., Philadelphia, 1966.

Shaw, D., "Anticoagulants and the Completed Stroke," *Mod. Treatm.*, 2:64, Jan. 1965.

Sister Marie Francis, "Nursing the Patient with Internal Hip Fixation," *Amer. J. Nurs.*, 64:111, May 1964.

Wilkinson, M., "Rehabilitation of Patients with Neurological Deficit," *Nurs. Times*, 63:315, Mar. 10, 1967.

UNIT IX

THE PATIENT WITH A PROBLEM IN CELLULAR NUTRITION

46

THE CULTURAL MEANING OF FOOD

FOOD is more than calories. It is essential for body and spirit, and a continuous supply of food and oxygen is required by cells if they are to survive and carry out their functions. Food calls forth thinking and emotion and is endowed with meaning and attitudes that may be referred to as the "body and soul" of the person.

The ability of the body to utilize food changes within a person in the face of any stress (physical, social, or emotional).[1*] In other words, as a person is healthy or less healthy, food attitudes, needs, and uses change. Needs also change with age, the older person requiring less than the younger.

From the day of birth, food is associated with intimacy. It carries with it the feelings of love, protection, security, and developing strength as well as pain, rejection, deprivation, and possibly the horror of starvation and death. In addition food carries with it power, such as we see in nations today that starve those they perceive as their enemies, hoping to starve them into submission.

In our culture foods are often blamed when otherwise healthy individuals complain of heartburn, hyperacidity, bloating, pressure, aching, "gas" pain, constipation, and diarrhea. Often these feelings lag far behind intellect, and if one experiences passing discomfort after eating a particular type of food, the tendency is to attempt to avoid that food thereafter; e.g., eating "onions" at night gives one bad dreams and thus must be completely eliminated from the diet.

Maintenance of an adequate food supply consumes the time of many thousands of workers each year in our farming industry. This maintenance involves many other areas such as land fertilization, conservation efforts, transportation, research, labor, and distribution. It also involves storing processes and use of surplus foods. In essence, food is involved in all aspects of life and work because all consumers need a continual supply. Our economy is also affected because the purchase of food takes a large part of the family budget, and prices vary according to the season, weather

---

* References for Unit IX are on pages 556–57.

conditions, place of purchase (supermarket versus neighborhood stores), and available supply.

The communications media continue to focus the consumer's attention on food through messages on the radio, in magazines, and on television. These messages are vivid (e.g., colored illustrations in magazines) and can be helpful because they assist individuals to learn that there is more about food than we know from our childhood experiences: There are facts about food to be understood and used. One fact is that learning to handle food is an art. For example, in pioneer times, the skill and art were more concerned with obtaining, preparing, and preserving food. Processed foods and a different kind of culinary skill and social structure demand an equal skill and art in the handling of food for sociability, ease, and health today.

Food takes on more meaning when people see that in its use there is great range, flexibility, and choice. This meaningfulness develops and expands as one learns the essential nutrients of a diet and that many foods can be used in a supplemental or complemental fashion. It is important to avoid, whenever possible, the cultural meaning attached to some foods that stimulate feelings of inadequacy or false pride, such as the concept that "salads" are only for ladies and "hot dogs" are only for teen-agers. What is age-appropriate must be respected as well as that which is nutrient-appropriate.

Proper nutrition helps to prevent illness as well as alter the course of illness when it does occur. Often the terms "nutrition" and "diet" are used synonymously. However, *nutrition* is a broader term that includes all the bodily processes involved in the use of food. The term "diet" is limited to the regimen of food required to support nutrition. A diet can be adequate but whether or not good nutrition follows depends on many other factors, such as digestion, absorption, transportation, and utilization within the cells.

Other terms requiring definition, which are related to nutrition and diet, are *appetite* and *hunger*. *Appetite* usually refers to a psychic desire for food and is a pleasant sensation. One's appetite may persist after sufficient food has been ingested to appease hunger. It is conditioned by habit and previous experiences as well as by the sight, smell, and taste of food.

Hunger is the most basic drive for food. When this feeling occurs, there is an awareness of the need to ingest food accompanied by increased salivation and food-searching behavior. Hunger is often associated with unpleasant or even painful contractions of an empty stomach or intestine. As hunger pangs increase, they occupy more and more attention of the individual. *Satiety* is a state of satisfaction or loss of desire for food following adequate ingestion of same.

Good nutrition is said to exist when calories (units of energy), water, and the nutrients (proteins, carbohydrates, fats, mineral, and vitamins) are adequately supplied and appropriately utilized by the body. These factors should come from the four basic food groups: (1) dairy foods, (2) meat group, (3) vegetables and fruits, and (4) breads and cereal group.[2]

Obesity

Obesity is still the principal nutrition problem in the Untied States.[3] Obesity is an excessive accumulation of adipose tissue. The factors involved are genetic, socioeconomical, metabolic, and psychologic. These factors aid in the production of obesity by contributing to the development of a prolonged imbalance between caloric intake and output (thermodynamic disequilibrium).[4]

Not all overweight persons are obese because *overweight* refers to body weight about 10 lb above a standard range. It does not differentiate between individual variations in body build, structure, or body composition. In obesity the excess weight is greater than 10 lb above the standard range, and the degree of fatness is sought; therefore, the amount of *fatness* should be measured.

Obesity can be measured by the use of a caliper.[5] This is an instrument that measures subcutaneous fat. A method of measurement of subcutaneous fat, using the triceps skinfold, was developed at the Harvard University School of Public Health. The skinfold at the back of the right upper arm is pinched and its full thickness is measured. It is thought that the triceps are most representative of total body fatness regardless of any disproportionate distribution of adipose tissue in various parts of the body.

One basic fact to remember is that the only way the body accumulates excessive fat is by having an energy intake in food and drink that is greater than its energy output, so that the excess calorie intake is laid down as body fat. Although the prevalence of obesity is difficult to document, it is implicated in many chronic diseases.

Additional factors to consider when obesity occurs are overall nutrition, exercise, occupation, climate, geographic location, social class, urban-suburban-rural residence, income, health, disease, and cultural and ethnic differences. There is also abundant evidence that genetic factors are responsible for certain forms of obesity in animals but this is *not* conclusive regarding humans.

There also appears to be a familial connection because fleshy parents do not usually produce slender offspring. Modern living favors a decreased energy expenditure relative to energy intake. Labor-saving devices at home and at work, short work weeks, spectator recreation, and small, well-heated homes and apartments have helped us to become lazier and lazier. These environmental factors contribute to the familial factors when present and tend to increase the possibility of obesity.

Poor people and primitives tend to value and admire obesity, and in many countries natives expect their leaders to be fat, e.g., Hawaii. Also, years ago it was necessary for the Chinese merchant to be fat. This "fatness" represented prosperity.

In addition, in our culture, hospitality is synonymous with the provision of food and drink, which adds to an environment conducive to the development of obesity. The provision of food has been extended from the home to include meetings, fund-raising events, celebrations, and so on.

Obese individuals have been grouped according to the causative factors:

1. The naturally obese—genetic factors "made" the individual "that" way.
2. Reactively obese—those individuals who eat in response to isolated psychic stress.
3. Chronically obese—those individuals who eat in response to chronic, continuous difficulties.
4. Addictive eaters—those who take food for the production of pleasure, and through this pleasure there is the reduction of tension and anxiety from whatever cause.[6]

Problems in Treatment

Treatment of the obese individual traditionally has not been successful. The results are even worse than for drug addicts. Success in treatment in men exceeds that in women. In the obese person the origin of excess fat is excess calories. Calories do count! A person is considered obese when his weight is 20 to 25 per cent above normal for his age and build.[7] The healthy adult male living in a moderate climate requires a minimum of 1,500 calories a day to maintain the basic functions of life.[8]

A calorie is a measure of heat. Heat produces energy. In obesity the energy equation looks like this:

1. Caloric intake is greater than the output and there occurs a buildup of body fat.
2. Intake greater than output yields increased body fat.

The converse equation would be as follows:

1. Caloric output is greater than intake and there occurs a decrease in body fat.
2. Output greater than intake yields decreased body fat.

It would appear that in obesity the equation could be reversed in three ways: [9]

1. Energy intake in the form of food and drink may be curtailed so that body fat must be burned to support the level of energy output.

2. Energy output may be increased by increasing physical activity or, in some few instances, by increasing the energy expanded for basal metabolic activity.

3. Energy intake may be decreased and energy output increased.

There are two stages of treatment in obesity: *the initial stage*—to effect progressive loss of weight until the desired weight is reached; and *the second stage*—to maintain weight at this new level.

In the past, obesity treatment via a reduction in food intake was frequently unsuccessful because (1) misinformation had been given to the patient; (2) the diet was complicated and difficult to understand; (3) the diet may have been unsuitable; (4) there had been several previous diet failures; or (5) there was inadequate motivation.

Dietary treatment of obesity can be *qualitative* (the patient is provided with lists of food he may or may not eat—caloric intake is not fixed) or *quantitative* (total daily calories are fixed). The patient needs to be instructed regarding food values, and with the exception of some artificial sweeteners, he should be discouraged from using the wide variety of special dietetic preparations. Liquid diets have no place in treatment when the objective is for slow, progressive, and permanent weight reduction. When one is constantly following a diet, a polyvitamin is indicated. Exercise is also an essential feature.

Drug therapy is sometimes used in the treatment of obesity. Anorexiant drugs such as dextroamphetamine sulfate (Dexedrine) and methylphenidate (Ritalin) may be used as adjuncts to low-calorie diets. These drugs improve the mood of the individual, and this action is thought to help the dieter because they make him feel better mentally.[10] There is also an increase in motor and speech activity, thus increasing the caloric output. These drugs are stimulants. They can be addictive and must be used carefully and with medical supervision.

Deficiency Correction

A deficiency disease is one in which lack of a specific nutrient in food is wholly or partly responsible. This kind of disease lowers resistance to infection. For instance, a protein-deficiency may occur anywhere and accompany other pathologic conditions. Children deprived of adequate food and with protein markedly deficient become emaciated, and growth is definitely retarded. Infection is common. After long periods of protein deficiency or starvation, many months may be required to restore depleted body tissues to normal.

Vitamin A deficiency with night blindness and beriberi due to thiamine deficiency are two extremes of vitamin-deficiency diseases. Beriberi is seldom encountered in North America, whereas night blindness has been discovered among children and adults in this country when instruments for detecting and measuring adjustment for dull light are used for routine examinations of large groups. Treatment in both cases is to assure the individuals with either condition an adequate intake of both vitamins via natural foods and vitamin supplements.

Mild forms of deficiency diseases seldom come to the attention of a physician unless more serious conditions develop. Although we seldom see signs of advanced deficiency diseases such as rickets, scurvy, and pellagra in the United States, severe protein deficiency has been revealed in some deprived areas. Our cereals and breads contain vitamin additives and many, if not all, American mothers supplement their family's diet with some form of multiple vitamin.

TABLE 46–1. SUMMARY OF DEFICIENCY DISEASES

Name	Deficiency
Protein deficiencies, edema, hypoproteinemia, kwashiorkor	Protein foods
Night blindness, glare blindness	Mild vitamin A deficiency
Conjunctivitis	Severe vitamin A deficiency
Beriberi (polyneuritis)	Thiamine
Pellagra	Niacin, thiamine, riboflavin
Scurvy	Ascorbic acid
Rickets	Vitamin D, calcium, phosphorus
Hemorrhagic disease of infants	Vitamin K
Nutritional anemia	Iron, protein, vitamins A and C
Common goiter	Iodine
Adult "rickets," osteomalacia	Vitamin D, calcium

For the individual who is obese and dieting to lose weight, it is important to see that foods supplying the required calories contain all the other essentials of a normal diet such as vitamins and minerals. If the total calories are very low, supplements of these vitamins and minerals are necessary.

47

ANATOMY AND PHYSIOLOGY OF THE GASTROINTESTINAL SYSTEM

The Nervous, Chemical, and Hormonal Activity in the Digestive Tract

As food travels down, an intricate and intriguing series of activities is set in motion. This process actually begins with the sight or smell of food [11,12] and gets into gear when the bolus moves down the esophagus. The esophagus is equipped with muscles (muscular layers) that work the food rhythmically downward. It is also the first contact point with the vagus nerves, or vagi.

The vagi supply sensory and motor fibers to the viscera. Motor fibers supply the muscles of the pharynx, larynx, esophagus, stomach, small intestine, pancreas, liver, spleen, ascending colon, and visceral blood vessels. The gastric and pancreatic glands are supplied with secretory fibers. Sensory fibers of the vagus are distributed to the mucous membrane of the larynx, trachea, lungs, esophagus, stomach, intestines, and gallbladder.[13] (See Fig. 47–1.)

The vagus nerves come into full play as the bolus descends into the stomach (see Figs. 47–1, 47–2, and 47–3), and the glands of the stomach get to work. Gastric juice containing hydrochloric acid is secreted. It provides an acid medium needed for digestive processes. Gastric juice combined with the churning action of the stomach reduces food to a semifluid consistency, and the churning action helps propel it forward. Alkaline mucus is also secreted. It helps balance the acid pH produced by the hydrochloric acid. Pepsinogen is secreted, too. In the presence of hydrochloric acid it is converted to pepsin. Pepsin is an enzyme [14] that catalyzes digestive processes. The gastric glands also produce a vital hormone called gastrin. Gastrin is carried by the blood to the fundic and pyloric glands and stimulates them to secretory activity.[15]

[*Text continued on page 515.*]

THE GASTROINTESTINAL SYSTEM   [513

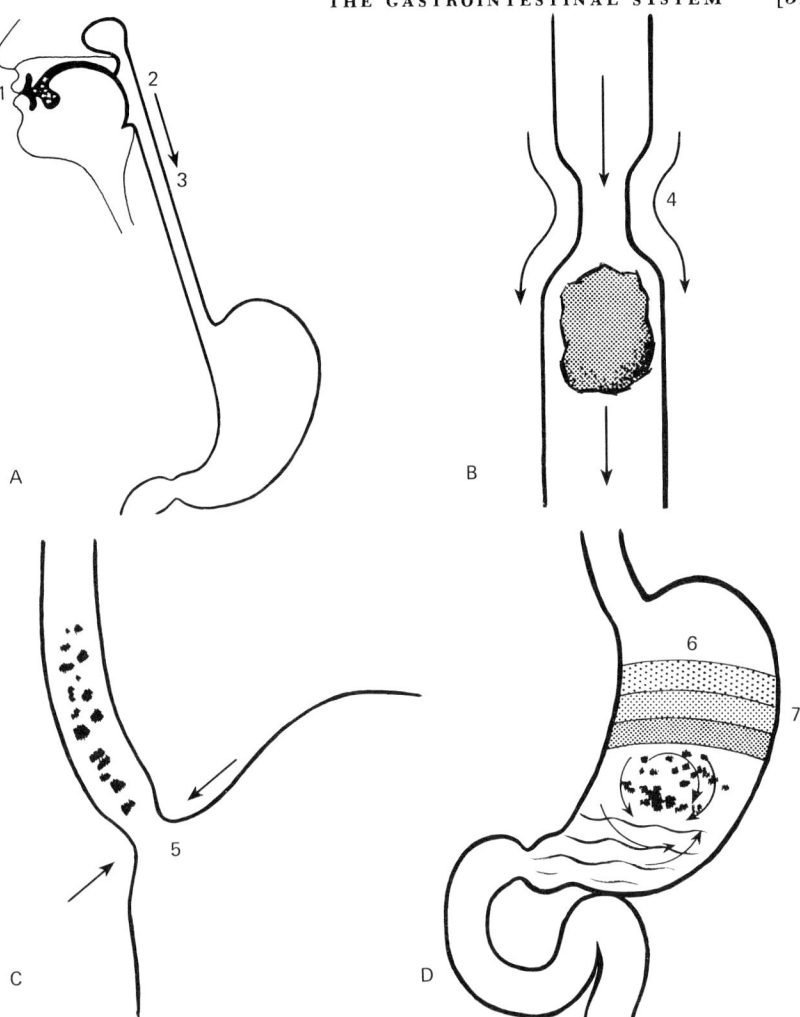

FIGURE 47–1. Salivary and gastric digestion. In the mouth (*1*), food is chewed and broken up for easy digestion. As food is being chewed, the salivary glands secrete saliva to moisten and soften it, making it easier for the tongue to roll it into a ball for swallowing.

When the bolus is swallowed, it passes through the pharynx (*2*). This first stage of the swallowing act is under voluntary control, but once the food reaches the pharynx, involuntary reflex control is established, and the food is forced into the esophagus (*3*). Here, circular muscles tighten behind the food, squeezing it along. As it is passed beyond the next band of circular muscles in line, they tighten, while the first set relaxes. This squeezing effect of the circular muscles is known as a peristaltic wave (*4*).

(*Continued*)

Fig. 47–1 (*Cont.*)

At the closed cardiac sphincter (5), the circular muscle that closes off the stomach, the bolus waits for a peristaltic wave to open the sphincter. When it opens, the bolus enters the stomach (6).

The stomach contains a three-layered coat of smooth, involuntary muscle (7). In this coat, the muscle fibers run in a longitudinal, circular, and oblique pattern. When food enters the stomach, these muscles are activated and a churning action results. In addition, the stomach secretes gastric juice containing a considerable amount of hydrochloric acid. The chemical action of this gastric juice, plus the churning action of the stomach, reduces the food to a semifluid consistency and propels it along the intestine. The stomach also acts as a temporary storehouse so that not too much food will enter the intestine at one time. (Courtesy, Geigy Pharmaceuticals, Division of Geigy Chemical Corp., Ardsley, N.Y., from *Bowel Evacuation: A Teaching and Reference Manual*, 1966.)

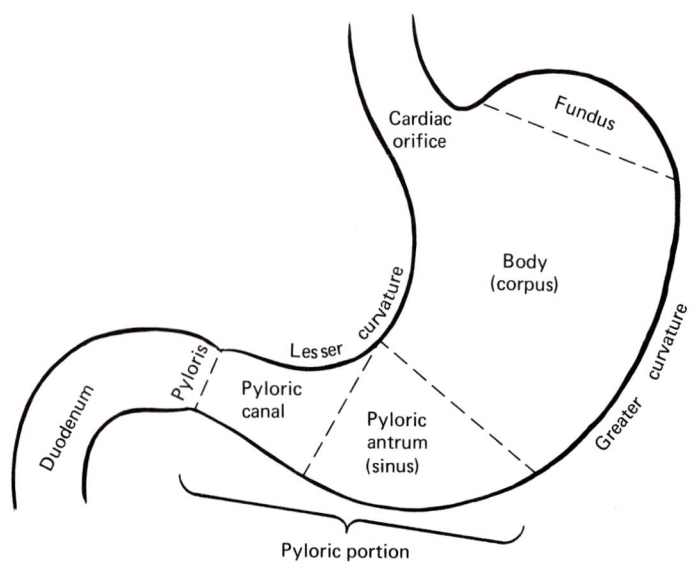

FIGURE 47–2. The stomach with regions, orifices, and curvatures indicated.

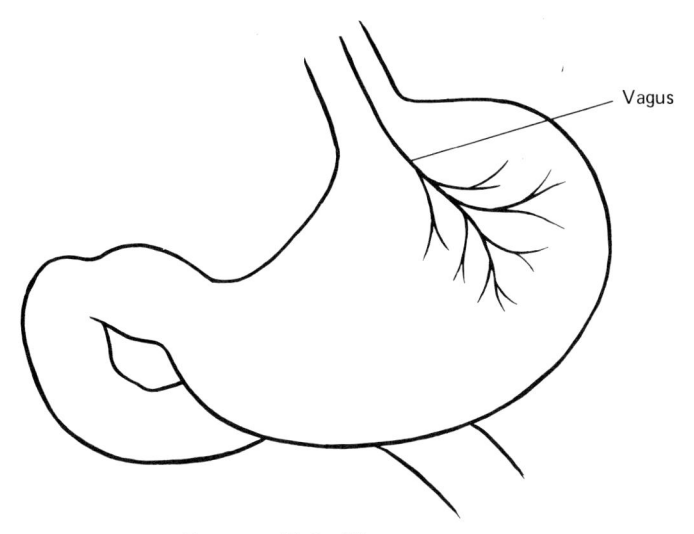

FIGURE 47–3. The vagus nerve.

The Duodenum (Figs. 47–4 and 47–5)

The duodenum is a sensitive organ and the beginning of the small intestine. It measures about 10 in. and is protected by a coating of mucus,

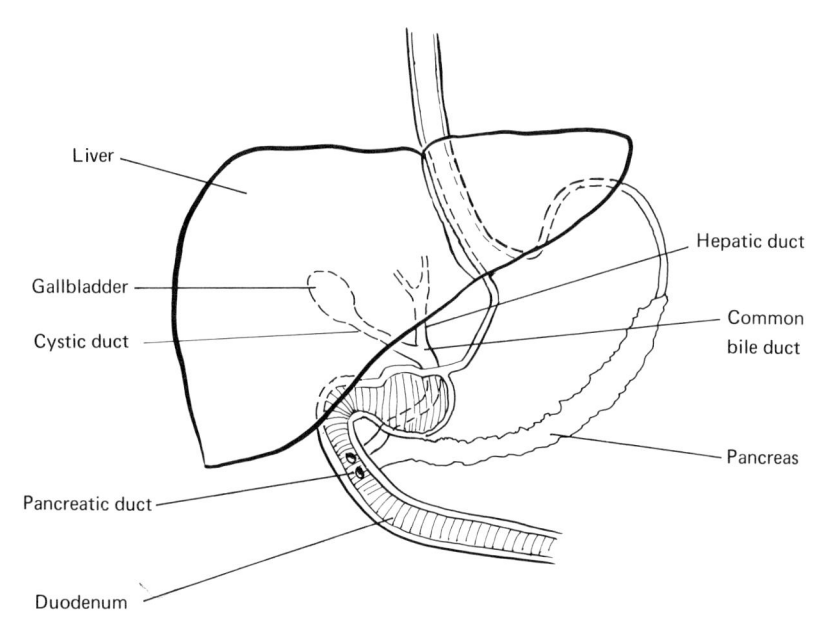

FIGURE 47–4. Structures surrounding and including the duodenum. *Note:* Both pancreatic and the common bile ducts empty into the duodenum.

516] CELLULAR NUTRITION

an alkaline substance. It needs this protection because the chyme (food digested in the stomach) is saturated with acid. As chyme enters the duodenum, a hormone called secretin is released and that retards the secretion of acid in the stomach—as well as activating the flow of bile from the liver, pancreatic juice from the pancreas, and duodenal juice from the duodenum. These juices flow into the duodenum in equal measure to the chyme.[16] Despite all this protection, the duodenum is the location of the most common form of peptic ulcer, which is called the duodenal ulcer.

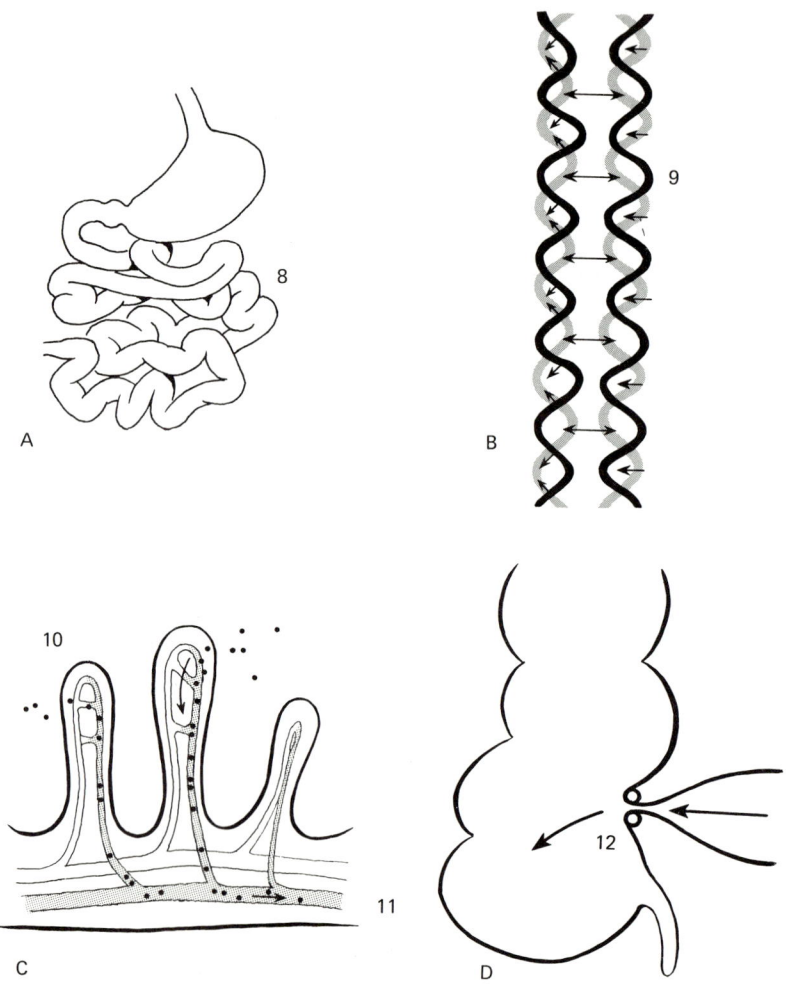

FIGURE 47–5. The small intestine—intestinal digestion. In the small intestine (8), which consists of the duodenum, the jejunum, and the ileum, the major process of digestion and absorption of food occurs. As the food enters the intestine, it is churned by sharp contractions of

the circular muscle of the intestinal wall at regularly spaced intervals. This is called rhythmic segmentation (9). When this occurs, the food is thoroughly mixed with secretions from the liver, the pancreas, and the intestinal mucosa, which break it down into substances that can be absorbed into the blood.

The digestive secretions include:
(1) bile, which is a brownish or greenish-yellow fluid secreted by the liver to aid in the production of an alkaline condition in the intestine and in the emulsification and absorption of fats;
(2) pancreatic juices, which are secreted by the pancreas and are rich in enzymes, including trypsin, that breaks down proteins; amylopsin, which converts starch into sugar; and lipase, which acts on fats, splitting them into fatty acids and glycerol;
(3) intestinal juices, which are secreted by the mucous glands of the intestine and contain many enzymes that complete the digestive processing of food prior to absorption.

Absorption is the final step in supplying to the body the sugars, fatty acids, amino acids, vitamins, salts, and water obtained from food. Most absorption results from the churning action of food in the small intestine and contact with the villi (10), small threadlike projections of the mucosa of the small intestine. In each villus are a small blood capillary and a lymph vessel, which absorb nutrients and carry them into the bloodstream (11). The capillaries absorb sugar and amino acids, and the lymph vessels absorb fatty acids and glycerol.

After the digestive process in the small intestine, the remaining contents, which are quite liquefied, move along the length of the small intestine by peristaltic waves through the ileocecal valve (12) into the large intestine. This valve permits the slow passage of the contents of the small intestine, at intervals, into the large intestine and prevents the return of the material into the ileum. (Courtesy, Geigy Pharmaceuticals, Division of Geigy Chemical Corp., Ardsley, N.Y., from *Bowel Evacuation: Teaching and Reference Manual*, 1966.)

The Small Intestine

The small intestine consists of the duodenum, jejunum, and the ileum. The jejunum is about 8 ft. long and is often called the "empty intestine" because it is always found empty after death.[17] The ileum is about 12 ft. long and consists of numerous coils that extend from the jejunum to the large intestine. In the small intestine the greatest amount of digestion and absorption takes place. The rugae of the intestines delay food in the intestine slightly to present greater surface area for digestion. The villi are located throughout the entire length of the small intestine (Fig. 47–5). Capillaries and lymph vessels in villi absorb nutrients; then the remaining contents are moved through the small intestines by peristalsis.

The Large Intestine (Fig. 47–6)

The large, or thick, intestine is about 5 ft. long but is wider than the small intestine. It extends from the ileum to the anus. It receives undigested residue and some water from the small intestine and propels it through the colon for excretion.

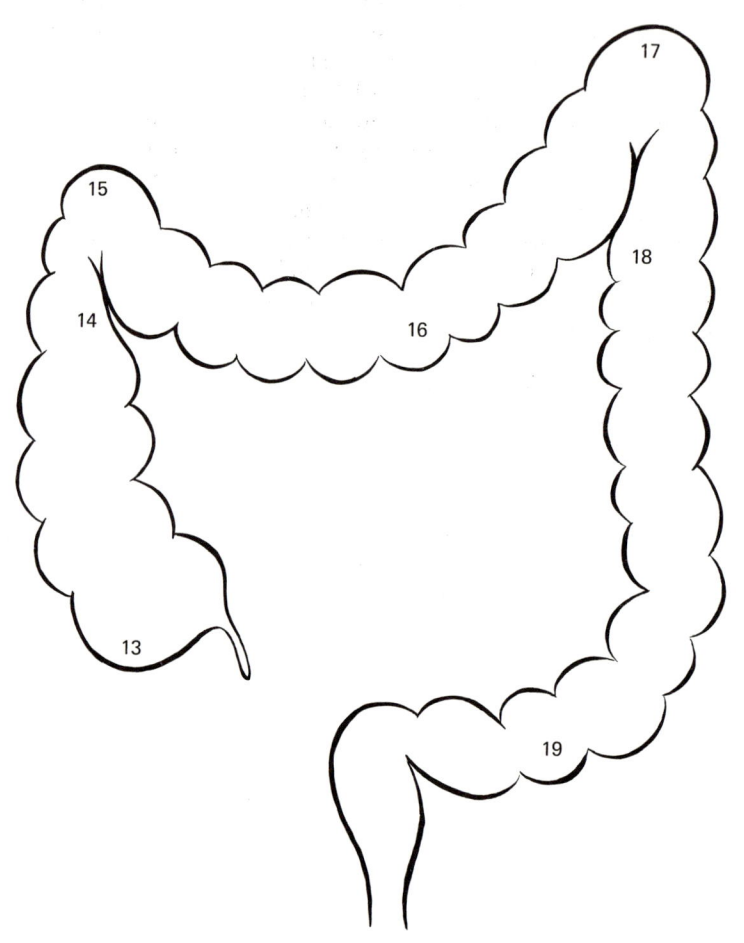

FIGURE 47–6. The large intestine—intestinal digestion. The large intestine receives the semiliquid material from the small intestine, after digestion has been completed. This material generally consists of undigested or undigestible residue (such as cellulose), fluids that have escaped absorption in the small intestine, bacteria, and discarded epithelial cells. The large intestine consists of the cecum (*13*), the ascending colon (*14*), the hepatic flexure (*15*), the transverse colon

(*16*), the splenic flexure (*17*), the descending colon (*18*), and the sigmoid colon (*19*).

In the cecum and the ascending colon, churning movements aid in the absorption of water so that by the time the contents have reached the transverse and descending colon, they are fairly solid. This fecal material is propelled through the colon by peristaltic-like mass movements. These mass movements occur relatively infrequently, perhaps three or four times a day, and are often stimulated by the entrance of food into the stomach. This is known as the gastrocolic reflex. The fact that food stimulates this reflex is one of the reasons that people are trained to evacuate after mealtime; after breakfast, for example.

Fecal masses, pushed forward by mass movements of the colon, are stored in the sigmoid or pelvic colon, and not in the rectum. Defecation is stimulated by the passage of fecal material from the large intestine into the rectum. Eating is also a stimulus for defecation; however, drinking a cup of coffee or a glass of water or smoking a cigar or cigarette may also be effective in initiating this reflex.

Although it is not normally recommended, particularly for older patients, defecation may be stimulated by straining to raise the abdominal pressure and force the feces into the rectum. (Courtesy Geigy Pharmaceuticals, Division of Geigy Chemical Corp., Ardsley, N.Y., from *Bowel Evacuation: A Teaching and Reference Manual,* 1966.)

48

PRINCIPLES IN THE CARE OF ANY PATIENT WITH IMBALANCE IN CELL NUTRITION; SOME COMMON DIAGNOSTIC PROCEDURES

1. Respect the patient's cultural and religious preferences for foods. Make every attempt to provide for these needs.
2. Realize the individuality of eating patterns and allow the patient whatever latitude possible in this area.
3. Most patients with alimentary tract imbalance will have some dietary modification. Make sure the proper foods are brought to the patient by checking the hospital's diet manual and the patient's tray. Teach the patient about his diet.
4. Observe the patient's tray after he has eaten and record pertinent information. Be specific. "Appetite good" is not adequate.
5. Observe and report subjective and objective symptoms, e.g., "patient states 'It hurts after I eat,'" or "legs were drawn up to the chest and patient stated he was in severe pain."
6. Realize the individuality of bathroom habits and respect the patient's right for privacy.
7. Realize that cleanliness and avoidance of contact with stool are acceptable standards in the United States. Help the patient to stay clean. If he must have contact with stool help him to accept this by being nonjudgmental. Keep the room well ventilated.
8. If a tube must be irrigated, know what cavity is being intubated, what solution has been ordered for the irrigation, the quantity of solution to use, and the frequency of irrigation.
9. Only suction the lower tract with physiologic (e.g., saline) solution so that electrolytes are not "washed out."
10. Observe and record amount, consistency, color, and odor of all alimentary tract discharge.
11. Realize that water and electrolyte imbalances are common sequels to alimentary imbalance. Observe and record symptoms. (See Chap. 17.)

12. Realize that many procedures involving the alimentary tract are extremely distasteful (e.g., nasogastric intubation, enemas). Stay with the patient and support him through the procedure.

Some Commonly Used Diagnostic and Therapeutic Procedures

In the GI series (gastrointestinal series) barium, a radiopaque substance, is swallowed and/or administered by enema, depending on the area of the digestive tract to be studied. A complete GI series includes barium swallow as well as barium enema. The barium is a chalky substance which is usually flavored and is often mixed in a blender to give it a milkshake consistency. It is administered in the x-ray department. The patient is allowed nothing by mouth for six to eight hours prior to the test. The patient is examined by fluoroscopy and several roentgenograms are taken by the physician as the barium is swallowed and about six hours later so that stomach emptying can be evaluated. The physician looks for spasms, overactivity of the gastrointestinal tract, rapid or delayed transit of barium and abnormalities in the contour of the stomach or duodenum. Constipation often results after a barium swallow. Because of this, the physician may order a cathartic. Enemas are usually administered after a barium enema.

A gastric analysis may be ordered to determine the acid level in the stomach of the patient. The gastric analysis with histamine is performed after the patient has had nothing by mouth for six to eight hours before the test. A Levin tube is inserted (this is a very uncomfortable procedure), and a fasting sample of gastric fluid is removed. Then, histamine phosphate, 0.5 mg, a gastric stimulant, is injected subcutaneously. Additional samples of gastric fluid are aspirated at regular intervals and tested for acidity in the laboratory. Histamine phosphate causes vasodilation and may make the patient feel flushed and warm. This does not last long. However, some patients react very strenuously to the action of the drug and may develop symptoms of shock. Epinephrine should be on hand to meet this emergency. When a duodenal ulcer is present, there is a high acid level. Hydrochloric acid is not increased when cancer is present. When the test is completed, the tube is clamped and quickly withdrawn by the nurse.

A tubeless gastric analysis can also be performed. It is useful for initial screening. It indicates the presence of free hydrochloric acid but not the amount. This tubeless gastric analysis is called the *azuresin test*. Caffeine sodium benzoate tablets are given to stimulate gastric secretions. One hour later a resin indicator, compound azure A, Azuresin (Diagnex Blue), is given with water on an empty stomach. If free hydrochloric acid is present, its hydrogen ions displace the azure A in the resin, and the dye imparts a blue color to the urine within two hours. This is visually compared with color standards.

Cytologic examinations of gastric mucosa are performed to determine the presence of benign or malignant cells. A Levin tube is inserted, and the stomach is vigorously lavaged with saline or a tube is passed which has a gastric brush or abrasive balloon attached to collect pieces of mucosa. All the aspirated solution, cells, and tissue obtained are sent to the laboratory for study.

Stool examination for occult (hidden) blood is often part of the diagnostic work-up of patients suspected of having a gastric ulcer. One complication of gastric ulcer is perforation with bleeding. Sometimes this bleeding is a slow process and can be detected through this examination. Stool specimens, usually three, are collected and taken immediately to the laboratory for gross, microscopic, chemical, and bacterial examination. The specimen should be warm and not permitted to sit at the bedside or in the utility room. Red meat should be eliminated from the diet for 24 hours before the specimen is collected. Animal protein in stool confuses the chemical reaction in some tests.

"Oscopy" Examinations

These are visual examinations of the gastrointestinal tract utilizing a "scope" instrument. For instance, a gastroscope is inserted through the esophagus to view the stomach. A proctoscope is inserted through the rectum to view the rectum and lower colon. When a gastroscopy is done, the patient is not permitted anything by mouth for eight hours before the test. A gastric tube is inserted to remove stomach secretions. A local anesthetic agent is sprayed on the pharynx, and the gastroscope is passed. The patient is allowed nothing by mouth for several hours after the test because of the danger of aspiration before the anesthesia has worn off. He may have a sore throat and be hoarse for a few days following the test. For sigmoidoscopy and proctoscopy, laxatives are administered the evening before the test, and enemas are administered until they are clear the morning of the test. This ensures a clear bowel. These tests are performed in specially assigned treatment rooms. Disposable equipment is available.

Gastrointestinal Decompression

Intubation, decompression, suction siphonage, and nasal suction are some of the terms used to indicate the introduction of a tube through the nose, down the esophagus, to the stomach. If intestinal decompression is needed, a special tube is used that is longer and has a device at one end that facilitates its passage along the intestinal tract.[18]

The therapeutic uses of decompression are:

1. Removal of gas and fluids in the prevention and treatment of distention following abdominal operations.
2. To study with x-rays the response of the alimentary tract to opaque liquids introduced through the tube.
3. To remove contents from the alimentary tract.
4. Removal of stomach contents as preparation for and during anesthesia.

The longer the tube and the greater the distance from the tubing to the drainage bottle, the greater the suction. The Levin tube, No. 16 French, is a rubber or polyethylene tube that has openings along the side. It is most frequently used.

The Miller-Abbott tube is a single, double-lumen (tube within a tube) tube with an air-weighted tip. The tube is passed with the balloon deflated, and it is not inflated until the tip of the tube has been carried through the pyloric valve of the stomach. This tube goes into the intestine. Because it is a double-lumen tube the balloon can be inflated without disturbing the suction function. The Miller-Abbott tube has an adapter on the part of the tube that remains outside the patient's body. The adapter has two openings, one for suction and one for air leading to the balloon.

The Cantor tube is usually a No. 18 French catheter that has a sufficient series of large holes to provide decompression of the intestinal tract. The Cantor tube has just one lumen. Five to ten milliliters of mercury is injected directly into the bag at the end of the tube. It helps to propel the tube along. This mercury is injected before the tube is passed. It does not seep out because the puncture hole is small.

When the physician has inserted a tube for gastrointestinal decompression of the intestines, he may order that the patient be turned to various positions to facilitate the passage of the tube. The goal is to increase peristalsis to carry the tube down.

Patients need to be prepared psychologically and physically for a decompression procedure. There may be fear and anxiety as a result of difficulty in trying to pass the tube, or nausea and vomiting may occur. It is helpful to keep tissues and an emesis basin nearby. The nurse can tactfully explain the procedure to the patient, and she should make sure she will be present when the tube is passed.

Tubing should be long enough to permit the patient to turn. No pins should be placed through the tube nor should traction be placed on the tube to further irritate the nose. The tube should be taped to the face in such a manner as not to obstruct the patient's view.

Distention caused by failure of the suction can occur, because the tube can become clogged and thus obstruct the lumen. It is essential that the nurse check the physician's orders carefully for irrigations and carry them out as ordered. An adequate intake-and-output record must also be kept. This record will serve as a guide for the physician as he orders or does not order parenteral fluids.

The tube is withdrawn gently when decompression is terminated. The nasogastric tube can be withdrawn quickly. To prevent aspiration of escaping fluid, the tube is pinched or clamped during its removal. As it is withdrawn, it is wrapped in a towel. Unless it is to be discarded, it should be rinsed with cool water immediately, washed well, and then sterilized.

49

THE PATIENT WITH PEPTIC ULCER

The Balance of Power

HYDROCHLORIC ACID is essential to normal digestion; mucus is necessary to dilute it and keep its destructive potential in check. The result is a kind of gastric balance of power.[19] When the lining of the stomach or of the duodenum is deeply penetrated at any point by acid, an ulcer develops: a *peptic ulcer* is called *gastric* if it occurs in the stomach and *duodenal* if it occurs in the duodenum. The least common form of the peptic ulcer is the *esophageal* ulcer, caused by the backwash of gastric juice into the lower esophagus. (See Fig. 49–1.) Most gastric ulcers occur on the lesser curvature of the stomach. Most duodenal ulcers occur in the first part of the duodenum.

Peptic ulcer is a sharply circumscribed loss of tissue resulting from acid

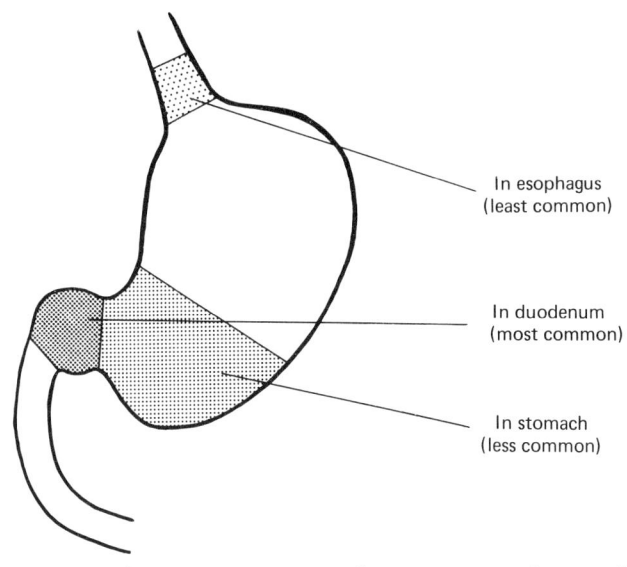

FIGURE 49–1. The most common ulcer areas in the esophagus, stomach, and the duodenum.

erosion. What happens is that the balance between acid and mucus breaks down. This imbalance may be due to one or more of the following causes: (1) high production (overproduction) of hydrochloric acid, (2) irritation of gastric mucosa, (3) poor blood supply, (4) inadequate secretion of alkaline mucus, (5) infection, (6) hereditary factors, (7) hormonal irregularities, and (8) psychological "hang-ups."[20] Drugs such as the adrenocorticosteroids, the salicylates, and phenylbutazone are known to be ulcerogenic.

It is popular to consider duodenal ulcers as a psychosomatic condition, and there is evidence to support this contention. Feelings of anger and hostility cause gastric mucosal engorgement, erosion of mucosa, and increased hydrochloric acid secretion.[21]

Predisposing factors leading to the development of gastric ulcers include worry, irregularity of eating, and hurried eating. The usual "ulcer individual" is described as tall, thin or fat, between 20 and 50 years of age with the highest number of cases occurring between 45 and 55, a perfectionist, conscientious, ambitious but not a sharing type, and male.

Ulcer Symptoms

Nearly every ulcer is the climax in a long series of gastric upsets occurring over an extended period of time in a rather definite pattern. These recurring gastric upsets include:

Heartburn

Caused by an acid spasm of the esophagus, heartburn is usually cleared up with the usual patent medicines or plain baking soda dissolved in water. When this occurs repeatedly over weeks or months, an examination is indicated.

"Water Brash"

A swelling up of sour or burning fluid in the mouth is again a common discomfort. If this becomes a frequent annoyance, a physician should be seen.

Eructation (Belching)

When this occurs regularly after meals, it can become a social inconvenience. When followed by stomach upset, it may be a sign that something has gone wrong in the digestive tract. Most ulcer patients have experienced this ailment before the ulcer actually developed.[22]

Pain

Typical ulcer pain is described as being of the gnawing, burning, or aching type at the pit of the stomach. It may radiate to the back. It is not constant, but comes and goes. It may last from 20 to 30 minutes with varying severity. It usually starts one to two hours after eating when the stomach empties. It is usually relieved by ingestion of food and by the taking of an antacid.

Ulcer pain is peculiar in that it is tied up with the seasons. Ulcer incidence reaches its peak in spring and autumn with September to January recognized as the ulcer hemorrhage high period.[23]

Acute peptic ulcers are superficial and occur in the mucosal layer. They usually heal in a short time but may bleed, perforate, and become chronic. Chronic ulcers are deep craters with sharp edges and a "clean" base invading mucosal and submucosal layers.

Additional symptoms indicative, in some cases, of peptic ulcer include tarry stools, constipation, and flatulence. Occasionally there are nausea and vomiting.

Cancer and Peptic Ulcer

Duodenal ulcers do not seem to have malignant potential. However, gastric ulcers present a more complex problem. The important question is how often an ulcer of the stomach is cancerous from its very inception because the cancer precedes the ulcer. It is thought that, if an ulcer is malignant, discomfort arrives earlier after meals and a constant dull pain may appear. Appetite diminishes and nausea becomes frequent. If unchecked, gastric ulcers may become malignant. A thorough diagnostic appraisal is necessary.

Diagnostic Measures

X-rays, gastric analyses, laboratory studies, cell examination, and biopsy are measures used in making a diagnostic appraisal of presence and state of a patient's ulcer. These measures are used to diagnose any condition of the alimentary tract.

Today about 90 per cent of all ulcers can be confirmed and located by x-rays.[24]

Medical Management of Peptic Ulcer

A trial of medical therapy is instituted. Many ulcers heal in a few weeks or months with an adequate medical regimen. The ulcer is "healed" when it is covered with normal mucosa. Surgery is resorted to when the crater of the ulcer has not healed.

Medical management of the patient with peptic ulcer focuses on the following:

1. Rest—patient is to avoid rushing, noise, worry.
2. Sedation—to ensure a "kind of" rest.

3. Diet—a chemically, thermally, mechanically nonirritating and nonstimulating diet (bland diet, Sippy regimen).
4. Restriction of irritating substances such as alcohol, coffee, and tobacco.
5. Antacids and anticholinergic medications.
6. Avoidance of situations that activate the ulcer.

Dietary Control

Food passes through the pyloric sphincter according to:

1. The size of the opening.
2. Gastric motility.
3. Type of food (carbohydrates pass through most rapidly, proteins next, fatty foods take the longest time).
4. The consistency of the food—the more liquid the food, the faster it passes through.[25]

The stomach is emptied in three and one-half to four hours after a normal-sized, mixed meal. Some physicians order a liberal but bland diet, restricting those specific foods that cause distress. The bland diet follows.

TABLE 49-1. BLAND DIET

PRINCIPLES:
1. Low or soft residue
2. Low in acid content
3. Little or no condiments, except salt in small amounts
4. Foods simply prepared

FOODS ALLOWED:

Milk	Milk, cream
Cheese	Cream, cottage, and other soft, mild cheeses
Fats	Butter, margarine
Eggs	Boiled, scrambled, poached
Meat	Roast beef and lamb, lamb or veal chops
Fish	Boiled, broiled, or baked
Fowl	Roast, baked, or boiled chicken
Soups	With milk or cream sauce
Bread	White bread, rolls, or crackers
Cereals	Cereals, macaroni, spaghetti, noodles
Vegetables	Potatoes, peas, squash, asparagus, carrots, beets, spinach, string beans (may be puréed if necessary)
Fruits	Apples, applesauce, apricots, peaches, pears, plums, purée of dried fruit (all without core, skin, or seeds)
Fruits	Ripe—avocados, bananas, peaches, pears
Desserts	Custards, junket, ice cream, tapioca, gelatin desserts
Beverages	Milk, cocoa, malted milk, fruit juices (if tolerated), coffee or tea if allowed

Table 49-2 Typical Menu for Bland Diet

BREAKFAST	DINNER	SUPPER
Ripe banana	Roast lamb	Cream of potato soup
Farina with milk	Mashed potatoes	Scrambled eggs
Egg (1) boiled	Peas	Fresh spinach
White-bread toast	White bread	Butter
Butter	Butter	Applesauce with cookies
Milk	Canned pears	Milk
	Cream (half milk)	Small glass of orange juice
	Small glass of tomato juice	

Some physicians believe that more rigid dietary control helps to heal the ulcer faster. The patient may be allowed only milk every hour initially. It may be dripped through a nasogastric tube to provide continuous neutralization of acid. Milk is a highly concentrated hypertonic solution. Unless it is balanced with sufficient intake of water, solute-loading occurs. There is extracellular water deficit plus sodium excess. Sometimes, the physician begins dietary control with six small feedings of soft, well-cooked bland foods daily. Meat proteins and coarse foods are omitted during the first stage of treatment because they stimulate acid secretions. Fatty foods are included to help slow down stomach motility and acid secretion.

The patient with a gastric ulcer who is receiving medical treatment is instructed to avoid excessively hot, cold, or spicy foods and carbonated drinks. Citrus fruits and juices are taken in diluted form and in moderation at the end of the meal.

The small feedings often include milk and milk derivatives between meals. Whole milk or skim milk is used. Flavorings such as maple may be added. If the patient is obese or allergic to milk, gelatin in water may be substituted for some of the milk feedings. Most often milk or milk and cream is placed at the patient's bedside to be taken every hour or every two hours. It must be kept on ice to remain fresh but not made so cold as to be irritating. Supplemental vitamins are given to make up for any deficiencies.

Table 49-3. Ulcer Diets

PRINCIPLES:

1. Foods that neutralize and inhibit acidity
2. Mechanically and chemically nonirritating foods
3. Frequent and small feedings
4. Gradual but ultimate restoration to an adequate diet

PROGRESSIVE PEPTIC ULCER REGIMEN

ACUTE STAGE (2–4 days)

Milk or milk and cream (Sippy mixture)	3 oz. every hour. Feedings are given from 7 A.M. to 7 P.M. and throughout the night if necessary and pain persists

Supplements (added one at a time, 3–5 days)

Eggs	Soft-cooked or poached, once or twice daily
Cereal	Cream of Wheat, rice, once or twice daily
Custard	Substituted for an egg

CONVALESCENT STAGE (5–15 days)

Milk	Milk, cream
Cheese	Cottage, cream, and other mild cheeses
Fats	Butter or margarine
Eggs	Soft-cooked, boiled, not fried
Vegetables	Puréed beets, string beans, peas, corn, squash, mashed or baked potatoes
Fruits	Canned, stewed, or purée of apples, peaches, pears, apricots
Meats	Minced, creamed chicken or fish, beef
Fish	Broiled, baked, boiled
Fowl	Boiled, baked, stewed

BLEEDING PEPTIC ULCER DIET

The patient is fed, from the very onset of hemorrhage, a full purée diet, supplemented by doses of iron. This is called a Meulengracht diet. The object is to keep suitable food in the stomach to neutralize acid and reduce pain. He is not fed by mouth if he is vomiting.

Example

6 A.M.	Tea, white bread, butter
9 A.M.	Oatmeal with milk, white bread, and butter
1 P.M. Dinner	This may include such food as soup, minced and boiled meats, plain cooked eggs, puddings, ice cream
3 P.M.	Cocoa
6 P.M.	White bread, butter, sliced meats, cheese, and tea

GENERAL RULES

1. Serve food warm, not hot or cold
2. The patient should eat slowly and chew food well
3. No other foods are allowed except when specified by the physician

Use of Drugs

Ulcer treatment and antacids go hand in hand. Antacids neutralize the hydrochloric acid and thus lessen its destructive potential. At times an antacid will form a temporary protective coating over the ulcer, thus preventing more erosion and the spasm of pain that goes with it.

Antacids are divided into two classes: systemic and nonsystemic. There are scores of *systemic antacids*. An example is sodium bicarbonate, which is ordinary baking soda.

One common side effect of the systemic antacids is alkalosis. Large doses of systemic antacid (alkali) prevent acid from entering the bloodstream but at the same time increase the alkalinity of the body.[26] Systemic antacids should be used with care, especially by older people as they can interfere with the functioning of the kidneys. Taken in excess they can cause self-induced alkalosis (headache, abdominal pain, nausea, and vomiting). They can also cause "acid rebound" in which larger amounts of acid are produced after the gastric acid is neutralized by the drug.

Another side effect is constipation. Constipation is infrequent or difficult evacuation of feces. Frequency must be viewed as "relative to the individual patient." Constipation exists when the period between bowel actions is too long, the fecal volume is too small, and the fecal consistency is too hard.[27] Common causes of constipation are failure to heed the defecation call, stress of modern life, neurotic habit of delay, reluctance of children to interrupt play, and modern travel with its changes in time and food.[28] Diet poor in bulk or fluid, strict diets for weight loss, and eating no food are additional factors that contribute to the development of constipation.

Treatment of constipation involves an intake of high-residue foods, adequate fluids, exercise, and laxatives and enemas when ordered.

The *nonsystemic antacids* include compounds of calcium, aluminum, and magnesium. The magnesium compounds have a laxative effect, whereas calcium and aluminum have a constipating effect. They come in tablet as well as liquid form. Examples of nonsystemic antacids are magnesium hydroxide mixture (Milk of Magnesia), precipitated calcium carbonate (Titralac, Dicarbosil), aluminum hydroxide (Amphojel). These drugs are a help, but they do not cure. Alkalosis is not a problem with nonsystemic antacids.

The anticholinergic drugs are used in ulcer treatment to depress the secretion of acid and modify the motility of the stomach. Examples of natural anticholinergic drugs are atropine, scopolamine, and other belladonna alkaloids. Tincture of belladonna given in water decreases gastrointestinal motility, muscle tone, and peristalsis. Pro-Banthine is an example of a synthetic anticholinergic drug.

Sedatives and Tranquilizers

Sedatives act as a "brake" on overactivity of the stomach and the flow of acid. Phenobarbital is excellent for this. Tranquilizers are useful when there is some exceptional strain. Meprobamate (Equanil), chlorpromazine (Thorazine), and chlordiazepoxide (Librium) have been found to be beneficial.

Complications of Ulcers

Perforation

The most common and the most hazardous complication of ulcer is perforation. When an ulcer perforates, the gastric contents of the stomach or duodenum are spilled into the peritoneal cavity, and life-threatening peritonitis may result. The patient experiences sudden sharp pain that spreads over the abdomen. To decrease the pull on the abdomen he usually draws his legs up to his chest and he breathes in a shallow manner. The abdomen feels boardlike and rigid and is exquisitely tender. Pain is severe. The patient may show symptoms of shock with profuse perspiration, rapid weak pulse, and apprehension. Perforations seem to occur most often when the patient is tired as at the end of a week's work. Antibiotics are administered to control infection; morphine or meperidine (Demerol) is administered to control pain. Surgical repair is essential. The longer the perforation exists without surgical repair, the higher the mortality. The stomach is constantly tube-drained to give the perforation a chance to seal over.

Peritonitis

The peritoneum is the serous sac that lines the abdominal cavity. If the stomach or intestines tear or rupture, their bacterial content spills out into the abdominal cavity and can infect its lining. This is a most serious inflammatory condition. The patient has severe abdominal pain especially in the areas of inflammation. There are tenderness, nausea, vomiting, fever, rapid weak pulse, and shallow respirations. The abdomen may become boardlike and rigid, and later soft. The patient may draw his knees up to lessen the pain. Paralysis of the intestines (paralytic ileus) often accompanies peritonitis. In this case peristalsis ceases, and intestinal content accumulates in the bowel. Gastrointestinal decompression is instituted to rid the intestine of gas and built-up intestinal material. Water and electrolytes are replaced. Antibiotics are used to control the infection and analgesics are used to control pain. The area may heal spontaneously, or surgery may have to be done to repair the ruptured area. A ruptured appendix often causes peritonitis. It must be removed as an emergency, immediate measure. The nurse must observe carefully for degree of distention, location of pain, rectal passage of stool or flatus that would indicate an open bowel, quantity and kind of vomitus, voiding, and vital signs. She must be very gentle.

Hemorrhage or Hematemesis and Melena

Hemorrhage may result as the ulcer erodes blood vessels. The incidence of hemorrhage is greater in the fall and early winter and when the person is physically or emotionally fatigued. The patient may vomit blood (hematemesis) or pass blood in his stools. Anticoagulant drugs used in the treatment of cardiovascular disease or ulcerogenic drugs (such as aspirin or cortisone) can precipitate bleeding.

One danger inherent in bleeding is that the patient may be considerably weakened and suffering from shock for some hours before he vomits any blood. Blood may have passed down the bowels and not show up for many hours. He must be observed carefully. Pulse, respiration, and blood pressure are taken frequently. Watch for rapid, weak pulse, fall in blood pressure, pallor, thirst, and faintness.

Melena, or the passing of blood in the feces, is usually indicative of hemorrhage in the duodenum. When black tarry stools are passed, it shows that the blood has moved through the intestines, has been partly digested, and has changed color from red to black. This color change shows that the blood has been passing through the intestinal tract for four to eight hours.[29]

Ulcer hemorrhage is a cause for anxiety. Pain may readily disappear and a sense of relief sets in. However, serious complications may follow. It is an established fact, however, that peptic ulcers heal quickly after a severe hemorrhage.[30] The patient is put to bed to rest. He may be fed intravenously or by small feedings of milk and cream. Blood may be administered. The patient may be taken to the operating room for ligation of the bleeding vessel. Sometimes a nasogastric tube with a balloon attached is passed. The balloon is filled with a cooling solution that provides cooling and pressure to the bleeding area.

Obstruction

This simply means that the passage of chyme is blocked. This obstruction is a physical barrier in the gastric tract and most often occurs at the pyloric opening or in the duodenum. It may be caused by edema, spasm, scar tissue, or inflammation. Obstruction is accompanied by uncomfortable symptoms: loss of appetite, a feeling of fullness, nausea and vomiting, halitosis, foul taste in the mouth, listlessness, thirst, weakness, dull headache, and decreased urination. Repeated vomiting of food eaten the day before is indicative of obstruction. Once an obstruction is suspected, the patient must be hospitalized and a gastric analysis is performed to help determine the degree of obstruction. X-rays are taken. If the obstruction is caused by an overgrowth of scar tissue, surgery is indicated. If it is caused by inflammation or edema, it usually subsides with a regimen of medical treatment. The stomach is drained of retained food and fluid by tube. (See p. 522.)

Subtotal Gastrectomy (Fig. 49-2)

In a subtotal gastrectomy the small bowel is linked to the upper part of the stomach, which has not been removed. One half to two thirds of

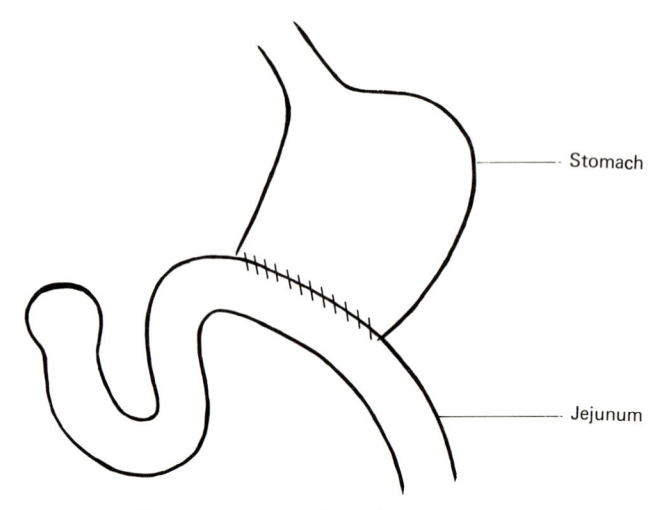

FIGURE 49–2. Subtotal gastrectomy.

the lower stomach is removed. Gastric juices can be secreted because some gastric glands remain. Although each individual operation for surgical treatment of peptic ulcer disease offers its own inherent advantages, there is no universally satisfactory procedure applicable to every patient. The operation is designed to prevent the complications of surgery and to ensure good long-term physiologic function.[31]

Preoperatively, the patient with a peptic ulcer needs to have care directed toward water and electrolyte regulation. Fluids may be given parenterally or orally. Usually a Levin tube is inserted and oral fluid intake is limited. This Levin tube is connected to suction to empty the stomach of food and secretions. As the food is removed from the stomach, electrolytes are also removed. Therefore, adequate fluid replacement is extremely important.

Postoperatively, the Levin tube is left in place as long as necessary. The nurse must note the drainage and record the output. If a small amount of blood shows up, this should not give rise to fear; if large amounts of bright red blood appear or if the drainage remains very blood-streaked, notify a physician at once. Drainage is dark red or brownish in the immediate postoperative period. This color is caused by the presence of "old blood." It should soon change to the normal greenish yellow of gastric fluid. Sometimes the physician orders irrigations of the Levin tube so that it will remain patent and clean. It is important to use the amount and kind of solution ordered. Normal saline is most frequently ordered, 30 ml being the average amount of solution used. Mouth and nose care must be given frequently. Mouth care relieves the dryness and the unpleasant odor that may exist. Nose care relieves the soreness on the external nares due to the pressure of the tube and prevents cracking and dehydration.

The patient is allowed nothing by mouth for one to two days. Beginning the second day he is given 30 ml water. If this is tolerated, the amount is increased to 60 and then 90 ml. Then he receives a soft diet and finally a regular diet. He may find that he is more comfortable if he eats six small meals rather than three large ones in the early postoperative period. Quantity can be gradually increased. *Repeated vomiting of small amounts of food means the food is not progressing along the alimentary tract successfully.* The physician should be notified. He may insert the Levin tube again.

The patient should be encouraged to cough and deep breathe. The high abdominal incision may make this difficult for him. He is allowed out of bed in a chair the day after surgery.

Total Gastrectomy

The stomach is removed. Gastrectomy and vagotomy are combined. Vagotomy tries to tackle the main causative factor: acid. The severing of the vagus nerves cuts down the flow of acid. In a total gastrectomy the patient loses all his acid cells. Bile and pancreatic juices are channeled into the improvised stomach to help dissolve the food and substitute for the acid.

Gastroenterostomy (Fig. 49–3)

This is an operative procedure that links the upper intestine to the stomach, so that the gastric juices bypass the duodenum. No portion of the stomach is removed. This procedure may be elected if the patient is too ill to withstand gastrectomy.

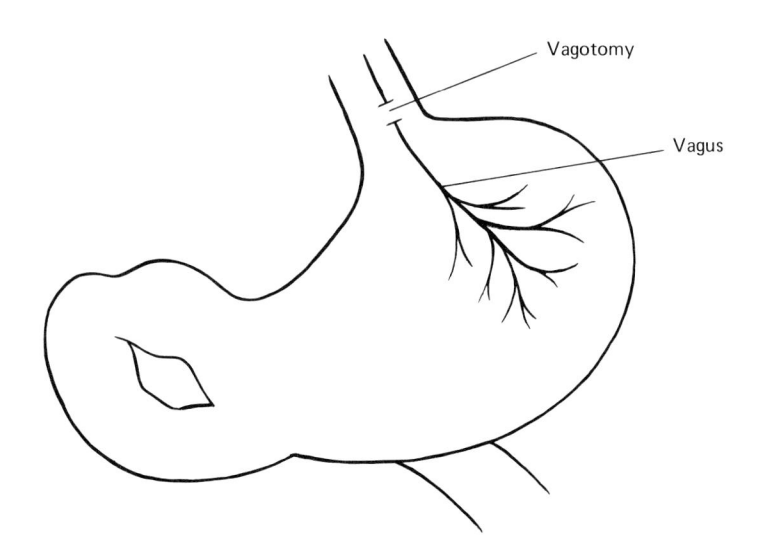

FIGURE 49–3. Gastroenterostomy and vagotomy.

Postgastrectomy Syndrome

The dumping syndrome is a common postoperative disturbance following a gastrectomy. This syndrome consists of transient feelings of weakness, fullness, sense of warmth, palpitations, fatigue, nausea, sweating, and pallor. The cause of the dumping syndrome is probably large volumes of food "dumped" directly into the jejunum and osmotic pull of the hypertonic content on surrounding water. The volume in the jejunum is increased; the circulatory volume is decreased. Thus, the shocklike symptoms. Patients who experience the dumping syndrome are instructed to eat small meals that are dry and have a low carbohydrate content, to lie down for about a half hour after eating, and to avoid sweet foods and liquids if they intensify symptoms.

The nurse needs to be aware that the stomach is essential for life, not because of its digestive function, but because it secretes the gastric *intrinsic factor* required for vitamin B_{12} absorption. In man this *intrinsic factor* is secreted by some unidentified cells in the body of the stomach. The person who lacks this needs parenteral administration of vitamin B_{12}.

50

THE PATIENT WITH INTESTINAL OBSTRUCTION

ANY disorder interfering with the forward movement of the contents of the alimentary canal is called an obstruction.[32] An obstruction in the esophagus interferes with the ability to ingest food; an obstruction in the stomach delays or prevents chyme from entering the duodenum. For the most part, the obstructions discussed will be related to blockage in the large or small intestine, resulting in failure of the bowel to propel intestinal contents and gas.

There are three kinds of disturbances that predispose to obstruction:

1. Mechanical blockage of the lumen
2. Reduced or absent peristalsis
3. Impaired circulation due to the occlusion of blood supply [33]

Examples of mechanical causes are neoplasms, volvulus (a twisting of intestines), and incarcerated hernia. Absent peristalsis may be the result of some disturbance in the autonomic nervous system. This is also called paralytic ileus. Impairment of circulation may be caused by a thrombosis.

Early symptoms of intestinal obstruction include anorexia, indigestion, flatulence, and a distaste for certain foods that previously were enjoyed. There may be changes in bowel habits, often with alternating periods of constipation and diarrhea. Later symptoms include severe pain, vomiting of blood, and passage of tarry stools. If the obstruction is complete, no gas or stool is passed; however, the patient may eliminate stool that remains beyond the obstruction. The patient has severe cramps as the body attempts to bypass the obstruction. A gurgling or bubbling sound may be heard. Vomiting may occur as food is eliminated by "reverse peristalsis." The vomitus may be thick and foul smelling if the stomach contents are "old." Sometimes there is no vomiting if the obstruction is very low in the intestinal tract. Severe water and electrolyte loss occurs, and the patient must have this fluid replaced intravenously. The severe distention may put pressure on blood vessels, and gangrene to that part of the bowel may result.

Adenocarcinoma of the colon and rectum is a leading cause of obstruction and of cancer deaths today. It occurs most often in men. It is sad that most patients have relatively advanced disease by the time they go to the physician, although a large percentage of the cancer in this part of the body occurs in that part of the colon that is directly accessible to examination and early treatment.[36]

Treatment

Treatment involves surgical excision of the tumor, the extent of which depends on the location of the tumor and the degree of metastasis. An artificial opening in the ileum (ileostomy) or in the colon (colostomy) through which feces are diverted is made. The procedure can be temporary to rest the bowel, or it can be permanent.

ABDOMINOPERINEAL RESECTION

An abdominal colostomy is established, and the lower portion of the bowel and the anus are removed through an opening made in the perineum. This is a permanent colostomy. In most instances the perineal opening is left open, and with the passage of time much of the area fills in and becomes solid. During the interim period perineal drainage can

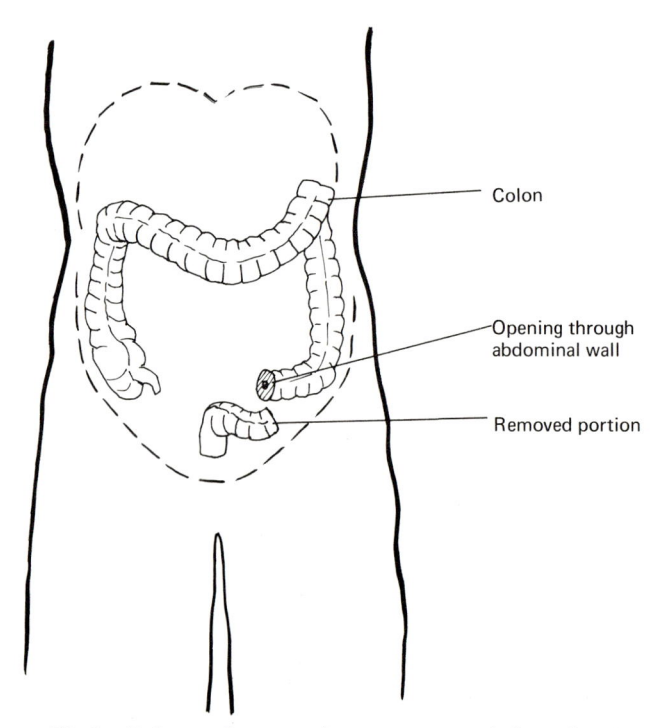

FIGURE 50–1. Abdominal perineal resection, single-barrel colostomy.

be a problem. Often dressings must be worn and changed frequently. (See Fig. 50–1.)

ABDOMINOPERINEAL PROCTOSIGMOIDECTOMY

In this procedure the sphincter is preserved. There is no colostomy because the upper colon is pulled down to unite with the upper margin of the anal sphincter.

RESECTION AND END-TO-END ANASTOMOSIS

The segment of the colon containing the cancer is resected and removed. Continuity of the bowel is re-established. There is no colostomy or opening in the perineum.

DOUBLE-BARRELED COLOSTOMY

In this procedure the transverse colon is divided and the ends brought out through the skin. There are two openings on the abdominal wall. The upper or proximal loop in the right margin of the incision is for stool outlet. The lower or distal loop in the left margin leads to the nonfunctioning lower bowel. This procedure is performed to divert feces and to relieve obstruction. It gives the bowel time to heal.

ILEOSTOMY

In this procedure a permanent opening is made in the small intestine. This is usually accompanied by removal of all or part of the remaining bowel. Drainage from an ileostomy is more liquid than that from a colostomy because absorption has not taken place. The drainage contains enzymes that are extremely irritating to the skin. They "digest" the skin if contact is allowed.

CARE OF THE NEW COLOSTOMY

The skin around the colostomy must be kept clean and dry. Therefore, the skin should be washed with soap and water and the dressings changed as often as necessary to prevent excoriation of skin and to prevent disagreeable odors. Montgomery straps may be used to hold the dressings in place and reduce possible trauma to the skin from frequent removal of adhesive tape. Ointments may be used as ordered by the physician. They should be used as sparingly as possible and removed at intervals in order to closely examine the skin under the protective coating. A colostomy may appear more objectionable to a patient when ointments are used.

Ample dressing supplies need to be kept at hand on the patient's bedside stand. As soon as the patient is psychologically and physically able, he should be encouraged to assist in changing the dressing. The facial as well as the verbal expressions of the nurse, as she changes the dressings, are important because the patient watches and takes clues from the nurse about how the colostomy appears to others. A temporary colostomy bag may be placed over the stoma. The nurse cuts an opening in it to fit the stoma. After healing has occurred, a permanent appliance is fitted. (See p. 203.)

Colostomy irrigations may be ordered, and it is the responsibility of the nurse to irrigate the colostomy. The nurse is also responsible for teaching the patient how to irrigate the colostomy. Equipment needed for the irrigation should be assembled and described to the patient. Equipment that may be used at home is also discussed, with substitutes suggested when necessary. See a text on nursing procedures for more detailed discussion. (See also p. 203.)

As soon as the patient is ambulatory the irrigation can be done on the toilet. Equipment must be organized and the room comfortably warm. Warm tap water is used for the irrigation (105° to 107° F.). The amount of water will vary with the patient. The catheter is inserted gently into the colostomy opening for 3 to 6 in. After the irrigation has been completed, the patient should be encouraged to stand up once or twice, massage his abdomen, or lean forward from side to side. This activity is carried out to hasten bowel discharge. Patience is needed because the patient should remain on the toilet until he is reasonably sure the drainage has ceased. When the drainage has ceased, clean the skin around the colostomy and dry it. Then apply a clean dressing. The equipment is cleaned immediately after use. It is first rinsed with cold water, then washed with soap and water. The equipment is then spread out to dry.

HOME CARE OF THE "OSTOMY" PATIENT

For the patient who has a permanent "ostomy," convalescence is usually long. After two weeks in the hospital the patient will be eager to go home. When he is at home, he must be patient and realize that healing is a rather slow process and that drainage will continue for several weeks, but eventually it will cease.

There is a period of adjustment, of conditioning and regulating bowel movements, of timing the desired intervals between irrigations, and of trial and error in food selection. Skin care and application of protective devices, i.e., plastic bags with belts, are time-consuming. Thus, schedules for daily activities are necessary. Fecal burns, which may occur at this time, can be controlled to a degree through dietary measures, e.g., avoiding spices, condiments, mustard, horseradish, pickles, alcohol, and so on.

In order to make home care realistic and safe for the patient with an "ostomy," the family can help by familiarizing themselves with equipment needed and used, its cost, and when the parts need to be replaced. The patient with an "ostomy" spends more time in the bathroom than he has been accustomed to in the past; thus the family can make sure he has everything he needs on a conveniently located shelf. Once in the bathroom, the patient should not have to rush out.

A good way of becoming familiar with nearly all the leading "ostomy" appliances and products is through the magazine *Ostomy Quarterly,* which for the past three years has been published by the United Ostomy Association, Incorporated, 111 Wilshire Boulevard, Los Angeles, California 90017.[34]

51

THE PATIENT WITH INTERFERENCE IN PRODUCTION AND/OR PASSAGE OF BILE

The Gallbladder

THE gallbladder is a little pear-shaped bag, about 3 in. long, attached to the undersurface of the liver. (See Fig. 47–3.) It is designed by nature to store bile ("chole" is Greek for bile) at night and between mealtimes when this fluid is not needed for the process of digestion.

Bile gets in and out of the gallbladder through a short tube, called the cystic duct. This connects with the common bile duct, which empties into the bowel at the papilla of Vater. The bile comes down from the liver to the common duct through the several hepatic ducts.

Bile is poured into the bowel at mealtimes to help in the digestion of fats. Between these times it is stored. In man the gallbladder capacity is 50 to 60 ml.[35] Bile salts promote the absorption of fat-soluble vitamins, A, D, E, K; they are mildly laxative; and they are absorbed through the upper bowel. Agents that cause the gallbladder to contract and empty most effectively are egg yolks, fat in any form, and meat.[36] If an agent promotes emptying of the gallbladder, it is called a cholagogue. The drug that best stimulates the musculature of the gallbladder to contract is magnesium sulfate (epsom salt).

Gallbladder Series

This is a series of x-rays taken to reveal the gallbladder and its ducts. A radiopaque dye such as iopanoic acid (Telepaque) is given orally following a low-fat evening meal after which no food is given.

Roentgen rays cannot penetrate the dye; thus the dye-filled gallbladder shows up as a dense shadow on examination. A satisfactory gallbladder shadow indicates a functioning gallbladder. An absence of opaque material in the gallbladder suggests a nonfunctioning gallbladder. After ingestion of a fatty meal, a functioning gallbladder should contract, and the radiopaque dye is expelled along with the bile through the common bile duct into the duodenum. X-ray examination at this point would outline the bile ducts.

The dye causes nausea, vomiting, and diarrhea in some people. Dosage must be checked carefully, and if any untoward signs occur, the physician should be notified immediately. The dye is contraindicated in gastrointestinal disorders and acute nephritis.

On the morning of the examination the patient may have black coffee, tea, or water only. Enemas may be ordered to help remove gas from the intestinal tract so that it will not interfere with the examination.

Examination may reveal calculi (gallstones), inflammation (cholecystitis), or tumors. These are common conditions that interfere with the normal function of this system of ducts. Biliary tract disease is common and accounts for a very high percentage of the abdominal operations performed in most general hospitals.

Cholelithiasis (Biliary Calculi)

Biliary calculi form, as a rule, in the gallbladder. The cause of their formation is not clearly understood. It is thought that alterations in the concentrated bile cause its solutes to be precipitated. Cholesterol, bile pigments, and calcium, which are concentrated in the bladder bile by the reabsorption of water, frequently precipitate to form gallstones. Stones may also form in the hepatic duct and its branches. Pregnancy, diets high in cholesterol and fats, and infections are thought to be important factors that may encourage stone formation. Biliary stasis and tumors are also implicated. Stones vary as to size, number, and shape. Cholecystitis and cholelithiasis are usually seen together.

Patients usually complain of indigestion and have severe discomfort after a meal that contains fat. A stone in the cystic duct tends to obstruct the lumen and may cause a severe type of colicky pain. This pain often begins in the right upper quadrant of the abdomen and radiates to the back. Passage of the stone results in sudden cessation of pain. This pain is often accompanied by nausea and vomiting, tachycardia, and profuse diaphoresis. Obstruction to passage of bile and/or spasm of the common bile duct results in jaundice. Stools lacking bile are lighter in color.

TREATMENT

The only cure is removal of the stone or stones. This should include removal of the gallbladder whenever possible, to prevent additional stone formation. If the gallbladder is only drained, additional stones are likely to form.

Cholecystectomy is the surgery of choice. Removal of a stone or stones from the common bile duct is called a *choledocholithotomy*.

FOCUS IN NURSING INTERVENTION

The care of those patients who have operations on the biliary tract does not differ from that for patients with other abdominal operations. The wound is high in the abdomen, breathing is painful, and the patient may hold his breath or take shallow ones. The patient should be assisted to deep breathe with the nurse splinting the incision.

In the immediate postoperative period a soft, low-fat diet may be given until bile salts are passed in sufficient amounts. The diet should be plentiful in carbohydrates. The liver stores glycogen and needs it to supply energy when the diet is curtailed after surgery. If the patient is not able to take large amounts of carbohydrates by mouth, glucose can be supplied by vein. The special diet is usually discontinued prior to discharge so that the physician can observe the patient's tolerance to regular diet. The patient may be advised to avoid excessive fat intake when he goes home.

If the common bile duct is to be drained, a drainage set should be available. The drainage must be measured carefully and observed for color, viscosity, and amount. A T tube may be inserted with the short ends placed into the common duct. The long end of this soft rubber tube is brought through the wound and sutured to the skin. The T tube is inserted to preserve patency of the common duct to ensure drainage of bile until edema in the common duct has subsided. The purpose of this tube should be explained to the patient, and he should be told why it must not be clamped, pulled, or kinked. Drainage must be checked frequently. This tube may be attached to a small drainage bottle to permit greater freedom of movement. Outer dressings are changed frequently because this drainage (bile) is irritating to the skin, and wet dressings interfere with the patient's rest and comfort. Sterile petrolatum gauze may be used. A low sitting position helps gravity drainage.

Vitamin K is given after surgery as indicated by measurement of the prothrombin activity of the blood. Bleeding may develop and vital signs should be checked. Bile salts may be given until bile is passed in sufficient amounts into the digestive tract. The patient's skin should be observed for jaundice. His stool should be observed for color.

Usually the patient is advised to continue a low-fat diet for six months to a year. After surgery, shock, hemorrhage, and pulmonary complications are to be watched for and prevented if possible. Other complications are infection, liver damage from long-standing gallbladder disease, pancreatitis, and scarring.

The Liver [37]

The liver, located on the right side beneath the diaphragm, is the largest gland in the body. It is divided into four lobes: right, left, quadrate, and caudate. (See Fig. 47–3.) The liver has five sets of vessels:

1. Branches of the portal tube
2. Bile ducts
3. Branches of the hepatic artery
4. Hepatic veins
5. Lymphatics

The liver has many functions. Among them are the following:

1. Secretes bile
2. Stores fat and glycogen
3. Detoxifies poisons
4. Modifies fat by desaturation
5. Helps to regulate blood volume
6. Produces antibodies
7. Forms prothrombin and fibrinogen concerned with the clotting of blood
8. Forms heparin, an anticoagulant of the blood
9. Stores vitamins A and D
10. Forms vitamin A from carotene
11. Stores iron and copper
12. Converts amino acids into glucose

TABLE 51–1. FUNCTIONS OF THE LIVER AND SYMPTOMS OF DYSFUNCTION

Function of the Liver	Symptoms Caused by Its Impairment
Production of bile; removal of bile pigments and salts	Jaundice. Faulty digestion of fats; decreased peristalsis; stool pale, frothy, foul-smelling. Pruritus. Loss of fat-soluble vitamins in stool; decreased vitamin K; increased bleeding tendency
Conversion of glucose to glycogen; storage of glycogen	Hypoglycemia; weakness
Production of plasma proteins: albumin, fibrinogen, prothrombin	Decreased pull of interstitial fluid back into circulation; generalized edema; ascites; faulty coagulation of blood; bleeding tendency
Desaturation of fatty acids	Increased level of circulating cholesterol; saturated fats
Detoxification	Toxic symptoms: lethargy, confusion
Deamination	Build-up of nitrogenous wastes; build-up of ammonia; hepatic coma with tremors of hands, lethargy, etc.
Production of antibodies; phagocytosis	Increased susceptibility to infection; low-grade fever

Liver disease is suspected whenever there is a history of jaundice, dietary imbalance, alcoholism, exposure to hepatotoxins, or direct injury. Diagnostic measures include:

1. Physical examination; this is the best method for evaluating the size of the liver.
2. X-ray studies; these are helpful as a supplement to physical examination. Chest x-rays may show an elevated diaphragm.
3. Special radiologic techniques permit reliable estimates of liver size. These special techniques include the gallbladder and gastrointestinal series. A liver scan may be ordered.
4. History taking may reveal that, with the gradual increase in liver size, the patient has sensations of abdominal fullness, not necessarily pain.
5. Liver biopsy and specific liver function tests may be ordered (see p. 548).

Physical Signs of Liver Disease

JAUNDICE

Jaundice is often the presenting sign of liver disease. This sign reflects an increase in circulating bilirubin or biliglobin. Blood is cleared of bilirubin as long as there is a normal functioning liver. Jaundice can be detected and confirmed from a serum bilirubin test when the level reaches 2.0 mg per 100 ml. With jaundice, the sclera appear yellow and there is discoloration of the skin—it takes on a yellow to gold color—and there is pruritus (itch) because of the accumulation of bile salts in the blood.

SPIDER ANGIOMAS

Spider angiomas are skin capillaries that have become prominent. These are observed around the face, neck, shoulder, and upper extremities. Their cause is unknown, and they may also occur in pregnancy, rheumatic disease, and endocrine disorders.

HEPATIC FETOR (LIVER BREATH)

This is a sweetish, musty odor resembling that of decayed fruit. It is often noted in patients with hepatic insufficiency.

MENTAL CHANGES

Depression, somnolence, apathy, disorientation, agitation, delirium, and coma may be seen in the patient with liver disease. These changes may be due to drugs, alcoholism, uremia, hypoglycemia, or a functional psychosis. They result from the liver's failure to adequately detoxify substances.

Nonspecific Signs of Liver Disease [38]

ASCITES

Ascites is the presence of fluid in the peritoneal cavity. This accumulation of fluid occurs when there is vascular obstruction that results in congestion of the entire area drained by the portal system. Ascites decreases respiratory reserve and predisposes the patient to pulmonary infection. A paracentesis is usually performed to remove the fluid that has accumulated in the peritoneal cavity. The patient should void before the procedure is begun. The patient is placed in a sitting position with support given by pillows as necessary. He may be seated at the side of the bed or on a treatment table with his feet supported on a chair. A chair is most comfortable because it offers good back and arm support. This is important because this procedure may take a long time. After the patient is in position with the legs slightly separated so that the site of entry is readily accessible, he should be covered adequately for warmth and to prevent unnecessary exposure. The physician cleanses the site of insertion and inserts the trocar. Tubing from the trocar is placed into a container for the collection of fluid. If fluid is draining too rapidly, the container should be elevated on a stool. Rapid drainage may produce symptoms of shock. During the procedure the nurse observes the patient for untoward reactions. His color and respiratory and pulse rates are noted.

The patient may soon begin to experience relief from the pressure of the fluid, which is desired. After the needle has been withdrawn, a sterile dressing is placed over the stab wound. This dressing is checked at frequent intervals and changed as necessary. Leakage usually occurs.

ANEMIA OR HEMORRHAGE

Anemia or hemorrhage occurs in many cases of chronic liver disease. Anemia is the result of a decreased production and an increased loss or excessive destruction of erythrocytes. Bleeding tendencies found in patients with liver diseases are due to increased capillary fragility, hypoprothrombinemia, thrombocytopenia, or low fibrinogen. These tendencies are evidenced by petechiae, purpura, epistaxis, bleeding gums, and melena. Capillary fragility is related to a vitamin C deficiency. Hypoprothrombinemia is related to an inability to produce prothrombin or the labile factor. The manufacture of prothrombin requires an adequate amount and supply of vitamin K and functional integrity of liver cells. Thrombocytopenia is reflected in an abnormal bleeding time, clot retraction, and prothrombin consumption.

HYPOVITAMINOSIS

Hypovitaminosis is primarily the result of an inadequate diet and interference with absorption of fat-soluble vitamins if bile is obstructed.

Thiamine hydrochloride deficiency is most frequently encountered. This deficiency contributes to the fatigue, weakness, and lethargy responsible for and seen in peripheral neuritis. Vitamin A and C deficiencies result in night blindness and poor dark adaptation. These are encountered in a large number of alcoholics.

REACTIONS TO INFECTIONS

In liver disease there is an increased susceptibility to infections. The liver normally helps control systemic infections by removing bacteria from portal venous blood and producing antibodies. An intact liver is necessary for the production of immune bodies and antitoxins.

Liver Function Tests [39]

There are more than 100 liver function tests. The following are a few of the more common.

SERUM BILIRUBIN (VAN DEN BERGH'S TEST)

Serum bilirubin is a byproduct of the catabolism of hemoglobin. Red blood cells break down to release hemoglobin, which is converted into bilirubin, iron, and globin. Iron is split off from this complex, and the liver takes up the other two agents. Only minute amounts of bilirubin are found in the blood of well persons. When hepatic and biliary ducts become blocked for any reason, bilirubin is no longer excreted into the bowel. It is then absorbed into the blood (jaundice) and excreted by the kidneys.

URINE BILE (UROBILINOGEN)

An elevated level of bile in the urine indicates liver damage. It is seen in patients with primary liver disease or obstructive jaundice. A 24-hour specimen may be requested. It should be saved in an amber bottle.

ICTERUS INDEX

This is used to determine the amount of bile pigment in blood serum. The normal reading is 4 to 6 units, but it may reach as high as 20 units before jaundice is evident.

BROMSULPHALEIN EXCRETION

One of the functions of the liver is excretion, and this test measures the rate at which a dye is removed from the bloodstream. This is the least toxic of the dyes. For this procedure the patient must fast from midnight on, and he must be weighed. The dosage of the dye is calculated on the basis of 5 mg per kilogram of body weight. The dye is injected slowly into the vein, and a blood sample is taken 45 minutes after injection from the opposite arm. The chief value of this test is that it helps determine when acute liver disease is healed. Because it may place additional strain on the liver, it is usually not ordered when acute disease is suspected. Normally, there is less than 5 per cent retention of the dye one hour after injection.

ALKALINE PHOSPHATASE

This test of blood serum is significant in that the level of this enzyme is only slightly elevated in liver disease, but it is markedly elevated in biliary obstruction. Alkaline phosphatase is normally excreted in bile. Normal range is 2 to 5 Bodansky units. Serum transaminase levels are also increased when liver tissue is damaged.

BIOPSY OF THE LIVER

This is done to establish a diagnosis. A specially designed needle is inserted through the chest or abdominal wall, and a piece of liver tissue is removed for study. Bleeding time, clotting time, capillary fragility, and prothrombin time should be evaluated before this procedure is carried out. To avoid hemorrhage vitamin K may be given parenterally. This procedure is performed with the patient lying on his back, very still in bed. The dangers of this sterile procedure are:

1. There can be accidental penetration of other vessels or organs.
2. Hemorrhage may follow the procedure.
3. Chemical peritonitis may occur from leakage of bile into the peritoneal cavity.

Vital signs should be checked frequently following this procedure. Drainage on the dressing should be reported.

The normal liver is reddish-brown; in obstructive jaundice green; the fatty or fibrous liver is yellowish-brown; the neoplastic liver is white.

Cirrhosis of the Liver

This is a condition in which the cells of the liver degenerate. It can develop as a result of obstruction to bile flow, viral hepatitis, drug reaction, or chronic alcoholism. The organ hypertrophies as its cells attempt to regenerate. Signs and symptoms include anorexia, nausea, vomiting, flatulence, and ascites. There may be abdominal pain, epistaxis, hematemesis, "black and blue marks," and jaundice. As the abdomen enlarges, breathing becomes shallow, pulse rapid. The patient is especially prone to bleeding. This may come from distended esophageal veins (esophageal varices). He is prone to secondary infection because of interference with production of antibodies and phagocytosis. Uncontrolled cirrhosis leads to increased circulating ammonia that produces a toxic condition called hepatic coma. The patient is confused and drowsy. He may develop tremors of his hands when he extends them. He eventually becomes comatose. Hepatic coma and delirium tremens associated with chronic alcoholism must be differentiated. Treatment is mainly supportive. The patient must have bed rest. His diet is often high in protein, carbohydrate, and vitamins with some fat included to make the diet palatable. Protein may be restricted if there is fear of liver decompensation because it makes the liver work harder. Appetite is poor, and the nurse's ingenuity is challenged because it is essential that the patient get nourishment. Meals should be small and served attractively. Frequent mouth care should be administered. The patient is allowed no alcohol or tobacco. Supplementary vitamins and bile salts may be ordered.

If pruritus is present, starch baths may be given. Medication includes use of diuretics to control ascites, corticosteroids to decrease the inflammatory response, and antibiotics such as neomycin to interrupt the normal intestinal bacterial flora that break down protein and thereby increase ammonia. Opiates and barbiturates that are detoxified by the liver are avoided.

If coma develops, focus is on maintaining adequate water and electrolyte balance intravenously. Ascites may be relieved by paracentesis (see p. 547). Infusions of whole blood are given for hemorrhage. If portal hypertension is present from blockage of free flow of blood from the liver to the vena cava (e.g., from thrombosis), a portacaval shunt may be done. This is a surgical procedure in which blood is diverted from the portal vein by direct anastomosis of the portal vein and the vena cava. This helps prevent the back-up of blood that leads to varices and hemorrhage. A Sengstaken-Blakemore tube may be passed if esophageal bleeding occurs. This tube contains a rubber balloon that is inflated when in place. It puts pressure on the bleeding vessels.

Toxicopathic Liver Disease

Toxicopathic is used to refer to liver disease caused by viruses, bacteria, spirochetes, or protozoa.[40] Viral hepatitis will be discussed as an example.

VIRAL HEPATITIS

Viral hepatitis is caused by two immunologically distinct agents: virus A or IH (infectious hepatitis) which is responsible for the naturally occurring disease, and virus B or SH (serum hepatitis; homologous serum jaundice) transmitted by parenteral injection of human blood or its products. Hepatitis is a reportable disease in most states.

Viral hepatitis A usually occurs in young adults and children, although anyone can contract the disease. It is prevalent in low-income areas and in schools, housing projects, and orphanages. This disease is more prevalent in the fall and winter months and has been attributed to closer contact during cold weather. It can be spread by infected stool, contaminated food and water, as well as infected parenteral equipment or contaminated blood. Man is the reservoir. Its incubation period is 15 to 50 days with an average of 25 days. Viral hepatitis B is transmitted through human blood, plasma, serum, or thrombin infused parenterally. The person donating the blood may not exhibit symptoms of the disease but may be a carrier. The incubation period is 50 to 160 days, with an average of 80 to 100 days.

Either form of viral hepatitis is diagnosed from biochemical liver function studies and liver biopsy. Bilirubin is found in the blood and urine. Symptoms are the same for both types of hepatitis. They include malaise, fatigue, fever, headache, anorexia, distaste for food, nausea and vomiting, sensorial changes, jaundice, chills, pruritus, dark urine, light stools, constipation, and diarrhea.

The natural course of viral hepatitis varies with age, complicating conditions, and general immunity. In most cases recovery is complete within two to three months. Chronic hepatitis, when it occurs, has been noticed in a large number of older patients.

TREATMENT

Basic treatment of liver disease is concerned with:

1. Elimination of causative factors
2. Judicious program of rest, especially during the acute stage
3. Appropriate dietary therapy
4. Management of secondary clinical complications
5. Treatment with broad-spectrum antibiotics
6. Use of adrenal steroids in some cases

Rest. The justification for rest regimes is based on the fact that physical activity increases energy needs and reduces hepatic blood flow. It is recommended that patients with hepatitis be hospitalized at once during the acute phase because activity to the point of fatigue may be harmful.

Diet. Food should be palatable with medications ordered to control the nausea that often accompanies eating. Sweetened hard candy is used to supplement the carbohydrate content of regular feedings. It is often necessary to divide the starches into four feedings to provide extra intake in patients with poor glycogen stores. Protein must be given in amounts sufficient to maintain nitrogen balance. Large quantities cannot properly be metabolized by the malfunctioning liver. Fat should be provided in amounts sufficient to provide palatability. Normal fat contained in meat, eggs, and dairy products is sufficient if there is no bloating or gaseous feeling.

Vitamin Therapy. Vitamin intake is inadequate; there is disturbance of absorption and increased destruction in the patient with hepatitis. Therefore, vitamins must be given. Vitamins A, D, E, and K may be ordered and administered orally or parenterally.

Constipation. Constipation is prominent in patients with liver disease owing to the disturbance of bile metabolism, the type of food ingested, and/or the amount of activity the patient carries out. Bulk cathartics such as Metamucil are preferred. These bulk cathartics are the most natural and least irritating. They must be taken with water, especially the dry seeds or granules. Saline and emollient cathartics may also be used.

CONTROL

1. Education of health personnel.
2. Proper handling of dishes.
3. Proper disposal of feces. Break the feces-to-hand-to-mouth cycle.
4. Immune gamma globulin may be advisable for patients exposed to hepatitis; 0.02 to 0.05 ml per kilogram body weight is given intramuscularly within one week of exposure. It apparently provides passive protection for six to eight weeks.
5. Serum hepatitis is difficult to avoid but its increase has been reduced by avoiding use of pooled plasma and by using blood substitutes such as Dextran when possible.
6. Adequate sterilization of parenteral equipment.

One attack of viral hepatitis confers immunity for that strain of virus infection but does not protect against attack by the other virus. The nurse can best make a contribution by careful hand washing with soap and running water. Proper disposal of needles and syringes is essential.

Since there are carriers of IH and SH viruses, all needles and equipment that have penetrated the skin of any patient should be handled with great care. All patients with hepatitis should have individual thermometers, tissues, and cups or a glass. During the acute phase the nurse encourages fluids and records intake and output. Isolation technique should be adhered to.

52

SOME FREQUENTLY OCCURRING GASTROINTESTINAL DISORDERS

Hemorrhoids

THE wall of the large intestine contains many networks of small veins. These veins may become dilated and form hemorrhoids: dilatations of the veins of the rectum and anal canal. These are "varicose veins" of the rectum. Hemorrhoids are *internal* if they occur above the internal sphincter, a thickening of the muscle layer of the large intestine. Internal hemorrhoids cause distress only if they become so large that they protrude through the anus. They often bleed when the patient defecates. Chronic loss of blood can lead to anemia. Hemorrhoids are *external* if they occur outside the external sphincter, a cylinder of skeletal muscle around the lower two thirds of the anal canal. They rarely bleed but do itch and cause severe pain if a vein ruptures and blood becomes clotted within it. This is called thrombosis. A patient may have both internal and external hemorrhoids.

Development of hemorrhoids seems related to a hereditary factor, occupations requiring long periods of standing or sitting, and increased intra-abdominal pressure caused by pregnancy, tumors, constipation, and straining at defecation. External hemorrhoids are seen during examination of the rectum; internal hemorrhoids are seen with a proctoscope. Symptoms should be examined with a proctoscope.

Conservative medical treatment includes local application of ice, warm magnesium sulfate compresses, Sitz baths, and use of analgesic-anesthetic ointments such as dibucaine (Nupercaine) and stool softeners such as mineral oil. A thrombosed external hemorrhoid may be incised at the bedside to release trapped blood, or a sclerosing drug such as 5 per cent phenol in oil may be injected under the mucosa (not into the hemorrhoid) where it causes an inflammatory response. Scar tissue develops and occludes the lumen of the vein, and the hemorrhoid shrinks.

Hemorrhoidectomy

Hemorrhoidectomy is the surgical removal of hemorrhoids. It is the most common rectal procedure done surgically for adults. Preoperatively the patient is given a laxative and is encouraged to eat until a few hours before anesthesia. After surgery the area is extremely sore. Analgesics, warm wet compresses, and ice bags are used for discomfort. Sitz baths also give relief and help to keep the area clean. There may be no postoperative dressings over the area. The patient may be more comfortable lying on his stomach or on his back with a rubber ring under his buttocks. He usually dreads the first bowel movement after surgery. It is very painful. If the male patient has difficulty voiding after surgery, he is usually permitted to stand at the bedside. In any case, the patient is out of bed the evening of surgery or the day after. A regular diet is permitted. The patient is advised to avoid constipation by eating a diet containing fresh fruits and vegetables, and so on; by drinking enough water; by getting enough exercise; and by making sure he takes enough time to have a regular bowel movement. The physician may prescribe a laxative.

What Is a Hernia?

Commonly called a "rupture," this condition involves the protrusion of any organ through its normal cavity. A lump or swelling can be felt where the organ protrudes. Intestinal hernias often protrude through the umbilicus or through the susceptible inguinal or femoral rings; these are "weakened" areas in the abdominal wall caused by the pressure of the weight of the abdominal viscera on the ventral part of the abdominal wall in the upright position. Inguinal hernias are most frequent in men.

Hernias develop as a result of congenital defect or weakened muscles, especially associated with the aging process. They are exacerbated when abdominal pressure is increased, e.g., in coughing, sneezing, and heavy lifting. They frequently develop and recur in the obese.

There may be no symptoms other than the protruding "lump," or there may be some pain especially after the patient stands for long periods of time or lifts something heavy. Treatment involves reduction (replacing the organ in its cavity) of the hernia. This can sometimes be done by placing manual pressure over the area with the patient recumbent. The hernia is irreducible if it becomes incarcerated. Incarceration means that the swollen, edematous protruded organ gets "stuck" in the opening. If the condition is not corrected, the organ becomes strangulated. Its blood supply is cut off and gangrene develops. Surgical reduction is the "surest" means of treatment. It is usually advised early to prevent the possible complications of hernia. The herniated part is put back in its cavity, and the weakened abdominal wall is repaired. This procedure is called *herniorrhaphy*. The patient is usually allowed out of bed the day after surgery. Diet is regular. Any coughing or sneezing should be reported to the physician because of the increased intra-abdominal pressure it creates. The patient is encouraged to move about freely as long as he does not do anything that would strain the operative area. Male patients who have inguinal hernias repaired may have pain and edema of the scrotum. This is relieved with ice bags and drugs.

Hiatus Hernia (Esophageal Hernia, Diaphragmatic Hernia)

This is a hernia in the upper gastrointestinal tract. It involves protrusion of part of the stomach up along the normal path of the esophagus through the hiatal opening in the diaphragm. Part of the stomach actually protrudes into the thorax. There is a back-up of unneutralized gastric juices into the esophagus.

The disease can be caused by trauma or by defects in the musculature associated with the aging process. Symptoms may be very mild or quite severe. They usually begin with epigastric distress during or shortly after meals, especially in the recumbent position. The patient frequently complains of hiccups and gaseous eructations. If the hernia progresses, there may be severe pain, exacerbated when food is taken. Misdiagnosis is a problem because there may be chest pain that mimics the pain of a cardiac condition. There may be vomiting with hematemesis and melena if the hernia becomes incarcerated.

Many hiatal hernias are small and are managed conservatively with small meals, moderate exercise, avoidance of recumbency after meals, and sometimes a bland diet. Surgery is indicated if one third or more of the stomach is involved. The condition is diagnosed by an upper gastrointestinal series.

Ulcerative Colitis

This is a serious condition in which the large intestine is inflamed and develops ulcers. Large areas may be denuded. Infection, allergy, autoimmunity, and emotional stress seem to be implicated as causative factors. Many authorities believe that the patient experiences severe hostility and, instead of letting it out, internalizes it and develops ulcerative colitis.

The disease can occur at any age. Symptoms include anorexia, nausea, vomiting, weakness, and severe diarrhea (sometimes 20 watery stools a day) with blood and mucus in the stool. There are weight loss, fever, and life-threatening electrolyte imbalance. Hemorrhage and peritonitis are often causes of the death from ulcerative colitis complications. Cancer of the colon is more frequent in patients with this condition.

Treatment includes rest, a bland diet, infusions of whole blood and oral iron preparations to improve anemia, and drugs that decrease symptoms. Examples include sedatives and tranquilizers to quiet the patient and decrease anxiety; atropine to decrease peristalsis; kaolin and pectin to coat and soothe the mucosa and adsorb toxins; and corticosteroids if the disease proves unresponsive to other drug intervention. Psychotherapy is suggested. Radical surgical procedures to remove involved areas (e.g., removal of the colon and rectum) with formation of permanent ileostomies are sometimes done for intractable colitis.

The disease may be mild and cause little distress for many years, or it may be rapid, fulminating, and potentially dangerous. The enlarged hiatus is closed around the esophagus and the stomach is anchored to the diaphragm.

REFERENCES

1. Babcock, C., "Attitudes and The Use of Food," *J. Amer. Diet. Ass.*, **68**: 546–57, June 1961.
2. Shafer, K., Sawyer, J., McCluskey, A., and Beck, E., *Medical-Surgical Nursing*. C. V. Mosby Co., St. Louis, 1967, pp. 114–16.
3. Young, C., "The Prevention of Obesity," *Med. Clin. N. Amer.*, **48**: 1317, Sept. 1964.
4. Seltzer, C., "Simple Criterion of Obesity," *Postgrad. Med.*, **38**:101–107, 1965.
5. *Ibid.*, p. 103.
6. Seltzer, C., "Body Build and Obesity —Who Are Obese?" *J.A.M.A.*, **189**: 677–84, 1964.
7. *Ibid.*, p. 680.
8. Shafer *et al., op. cit.*, p. 87.
9. Young, *op. cit.*, p. 13–18.
10. Rodman, M., and Smith, D., *Pharmacology and Drug Therapy in Nursing*. J. P. Lippincott, Co., Philadelphia, 1968, p. 208.
11. *Bowel Evacuation: A Teaching and Reference Manual*. Geigy Chemical Corp., New York, 1967, pp. 7–13.
12. Serino, G., *Your Ulcer—Prevention, Control, Cure*. J. B. Lippincott Co., Philadelphia, 1966, p. 29.
13. Kimber, D., Gray, C., Stackpole, C., and Leavell, L., *Anatomy and Physiology*, 14th ed. The Macmillan Co., New York, 1961, p. 491.
14. *Ibid.*, p. 487.
15. *Ibid.*, p. 486.
16. *Ibid.*, p. 491.
17. *Ibid.*, p. 487.
18. Harmer, B., and Henderson, V., *Textbook of the Principles and Practice of Nursing* 5th ed. The Macmillan Co., New York, 1955, p. 823.
19. Serino, *op. cit.*, p. 31.
20. Guyton, A., *Textbook of Medical Physiology*. W. B. Saunders Co., Philadelphia, 1964, p. 919.
21. *Ibid.*, p. 921.
22. Serino, *op. cit.*, p. 36.
23. *Ibid.*, p. 38.
24. *Ibid.*, p. 39.
25. *Bowel Evacuation, op. cit.*, p. 14.
26. Serino, *op. cit.*, p. 91.
27. *Bowel Evacuation, op. cit.*, p. 7.
28. *Ibid.*, p. 14.
29. Nordmark, M., and Rahweder, A., *Scientific Foundations of Nursing*. J. B. Lippincott Company, Philadelpia, 1964, p. 87.
30. Serino, *op. cit.*, p. 104.
31. Rosemond, G., and Riechle, F., "The Operation of Choice for Peptic Ulcer," *Amer. J. Gastroent.*, **48**:392, Nov. 1967.
32. Beland, I., *Clinical Nursing*. The Macmillan Company, New York, 1967, p. 807.
33. *Ibid.*, p. 807.
34. Happenie, S., *Colostomy, A Second Chance*. Charles C Thomas, Publisher, Springfield, Ill., 1968, p. 68.
35. Davenport, H., *Physiology of the Digestive Tract*. Year Book Publishing Co., Chicago, 1961, p. 135.
36. *Ibid.*, p. 136.
37. Kimber, *op. cit.*, p. 497.
38. Leevy, C., *Practical Diagnosis and Treatment of Liver Disease*. Hoeber-Harper, New York, 1957, pp. 42–61.
39. *Ibid.*, pp. 67–101.
40. *Ibid.*, p. 232.

ADDITIONAL READINGS

BARTON, K., and KIRSNER, J. "Gastric Ulcer—Individualization in Diagnosis and Therapy," *Med. Clin. N. Amer.*, **64**:103–15, Jan. 1964.

DAVIS, L. (ed.), *Christopher's Textbook of Surgery*, 8th ed. W. B. Saunders Co., Philadelphia, 1964.

DERECKS, V. C., "Rehabilitation of Patients with Ileostomy," *Amer. J. Nurs.*, **61**:48–51, May 1961.

DRUMMOND, E., and ANDERSON, M., "Gastrointestinal Suction," *Amer. J. Nurs.*, **63**:109–113, Dec. 1963.

GABRIEL, W., *The Principles and Practice of Rectal Surgery*. Charles C Thomas, Publisher, Springfield, Ill., 1963.

INGLES, T., and CAMPBELL, E., "The Patient with a Colostomy," *Amer. J. Nurs.*, **58**:1544–46, 1958.

KATONA, E., "Learning Colostomy Control," *Amer. J. Nurs.*, **67**:534–41, Mar. 1967.

KLUG, T., MAGRUDER, L., et al., "Gastric Resection—and Nursing Care," *Amer. J. Nurs.*, **61**:73–77, 1961.

LITTMAN, A., and DUMPHY, J., "Management of the Complications of Duodenal Ulcer," *Med. Clin. N. Amer.*, **48**:93–102, Jan. 1964.

RYNBERGEN, H., "In Gastrointestinal Disease—Fewer Diet Restrictions," *Amer. J. Nurs.*, **63**:86–89, Jan. 1963.

SECOR, S., "Colostomy Care," *Amer. J. Nurs.*, **64**:127, Sept. 1964.

SMITH, D., and GIPS, C., *Care of the Adult Patient*. J. B. Lippincott Co., Philadelphia, 1966.

STEIGMANN, F., "Are Laxatives Necessary?" *Amer. J. Nurs.*, **62**:90–93, Oct. 1962.

WHITE, D., "I Have an Ileostomy," *Amer. J. Nurs.*, **61**:51–52, May 1961.

Appendix A

MEDIC ALERT

The Medic Alert Foundation International is a charitable, nonprofit organization that provides a medical protection service for persons with any hidden

TABLE A–1 * MEDIC ALERT

If your medical problem is not listed below, state it clearly and concisely on the lines provided. The engraving of any one medical problem is included with your membership fee. Additional medical problems, or other engravings are charged at 75 cents a line (4 lines maximum with 14 letters or spaces per line).

Allergic to:

☐ Horse serum † ☐ Diabetic ☐ Heart condition ☐ Multiple
   (tetanus antitoxin) ☐ Epilepsy ☐ Taking anti-   sclerosis
☐ Tetanus toxoid ☐ Glaucoma   coagulants ☐ Scuba diver
☐ Penicillin ☐ Hemophilia ☐ Myasthenia ☐ Wearing
☐ Insect stings ☐ Neck breather   gravis   contact lenses
☐ Other . . . . ☐ Implanted pacemaker
☐ I am taking . . . .
☐ Medical condition or problem . . . .
. . . .
☐ Organ donor (Eyes) . . . . (Other) . . . .
   (Where to, if possible) . . . .
☐ Blood type (optional) AB ☐ A ☐ B ☐ O ☐; Negative ☐ Positive ☐
☐ Religion . . . .
☐ Other medical information, immunization records, etc. . . . .
. . . .
Blood type & immunization information checked for accuracy by doctors:
                                                                                     Yes ☐   No ☐
Signature of person submitting application . . . .

We suggest diabetics order stainless steel as they usually have an acid condition which can cause silver or gold to discolor.

All information will be filed in the Central Answering File and will appear on the medical wallet card presented with your emblem. The emblem will state only your MAJOR medical problem(s).

   † Horse serum is the allergen in tetanus antitoxin. Please check with your physician to verify whether you are allergic to tetanus antitoxin or tetanus toxoid or both.

   * Reprinted with permission of Medic Alert Foundation, Turlock, Calif. 95380.

medical problems that should be known in an emergency. Its purpose is to prevent tragic, even fatal mistakes in the course of administering aid to these people. The person wears a bracelet or pendant stating his immediate medical problem. He also carries a wallet card containing pertinent medical information. Medic Alert maintains a central file in its Turlock, California, headquarters with more detailed medical information and addresses of physicians and nearest relative of every member. The information is available to physicians and other

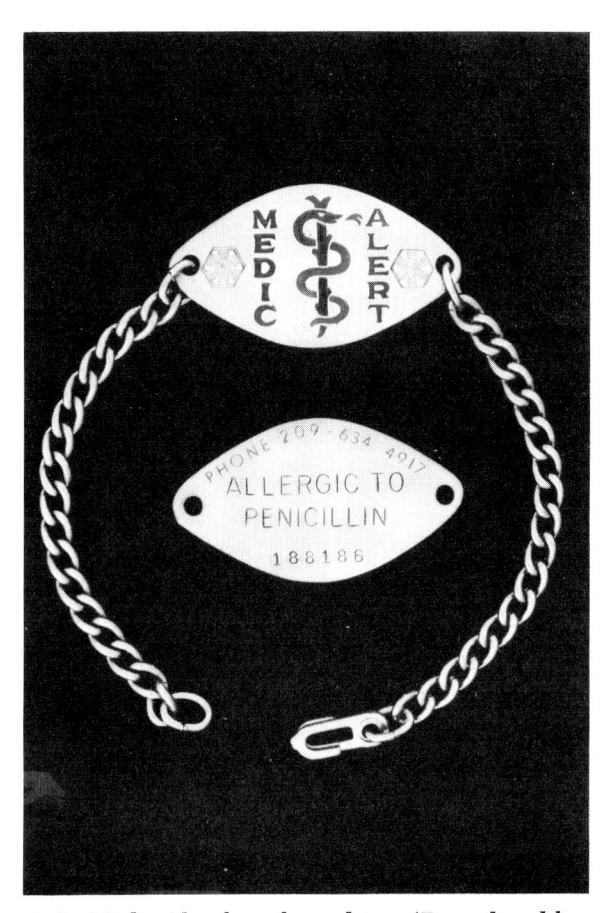

FIGURE A–1. Medic Alert bracelet and tag. (Reproduced by courtesy of Medic Alert Foundation, Turlock, Calif. 95380.)

authorized personnel 24 hours a day via collect telephone call. Medic Alert's telephone number is engraved on the bracelet or pendant. The foundation also maintains an organ-donor file. A potential donor wears a bracelet or pendant stating the organ he wishes to donate in case of emergency death.

Medic Alert's services are maintained through a one-time-only membership fee of $7.00. It is free to persons in need.

Appendix B

CLASSIFICATION OF MENTAL ILLNESS *

ACUTE BRAIN DISORDERS

THESE are the result of temporary, reversible, diffuse impairment of brain tissue function from which the patient recovers. The basic disturbance of the sensorium may release other disturbances, such as hallucinations, poorly organized, transient delusions, and behavior disturbances of varying degree.

1. Acute brain syndrome associated with intercranial infection
2. Acute brain syndrome associated with systemic infection
3. Acute brain syndrome, drug or poison intoxication
4. Acute brain syndrome, alcohol intoxication
5. Acute brain syndrome associated with trauma
6. Acute brain syndrome associated with circulatory disturbance
7. Acute brain syndrome associated with convulsive disorder
8. Acute brain syndrome associated with metabolic disturbance
9. Acute brain syndrome associated with intracranial neoplasm
10. Acute brain syndrome with disease of unknown or uncertain cause
11. Acute brain syndrome of unknown cause

CHRONIC BRAIN DISORDERS

These brain syndromes result from relatively permanent, more or less irreversible, diffuse impairment of cerebral tissue function.

1. Chronic brain syndrome associated with congenital cranial anomaly, congenital spastic paraplegia, mongolism, prenatal maternal infectious disease, birth trauma
2. Chronic brain syndrome associated with central nervous system syphilis (meningoencephalitic)
3. Chronic brain syndrome associated with central nervous system syphilis (meningovascular)

* Condensed from *Diagnostic and Statistical Manual: Mental Disorders,* American Psychiatric Association Mental Hospital Service, 1785 Massachusetts Avenue, N.W., Washington, D.C., 1952.

4. Chronic brain syndrome associated with other central nervous system syphilis
5. Chronic brain syndrome associated with intracranial infection other than syphilis
6. Chronic brain syndrome associated with intoxication
7. Chronic brain syndrome associated with brain trauma
8. Chronic brain syndrome associated with cerebral arteriosclerosis
9. Chronic brain syndrome associated with circulatory disturbance other than cerebral arteriosclerosis
10. Chronic brain syndrome associated with convulsive disorder
11. Chronic brain syndrome associated with senile brain disease
12. Chronic brain syndrome associated with other disturbance of metabolism, growth, or nutrition
13. Chronic brain syndrome associated with intracranial neoplasm
14. Chronic brain syndrome asociated with diseases of unknown or uncertain cause (includes multiple sclerosis, Huntington's chorea, Pick's disease, and others)
15. Chronic brain syndrome of unknown cause

MENTAL DEFICIENCY

Classified here will be cases presenting primarily a defect of intelligence existing since birth, without demonstrated organic brain diseases or known prenatal cause. Degree of intelligence will be specified as mild, moderate, or severe.

DISORDERS OF PSYCHOGENIC ORIGIN OR WITHOUT CLEARLY DEFINED PHYSICAL CAUSE OF STRUCTURAL CHANGE IN THE BRAIN

PSYCHOTIC DISORDERS

1. Involutional psychotic reactions
2. Affective reactions
   a. Manic depressive reaction, manic type
   b. Manic depressive reaction, depressed type
   c. Manic depressive reaction, other
   d. Psychotic depressive reaction
3. Schizophrenic reactions

A group of psychotic reactions characterized by disturbances in reality relationships and concept formations, with affective, behavioral, and intellectual disturbances in varying degrees.

   a. Schizophrenic reaction, simple type
   b. Schizophrenic reaction, hebephrenic type
   c. Schizophrenic reaction, catatonic type
   d. Schizophrenic reaction, paranoid type
   e. Schizophrenic reaction, acute undifferentiated type
   f. Schizophrenic reaction, chronic undifferentiated type

APPENDIXES

g. Schizophrenic reaction, schizoaffective type
h. Schizophrenic reaction, childhood type
i. Schizophrenic reaction, residual type

PARANOID REACTIONS

Characterized by persistent delusions, usually persecutory or grandiose. Emotional responses and behavior are consistent with the ideas held.

1. Paranoia
2. Paranoid state

PSYCHOPHYSIOLOGIC AUTONOMIC AND VISUAL DISORDERS

These reactions represent the visceral expression of affect that may be largely prevented from being conscious. There is involvement of organs and viscera innervated by the autonomic nervous system and not under voluntary control.

1. Psychophysiologic skin reaction
2. Psychophysiologic musculoskeletal reaction
3. Psychophysiologic respiratory reaction
4. Psychophysiologic cardiovascular reaction
5. Psychophysiologic hernia and lymphatic reaction
6. Psychophysiologic gastrointestinal reaction
7. Psychophysiologic genitourinary reaction
8. Psychophysiologic endocrine reaction
9. Psychophysiologic nervous system reaction
10. Psychophysiologic reaction of organs of special sense

PSYCHONEUROTIC DISORDERS

The chief characteristic of these disorders is "anxiety." Patients with psychoneurotic disorders do not exhibit gross distortion or falsification of external reality and they do not present gross disorganization of the personality.

1. Anxiety reaction
2. Dissociative reaction
3. Conversion reaction
4. Phobic reaction
5. Obsessive compulsive reaction
6. Depressive reaction
7. Psychoneurotic reaction, others

PERSONALITY DISORDERS

These disorders are characterized by developmental defects or pathologic trends in the personality structure, with minimal subjective anxiety, and little or no sense of distress.

1. Personality pattern disturbance
   a. Inadequate personality
   b. Schizoid personality
   c. Cyclothymic personality
   d. Paranoid personality
2. Personality trait disturbance
   a. Emotionally unstable personality
   b. Passive-aggressive personality
   c. Compulsive personality
   d. Personality trait disturbance, other
3. Sociopathic personality disturbance
   a. Antisocial reaction
   b. Dyssocial reaction
   c. Sexual deviation
4. Addiction
   a. Alcoholism
   b. Drug addiction
5. Special symptom reactions
   a. Transient situational personality disturbance
   b. Gross stress reaction
   c. Adult situational reaction
   d. Adjustment reaction of infancy
   e. Adjustment reaction of childhood
   f. Adjustment reaction of adolescence
   g. Adjustment reaction of late life

INDEX

INDEX

Abdominal distention, 523
Abdominoperineal resection, 538
Abducens nerve, 420
Accommodation, 480
Acetone, urine, 374
Acid ash diet, 198, 408
Acid-base regulation, 119–25
  buffers, 121
  carbonic acid:base bicarbonate, 121
  kidney regulation, 122
  metabolic regulation, 122
  respiratory regulation, 122–23
  tests, 125
Acid-citrate dextrose, anticoagulant, 144
Acidifiers for urine, 190, 198
Acidosis, 122
  calcium ionization, 134
  diabetes mellitus, 370–72, 387–88
  metabolic, 122
  respiratory, 123
  shock, 214
  symptoms, 123
  uremia, 178
Acoustic nerve, 422
Acromegaly, 346–47
Actinomycin C, 209
Action for Mental Health, 61
Activities of daily living, 398
Adaptation, eye, 480
Addiction, 53–58
  alcohol, 53–55
  drugs, 54–58
Addison's disease, 351–52
Adenocarcinoma, 91, 538
Adenosine triphosphate (ATP), 214
Adjunctive therapies, 44–46
  art, 46
  music, 45
  nursing responsibilities, 45–46
  occupational, 45

Adjunctive therapies (cont.)
  recreational, 45
Adler, Alfred, 64
Adrenal cortex, 349–53
Adrenal crisis, 351–52
Adrenal glands, 342, 343, 346, 349–53
  stress, 119
Adrenal medulla, 349
Adrenalectomy, 105
Adrenarche, 357
Adrenergic nervous system, 416–17
Adrenocorticotrophic hormone, 342, 343, 345, 346, 352
Adrenosterones, 350, 351
Affective disorders, 32
  nursing expectations, 32
Agglutinins in blood, 142
Agnosia, 403
Airway, maintenance in unconscious patient, 428
Albuminuria, glomerulonephritis, 187
  nephrotic syndrome, 188
Alcoholism, 53–55
  antabuse therapy, 55
  magnesium deficit, 134
  treatment, 54
Aldosterone, 119, 350–51
Alkali, 267
  absorption and alkalosis, 122
Alkaline ash diet, 198, 408
Alkalosis, 122
  calcium ionization, 134
Allergy, 326
Alpha-chymotrypsin, 491
Aluminum hydroxide gel (Amphogel), 198
Ambivalence, 29
Ambulation in heart disease, 259
Amenorrhea, 365
American Cancer Society, 92, 99, 105

567

INDEX

American Public Health Association, 80
Ametropia, 482
Amphetamines, 57
Amputation, 469–71
Anabolism, 88
Analgesics, burns, 151
   myocardial infarction, 265
   respiratory diseases, 337
Androgens, 343, 351, 389
Anemia, 293–95
   burns, 154, 160
   hemolytic, 295
   liver disease, 547
   nutritional, 293
   pernicious, 294
   uremia, 178
Anesthesia for eye surgery, 488
Aneurysm, cerebrovascular disease, 242, 446, 447
Angina pectoris, 244–46
Angiocardiography, 237
Angiography of cranial vessels, 425
Anions in fluid phases, 117
Ankylosis in neurologic-orthopedic difficulty, 405
Antacids, nonsystemic, 531
   systemic, 531
Anterior chest wall syndrome, heart disease, 260
Antiarrhythmic drugs, 270
Antibiotics, burns, 161
Antibodies in blood, 142
Anticancer drugs, 93–95
   alkylating agents, 95
   antimetabolites, 94
   hormones, 94
Anticoagulants, 267–68, 270–72, 533
   management of hypertension, 446
Anticonvulsants, 441–42
Antidepressants, 50–52
Antidiuretic hormone, 119, 347–48
Antigen-antibody response, 74–75
Antigens in blood, 142
Antihistamines, 184, 327
Antilymphocytic-globulin and kidney transplant, 207, 209
   heart transplant, 277
Antimetabolites for leukemia, 297
Antispasmodic drugs, disk problems, 476
   Parkinson's disease, 452
   prostate surgery, 194
   urinary colic, 197
Antistreptolysin titer, 241

Antithyroid drugs, 359–60
Antitoxin, tetanus, 152
Anuria, 169
Anxiety, degrees, 7–8
   psychoneuroses, 25–28
Apathy, 29
Aphakic eye, 491
Aphasia, 403
   increased intracranial pressure, 432
   receptive, 422
Apical pulse, cardiotonic glycosides, 269
Apnea, 315
Apoplexy. See Cerebrovascular disease
Appetite, 507
Apraxia, 403
Aqueous humor, 479
   glaucoma, 488
Arachidonic acid, 264
Arachnoid, 414
Aramine (metaraminol bitartrate), shock, 216
Armchair therapy, 257
Arrhythmias, 219–21
Arterial blood pressure, 231
Arterialization of veins, hemodialysis, 174
Arteriography, coronary arteries, 246
   kidneys, 189
   peripheral vascular disease, 285
Arteriosclerosis, 242
Arteriosclerosis obliterans, 278–80
Arteriotomy, 290
Arthritis, 471–74
Arthrodesis, 474
Arthroplasty, 474
Arthrotomy, 474
Artificial dialysis. See Hemodialysis; Peritoneal dialysis
Artificial eye, 486–87
Artificial kidney. See Hemodialysis
Ascites, 547, 550
Aspiration of bone marrow, 295
Associative looseness, 29
Asthma, 326–27
   cardiac, 251
Astigmatism, 482
Ataractic drugs, 47–50
   major tranquilizers, 48
   minor tranquilizers, 50
   side effects, 49–50
   tranquilizing effects, 47
Ataxia, interference in cerebellum, 417
Atelectasis, 328–29
   following urinary tract surgery, 202

Atherosclerosis, 242
Atrial fibrillation, 220
Aura, 437
Autistic thinking, 29
Autografts, burns, 163
　vascular surgery, 290
Automatic bladder, 409–10
Automatic nervous system, 416–17
　cardiac control, 219
Autonomous bladder, 409–10
Azathioprine (Imuran), heart transplant, 277
　kidney transplant, 207, 209
Azotemia, 172
Azuresin test, 521

Babinski sign, 420
Backache, pyelonephritis, 189
　slipped disk, 474
Bacteriuria, 181
Balanced traction, 464
Banish, 203
Barium enema, 521
　swallow, 521
Barnard, Christian, 276
Bartholin's glands, 84
Basal ganglia, 416
　Parkinson's disease, 452
Basal metabolic rate, 356
Basedow's disease, 358
Bathing, heart disease, 258
Beers, Clifford, 64
Behavior, 4
Belching, 526
Bell's palsy, 421–22
Bennett pressure cycled respirator, 277
Benzedrine, 57
Bicarbonate, deficit, 122
　excess, 122
　plasma, 125
Biceps reflex, 420
Bifocal lenses, 483
Bile, 517, 535, 542–43, 545
Biliary calculi, 543
Bini, 41, 64
Biochemical regulators, 342–92
　general suggestions for care, 345
　hormones, 342–45
　malfunction of endocrine glands, 346–88
Biopsy of prostate, 196
Bisacodyl (Dulcolax), 184

Bladder (urinary), 165
　autonomous, 409–10
　decompression, 192
　external sphincter, 170
　flaccidity, 409
　internal sphincter, 170
　irrigation, 409
　kidney transplant, 207
　reflex, 409–10
　removal, 202
　sphincter, 170–71
　training, 409
Blepharitis, 481
Bleuler, Eugene, 64
Blind spot, 480
Blindness, 491–95
Blood, administration, 141–45
　allergic reactions, 144
　anticoagulants, 144
　circulatory overloading, 144
　groups, 142
　hazards, 142
　hepatitis, 144
　incompatibility, 143
　potassium excess, 144
　clotting, 271
　cross matching, 143
　dyscrasias, 293–99
　filter unit, 140
　to kidneys, 165
　pH, 125
　prostate surgery, 194
　simultaneous multiple analysis, 137
Blood pressure, arterial, 231
　venous, 232
　See also Hypertension
Blood sugar, postprandial, 372
Blood urea nitrogen (B.U.N.), 182
Body cast, 459
Bone healing, 460
Bone marrow aspiration, 295
Bones of the ear, 496
Bowel training in neurologic-orthopedic difficulty, 410–11
Bowman's capsule, 166
Brain, 415–17
　circulation to, 415, 445
　scan, 425
　surgery, 432–36, 447
　thrombosis, 445
　vascular diseases, 444–50
Brainstem, 417
　surgery, 434

570] INDEX

Breast cancer, 101–108
  incidence, 101
Breast self-examination, 102–103
Bright's disease, 187–88
Bronchiectasis, 328
Bronchitis, 329
Bronchodilators, 326–27
Bronchogram, 313
Bronchoscopy, 313
Bronchospirometry, 313
Brown electric dermatome skin grafting, 163
Brudzinski's sign, 419
Buck's extension, 463
Buerger's disease, 280
  exercises in peripheral vascular disease, 287–88
Buffalo hump, Cushing's disease, 353
Buffers, 121
Burns, 148–64
  Brooke Army Medical Center formula in burn treatment, 155
  contractures, 164
  debridement, 161
  depth, 148
  dietary control, 158
  emergency care, 149, 152–53
  eschar, vaporization, heat loss, 159
  exposure, 162
  ice water treatment, 150
  infection, 160
  kidney output, 157
  negative nitrogen balance, 159
  occlusive dressings, 162
  percentage of involvement, 149
  phases, 154–64
  positioning, 159
  relief of pain, 160
  skin grafting, 163
  silver nitrate, 161
  tetanus immunization, 151
Busher automatic insulin injection, 386
Butter-sugar balls, 179

Cadaver, kidney, 207
Caffeine, 52
Caffeine sodium benzoate, 424, 432
Calcium, 133–34
  deficit, 133
    uremia, 178
  excess, 134
  restriction, calculi, 198

Calcium (cont.)
  stone, 198
Calcium phosphorus level in blood, 365
Calcium salts for tetany, 365–66
Calculi, 196–99
  calcium-containing, 198
  diagnosis, 197
  factors in formation, 197
  management, 198–99
  phosphate-containing, 198
  staghorn, 198
  symptoms, 197
  uric acid-containing, 198
Caloric test of equilibrium, 422
Calories, 506–10
Calycectomy, 199
Cancer, 88–109
  breast, 93–98
  peptic ulcer, 527
  prostate, 196
  thyroid, 358
Cancer detection, 92
  meaning to patient, 98–99
  Pap smear, 92
  seven warning signals, 93
Cannula and peritoneal dialysis, 176
Cannulation and hemodialysis, 173
Cantor tube, 523
Capillary fragility test, 295
Carbohydrate, solutions for venoclysis, 141
  uremia, 179
Carbon dioxide, combining power in diabetes mellitus, 373
  content in blood, 125
  pressure, 125
Carbonic acid:base bicarbonate buffer system, 121
Carcinoma, 91
Cardiac arrest, 216
Cardiac catheterization, 238
Cardiac disease, 214–76. See also Coronary disease
  cardiac surgery, 273–77
  coronary disease and proneness, 234–54
  emergency care, 216–33
  management, 255–72
  shock, 214–15
Cardiac monitor, 228, 230–31
Cardiac surgery, 273–77
Cardiogenic shock, 214
  myocardial infarction, 246

Cardiopulmonary bypass 273–77
Cardiopulmonary emergency, 214–33
Cardiotonic glycosides, 266, 269–70
Cardioversion, 223–26
Carpopedal spasms and calcium, 134
Castration, 196
Casts, 457–60
Catabolism, 88
Cataract, 490–91
Catecholamines, 241
  propranolol, 270
Cathartics, 268
Catheter, burns, 151
  care, 409
  Foley, 194
  suprapubic, 195
  three-way, 194
  uremia, 180–200
  ureteral, 197
Catheterization, burned patient, 157
  heart, 238
  infection, 181
  following urinary tract surgery, 201
Cation exchange resins, 178
Cation in fluid phase, 117
Cells, 88–90
  function, 88
  types, 88
Cell nutrition, principles of care, 520–21
Central hearing loss, 500–501
Cerebellum, 417
  surgery, 434
Cerebrospinal fluid, 415, 423
  leakage after craniotomy, 434
Cerebrovascular disease, 444–50
  causes, 445
  management, 446–50
  symptoms, 446
Cerletti, 41, 64
Cerumen, 496
Chalazion, 492
Chancre, 82
Charcot, Jean, 64
Chemical regulators, hormones, 342–45
Chest surgery, 337–39
  nursing observations, 338–39
Chest x-ray, 312
Cheyne-Stokes respirations, 251, 315
  increased intracranial pressure, 431
  stroke, 446
Chloride, reabsorption in ureteral intestinal anastomosis, 206
Choked disc, 420, 431

Cholecystectomy, 543
Choledocholithotomy, 543
Cholelithiasis, 543
  nursing care, 544
Cholesterol, 263–64
  blood, 241
  thyroid disease, 356
Cholinergic nervous system, 416–17
Choloxin, 358
Chordotomy, 477
Choroid, 479
Choroid plexuses, 415
Chvostek sign and tetany, 134, 365
Cigarette smoking and coronary artery disease, 235
Ciliary body, 479
Circ-O-Lectric bed, 164, 199, 404
Circulation time, 239–40
Circulatory overloading, 144
Cirrhosis of the liver, 549–50
Cisternal puncture, 424
Classification of mental illness, 560–63
Claudication in peripheral vascular disease, 283
Clean-catch urine specimen, 180
Clinitest tablets, 376
Clonic phase of convulsion, 437–38
Closed-angle glaucoma, 489
Closed-chest cardiac massage, 216–18
Clostridium botulism, 78
Clostridium tetani, 151
Codeine, 55
Colic and urinary calculi, 197
Collagen disease, 471
Collateral circulation, angina pectoris, 245–46
  myocardial infarction, 248
  peripheral vascular disease, 286
Colloids, burns, 155
  edema, 130
  solutions for venoclysis, 141
Color-blindness, 484
Colostomy, 538–41
  care, 537–41
  diet, 540
  double-barreled, 539
  home care, 540
  irrigations, 540
  urinary diversion procedures, 203–206
Coma, 419
Communication, neurologic-orthopedic difficulty, 402

Communication (cont.)
  process, 2–5
    nonverbal, 2
    verbal, 2
Compazine (prochlorperazine), 48
Compound fracture, 455
Compression of brain, 427
Compulsion, 27
Concussion, 427
Conductive hearing loss, 500
Cones, 479
Conflict, 9
Congestive heart failure, 250–54
  aldosterone, secretion, 250
  complication of myocardial infarction, 248
  events leading to, 250
  management, 255–72
  pulmonary edema, 251–53
  symptoms, 251–54
Coning, 424
Conjunctivitis, 480, 492
Conscious, 20
Consciousness, levels, 418–19
Constipation, 531
  barium enema, 521
  rejection crisis, 209
  treatment, 531
Contact lenses, 484
  cataract removal, 491
Contraction of fluid phase, 114
  uremia, 178
Contractures, amputations, 470
  burns, 159
  neurologic-orthopedic difficulty, 405
  prevention for the unconscious patient, 429
Contusion, 427
Conversion, 21
Convulsions, 428, 437–43
  uremia, 172
Convulsive disorders, 437–43
Corneal abrasion, 481
Corneal transplant, 492
Coronary arteriography, angina pectoris, 246
Coronary artery, occlusion, 246
Coronary care unit, 230–33
Coronary disease, 234–72. See also Cardiac disease
  angina pectoris, 244–46
  congestive heart failure, 250–54
  management, 255–77

Coronary disease (cont.)
  myocardial infarction, 246–50
  proneness, 242–44
Coronary insufficiency, 244
Corpus luteum, 389
Corticospinal tract, 417
Corticosteroids. See Steroids
Corticosterone, 350
Cortisol, 350
Cortisone, 350
Cough, 275, 315, 338
  congestive heart failure, 251
  medicine, 315
  technique, 275
Coumarin derivatives and anticoagulants, 271–72
Cranial nerves, 417, 420–22
Craniotomy, 433–36
Cranium, increased pressure, 430
Creatine phosphokinase (CPK), 241
Crutch walking, 467–69
Crutchfield tongs, 426
Cryogenic surgery, 453
Cryosurgery, cataract, 491
  retinal detachment, 493
Culture and food, 506–508
Culture of urine, 190
Cushing's disease, 352–53
Cushingnoid features, 353
Cutaneous transplant for urinary diversion, 205
Cutaneous uterostomy appliance, 205
Cycle of infection, 79
Cycloplegia, 482
Cycloplegic drugs, 487
Cystectomy, 200, 202
Cystitis, 191
Cystogram, 185
Cystolithotomy, 198
Cystoscope, 186
Cystoscopy, 185
  calculi, 197
Cystostomy tube, 195
Cytomel, 358

Deafness, 500–501
Debridement in burns, 161
Decompression drainage, bladder, 192
Decortication, 337
Decubitus ulcers, neurologic-orthopedic difficulty, 403–404
Dederick, Chuck, 56

Defense mechanisms (mental mechanisms), 21-22
Defibrillator, 223-26
Deficiency diseases, 511
Degenerative arthritis, 472
Degenerative kidney disease, 186
Dehydration, 114, 126
　increased intracranial pressure, 432-33
　ketoacidosis, 371
　peritoneal dialysis, 177
　uremia, 178
Delirium tremens, 54
Delusion, 28
Demerol (meperidine), 55
Denial, 21
Dependent edema, 131
Depressants, 56
Depression, 33
　endogenous, 34-35
　neurotic, 34-35
　reactive, 34-35
Dermis, burns, 148
Desiccated thyroid, 358
Developmental tasks, 11-19
Dexedrine, 51
Dextran for burns, 155
Diabetes insipidus, 348
Diabetes mellitus, 367-88
　description, 368
　diabetic emergency, 387-88
　diagnosis, 372-74
　diet, 377-80
　distribution, 369
　insulin, 380-99
　management, 375-83
　special needs, 387-88
　stages, 369-71
　teaching the patient, 374-88
Diabetic acidosis, 387-88
Diabetic coma, 370-72
Diabetic microangiopathy, surgical treatment, 351
Dialysate for peritoneal dialysis, 173, 176
Dialysis. See Hemodialysis; Peritoneal dialysis
Dianeal, 176
Diarrhea and rejection crisis, 209
Diet, heart disease, 261-65
　peptic ulcer, 528-30
　　bland, 528-29
　　Meulengracht, 530
　　Sippy, 530
Dietetic foods, 380

Diffusion, 118
　dialysis, 173
Digitalis, 266
　preparations, 269-70
　cardiotoxicity, 269
Digitalization, 269
Dilantin, 270, 441
Diplopia, 421, 449
Dip-stick test of urine, 182
Disk, rupture, 474-78
Disposable bags, urinary diversion procedures, 203
Diuresis, burns, 160
　following kidney transplant, 208
Diuretic phase of uremia, 178
Diuretics for uremia, 178
Diversion, heart disease, 260
　urinary procedures, 202-206
Dix, Dorothea, 64
Donor, kidney transplant, 206
Draft Act, 59
Drains for serous drainage, 201
Drug addiction (abuse), 55-58
　categories of substances, 55
　factors in addiction, 53-55
　nursing implications, 57
Dumping syndrome, 536
Dura mater, 414
Dysphagia, 403
Dyspnea, 315
　congestive heart failure, 251
　congestive heart syndrome, 257
Dysuria, 169

Ear, 496-501
　anatomy, 496
　care of patient, 499-500
　foreign bodies, 497
　surgery, 497-501
Ear drum, 496
Echoencephalography, 425
Ecology, 72
Ectopic beat of heart, 220
Edema, 130-31
　burns, 154, 160
　cerebral, 434, 445
　congestive heart failure, 253-54
　Cushing's disease, 353
　glomerulonephritis, 187, 188
　nephrotic syndrome, 188
　refractory, 131
　respiratory tract, 151-52

Edema (cont.)
  uremia, 179
Edema control in heart disease, 257
Ejaculate, 191
Elavil (amitriptyline hydrochloride), 51
Electrocardiography, 221–23
Electroencephalography, 425, 441
Electrolyte, 112
  body secretions and excretions, 135
  chemical combining, 116
  measurement, 115–16
  milliequivalent value, 116
  movement, 118
Electrolyte hormone, 350
  stress response, 119
Electrolyte ice chips, 158
Electrolyte solutions, oral for burns, 158
  venoclysis, 141
Elimination in heart disease, 258–59
Embolism, air, 142
  brain, 445
  defibrillation, 225
Emmetropia, 482
Emphysema, 329–33
  barrel chest, 330
  complications, 331–32
  exercises, 332
Endarterectomy, 447
  angina pectoris, 246
  peripheral vascular disease, 290–92
Endocrine glands, 342–92. See also
  Biochemical regulators
Endometrium, 389
Enemas, craniotomy, 435
  heart attack, 259
Enteral fluid replacement, 139
Enucleation, 486
Enzyme tests in heart disease, 241–42
Epidermis in burns, 148
Epilepsy, 439–43
Epinephrine, 349
Epistaxis in uremia, 172
Epitheliazation and burn healing, 155, 161
Equanil (meprobamate), 50
Equilibrium, water and electrolytes, 112
Equivalent value of electrolytes, 116
Eructation, 526
Erythrocyte binding, 355
Eschar in burns, 148, 155, 161
Estradiol, 351
Estrogen, 343, 389
Eustachian tube, 496

Exchange list plan in diabetes mellitus, 377–80
Excretory urography, 184
Exercises, amputation, 470
  bedridden patients, 466–67
  burns, 164
  following mastectomy, 106–107
  peripheral vascular disease, 287
Exophthalmic goiter, 358
Exophthalmos, 359
Expansion of fluid phase, 114
Expressive aphasia, 403
External respiration, 309
Extracellular fluid, 114
Extracellular phase, 126, 127, 130
Extracorporeal circulation, 273
Extradural hematoma, 427
Extrapyramidal tract, 416
Extrinsic factor, 293
Extrinsic muscles, 479
Exudate from burns, 115
Eye, 479–95
  accommodation, 480
  anatomy, 479
  care, 485
  diseases, 488–94
  emergency, 485
  examination, 420, 480
  surgery, 487
  unconscious patient, 429

Facial nerve, 421
Farsightedness, 482
Fat, allowance in uremia, 179
  dietary restriction, 263–65
  polyunsaturated, 263
  saturated, 263
Fat-soluble vitamins, 542
Fatty plaques, 242
Fear, 8
Federal Bureau of Narcotics, 55
Feedback mechanism, 343–45, 351
Feeding, heart disease, 258
Fibrillation, 220
Field of vision, tests, 484
Fingerprinting, 129
First-degree burns, 148
Fishberg concentration test, 183
Fistulation and hemodialysis, 173
Fixed traction, 464
Flank incision, shave, 199
Flatus, 532

Fluid allowance, calculi, 198
  chronic renal disease, 178
  glomerulonephritis, 187
  pyelonephritis, 190
  unconscious patient, 429
  urinary diversion procedures, 205
Fluid and electrolyte, 112–212
Fluid phase, cations and anions, 117
  contraction, 114
  expansion, 114
Fluid replacement, 137–47
Fluid shift in burns, 154
Follicle-stimulating hormone, 347
Fomite, 72
Food poisoning, 78
Foot care and peripheral vascular disease, 286
Foot drop, 407
Foreign bodies, eye, 486
  ear, 497
Four-point gait, 468
Fovea centralis, 480
Fractures, 455–56
  emergency treatment, 456
  immobilization, 457
  skull, 427
Franklin, Benjamin, 63
Freezing techniques for surgery, 453
Frequency of urination, 169
Freud, Sigmund, 43, 64
Frontal lobe, 416
Functional hearing loss, 500
Fundus of eye, 420, 481
Fusion of spinal vertebrae, 477

Gaits and crutch walking, 468
Gallbladder, 542–44
Gallbladder series, 542
Gangrene, diabetes mellitus, 368
  peripheral vascular disease, 283
Gastric analysis, 521
Gastric gavage, 139
Gastric obstruction, 533
Gastroenterostomy, 535
Gastrointestinal decompression, 522
  therapeutic uses, 523
Gastrointestinal series, 521
Gastrointestinal tract, anatomy and physiology, 512–19
Gastrointestinal ulcers in uremia, 172
Gastroscopy, 522
Gigantism, 346

Glaucoma, 488–90
Glioma, 430
Global aphasia, 403
Glomerular filtration, 168
Glomerulonephritis, 187–88
Glomerulus, 166
Glossopharyngeal nerve, 422
Glucagon, 367, 368
Glucocorticoids, 243, 350
Glucola, 373
Gluconeogenesis, 367
Glucose, effect of insulin, 367
  protein sparer, 127
  urine, 374
  by vein for burns, 155
Glucose tolerance tests, 372–73
Glycolipids (triglycerides), 263
Glycosides, cardiotonic, 269–70
Goiter, 356–57
Goldblatt phenomenon, 188
Gonadotropic hormone, 347, 389
Gonorrhea, 84
Gout, 198
Gouty arthritis, 473
Grafting, burns, 155, 161
  decubitus ulcers, 405
  vascular surgery, 290–91
Grand mal convulsion, 437
Granulation tissue, bone healing, 460
  burns, 155
Grave's disease, 356
Gray matter of brain, 415
Greenstick fracture, 455
Grief, 9–10
  neurologic-orthopedic disability, 401–402
Group therapy, 43–44
Growth hormone, 346–47

Hallucination, 28
Hallucinogens, 57
Havinghurst, Robert, 11
Head injuries, 427
Headache, craniotomy, 435
  increased intracranial pressure, 431
Heaf test, 334
Hearing impairment, 500–501
Hearing scotomas, 422
Heart attack. *See* Myocardial infarction
Heart blocks, 220
Heart disease, 234–72. *See also* Coronary disease

Heart-lung machine, 273
Heart transplant, 276
Heartburn, 526
Heat exhaustion, 128
Heatstroke, 129
Heberden's nodes, 472
Hematogenic shock, 214
Hematoma, extradural, 427
   subdural, 427
Hematuria, 172
   malignant growth, 185
   prostate surgery, 194
Heminephrectomy, 199
Hemiparesis and cerebrovascular disease, 432, 444
Hemispheres of the brain, 415
Hemodialysis, 173–76
Hemodilution and prostate surgery, 194
Hemolysis from blood administration, 141–43
Hemolytic anemia, 295
Hemophilia, 295
Hemorrhage, gastric, 532
   liver disease, 547
   thyroid surgery, 363
   urinary surgery, 201
Hemorrhoidectomy, 553–54
Hemorrhoids, 553
Hemostatic device for prostate surgery, 195
Heparin, 271, 545
Hepatic fetor, 546
Hepatitis, viral, 144, 550–52
Hernia, 554–55
Herniation, brain stem, 424
   nucleus pulposis, 475
Heroin, 55
High-threshold substances, 168
Hirsutism and Cushing's disease, 353
Histamine, inflammatory response, 153
   tests, peripheral vascular disease, 284
   pheochromocytoma, 349
History, care of the mentally ill, 63–65
Hodgkin's disease, 298
Homan's sign, 281
Homeokinesis, 112
Homeostasis, 112
Homograft, kidney transplant, 206
   bed, 208
   burns, 64
Homologous serum jaundice, 144
Hordeolum, 492

Hormone, imbalance, 342–92
   male and orchiectomy, 196
Hospitalization of the mentally ill, 59–60
Hubbard tank, 404
Human chorionic gonadotropin, 348
Hunger, 507
Hyaluronidase with hypodermoclysis, 139
Hydraulic lift, 400
Hydrochloric acid, 512
   gastric analysis, 521
   peptic ulcer, 525–26
Hydrocortisone, 350
Hydrogen, acid base regulation, 119–22
Hydrogen acceptor, 120
Hydrogen donor, 120
Hydronephrosis, 190
Hydroureter, 190
Hypercalcemia, 366
Hyperglycemia, 387
Hyperopia, 482
Hyperparathyroidism, 366
Hyperplasia of endocrine glands, 345
Hypertension (renal), 188
   coronary artery disease, 244
   Cushing's syndrome, 353
   Goldblatt phenomenon, 189
   glomerulonephritis, 187
   kidney transplant, 208
Hyper-Tet, 152
Hyperthermia following craniotomy, 435
Hyperthyroid crisis, 363–64
Hyperthyroidism, 358–64
Hypertonic solutions, 119
   dehydrating regime, 432
   eye surgery, 487
   glaucoma, 489
Hypertrophic arthritis, 472
Hypertrophy of endocrine glands, 345
Hypocalcemia, 132, 134, 365
Hypodermoclysis, 139
Hypoglossal nerve, 422
Hypoglycemia, 383
Hypoglycemic drugs, 386–87
Hypogonadism, 390
Hypoparathyroidism, 365
Hypophysectomy, 106, 348
   diabetes mellitus, 368
Hypophysis, 346–48
Hypoplasia of endocrine glands, 345
Hypostatic pneumonia, 202
Hypothalamus, 416
   hormone production, 344
   stress response, 119

Hypothermia, 273, 447
  blanket, craniotomy, 435
  thyroid storm, 363
  cold blood, 145
Hypothyroidism, 357–58
Hypotonic solutions, 119
Hypovitaminosis, 547–48
Hypovolemic shock, 215

Ice chips (electrolyte), 158
Ice water treatment for burns, 150
Idiopathic epilepsy, 439
Ileal bladder, 202
Ileal conduit, 202
Ileostomy, 539
Illusion, 28
Imferon, 294
Immobility, complication, 197, 259, 408, 435
Immunity, 75
Immunization for tetanus, 151
Immunologic agents, 75–76
Immunologic kidney disease, 186
Immunosuppressive drugs, heart transplant, 277
  kidney transplant, 207–209
Impersol, 176
Imuran, 207, 209, 277
Incontinence of urine, 172
  unconscious patient, 429
Incus, 496
Indanedione derivative, 271–72
Infarction, brain, 444
  myocardium. *See* Myocardial infarction
Infection, 73
  burns, 160
  endemic, 76
  epidemic, 76
  peritoneal dialysis, 177
  urinary tract with calculi, 199
Infectious kidney disease, 186
Infectious mononucleosis, 298
Inflammation, steroid suppression of, 350
Inflammatory process, 74
Inflammatory response, 153
  myocardial infarction, 247
Influenza, 327
Infratentorial structures, 415
  tumors, 430, 433
Insensible water loss, 114

Insulin, 343, 367–68, 380–88
  administration, 381–86
  antagonists, 368
  exercises, 382
  reaction, 383
  stress, 382
  syringe, 383–84
    automatic injector, 386
Intake and output record, 158
  burns, 158
  uremia, 178
Intensive care unit. *See* Coronary care unit
Intermittent claudication in peripheral vascular disease, 283, 287
Internal capsule, 416
Internal fixation of bone, 461
Internal respiration, 309
Interstitial cell–stimulating hormone, 347
Interstitial fluid, 114
Intestinal obstruction, 537–41
Intoxication from water, 129
Intracellular fluid, 114
Intracellular phase, magnesium, 134
  potassium, 131–33
Intracranial pressure, increased, 430–36
Intracranial surgery, complications, 435
Intraocular pressure, 482
  glaucoma, 489
Intravascular fluid, 114
Intravenous fluids for burns, 155
Intravenous glucose tolerance test, 373
Intravenous pyelography, 184
Intravenous replacement, 139
  air embolism, 142
  calculation, 139
  hazards, 141–45
  speed shock, 141
  systemic reactions, 141
  thrombophlebitis, 141
  types of solutions, 141
Intrinsic factor, 293, 536
Intrinsic muscles, 479
Iodide in dyes, 184
Iodine, angina pectoris, 246
  goiter, 357
  hyperthyroidism, 359
  protein-bound iodine, 354
  radioactive uptake test, 354–55
  thyroid disease, 353
  trapping by thyroid gland, 354
Ionization, 95–96
  alpha, beta, gamma rays, 95

578]   INDEX

Ionization (cont.)
　control, 96
　hazard, 96–97
　nursing instructions, 97–98
Iridectomy, 490
　cataract, 491
Iridencleisis, 490
Iris, 479
Iron content in foods, 293
Iron-deficiency anemia, 293
Iron-dextran injection, 296
Iron preparations, 294
Irradiation of thyroid, 360
Ischemia, 243
　angina pectoris, 244
　brain, 444
　Goldblatt phenomenon, 189
　myocardial infarction, 246
Ischemic injury to cadaver kidney, 207
Ischemic nephrosclerosis, 186
Isolation, burns, 162
　kidney transplant, 208
Isolator, Life-Island, 209
Isoniazid, 334–35
Isotonic solutions, 119
Isotopes, 96
　half-life, 96

Jacksonian convulsions, 438
Jaundice, 546
Joint range of motion, 465–66
　burns, 164
Jones, Maxwell, 6
Jung, Carl, 64

Kayexalate, 178
Kennedy, John F., 61
Keratitis, 492
Keratoplasty, 492
Kernig's sign, 419
Ketoacidosis, 387–88
　diabetes mellitus, 370–72
Kidneys, 165–66
　disease, 186–90
　drugs toxic, 190
　involvement in neurologic-orthopedic
　　difficulty, 408–409
　ischemia, 188
　transplants, 173, 206
Kiil artificial kidney, 174
Kline and Kahn test, 83

Knee-jerk reflex, 420
Kolff artificial kidney, 174
Korsakoff's psychosis, 55
Kraepelin, Emil, 64

Lactic dehydrogenase enzyme (LDH),
　241
Lactogenic hormone, 347
Laminectomy, 477–78
Large intestine, 518–19
Laryngeal nerve, 353
　injury, 363
Laryngectomy, 324
Lasègue's sign, 475
Lateral position in bed, 408
Laws of physics, 311
L-dopa, 452
Leads for electrocardiography, 221
Lee-White test and use of heparin, 271
Lenses, 483–84
Leukemia, 91, 296
Levin tube, 521
　cytologic examination, 522
　decompression, 623
　irrigation, 534
　postoperative use, 534
Levophed (levarterenol bitartrate), 216
Librium (chlordiazepoxide), 50
Lidocaine (Xylocaine), 270
Life-Island isolator, 209
Ligation of veins, 289
Linoleic acid, 264
Lip reading, 501
Lipids, 263
Lipoproteins, 263
Liquid ostomy soap, 204
Lithium carbonate, 52
Litholopaxy, 198
Lithotrite, 198
Liver, 544–52
　biopsy, 549
　functions, 545
　tests, alkaline phosphatase, 549
　　bromsulphalein, 548–49
　　icterus index, 548
　　urobilinogen, 548
　　van den Berg's test, 548
Lobectomy, 337
Lockjaw, 151
Low back pain, 475
Low-residue diet, 184–85
Lues, 81

Lugol's solution, 360
Lumbar air encephalography, 424
Lumbar puncture, 423-24
Lumbar sympathectomy, 289
Luteinizing hormone, 347
Luteotropic hormone, 347
Lymphedema, 105
Lymphocytic leukemia, 296

Magnesium, 134-35
  deficit, 134
  excess, 135
Magnesium sulfate, saturated solution, 432
Malleus, 496
Mammeotropic hormone, 347
Mammography, 101
Mandelic acid, 408
Mannitol, 432
Mantoux tests, 334
Manual manipulation of spine, 477
Margarine, 264
Marihuana, 55
Marplan (isocarboxazide), 51
Mastectomy (radical), 103-105
  postoperative care, 104
  preoperative care, 104
  prosthesis, 105
Mastoid cell infection, 498
Mastoidectomy, 498
Mechanical pumps and cardiac surgery, 277
Mechanical traction, 461
Medic Alert, 555
Medic Alert Foundation, 556
Meduna, 41, 64
Melanocyte-stimulating hormone, 347
Melanoma, 91
Melena, 532-33
Mellaril (thioridazine), 48
Mendelian trait in diabetes mellitus, 369
Meningeal irritation, 419
Meninges, 414-15
Meningioma, 430
Menninger, Karl, 33
Menopause, 390
Menstrual cycle, 389
Menstruation, 365
Mental health, criteria, 19
Mental illness, 19, 25-39
Mental status, 419
  increased intracranial pressure, 432

Mesantoin, 441
Mesmer, Franz, 63
Metabolic acidosis. *See* Acid-base regulation
Metabolic alkalosis. *See* Acid-base regulation
Metabolic basal rate, 356
  diabetes mellitus, 368
Metastases, 90
Methadone, 55
Methionine, 198
Methylphenylethyl hydantoin, 441
Metrazol (pentylenetetrazol), 41
Microangiopathy in diabetes mellitus, 368, 376
Microorganisms, 73
Midstream collection of urine, 181
Miller-Abbott tube, 523
Milliequivalent value of electrolytes, 116
Mineralocorticoids, 343, 350
Miotic drugs, 487
Mixed aphasia, 403
Monitor, 228, 230-31
Moniz, Egas, 64
Monoamine oxidase, 241
Monocytic leukemia, 296
Mononucleosis, 298
Mood lability, 419
Morphine sulfate, addiction, 55
  brain involvement, 433
  after brain surgery, 434
  burns, 160
Motor aphasia, 403
Motor function tests, 419
Motor neuron, flaccidity, 411
  spasms, 411
Motor strip of brain, 416
Mouth-to-mouth breathing, 216-18
Multiple glass test for urine, 180
Multiple sclerosis, 453-54
Mydriatic drugs, 482, 487
Myelocytic leukemia, 296
Myelography, 424-25, 476
Myocardial infarction, 246-50, 255
  complications, 249
  drugs, 265-72
  electrocardiogram, 248-49
  laboratory studies, 248
  management, 255-72
  pain, 247
  symptoms, 247
Myocardium, 132
Myopia, 482

INDEX

Myringoplasty, 498
Myringotomy, 498
Myxedema, 357, 364

Narcotic abuse, 55–56
Nardil (phenylzine dihydrosulfate), 51
Nasogastric feeding, 140
    after brain surgery, 434
National Association of Mental Health, 65
Nearsightedness, 482
Necrotic tissue, burns, 163
    myocardial infarction, 248
Negative nitrogen balance, 159
    steroids, 350
Nembutal (pentobarbital), 56
Nephrectomy, 199, 202
Nephrolithotomy, 198
Nephron, 166
Nephropathy, diabetes mellitus, 368
Nephroptosis, 165
Nephrostomy tube, 200
Nephrotic syndrome, 188
Nerve(s), autonomic, 416–17
    cranial, 417, 420–22
    deafness, 500
    regeneration, 413
Nervous system, anatomy, 413–18
Neurillema, 412
Neurohormone, 344
Neurologic disease, 451–54
Neurologic emergency, 425–28
Neurologic evaluation, 418–25
Neurologic-orthopedic continuity, 396–504
Neurology, 396–454, 479–504
Neuron, 413
Neuropathy in diabetes mellitus, 368
Niamid (nialamid), 51
Nitroglycerin, angina pectoris, 244, 245
Nocturia, 169
Nonelectrolytes, 112
Nonprotein nitrogen test (N.P.N.), 182
Norepinephrine, 349
Nuchal rigidity, 419, 428
Nurse-patient relationships, 5
Nutrament, 159
Nystagmus, 421–22

Obesity, 508
    treatment, 509–10

Obligatory water loss, 114
Obsession, 27
Obstructive uropathy, 190–99
Occipital lobe, 416
Occlusive dressings, burns, 162
Occult blood, 522
Oculist, 40
Oculomotor nerve, 420
Olfactory nerve, 420
Oligomenorrhea, 365
Oliguria, 169
    phase of uremia, 172, 178
Oophorectomy, 105, 199
Open-angle glaucoma, 489
Ophthalmologist, 480
Optic nerve, 420, 480
Optician, 480
Optometrist, 480
Oral contraceptives, 391–92
Oral hygiene, 297, 320, 534
Orchiectomy, 196, 199
Organ of Corti, 496
Organic brain disorders, 37–39
    acute, 37
    nursing expectations, 38–39
    organic, 37
Orthopedics, 455–78
    amputation, 469
    arthritis, 471
    casts, 457
    crutch walking, 467
    emergency treatment, 456
    injury, 455
    joint range of motion, 467
    ruptured intervertebral disk, 474
    traction, 461
Orthopnea, congestive heart syndrome, 257
Oscillometer, measurement of pulse volume, 285
Oscilloscope, 231
Osmitrol, 432
Osmosis, 118
    dialysis, 173, 174
Osmotic pressure, 118
Ossiculoplasty, 498
Osteoarthritis, 472
Osteoporosis, 461
Otitis media, 496
Otologist, 496
Otosclerosis, 498
Ototoxic drugs, 497
Ovariectomy, 105

Ovaries, hormone production, 347, 389
  hyperthyroidism, 358
  menstruation, 365
  panhypopituitarism, 348
Overhydration, 130
  peritoneal dialysis, 177
Oxidation, 113
Oxygen, cardiac disease, 257
  respiratory illness, 316
Oxytocin, 343, 347

Pacemaker, 226–30
Packing for prostate surgery, 195
Pain, intractable, 100
  ulcer, 526
Palsy, 451–53
Pancreas, 343, 367
Pancreatic enzymes, 517
Panhypopituitarism, 348
Papilledema, 420
  increased intracranial pressure, 431
Para-aminosalicylic acid, 334–35
Paracentesis, congestive heart failure, 253
  liver disease, 547, 550
Paraffin treatment, 473
Paraldehyde, 47
Paralysis agitans, 451
Paralytic ileus, gastric surgery, 532
  urinary surgery, 202
Paraplegia, 408
Parasympathetic nervous system, 416–17
  myocardial infarction, 247
Parathyroid gland, 365–66
  thyroid surgery, 363
Parenchyma, 166
Parenteral replacement, 139
Parietal lobe, 416
Parkinson's disease, 416, 451–53
Paroxysmal nocturnal dyspnea, 251
Pathologic fracture, 455
Pearly plaques, 242
Pectoralis muscles, 103
Pelvic belts, 461
Penrose drain, 201
  prostate surgery, 195
Peptic ulcer, 525–36
Perforation, gastric, 532
Pericardial sac, tapping, 253
Pericarditis, 248
Perineal prostatectomy, 196
Peripheral vascular disease, 278–92
  description, 278–83

Peripheral vascular disease (cont.)
  diagnostic tools, 283–85
  management, 285–92
  symptoms, 283–85
Peripheral vision, tests, 484
Peritoneal dialysis, 176
Peritonitis, 204, 532
Pernicious anemia, 294
Personality development (psychosocial, psychosexual), Erikson, 22
  Freud, S., 22
  Sullivan, H., 22
Personality structure, id, ego, superego, 20–21
Petit-mal convulsions, 438
pH, 119–24
  alkaline of body, 165
  urine, 181
  calculi, 196
Phantom sensation, 470
Phenobarbital, 441
Phenolamines, 343
Phenolsulfonphthalein test (P.S.P.), 182
Phenothiazines, 48–50
Pheochromocytoma, 349
pHisoHex for burns, 161
Phlebothrombosis, 280
Phlebotomy, congestive heart failure, 253
Phobia, 27
Phosphate-containing stone, 198
Phthisis, 333
Physiatrist, 396
Physical examination for heart disease, 237
Pia mater, 414
Pill rolling and Parkinson's disease, 451
Pinel, Philippe, 63
Pink eye, 492
Pitting edema, 131
Pituitary gland, 342, 343–44, 346–48
  excision in diabetes mellitus, 368
  gonadotropic hormones, 389
  stress response, 119
Plantar reflex, 420
Plaques, 242
Plasma and viral hepatitis, 144
Pleurisy, 309
Pneumoencephalogram, 424
Pneumonectomy, 337
Pneumonia, 329
Polypeptides, 343
Polyunsaturated fats, 264
Polyuria, 170

Pomeroy syringe and ear infection, 497
Pons, 418
Position, peripheral vascular disease, 287
 test, 284
Positions for bed, 407–408
Postprandial blood sugar test, 372
Postshock phase in burns, 160
Postural drainage exercise, 317–19
Potassium, alkalosis, 122–23
 burns, 155
  depletion, 160
 deficit, 132
 elevation, inflammatory process, 154
  uremia, 178
 excess, 133
 loss following surgery, 206
Potassium salts, 270
Prednisone, heart transplant, 277
 kidney transplant, 277
Pressure changes, intrapulmonic, 310
 intrathoracic, 310–11
Pressure dressings for burns, 162
Probenecid (Benemid), 198
Procaine amide (Pronestyl), 270
Proctoclysis, 139
Profound hypothermia, 273
Progesterone, 351, 389
Progestins, 343, 351
Progressive neurologic disease, 445–54
Projection, 22
Prolactin, 347
Proliferation, 88
Prone position, 407
Propranolol (Inderal), 270
Proptosis, 359
Prostate hypertrophy, diagnosis, 191–92
 symptoms, 191
 treatment, 192–96
Prostate surgery, 195
Prostatectomy, radical for malignancy, 196
 surgical procedures, 192–96, 200
Prostatic secretion, 191
Prostatic washings, 180
Prostatism, 191–96
Prosthesis, amputation of limb, 471
Protein allowance, liver disease, 551
 restriction in glomerulonephritis, 187
 solutions for venoclysis, 141
 sparer, 127
 uremia, 179
Protein-bound iodine, 354
Proteins in hormones, 343

Prothrombin time, 271
 heart disease, 241
Protoscopy, 522
Psychiatric nursing, general principles, 23–24
Psychoanalysis, 43
Psychomotor convulsion, 438–39
Psychoneuroses, 25–28
Psychophysiologic autonomic and visceral disorders, 36–37
Psychoses, 28–33
Psychotherapy, 42–43, 327, 555–56
Psychotropic drugs, 46–52
Ptosis, 221, 481
Pulmonary artery, veins, 309
Pulmonary edema, burns, 160
 congestive heart failure, 251–53
Pulmonary volumes, 313
Pulp traction, 462
Pulse rate, increased intracranial pressure, 431
 peripheral vascular disease, 284–85
Pump oxygenation, 273
Pupil, 479
Puritus, uremia, 173, 180
Pyelolithotomy, 198
Pyelonephritis, 189–90
Pyramidal tract, 417
Pyuria, 172

Quadriplegia, 408
Queckenstedt test, 423
Quinidine sulfate, 270

Radiation sickness, thyroid gland irradiation, 360
Radical perineal prostatectomy, 203
Radioactive iodine uptake test, 354
Radioactive isotopes, brain tumors, 433
Radioactive materials, safety precautions, 95–98, 361
Radioactive triiodothyronine erythrocyte uptake test, 355
Radioiodine (I^{131}) and urinary function, 184
Radioisotope uptake of brain, 425
Radiologic examination, 237
Radiorenography, 184
Range-of-motion exercises, 465–66
 burns, 164
 calculi, 198

Rationalization, 21
Rauwolfia derivatives, 47–48
Raynaud's disease, 280
Reach to recovery, 105
Reaction formation, 22
Reactive hyperemia test, peripheral vascular disease, 284
Receptive aphasia, 422, 430
Reciprocal arm movement, 448
Rectal examination, 191
Reflex, 412, 420
Reflex bladder, 409–10
Refraction, 482
Refractory edema, 131
Regression, 21
Regitine test for pheochromocytoma, 349
Regression, 21
Regular insulin, 381
Rehabilitation, 396–412
 cerebrovascular disease, 447–50
Rejection of kidney, 206, 209–10
Renal arteriography, 189
Renal disease, chronic, 178
Renal function tests, 182–86
Renal hypertension, 188
Renal involvement in neurologic-orthopedic difficulty, 408
Renal parenchyma, 166, 201
Repression, 21
Reserpine (serpasil), management of hypertension, 446
 treatment of mental illness, 48
Respirations in uremia, 173, 178
Respirator, Bennett, 277
Respiratory arrest, 216
Respiratory interference, 315
 general measures, 324–25
 nursing care, 315
Respiratory obstruction, burns, 151
 thyroid surgery, 363
Respiratory rate, 309
Respiratory system, 306–40
 structures, 306–307
Resuscitation, 216
Retention catheter, neurologic-orthopedic difficulty, 409
Retina, 479
Retinal detachment, 493–94
Retinopathy in diabetes mellitus, 368
Retrograde pyelography, 186
Retropubic prostatectomy, 195
Reusch, Jurgen, 2

Reverse isolation, burns, 162
 kidney transplant, 208
Rh-Hr system in blood, 142
Rheumatic heart disease and antistreptolysin titer, 241
Rheumatoid arthritis, 471
Rhizotomy, 477
Ringer's solution for burns, 155
Ritalin, 51
Rods, 479
Roentgens, 96
Role, modification, 402
Romberg test, 419
Rotating tourniquets, 251–53
Rule of nines in burns, 149–50
Rumpel-Leede phenomenon, 295
Rupture of heart muscle, 249
Ruptured intervertebral disk, 474–78
Rush, Benjamin, 63
Russel's traction, 464

Sakel, Manfred, 40, 64
Salicylates for arthritis, 473
Salt, dietary restriction, 261–63
 edema, 131
 electrolyte, 112
 solutions with silver nitrate, 162
 substitutes, 263
Sarcoma, 91
Satiety, 507
Saturated fats, 263
Scar tissue, burns, 155
 myocardial infarction, 248
Schizophrenia, 29–32
 incidence, 29
 major types, 30–31
 nursing expectations, 31–32
Sclera, 479
Scrotal incision, shave, 199
Seawater ingestion, 127
Seconal (secobarbital), 56
Second-degree burns, 148
Sedatives and myocardial infarction, 265
Seizure. See Convulsions
Semen, 191
Semicoma, 419
Sensation tests, 420
Sensible water loss, 114
Sensitivity test, 190
Sensorineural hearing loss, 500
Sensory aphasia, 403
Septic shock, 214

Serum cholesterol, 241
Serum glutamic oxaloacetic transaminase (SGOT) (GOT), 241
Sewel procedure for angina pectoris, 246
Sex steroids, 389
Shock, 214–16
  assessment of patient, 215
  circulatory from burns, 154
  congestive heart failure, 251
  hemodialysis, 175
  management, 215
  spinal, 409
Shoulder-hand syndrome, congestive heart failure, 253
  heart disease, 259–60
  prostate surgery, 194
  uremia, 178
Sodium acid phosphate, 198
Sodium bicarbonate, alkalinize urine, 198
  alkalosis, 122
Sodium chloride, 112
  unconscious patient, 429
Sodium dextrothyroxine (Choloxin), 358
Sodium dietary restrictions, 261–63
Sodium iodide for thyroid gland, 360
Sodium lithyronine (cytomel), 358
Sodium phytate (rencal), 198
Sodium restrictions, glomerulonephritis, 187
  uremia, 179
Solute loading, 127
Solvents, 57
Somatic therapies, 40–42
  electroconvulsive therapy, 41–42
  insulin coma therapy, 40
  nursing expectations, 44
Somatotropic hormone, 346–47
Somnolence, 419
Spasms in neurologic-orthopedic difficulty, 411–12
Speech center, 442
Speech reading, 501
Shuffling gait, Parkinson's disease, 451
Sickle-cell disease, 57
Sigmoidoscopy, 522
Silver nitrate, solution and vaporizational heat loss, 159
  treatment for burns, 161
Simultaneous multiple analysis of blood, 137
Sinus bradycardia, 220
Sinus tachycardia, 220
Sitz bath following cystoscopy, 186

Skeletal traction, 461
Skene's glands, 84
Skin-Band Cement, 203
Skin breakdown in neurologic-orthopedic difficulty, 403
Skin destruction in burns, 148
Skin grafting, 163
Skin testing, 160
Skin traction, 461
Skull fracture, 427
Slipped disk, 474–78
Slit lamp, 481
Small intestine, 515–17
Snellen chart, 420, 482
Sociopathic personality disturbances, 39, 53–58
Sodium, 126–30
  burns, 154, 160
  deficit, 127–28
  excess, 126, 130
Speed shock, 141
Spica cast, 459
Spider angiomas, 546
Spinal accessory nerve, 422
Spinal cord, 414
  circulation to, 415
  injury, 425
  lumbar puncture, 423
Spinal shock, 409
Spinal tap, 423–24
Spinothalamic tract, 47
Spleen, removal, 207
Sputum examination, 312
Staghorn calculus, 198
Stapedectomy, 498
Stapes, 496
  mobilization, 498
Staphcillin, 78
Staphylococcus aureus, 77
  treatment with antibiotics, 78
Status epilepticus, 438
Stelazine (trifluperazine), 48
Stem cell leukemia, 296
Sterilization, 199
Steroids, 343, 346, 349–51, 352–53, 389
  carcinoma, 390
  combinations to prevent conception, 391
  cerebral edema, 442
  diabetes, 350
  exophthalmos, 359
  leukemia, 297
Sterols, 263

Stokes-Adams attack, 220, 230
Stoma, ileal bladder, 203
Stomach, 514
Stone, calcium-containing, 198
 phosphate-containing, 198
 renal system. See Calculi
 uric acid-containing, 198
Stool, examination, 522
 manual removal, 410
Strabismus, 421
Strain gavage for arterial blood pressure, 232
Streptomycin, 334–35
Stress, response, 119
 steroids, 350, 351
Streptococcus, glomerulonephritis, 187
 rheumatic heart disease, 241
Streptokinase to dissolve clots, 272
Stripping of veins, 289
Stroke. See Cerebrovascular disease
Stryker frame, 164, 404
Stump, 469–71
Stupor, 419
Stye, 492
Subarachnoid hemorrhage, 427
Subarachnoid space, 414
Subconscious, 20
Subcutaneous pocket for pacemaker, 229
Subdural hematoma, 427
Subtotal gastrectomy, 533–34
Sucrose for circulation time, 239
Suctioning, loss of electrolytes, 127
Suicide, 33–36
 dynamic theory, 33
 factors in evaluation, 35
 prevention, 36
Sullivan, Harry, 64
Supine, position for bed, 407
Suprapubic incision, shave, 199
Suprapubic prostatectomy, 195
Supratentorial structures, 415
 tumors, 430, 433
Surface hypothermia, 273–74, 275
Surgery and stress response, 119
Sustagen, 159
Swing-through gait, 468
Sympathectomy, angina pectoris, 247
 peripheral vascular disease, 289
Sympathetic nervous system, 416–17
Sympathetic ophthalmia, 486
Symptomatic epilepsy, 439
Synanon, 56

Syphilis, 81–84
 diagnosis, 83
 stages, 82
 treatment, 83–84

Talipes equinus, 407
Target organ, endocrinology, 342–45
Tarsal plate, 479
Temporal lobe, 416
Tentorium, 430
Testape, 374
Testosterone, 347, 351, 389, 390
Tetanus antitoxin, 152
Tetanus toxoid, 151
Tetany, 133, 178, 363, 365–66
Therapeutic environment, 6–10
Thiouracil derivative drugs, 360
Third-degree burns, 148
Thomas splint, 459, 464
Thoracentesis, 312
Thoracoplasty, 337
Thoracotomy, 337
Thorazine (chlorpromazine), 48–50
Three-point gait, 468
Thromboangiitis obliterans (Buerger's disease), 280
Thromboemboli in myocardial infarction, 249
Thrombophlebitis, 141, 280
Thrombosis of brain, 445
Thymus gland, 366
Thyroglobulin (Proloid), 358
Thyroid, 358
Thyroid gland, 352–65
 cancer, 356–61
 drugs to suppress, 359–60
 goiter, 356–57
 hyperthyroidism, 358–64
 hypothyroidism, 357–58
 irradiation, 360
 management, 361–63
 safety precautions for use of radioactive material, 361
 surgery, 361–64
 tests of function, 354–56
Thyroid hormone in angina pectoris, 246
Thyroid scan, 355
Thyroid-stimulating hormone, 354
Thyroid storm, 363–64
Thyroid suppression test, 356
Thyrotoxic goiter, 358
Thyrotropic hormone, 343, 347

Thyroxin, 343, 353
Thyroxin binding, 354
Tic douloureux, 421
Tidal drainage, 410
Tilt table, 199, 408, 424
Tincture of benzoin spray, 203
Tine test, 334
Tinnitus, 422
Tissue protection, peripheral vascular disease, 285
Tobacco, 286
Tofranil (impiramine), 51
Tonic phase of convulsion, 437–38
Tonicity, 119
　solute loading, 127
Tonography, 482
Tonometer, 481, 482
Torkildsen procedure for ventricular tumors, 431
Torticollis, 476
Total gastrectomy, 535
Toxic nodular goiter, 358
Toxoid, tetanus, 151
Tracheostomy, 321–23
　care, inner cannula, 322
　dressings, 321
　suction, 323
Tracheotomy, burns, 151
　respiratory illness, 320
Traction, 461–65
　disk problems, 476
Tranquilizers, 47–50
　myocardial infarction, 265
　peptic ulcer, 531
Transaminase, 241
Transcellular fluid, 114
Transfer procedures, activities of daily living, 399
Transference, 43
Transmural infarction, 247
Transplant, cornea, 492
　heart, 276–77
　kidney, 173, 206
Transurethral resection, 192
Traumatic arthritis, 472
Trendelenburg position, 215
Trephination, 490
Treponema pallidum, 81
Tridione, 441
Trifocal lenses, 483
Trigeminal nerve, 421
Trigeminal neuralgia, 421
Triglycerides, 263

Triiodothyronine, 353
Trilafon (perphenazine), 48
Trimethadione (Tridione), 441
Trochlear nerve, 420
Trousseau sign in tetany, 134, 365
Tube feedings, 139, 159, 201
Tuberculosis, 333
　complications, 336
　diagnosis, 334
　immunization, 75, 335–36
　incidence, 333
　pathology, 333–34
　treatment, 334–35
Tubular excretion, 169
Tubular function test, 184
Tubular reabsorption, 168
Tubular secretion, 169
Tumor, 89–90
　brain, 430–32
Tympanic membrane, 496
Tympanoplasty, 498

Ulcerative colitis, 555–56
Ulcers, varicose, 289
Ultraviolet treatment for decubitus ulcers, 404
Unconscious, 20
Uni-Solve, 203
United Ostomy Association, Inc., 541
Unna's paste boot, 289
Urea, clearance test, 183
　protein breakdown, 179
　splitters, 197
Uremia, 172
　diuretic phase, 178
　frost, 173, 180
　gastrointestinal ulcers, 172
　management, 173–80
　oliguric phase, 172, 178
　potassium elevation, 178
　pyelonephritis, 189
Ureteral intestinal anastomosis, 206
Ureteroileostomy, 206
Ureterosigmoidoscopy, 206
Ureterostomy, tube, 200
Ureterotomy, 200
Ureters, 165
　cutaneous transplant, 205
　transplantation for urinary diversion, 202
Urethra, 165
Urethrogram, 185

Urgency, 169
Uri Kleen, 203
Uric acid stones, 198
Urinary diversion procedures, 202–206
Urinary output in burns, 157
Urinary system, infections and calculi, 199, 408
 obstruction, 190–99
 surgery, 199–210
Urine, acetone in diabetes mellitus, 374
 acid, 408
 acidifiers, 198
 collection bag, 157
 culture, 190
 drainage, 200–201
 examination, 180–82
 interference in manufacture or transportation, 169–72
 pH, 181
 production and excretion, 165, 168–69
 protein, 182
 residual, 192
 retention, 429
 schematic representation, 169
 specific gravity, 181
 specimens, 180–81
 straining for calculi, 198
 tests in diabetes mellitus, 373
 turbidity, 182
Urokinase, 272
Urolithiasis, 196–99
Urologic dysfunction, 165–212
 diagnosis, 180–86
 renal function tests, 182–86
Uterine lining, estrogen levels, 389
Uveitis, 486, 492

Vaccines, 75
Vagal stimulation in myocardial infarction, 247
Vagus nerve, to heart, 219
 to gastrointestinal tract, 512, 535
Valence, 116
Valium (diazepam), 50
Valsalva maneuver, 239
Vaporizational heat loss in burns, 159
Varicose ulcers, 289
Varicose veins, 280–82, 285–92
Vascular disease of the brain, 444–50
Vascular surgery, 290–92
Vasopressin, 347–48
Vasopressors, 266

VDRL, 83
Vector, 72
Vein ligation for varicose veins, 289
Venereal disease, 81–84
Venesection for congestive heart failure, 253
Venoclysis, 139
 solutions, 141
Venous blood pressure, 232
Venous pressure time, 240
Ventricle and cerebrospinal fluid, 415
Ventricular fibrillation, 220
 pacemaker, 230
Ventriculography, 424
Vertebral column, 414
Vessel deterioration, 242–50
Vineberg procedure for angina pectoris, 246
Viral hepatitis, 144
Vital capacity, 313
Vital signs and observations of neurologic emergencies, 428
Vitamin A deficiency, calculi, 196
Vitamin K, anticoagulant drugs, 271
Vitreous humor, 479
Voiding changes, 169
Vollmer patch test, 334
Vomiting and increased intracranial pressure, 431

Wassermann and Kolmer test, 83
Water, 112–14
 deficit, 126–28
 excess, 129–30, 178
 insensible loss, 114
 intoxication, 129
 movement, 118
 obligatory loss, 114
 percentage in adult, 113
 reabsorption by kidneys, 168
Water brash, 526
Water and electrolytes, 112–212
 imbalances, 126–36
 needs in 24 hours, 137
 observations, 145
 replacement, 137–47
 surgery of the urinary tract, 199
 unconscious patient, 429
 urologic dysfunction, 172
Wax in ear, 496
Weight record, hemodialysis, 174
 peritoneal dialysis, 176

Wernicke's aphasia, 403
Whiplash, 475
Whirlpool bath, 161, 404
White matter, 415
Withdrawal in schizophrenia, 29
Wolff's law, 460

Yttrium implantation, 348

Zephirin for bladder instillation, 409
Zonules of Zinn, 479